COMMONLY USED CHINESE HERB FORMULAS WITH ILLUSTRATIONS

by

Dr. Hong-yen Hsu
Dr. Chau-shin Hsu

ORIENTAL HEALING ARTS INSTITUTE
8820 SOUTH SEPULVEDA BOULEVARD, SUITE 218
LOS ANGELES, CALIFORNIA 90045 U.S.A.

COMMONLY USED CHINESE HERB FORMULAS WITH ILLUSTRATIONS

NOTICE

The following is a summary description of some of the natural herbal formulas widely used throughout Asia. The information compiled from traditional medical texts and from the observations of modern authorities on Chinese medicine is presented here for its educational value and should not be used for diagnosis, treatment, or prevention of disease without the advice of a Chinese physician or other medical authority.

ISBN: 0-941 942-03-1
Printed in the Republic of China

Contents

Foreword vii

Part I General 1

The Constitution of Chinese Herbal Formulas 3

Variations of Chinese Herb Formulas 6

Classification of Chinese Herb Formulas 12

The Nomenclature of Chinese Herbal Formulas 22

Dosage Forms and Uses of Chinese Herbal Formulas . 23

Changes in the Weighting and Measuring Units of Herbs 27

Scientific Chinese Herb Preparations 29

Part II Detailed Discussion of Formula Types 31

1. *Chieh Piao Chi* 33
2. *Ho Chieh Chi* 84
3. *Piao Li Shuang Chieh Chi* 116
4. *Yung Tu Chi* 132
5. *Kung Li Chi* 138
6. *Ching Je Hsieh Huo Chi* 158
7. *Hsiao Tao Chi* 202
8. *Ching Shu Chi* 216
9. *Pu I Chi* 224
10. *Chu Han Chi* 276
11. *Kai Chiao Tung Kuan Chi* 329
12. *Chen Ching Chi* 339
13. *Sho She Chi* 357
14. *Li Ch'i Chi* 364
15. *Li Hsieh Chi* 413
16. *Chu Feng Chi* 442
17. *Chu Shih Chi* 463
18. *Jun Tsao Chi* 528
19. *Chu Tan Chi* 542
20. *Chu Chung Chi* 564
21. *Ching Chan Chi* 571
22. *Tou Ma Chi* 590

23. *Ming Mu Chi* 597
24. *Yung Yang Chi* 602

Where You Can Buy Chinese Herb Formulas 635

Bibliography 637

Index 650

Chinese Index 661

FOREWORD

In China and Southeast Asia, diseases are treated by both Western and Chinese therapies. Western medicine adopts an objective approach: first it establishes the name of the disease, and then prescribes treatment specific to that disease. Chinese therapy, on the other hand, pays special attention to the patient's symptoms and prescribes a general treatment on a subjective basis based on the lifestyle and physical constitution of the patient and the determined cause. Although both systems aim to alleviate pain, their theories as to cause and therapies vary considerably. Western medicine uses mainly synthetic chemicals, while Oriental medicine employs herbs and natural materials. Herbal formulas generally contain several components, except Ginseng Combination and Licorice Combination, which are plant simples.

Chinese herbal formulas generally are composed of eight to twelve different herbs. The combination of these component herbs is called an "herbal formula" and the science of the composition, actions, indications, dosage, and clinical uses of these herbal formulas is called "herbal pharmaceutics." Hence before one can have a good command of herbal formulas, he or she must thoroughly study the properties of the component herbs.

A Chinese herbal formula is generally composed of four classes of herbs, namely, imperial, ministerial, assistant, and servant herbs. The imperial herb is the chief herb of a formula; the ministerial herb is ancillary to the imperial herb; the assistant herb augments the actions of the preceding two herbs or diminishes their side effects; the servant herb coordinates and directs the actions of all the herbs comprising the formula. From long term clinical practice, some standard formulas have emerged which are called "basic formulas." The addition or omission of herbs to or from these basic formulas results in different effects. For example, in the table that follows, *Ma-huang-tang* (麻黃湯 *Ma-huang* Combination) is listed as the basic formula to induce sweating and suppress coughing. However, *Ma-hsing-kan-shih-tang* (麻杏甘石湯 Apricot Seed and *Ma-huang* Combination) is an alternative formula in which Cinnamon is omitted and Gypsum added. The new formula suppresses sweating and coughing. When Atractylodes is added to *Ma-huang-tang*, the formula becomes *Ma-huang-chia-chu-tang,* (麻黃加朮湯 *Ma-huang* and Atractylodes Combination) a diuretic. (See table 1.)

These variations of basic formulas were introduced by Otsuka Keisetsu, an authority on Chinese medicine in Japan in his book *The Characteristics of Chinese Herb Medicine* in the chapter "Characteristics and Constitution of Chinese Herb Formulas." They are included also in *Chinese Herb Therapies for the Recalcitrant Diseases,* Volume One. Over half of these combinations were formulated 1800 years ago. After centuries of clinical use by herbal physicians, these formulas are still in wide use today.

The pharmacological effects of herbal combinations on the human body are very complex. Three types of interactions take place.

1. Between the individual herbs.
2. Between the constituents of the individual herbs.
3. Between the constituents of different herbs.

The pharmacological interaction between herbs occurs in several ways:

1. Synergism: When two constituents are mixed, their pharmacological actions increase or double. This action is differentiated into addition and the potentiation.

Table 1. Basic Formula of *Ma-huang-tang* and Its Variations

Formula	*Ma-huang*	Licorice	Apricot seed	Cinnamon	Gypsum	Atractylodes	Action
Ma-huang-tang (*Ma-huang* Combination)	5g	1.5g	5g	4g			Diaphoretic, cough suppressant
Ma-hsing-kan-shih-tang (*Ma-huang* and Apricot Seed Combination)	4g	2.0g	4g		10g		Anhidrotic, cough suppressant
Ma-huang-chia-chu-tang (*Ma-huang* and Atractylodes Combination)	5g	1.5g	5g	4g		5g	Diuretic

2. Antagonism: When two constituents are combined, their pharmacological actions may be reversed or antagonistic. This condition is subdivided into competing and non-competing.
3. Transition: The combined constituents may affect the same or different sites.

Using modern scientific methods to establish the pharmacological properties of Chinese herbal formulas is extremely difficult. Yet based on centuries of empirical use of herbal remedies, Chinese herbalists are able to diagnose and prescribe the correct treatment and to predict the action a formula will have on the human body. Likewise, lengthy experience using formula modifications has resulted in the ability to prescribe the right drug for the right symptom. Take headache for example: based on his experience, a Chinese herbal physician prescribes Evodia and Cnidium for a headache that has a chill character; Chrysanthemum and Perilla for a feverish headache; *Chianghuo* and *Mahuang* for posterior encephalgia; Angelica and Pueraria for anterior encephalgia; Vitex, white Peony, and Tribulus for bilateral headache; *Kao-pen* and Achyranthes for headache on the crown of the head; and bleached dead Silkworm and Scorpion for a stubborn headache. (For further information, please refer to my paper "The Difference Between Chinese Herb Medicine in China and Chinese Herb Medicine in Japan" in *Practical Kanpo,* (漢方之臨床) Vol. 25, No. 11 and 12, 1978).

Based on the experiences of our ancestors, Chinese herbal formulas are classified as major and minor or for treating mild and acute types of diseases. Altogether there are seven types of formulas: major formulas (such as Major Rhubarb Combination); mild formulas (such as Four Major Herb Combination); acute formulas (those having a strong action such as Aconite and G. L. Combination); odd formulas (those containing only one single herb, such as Ginseng Combination); even formulas (those containing over two herbs, such as Rehmannia Eight Combination); and compound formulas (the combined formula of two to three basic formulas like Bupleurum and Cinnamon Combination).

According to their actions, Chinese herbal formulas are further subdivided into ten categories: *hsuan* (宣, dispersant), *tung* (通, channeling), *pu* (補, nutritive), *hsieh* (泄, purgative), *ching* (輕, light), *chung* (重, heavy), *hua* (滑, slippery), *she* (濇, harsh), *tsao* (燥, arid), and *shih* (溼, moist). Also, based on the therapeutic usage, formulas are classified as one of the eight classes: *pu* (補, nutritive), *ho* (和, harmonizing), *san* (散, dispersant), *han* (寒, chilly), *je* (熱, hot), *ku* (固, solidifying), *kung* (攻, attacking), and *in* (因, guiding).

There are 113 formulas recorded in the *Shang han lun* (傷寒論) and 110 formulas in the *Chin kuei yao lueh* (金匱要略) of the Han dynasty; over 6,000 formulas in the *Wai tai mi yao* (外臺秘要) of the Tang dynasty; over 30,000 formulas in the *Tai ping sheng huai fang* (太平聖惠方) of the Sung dynasty; 61,739 formulas in the *Pu chi fang* (普濟方) of the Ming dynasty; and over 8,000 formulas in *Pen tsao kang mu* (本草綱目). These prescriptions together with formulas from other medical compendia such as *I fang chi chieh* (醫方集解), total in excess of 100,000. In *The Outlines of Conformation in Chinese Herb Medicine* (中醫辨證綱要) I have gathered about 1,200 frequently used Chinese formulas. The number of commonly used herbal formulas in Japan numbers only a little over 200. In the *Analysis of the Commonly Used Chinese Herb Formulas* (常用方劑分析)–written during my tenure as Director of the Bureau of Food and Drug Control of the National Health Administration, Republic of China, and published by the Committees of Chinese Herb Medicine of the National Health Administration–are more than 300 formulas which have been analyzed, classified, and logically arranged. Because of limited space, detailed descriptions of these formulas are omitted here. From the immense corpus of Chinese herbal formulas, some of which are out-dated, some oversimplified, some seldom used, I have selected 367 contemporary herbal formulas that are commonly prescribed. For each formula there is a short description of its origin, historical background, indications, action, and discrimination from similar formulas. To make this book useful for clinical application, original illustrations adopted from Nagakura Onzo's *The Catalogue of Drugs* (藥品目錄) or the Korean Li Tsai-hsi's *Illustrated Chinese Medical Diagnosis and the Important Herb Formulas* (圖說漢方診療要方) accompany each formula. The figures on abdominal diagnosis are taken from *Fu ku sho ki lan* (腹證奇覽. An Extraordinary Review on Abdominal Conformation) and *Fu ku sho ki lan yoku gen to* (腹證奇覽翼 Supplementary to an Extraordinary Review on Abdominal Conformation Attached with the Original Figures). I have collected as many commonly used Japanese formulas as possible. A few prevailing Korean formulas have also been included. It will bring me great pleasure if this book fosters interest in herb medicine.

Information concerning the origins of formulas and the works in which these formulas first appeared comes from the *Chinese Medical Dictionary* (中國醫學大辭典). References to Japanese practices have been obtained partly from *Chinese Therapeutic References* (漢方診療醫典) and partly from information provided by Dr. Otsuka Yasuo and Terashi Mokuso of Japan. In Part II, "Discussion of Formula Types," the prefaces with definitions and contraindications for each category of formulas have been taken verbatim from *The Analysis of the Commonly Used Chinese Herb Formulas* (常用方劑分析) by Professor Wu Kuo-ting and Hong-yen Hsu.

For any errors, incompleteness or oversights, I sincerely solicit suggestions from my readers in the hope that a revised edition will be greatly enhanced. The arrangement of the collection and proofreading for the entire book in Chinese have been done by Mrs. Lin Kuei-ying. I also wish to acknowledge Mr. Wang Su-yen and Mrs. Wang Shu-kuei for their translation and Judith Haueter and Jeannine Talley Ph.D. for their editorial work on the English version. Without their help the publication of this book would have suffered numerous delays. To them, my hearty thanks.

Hong-yen Hsu, Ph.D
Chau-hsin Hsu, Ph.D
January 15, 1981

PART I

GENERAL

The Constitution of Chinese Herbal Formulas

Each Chinese herbal formula contains four types of herbs: imperial, ministerial, assistant, and servant. The imperial herb is the chief component of the formula; the ministerial herb augments or promotes the action of the chief component; the assistant herb reduces side effects or restricts the actions of the chief herb, (for example, if the chief herb is poisonous, the assistant reduces its toxicity); and the servant herb harmonizes or coordinates all the herbs.

Ma-huang-tang (麻黃湯), recorded in the *Shang han lun* (傷寒論), is indicated for fevers, headaches. chillphobia, arthralgia, anhidrosis (absence of sweat), asthma, and a buoyant and tight or tense pulse. It is composed of the imperial herb *Ma-huang,* which promotes sweating; the ministerial herb Cinnamon, which also causes perspiration; the assistant herb Apricot seed, which augments the antiasthmatic action of *Ma-huang*; and the servant herb, Licorice which coordinates the other components.

Obviously many Chinese herbal formulas are composed of more than four herbs or less than four herbs. However, formulas of only two or three herbs also exhibit the imperial, ministerial, assistant, and servant relationships. For instance, the formula *Chieh-ken-tang* (桔梗湯), included in the lesser yin section of the *Shang han lun*, is indicated for sore throats. It is composed only of Platycodon and Licorice. Platycodon is an imperial herb that cleanses the throat and aids in alleviating soreness. It also acts as a servant herb, in that it carries all herbs upward. Licorice, a ministerial herb, acts as a throat lubricant and a ptyalogogue (an agent causing saliva to flow) and also as an assistant herb in expelling fevers and detoxifying poisons. *Tiao-wei-cheng-chi-tang* (調胃承氣湯 Rhubarb and Mirabilitum Combination), also from the *Shang han lun* under the section on greater yang diseases, is another example. This formula is taken for the mild condition of visceral firmness. It is composed of the imperial herb *Ta-huang* (Rhubarb) which has fever cleansing and "interior-attacking" actions. It also acts as a servant by entering into the stomach and intestines. The ministerial herb mirabilitum, characterized as salty and chilly, has a lubricating effect on dryness, or a softening action. The assistant herb, Licorice, mollifies the drastic cathartic action of Rhubarb, harmonizes the stomach, and moistens dryness.

From the preceding examples it is apparent that the incorporation of each herb must be given careful consideration for the possible harmful effects it might exert on the human body. Moreover, herbal practitioners are concerned with achieving the greatest therapeutic effect.

Since antiquity the Chinese have known about the interactions of herbs. In older medical treatises we find the phrase "seven conditions of incorporation." These are independent, dependent, assistant, subjugating, depriving, antagonistic, and antidotal. These seven conditions have been used for years and are the established rules by which a practitioner determines the properties and effects of herbs and judges their compatibility and incompatibility.

Variation in the combination of herbs results in different formulas. For example, *Ma-huang* (麻黃) combined with Apricot seed treats asthmatic cough; *Ma-huang* with Atracylodes exerts a diuretic effect and treats dysuria (painful or difficult urination), edema, and anhidrosis; *Ma-huang* with Cinnamon treats anhidrosis; *Ma-huang* with Gypsum promotes sweating; *Ma-hsing-kan-shih-tang* (麻杏甘石湯 Apricot Seed and *Ma-huang* Combination)– composed of *Ma-huang*, Apricot kernels, Licorice, and Gypsum– treats spontaneous sweating and asthmatic cough; *Yueh-pei-chia-*

chu-tang (越婢加朮湯Atractylodes Combination)–comprised of *Ma-huang,* Gypsum, Ginger, Jujube, Licorice and Atractylodes–treats dysuria, edema, and spontaneous sweating; *Ta-ching-lung-tang* (Major Blue Dragon Combination)–made up of *Ma-huang,* Apricot seed, Cinnamon, Ginger, Jujube, Licorice, and Gypsum–treats anhidrosis and the serious condition of a *Ma-huang-tang* conformation.

Herbal formulas are also governed by other rules concerning the proportions.

1. Odd system: imperial herb, one part; ministerial herb, two parts. Or imperial herb, two parts; ministerial herb, three parts.
2. Even system: imperial herb, two parts; ministerial herb, four parts. Or imperial herb, two parts; ministerial herb, six parts.
3. Small system: imperial herb, one part; ministerial herb, two parts.
4. Middle system: imperial herb, one part; ministerial herb, three parts; assistant herb, five parts.
5. Large system: imperial herb, one part; ministerial herb, three parts; assistant herb, nine parts.

The above rules come from prescriptions of the ancient school. Post-Sung Dynasty School prescriptions do not adhere to these rules.

Variations of Chinese Herb Formulas

An herbal formula is modified according to clinical change in condition, physique, and age of the patient. A formula is tailored to the individual exactly in order to achieve the best results.

A Chinese herbal formula made from the same component herbs may change its name when the amounts of its component herbs change in compliance with different goals of treatment. For example, *Hisao-cheng-chi-tang* (小承氣湯 Minor Rhubarb Combination), *Hou-pu-san-wu-tang* (厚朴三物湯 Magnolia Three Combination), and *Hou-pu-ta-huang-tang* (厚朴大黃湯 Rhubarb, Magnolia, and *Chih-shih* Combination) contain the same herbs. However, in accordance with changes in the proportions of the herbs to agree with the changes in their roles of being either imperial, ministerial, assistant, or servant herb, the name of the formula also changes so that the therapeutic effect may be distinguished. (See Table 2.)

The therapeutic effect of Chinese herbal formula changes when the number of herbs included change as demonstrated by *Hsiao-chai-hu-tang* (小柴胡湯 Minor Bupleurum Combination), a formula frequently mentioned in the *Shang han lun*.(See table 3.)

Table 2

<table>
<tr><th rowspan="2">Combination</th><th colspan="6">Composition</th><th rowspan="2">Chief Indication</th></tr>
<tr><th colspan="2">Imperial</th><th colspan="2">Ministerial</th><th>Assistant</th><th>Servant</th></tr>
<tr><td>Hou-pu-san-wu-tang (Magnolia Three Combination)</td><td colspan="2">Magnolia bark 8 liang</td><td colspan="2">Chih-shih 5 pieces</td><td>Rhubarb 4 liang</td><td>Rhubarb</td><td>Abdominal fullness, constipation</td></tr>
<tr><td>Hsiao-cheng-chi-tang (Minor Rhubarb Combination)</td><td colspan="2">Rhubarb 4 liang</td><td>Magnolia bark 2 liang</td><td>Chih-shih 3 pieces</td><td>Magnolia bark</td><td>Rhubarb</td><td>Visceral fullness of sunlight yang condition, constipation, tidal fever, and delirium</td></tr>
<tr><td>Hou-pu-ta-huang-tang (Rhubarb, Magnolia and Chih-snih Combination)</td><td>Magnolia bark 1 foot</td><td>Rhubarb 6 liang</td><td colspan="2">Chih-shih 4 pieces</td><td></td><td></td><td>Bronchial fluid stagnation and chest fullness</td></tr>
</table>

1 *liang*=31.2g

Table 3. Minor Bupleurum Variations

Basic Components	General Indications	Complications	Changes	
			Additions	Deletions
Bupleurum ½ *chin* Scute 3 *liang* Ginseng 3 *liang* Pinellia ½ *chin* Licorice 3 *liang* Jujube 12 pieces Fresh Ginger 3 *liang*	alternating chills and fever; rib and chest distress, general discomfort; nausea; bitter taste in mouth; dry throat; dizziness	binding and obstruction in the chest; nausea	Trichosanthes 1 piece	Pinellia Ginseng
		thirst	Ginseng 1.5 *liang*, Trichosanthes 4 *liang*	Pinellia
		abdominal pain	Peony 3 *liang*	Scute
		obstruction and hardening underneath the chest, dysuria, palpitations beneath the heart	Oyster shell 4 *liang*, Hoelen 4 *liang*	Jujube Scute
		no thirst but mild fever; cough	Cinnamon 3 *liang*, Schizandra ½ *chin* Dry ginger 2 *liang*	Ginseng

1 *liang*=31.2g
1 *chin*=500g

1. When Pinellia and Ginseng are omitted from Minor Bupleurum Combination and one piece of Trichosanthes added, the modified formula treats a feeling of binding and obstruction in the heart, and nausea
2. When Pinellia is deleted and Ginseng and Trichosanthes root are added, the modified formula stimulates saliva production and hence quenches thirst.
3. When Scute is omitted and Peony added, the modified formula treats abdominal pain.
4. When Jujube and Scute are omitted and *Ostrea testa* (oyster shell) and Hoelen added, the new formula attacks obstruction and hardening below the chest, painful or difficult urination, and palpitation below the heart.
5. When Ginseng is delected and Cinnamon, Schizandra, and dry Ginger added, the modified formula treats a mild fever and cough.

Another example is *Kuei-chih-tang* (Cinnamon Combination) composed of Cinnamon, Paeonia (Peony), Licorice, fresh Ginger, and Jujube. It relieves muscle tension, causes perspiration, and regulates skin and blood domains. Cinnamon Combination is used for externally contracted wind toxin and the accompanying surface conformation manifested by headaches, fever, spontaneous sweating, anemophobia, a buoyant and moderate pulse, and a tongue coated with white, thin, and slippery fur. Based on these indications, the recurrence of an old condition induced by the disease, such as asthma, should be treated with the modified formula to which Magnolia bark and Apricot seed have been added. Magnolia bark causes *ch'i* (vigor) to descend and relieves distention by purging the body; Apricot seed calms adverse upflushing *ch'i* and eases asthmatic breathing. The modified formula is named *kuei-chih-chia-hou-pu-hsing-jen-tang* (桂枝加厚朴杏仁湯 Magnolia, Apricot, and Cinnamon Combination). If the *Kuei-chih-tang* conformation is mistreated with a purgative and chest distention arises, Paeonia which is sour and astringent and contraindicated for chest distention must be removed from the formula. The formula then solely acts as a muscle relaxant and detoxifier. (This modified formula is called *Kuei-chih-chu-shao-yao-tang* (桂枝去芍藥湯) or Cinnamon Minus Peony Combination).

It should be stressed here that the addition or deletion of

one or more herbs from a basic formula is done only when the patient's basic conformation remains unchanged. A change in conformation necessitates changing treatment to another method or to a completely different basic formula.

Changes in the lesser herbs of a formula have a direct effect on the chief action of the formula. For example, for a surface firm conformation of *shang han* disease, the sweating method is indicated. *Ma-huang* induces sweating thereby dissolving surface fever. *Ma-huang* combined with Cinnamon, both acrid and warm herbs, makes an acrid and warm formula that is suitable only for a surface-firm conformation of the *shang han* disease. However, if a surface fever persists and an internal fever begins to thrive, then *Ma-huang* is combined not with Cinnamon but with Gypsum which is acrid and cool. The *Ma-huang* then disperses the surface toxins and the Gypsum cleans and purges the internal fever. The combination becomes a sweat-inducing as well as cooling formula that treats strong fevers with or without perspiration accompanied by a cough. If the patient manifests chillphobia, fever, and a submerged pulse–a lesser yin *shang han* condition–*Ma-huang* is then combined with Aconite. Chillphobia and fever are symptoms of a surface conformation, whereas a submerged pulse indicates deficient yang *ch'i* of the lesser yin stage. Hence *Ma-huang* is used to dissolve the surface fever and Aconite to warm the insides.

If the conformation is internal and firm, the method of treatment is purgation with Rhubarb as the chief herb. If the fever is thriving and the stools are not hard, the heart is acting irregularly, and there is distention in the abdomen, then Rhubarb is combined with salty, cold Mirabilitum to reduce the fever. The result is *Tiao-wei-cheng-chi-tang* (Rhubarb and Mirabilitum Combination). If the stools are hard and bowel movement difficult, the fever is not thriving and the abdomen is full, then Magnolia bark and *Chih-shih* are incorporated to purge the constipation–*Hsiao-cheng-chi-tang* (小承氣湯 Minor Rhubarb Combination). However, if both constipation and fever are severe or the condition develops to such an extent that there is watery diarrhea, Magnolia bark, Mirabilitum, *Chih-shih,* and Rhubarb (*Ta-cheng-chi-tang* 大承氣湯 Major Rhubarb Combination) are combined in order to effect prompt catharsis so that the yin fluids may be saved.

From the foregoing analysis of sudorific and purgative formulas, it is apparent that a relationship exists between the functions of a formula and the combination of its component herbs. This is especially true when the change involves the chief herb.

Dosage corresponds to the conformation of each disease. For chronic diseases, in which a quick cure is impossible, pills are given to achieve a slow curing effect. For example, the formula *Ti-tang-tang* (抵當湯 Rhubarb and Leech Combination) composed of Leech, Tabanus (snipe-fly), Persica and Rhubarb, is used in the decocted from in the *Shang han lun* but can be changed to pill form. Chang Chieh-ku changed *Chih-chu-tang* (枳朮湯 *Chih-shih* and Atractylodes Combination) into *Chih-chu-wan* (枳朮丸), a pill equivalent. Another example is *Hsieh-hsin-tang* (瀉心湯 Coptis and Rhubarb Combination), which in the pill form is called *San-huang-ting* (三黃錠) or *San-huang-wan* (三黃丸). When *Jen-sheng-tang* (人參湯) is made in pill form, the preparation is referred to as *Li-chung-wan* (理中丸 Ginseng and Ginger Formula).

Classification of Chinese Herb Formulas

Treatments are divided into fast and slow, and formulas into large or small. In ancient times Chinese formulas were divided into seven types: large, small, slow, fast, odd, even, and complex. Large formulas are taken in large amounts and are used to treat serious, injurious toxic conditions accompanied by another conformation; *Ta-cheng-chi-tang* (Major Rhubarb Combination) recorded in the *Shang han lun* is such a formula. Small formulas are indicated for mild illnesses without any accompanying sub-conformation; hence the doses required are small. *Hsiao-cheng-chi-tang* (Minor Rhubarb Combination) is a small formula. A slow-acting formula is prescribed for a weak fever since a quick cure is impossible; the treatment must be given over a lengthy period. A quick-acting formula is suggested for an acute condition which may worsen without proper emergency treatment, as represented by the formula *Szu-ni-tang* (四逆湯 Aconite, Ginger, and Licorice Combination). An odd formula contains a single herb and is indicated for simple conditions. An even formula contains two herbs and is for conditions more complicated than those of the odd formulas, for example *Shao-yao-kan-tsao-tang* (芍藥甘草湯 Peony and Licorice Combination)., A complex formula contains three or more herbs, for example *Chai-hu-kuei-chih-tang* (柴胡桂枝湯 Bupleurum and Cinnamon Combination).

Chen Tsang-chi of the Tang dynasty separated Chinese herb formulas into ten categories: *hsuan (* 宣 removing obstructions), *tung* (通 channeling), *pu* (補 tonic), *hsieh* (泄 purgative), *Ching* (輕 light), *chung* (重 heavy), *hua* (滑 lubricating), *she* (澀 harsh), tsao (燥 drying), and *shih* (濕 moistening). *Hsuan* formulas remove blockages as represented by *Kua-ti-san* (瓜蒂散 Melon Pedicle Formula). *Tung* channel stagnancy, like *Shih-tsao-tang* (十棗湯 Jujube Combination). *Pu* combat weakness as in *Szu-chun-tzu-tang* (四君子湯 Major Four Herb Combination). *Hsieh* eliminate constipation, for example *Ta-cheng-chi-tang* (Major Rhubarb Combination). *Ching* remove firmness, e.g., *Ma-huang-tang* (麻黃湯 *Ma-huang* Combination). *Chung* calm the emotions, example *Chu-sha-an-sheng-wan* (硃砂安神丸 Cinnabar Formula). *Hua* remove clinging or adhering substances, for example, *Mi-chieh-tao-hua* (蜜煎導法). *She* are absorbents such as *Chih-shih-chih-yu-yu-liang-tang* (赤石脂禹餘糧湯 Kaolin and Limonite Combination). *Tsao* dry excessive moisture as in the formula *Erh-miao-wan* (二妙丸 Phellodendron and Atractylodes Formula). *Shih* moisten as in the formula *Chung-yu-kao* (瓊玉膏 Rehmannia and Ginseng Ointment).

In the Ming dynasty Chang Ching-yuen divided formulas into eight groups according to therapeutic methods. They were *pu, ho, kun, san, han, je, ku,* and *yin*. *Pu* restore strength, the loss of which is caused by depletion or injury to *ch'i*. *Ho* harmonize the body. *Kun* attack acute symptoms of a firm conformation. *San* are used for a surface conformation. *Han* are used for a chill conformation or to control heat. *Je* are for a feverish conformation, or to aid yang in driving out chills. *Ku* are used for conditions which present incessant diarrhea. *Yin* are formulas whose compositions attack the actual cause of the disease.

Generally, current practitioners of Chinese herbal medicine have adopted the classification system of *I fang chi chieh* (醫方集解 A Collective Annotation to Medical Prescriptions) by Wang Ang of the Ching dynasty. Two additions have been accepted: *hsuan chaio* (smelling salts) and *chen ching* (sedatives), bringing the total categories to twenty-three. Twenty-four types of formulas exist if we include the formulas used for measles classified as pox remedies. These classifications are explained below.

1. *Pu yang chi* (補養劑 replenishing and tonic formulas). This type of formula treats weakness and debility by replenishing blood and *ch'i*. More specifically, this classification is divided into four subtypes: *pu hsieh* (hematinics); *pu ch'i* (*ch'i* tonics); *pu yang* (yang tonics); and *pu yin* (yin tonics). *Szu-chun-tzu-tang* (Four Major Herb Combination) is a *ch'i* tonic (regulates respiration). *Szu-wu-tang* (四物湯 *Tang-kuei* Four Combination) or *Tang-kuei-pu-hsieh-tang* (當歸補血湯 *Tang-kuei* and Astragalus Combination) is a yin tonic. *Kuei-pi-tang* (歸脾湯 Ginseng and Longan Combination) is a lung tonic as well as a hematinic (increases hemoglobin). *Liu-wei-ti-huang-wan* (六味地黃丸 Rehmannia Six Formula) is a yang tonic.

2. *Fa piao chi* (發表劑 sudorific formulas–promote sweating). A sudorific formula disperses external toxins and treats surface conformations. These formulas are divided into three sub-types: acrid, warm sudorifics; acrid, cool sudorifics; and lung sudorifics. *Ma-huang-tang* (*Ma-huang* Combination) and *Kuei-chih-tang* (Cinnamon Combination) are acrid, warm sudorifics. *Sang-chu-yin* (桑菊飲 Morus and Chrysanthemum Combination) and *Yin-chiao-san* (銀翹散 Lonicera and Forsythia Formula) are acrid, cool sudorifics. *Hsiang-su-san* (香蘇散 Cyperus and Perilla Formula) is a lung sudorific. Acrid, cool sudorifics are more effective against a pulmonary disorder or cough, while *Yin-chiao-san* (銀翹散 Lonicera and Forsythia Formula) is better in reducing surface fevers. A lung sudorific is more effective in treating *ch'i* obstruction and the *ch'i* conformation caused by a surface toxin.

3. *Tsui tu chi* (催吐劑 emetic formulas). An emetic formula induces vomiting as a means of removing injurious toxins. The representative formula is *Kua-ti-san* (瓜蒂散 Melon Pedicle Formula).

4. *Kung li chi* (攻裏劑 interior attacking formulas). As exemplified by *Ta-cheng-chi-tang* (大承氣湯 Major Rhubarb Combination), this type of formula is a laxative which cleans accumulations and obstructions in the stomach and intestines. *Hsiao-cheng-chi-tang* (小承氣湯 , Minor Rhubarb Combination) also belongs to this type. The difference between *Ta-cheng-chi-tang* (Major Rhubarb Combination) and *Hsiao-cheng-chi-tang* is that the former contains a greater amount of Rhubarb, caus-

ing the formula to have a more violent action. It treats four symptoms: obstruction, distention, dryness, and firmness. *Hsiao-cheng-chi-tang*, with a lighter dose of Rhubarb, treats only obstruction, distention, and firmness.

5. *Piao li chi* (表裏劑 surface-interior attacking formulas). As implied by the name, this type of formula treats both the outside and inside of the human body. In *Kuei-chih-chia-ta-huang-tang* (桂枝加大黃湯 , Cinnamon and Rhubarb Combination), Cinnamon treats external toxin on the surface while Rhubarb treats the insides. Another example is *Fang-feng-tung-sheng-san* (防風通聖散 Siler and Platycodon Formula) which lowers fever.

6. *Ho chieh chi* (和解劑, harmonizing formulas). A formula of this type, like *Hsiao-chai-hu-tang* (Minor Bupleurum Combination), generally acts by harmonizing, that is, by removing the toxins when the patient has entered into the lesser yang stage and cannot be treated by sweating, vomiting, or purging. Other examples are *Hsiao-yao-san* (逍遙散 Bupleurum and *Tang-kuei* Formula), and *Huang-lien-tang* (黃連湯 Coptis Combination).

7. *Li ch'i chi* (理氣劑 *ch'i* formulas). This type of formula dissolves stagnation, causes *ch'i* and adverse up-flushing of *ch'i* to descend, and replenishes *ch'i*. The symptoms are obstruction and depression below the chest, swelling pain, distention, vomiting, nausea, heartburn, *ch'i* adversity, and asthma. These symptoms may be treated with *Hsuan-fu-hua-tai-che-shih-tang* (旋覆花代赭石湯 Inula and Hematite Combination). *Pan-hsia-hou-pu-tang* (半夏厚朴湯 Pinellia and Magnolia Combination), or *Su-tzu-chiang-chi-tang* (蘇子降氣湯 Perilla Fruit Combination).

8. *Li hsieh chi* (理血劑 blood formulas). These formulas remove occluded blood, stop bleeding, and replenish the blood. Blood occlusion means blood loss due to the extravasation or stagnation that occurs in ordinary injuries. For acute, spontaneous symptoms with distention, extravasation, pain, fainting and mania, formulas that attack the extravasated or occluded blood are generally prescribed. Such formulas include *Tao-ho-cheng-chi-tang* (Persica and Rhubarb Combination) and *Ti-tang-tang* (Rhubarb and Leech Combination) whereas *Shih-hui-san* (十灰散 Trachycarpus and Biota Leaves Formula) and *Huai-hua-san* (槐花散 Sophora Flower Formula) stop bleeding.

9. *Chu feng ch'i* (去風劑 carminative formulas). Wind conformations are differentiated according to whether they are external or internal. External wind is a conformation caused by an external toxin that has penetrated the depths of the human body; in a severe condition, it is known as *chung feng* (wind stroke) and characterized by unconsciousness, convulsions of the muscles or vessels, contractions of the eyes and mouth, and blurred speech. Internal wind resembles the *chung feng* condition but further exhibits the symptoms of monoplegia, (partial paralysis), slobbering, and spasms of the mouth. The chief distinction between the two wind conformations is that internal wind does not exhibit any symptoms along the six meridians and must be treated with a carminative. Wind dispelling formulas are represented by *Hsiao-hsu-ming-tang* (小續命湯 *Ma-huang* and Peony Combination) and *Tu-huo-chi-sheng-tang* (獨活寄生湯 *Tu-huo* and Vaeicum Combination). The kidneys must be nourished and the wet phlegm treated with formulas such as *Ti-huang-yin-tzu* (地黃飲子 Rehmannia Formula).

10. *Chu han chi* (祛寒劑 chill dispelling formulas). This type of formula is chiefly used to dispell chills, warm the insides, and nourish the body with herbs such as aconite or ginger. Representative formulas are *Szu-ni-tang* (四逆湯 Aconite, Ginger, and Licorice Combination), *Chen-wu-tang* (眞武湯 Vitality Combination), and *Wu-chu-yu-tang* (吳茱萸湯 Evodia Combination).

11. *Ching shu chi* (清暑劑 heat dispelling formulas). Heatstroke is a summer condition treated by this type of formula. Representative formulas are *Liu-i-san* (六一散 Talc and Licorice Formula), *Liu-ho-san* (六和散 Cardamon Formula), *Huo-hsiang-cheng-chi-san* (藿香正氣散 Agastache Formula), and *Ching-shu-i-chi-tang* (清暑益氣湯 Astragalus and Atractylodes Combination).

12. *Li shih chi* (利濕劑 moisture dispelling formulas). These formulas expel moisture or liquid toxins by means of excretion. Moisture is divided into internal and external types. External moisture is sweating, rain falling on the body, or living in a humid environment. The liquid toxins invade the body through the pores. Internal moisture accumulates from excessive intake of water, fruit, and alcoholic beverages causing the spleen and stomach to function abnormally. Because such liquid toxins

develop internally, the condition is called internal moisture. Moist toxins in the upper portion of the body cause headaches and dizziness; on the surface, chills and fever, generalized heaviness and aching, and edema in the legs and arms; in the interior of the middle of the body, chest paralysis, vomiting, stomach distention, abdominal fullness, or jaundice; and in the lower portion of the body, swelling in leg muscles and turbid urine.

The methods of treatment include sudorific formulas for the fluid located in the upper body and on the surface, or stomachics, diuretics, and spleen-strengthening formulas for fluid in the lower and internal portions. In prescribing the formulas, attention must be paid to whether the condition is of a chill or hot nature. If it is a wet chill, then acrid, warm, and dry herbs such as Atractylodes, Magnolia bark, and Citrus are prescribed. If the condition is hot in nature, then bitter, cool, and dry herbs such as Coptis, Scute, and Phellodendron are used. Very severe fluid stagnation that causes edema must be treated according to whether the conformation is weak or firm. If the condition occurs in a person with a firm pulse and strong build, a water dispelling method is used. On the other hand, a weak person with a submerged and slow pulse requires formulas that strengthen the spleen. This type of formula is represented by *Wu-ling-san* (Hoelen Five Herb Formula), *Chu-ling-tang* (Polyporus Combination), *Wu-pi-yin* (五皮飲 Hoelen and Areca Combination), *Shih-tsao-tang* (十棗湯 Jujube Combination), *Ling-kuei-chu-kan-tang* (苓桂朮甘湯 Atractylodes and Hoelen Combination), and *Yin-chen-hao-tang* (茵陳蒿湯 Capillaris Combination). Both *Wu-ling-san* (Hoelen Five Herb Formula) and *Chu-ling-tang* (Polyporus Combination) are diuretics. They treat water stagnation in a yin-weakness condition or conformation with dysuria (difficult or painful urination). *Wu-ling-san* (Hoelen Five Herb Formula) is used for treating dysuria, a dry mouth, and regurgitation of water just drunk. *Wu-pin-yin* (五皮飲 Hoelen and Areca Combination) treats edema. *Shih-tsao-tang* (十棗湯 Jujube Combination) is a strong diuretic. *Yin-chen-hao-tang* (茵陳蒿湯 Capillaris Combination) reduces fevers, helps dispel moisture, and treats jaundice.

13. *Jun tsao chi* (潤燥劑 moistening formulas). This type of formula is used to remove externally contracted dry toxins, nourish swollen abdomens, produce saliva, and increase body

fluids. Aridity is both external and internal. External dryness is further classified into warm and cool. In late autumn when the weather becomes cool, the western wind ceases to blow and one catches cold. This type of cold is known as a cool-aridity cold. A warm-aridity cold is contracted on autumn days when it is clear and the air is dry. Cool aridity usually affects the lungs causing a cough, stuffy nose, headaches, chillphobia, and dry lips. Warm aridity may also attack the lungs but it causes headaches, generalized fever, a dry cough, scanty saliva, discomfort, a dry mouth, stagnation, and thin, white fur on the tongue with the apex and rim of the tongue red and the other areas white. A lack of internal fluid (dehydration) is often a serious condition. When aridity develops in the upper portion of the body, the nose and the throat become dry; when in the middle portion, thirst develops; and when in the lower portion, constipation results. The rule of treatment is to restore saliva for upper aridity, produce more fluids for middle aridity, and nourish the blood for lower aridity. Representative formulas of this type are *Hsiang-su-san* (香蘇散 Cyperus and Perilla Formula), a cool-aridity remedy, and *Ching-tsao-chiu-fei-tang* (清燥救肺湯 Eriobotrya and Ophiopogon Combination), a warm-aridity remedy.

14. *Hsieh huo chi* (瀉火劑 fire-purging formulas). Formulas that act to reduce heat or cool the blood, or detoxify are called *Hsieh huo chi*. There are four of these kinds of formulas: fire-cleansing formulas acting in the *ch'i* domain; fire-cleansing formulas acting in the blood domain; fire-cleansing formulas for restoring *ch'i* and blood; and miscellaneous fire-cleansing formulas.

In the *ch'i* domain fire purgatives are represented by *Pai-hu-tang* (白虎湯 Gypsum Combination), *Chu-yeh-shih-kao-tang* (竹葉石膏湯 Bamboo Leaf and Gypsum Combination), *Huang-lien-chieh-tu-tang* (黃連解毒湯 Scute and Coptis Combination), and *Liang-ke-san* (Forsythia and Rhubarb Formula). *Pai-hu-tang* (Gypsum Combination) is an acrid, chilly febrifuge for strong fever and extreme thirst. *Chu-yeh-shih-kao-tang* (Bamboo Leaf and Gypsum Combination) is a sweet, acrid, cooling fire purgative which has stronger ptyalogogue (causing saliva) and stomachic actions than *Pai-hu-tang* (Gypsum Combination). *Huang-lien-chieh-tu-tang* (Scute and Coptis Combination) is a bitter, chilly fire purgative. *Liang-ke-san* (Forsythia and Rhubarb Formula) cleanses fever and induces bowel movements.

In the blood domain, fire purgatives are formulas, such as *Hsi-chiao-ti-huang-tang* (犀角地黃湯 Rhinoceros and Rehmannia Formula), which treat a fever toxin that has invaded the blood causing high fever, depression, hallucinations, and other symptoms.

Fire-cleansing formulas for excessive *ch'i* and blood are represented by *Yu-nu-chien* (玉女煎 Rehmannia and Gypsum Combination), *Ching-wen-pai-tu-yin* (清瘟敗毒飲 Gypsum and Moutan Combination), and *Pu-chi-hsiao-tu-yin* (普濟消毒飲 Soute and Cimicifuga Combination)–all of which are modifications of *Pai-hu-tang* (白虎湯 Gypsum Combination) and are indicated for conditions in which fever attacks in the *ch'i* and blood. They act to cleanse the blood and remove stomach fever and are often prescribed for plagues, toothaches, hematemesis, and nosebleeds.

15. *Chu tan chi* (除痰劑 expectorant formulas). Formulas that render removal of sputum are called *chu tan chi*. The *tan* (or humor) diseases often rise and fall with *ch'i*. An ascending *ch'i* brings on asthma and coughing whereas descending *ch'i* causes diarrhea. Ascending *ch'i* also causes dizziness, vomiting, cardiac palpitation, or epilepsy.

Sputum is divided into moist and dry. Injuries to the spleen transform fluid into moist sputum. Insufficiency to liver yin transforms fluid into dry sputum. Sputum developed due to fever is called hot sputum, whereas the sputum caused by chills is called cold sputum. Sputum resulting from food stagnation is called food sputum, and sputum due to the obstruction of *ch'i* is called obstructed sputum. Thus the treatment for sputum disorders depends on the cause. For good sputum, digestives are indicated and for obstructed sputum, *ch'i*-dissolving expectorants. There are two chief representative formulas: *Erh-chen-tang* (二陳湯 Citrus and Pinellia Combination) and *Ching-chi-hua-tan-wan* (清氣化痰丸 Ginseng, Atractylodes, and Licorice Formula).

16. *Fang hsiang kai kung chi* (芳香開孔劑 aromatic inhalant formulas). The odor of an herb can treat unconciousness caused principally by internally entrapped fever toxin within the heart, or by sputum and saliva lodged in the throat. This type of formula removes fever toxins, induces expectoration,

and revives consciousness. The representative formulas are *Niu-huang-ching-hsin-wan* (牛黃清心丸 Bos and Musk Formula) and *An-kung-niu-huang-wan* (安宮牛黃丸 Bos Formula).

17. *Chen ching* or *chen tsing chi* (鎮靜鎮痙劑 sedative, spasmolytic formulas). This type of formula includes all combinations that have tranquilizing and convulsion-arresting actions. They are generally used for cardiac palpitations, insomnia, amnesia, hallucinations, epilepsy, and convulsions. The representative formulas are *Tien-wan-pu-hsin-tan* (天王補心丹 Ginseng and Zizyphus Formula) and *Suan-tsao-jen-tang* (酸棗仁湯 Zizyphus Combination).

18. *Hsiao hua chi* (消化劑 digestive formulas). These formulas act to dissolve accumulations, aid digestion, and strengthen functions of the spleen and stomach. The representative formulas are *Ping-wei-san* (平胃散 Magnolia and Ginger Formula), *Chien-pi-wan* (健脾丸 Ginseng, Coptis, and Atractylodes Combination), and *Pao-ho-wan* (保和丸 Crataegus and Citrus Formula).

19. *Shou she chi* (收澀劑 astringent formulas). These formulas astringe sperm and *ch'i* or stop excessive release of saliva and body fluids. Prolonged illnesses, a weak physique, erroneous treatment, or excessive intake of attacking herbs may cause over-excretion of stomach fluids and result in spontaneous sweating, night sweats, spermatorrhea, incontinence, frequency of urination, and metrorrhagia–symptoms which are treated with an astringent formula. There are three varieties of astringent formulas: intestinal, anhidrotic, and spermatostatic. The chief formulas of this type are *Tao-hua-tang* (桃花湯 Kaolin and Oryza Combination), *Mu-li-san* (牡蠣散 Oyster Shell Formula), and *Chin-sou-ku-ching-wan* (金鎖固精丸 Lotus Stamen Formula).

20. *Sha chung chi* (殺蟲劑 anthelmintic formulas). This type of formula is used to dispel parasites in the stomach and intestines of an infested patient who has a pale facial complexion with white spots, red or white spots in the mouth or on the lips, cardiac irregularity and abdominal pain, vomiting of water, grinding of the teeth, mental fatigue, and loss of appetite. The representative formulas are *Wu-mei-wan* (烏梅丸 Mume Formula), *Lien-mei-an-huei-tang* (連梅安蛔湯 Picrorrhiza and Mume Combination), and *Shih-chun-tzu-wan* (使君子丸 Quisqualis Formula).

21. *Ming mu chi* (明目劑 vision-improving formulas).

Formulas that treat any ophthalmic disease are collectively termed *ming mu ch'i*. Eye diseases are generally derived from visceral disorders. For example, excessive heart fire may cause mydriasis (abnormal dilation of the pupil) and should be treated with a blood-nourishing and fire-purging formula. Eye diseases that are due to weakness in the liver, kidneys, or *ch'i* should be treated by a liver-replenishing and kidney-nourishing formula. Representative formulas of this type are *Tzu-yin-ti-huang-wan* (滋陰地黃丸 Phellodendron and Ophiopogon Formula), *Ting-chih-wan* (定志丸 Hoelen and Polygala Formula), and *Puo-yun-tuei-i-wan* (撥雲退翳丸 Cnidium and Chrysanthemum Formula).

22. *Yung yang chi* (癰瘍劑 , carbuncle-dermatosis formulas). Skin ailments that are red, swollen, aching, and burning are named *yung* (carbunculosis). Therapeutics for this kind of disease is treatment of the skin and body surface and inducement of excretion if there is constipation. If the skin is white, indurated but without pain, and the condition progressing slowly, it is deemed *chu* (ulcer) which in most instances is a yin conformation. Chief formulas for this type are *Chen-jen-huo-ming-yin* (眞人活命飲 Angelica and Mastic Combination), *Tuo-li-tou-nung-tang* (托裏透膿湯 Cimicifuga and Gleditsia Combination), and *Ta-huang-mu-tan-pi-tang* (大黃牡丹皮湯 Rhubarb and Moutan Combination).

23. *Ching chan chi* (經產劑 gyneco-obstetric formulas). These formulas treat abnormal menstruation and leukorrhea, and pregnancy and delivery problems. Chief formulas of this type are *Chiao-ai-tang* (膠艾湯 Gelatin and Artemisia Combination), *Wen-ching-tang* (溫經湯 *Tang-kuei* and Evodia Combination), and *Tang-kuei-shao-yao-san* (*Tang-kuei* and Peony Formula).

24. *Tou ma chi* (痘麻劑 pox-measles formulas). This type of formula is most frequently given to children with measles. Clinically the treatment is carried out according to the stage of the disease. The chief formulas are *Sheng-ma-ko-ken-tang* (升麻葛根湯 Cimicifuga and Pueraria Combination), *Sha-shen-mai-tong-tang* (沙參麥冬湯 Adenophora and Ophiopogon Combination), and *Hsuan-tu-fa-piao-tang* (宣毒發表湯 Cimicifuga and Peucedanum Combination).

The Nomenclature of Chinese Herbal Formulas

Formulas are named in Chinese in several ways, according to: (1) the principal herb; (2) the effect; (3) the indicated symptom; (4) the number of herbs in the formula; (5) the origin of the formula (what classic the formula first appeared in); or (6) the addition or deletion of herbs from the basic formulas. The last syllable of a formula usually indicates whether the combination is in liquid form (tang), pill form (wan) or powder form (san). Sometimes "major" or "minor" is prefixed to the name.

Dosage Forms and Uses of Chinese Herbal Formulas

After many generations, Chinese herbal physicians have developed many dosage forms, each of which has specific therapeutic characteristics. Here only the more commonly used forms are described.

Tang chi (湯劑 decoctions). Herbs are boiled with water and the liquid is called *tang chi*, for example *Ma-huang-tang* (麻黃湯 *Ma-huang* Combination) and *Szu-ni-tang* (四逆湯 Aconite and G. L. Combination). Advantages of *tang chi* are easy absorption, fast action, and flexibility in adjusting the number or amount of the component herbs. Most acute conditions are treated with the *tang chi*.

San chi (散劑 powders). This dosage form is divided into internal and external powder. Internal powder is made by grinding all herbs into a powder that is taken with boiled water, rice gruel, or wine, as exemplified by *Wu-ling-san* (五苓散 Hoelen Five Herb Formula). External powder is likewise made by grinding all herbs into an extremely fine powder, but the powder is dusted on or applied to a wound, as exemplified by the surgical *Sheng-chi-san* (生肌散 Cuttlebone and Talc Formula).

Wan chi (丸劑 pill). This form is made by grinding all

herbs into a very fine powder and then blending and kneading the powder with water, honey, flour paste, or rice paste, and forming pills. *Wan chi* is often used: (1) for debilitating diseases that require treatment over a long period of time, for example, *Liu-wei-ti-huang-wan* (六味地黃丸 Rehmannia Six Formula); (2) for blood extravasation or occlusion, and abdominal neoplasm or ascites that cannot be treated with a more powerful decoction, for example, *Ti-tang-wan* (抵當丸 Rhubarb and Leech Formula); (3) in combinations which require herbs with high toxicity that cannot be incorporated into a decoction, for example, *Pei-chi-wan* (備急丸 Rhubarb, Ginger, and Croton Formula); and (4) in combinations which require special herbs such as borneol and musk that are not suitable for a decoction preparation, for example, *Chih-pao-tan* (至寶丹 Rhinoceros and Succinum Formula).

Kao chi (膏劑 unguents). This form is divided into internal and external types. Internal unguents are prepared by boiling sliced herbs repeatedly for a long time, then discarding the dregs. The solution is further condensed over a low fire and thickened into a salve by adding lumps of crystal sugar or honey. Such a dosage form can be taken over a long period of time and generally is the form in which most tonics are prepared. Hence tonics are also known as *kao tsu yao* (unguent tonics); an example is *Chuon-yu-kao* (瓊玉膏 Ginseng and Rehmannia Ointment). External unguents are ordinarily called plasters. They are made by boiling the herbs in oil, then discarding the dregs and adding cinnabar (red lead) and white vinegar. The ointment is finally heated and then spread over a piece of paper or cloth. The plaster so formed is placed on the surface of the body. They are often used for surgical carbunculosis or dermatosis, and for paralysis and aching due to winds and chills.

Tan chi (丹劑 pellets). *Tan chi* is also of two kinds, external and internal. *Tan chi*, a collective name, are mostly made of pure, refined, or very precious drugs. They are usually in fine powder form, sometimes bonded with glue or sticky herb juice. Examples are *chih-pao-tan* (至寶丹 · Rhinoceros and Succinum Formula), an internal, and *Hung-sheng-tan* (紅升丹 Cinnabar and Realgar Formula), an external.

Chu chi (酒劑 elixirs). Also known as *yao chu* (medicated liquor), elixirs are prepared by soaking the herbs in wine for a certain length of time or simmering them with wine in water, then removing the dregs. The remaining liquid is then drunk. One example of this form is *Hung-lan-hua-chu* (紅藍花酒 Carthamus Wine), generally indicated for rheumatic paralysis and aching.

Yao lu (藥露 medicated essence). These essences are primarily distilled from fresh herbs. They have a light odor and bland taste and are commonly drunk for a summer medication; example: *Chin-yin-hua-lu* (金銀花露 Lonicera Essence).

Ting chi (錠劑), *ping chi* (餅劑 tablets, cakes). Herbs for tablets and cakes are pulverized into fine powders and admixed with some kind of mucilaginous juice. The mixture is kneaded and formed into tablets, *ting chi*, or small cakes, *ping chi.*

Tiao chi (條劑 rods). A rod is made by gluing herb powder onto a thread or by rolling the herb powder into a rod which can then be inserted into a sore for the purpose of dissolving pus and removing fistulas.

Hsien chi (線劑 threads). A silk or cotton thread is immersed in a medicinal juice and boiled. Such a thread is used for tying up a fistula or polyp so that the latter withers and falls off.

Chin hsi chi (浸洗劑 washes). These are herbal decoctions used for soaking or washing either the whole or part of the body, for example, *ku-sheng-tang* (苦參湯 Sophora Combination).

Hsun chi (薰劑 fumigants). The required herbs are burned and a lesion fumigated with the smoke, for example, realgar. In ancient times a boiling decoction of herbs was placed in a wooden keg. The patient sat on the keg above the decoction so that sweating could be induced by the fumes and heat.

Suan chi (栓劑 suppositories). A suppository is made the same way as a pill or tablet is made or by wrapping the herb powder in a silk or linen cloth. Suppositories are placed in the vagina for the treatment of abnormal leukorrhea or pudendal pruritus.

Tao fa (導法 guide-method or enema). Readily dissolvable or soluble herbs are formed into tablets and inserted in the anus. As the tablet dissolves, it lubricates the rectum and colon, making dry stool soft and easy to discharge. One such preparation is *Mi-chien-tao* (蜜煎導).

Of all these dosage forms, decoctions, pills, powders, unguents, and elixirs are the most frequently used. Based on the patient's condition, the length of use varies. Generally speaking though, if an herbal decoction is to be taken for an extended time in order to exert a healing action on the diseases in the upper warmer area, then the formula is taken after a meal. For diseases of the lower warmer, the medicine must be taken before meals to expedite the herbs in reaching the lower warmer. Tonics are taken on an empty stomach.

Changes in the Weighing and Measuring Units of Herbs

The weighing and measuring systems of the various generations differed and conclusions reached by contemporary scholars are often contradictory. Here, we only use the measurements recorded in the ancient medical classics as a reference point. As these writings show, the proper dosage is based on the age, physical build, and condition of the patient. A table of weights and measurements of the various generations and the present-day system is given below.

Time	Ancient Weight Unit	Present Market System Equivalent	Ancient Volume Unit	Present Market System Equivalent
Chin dynasty	1 *liang*	0.5165 market *liang*	1 *sheng*	0.34 market *sheng*
West Han dynasty	1 *liang*	0.5165 market *liang*	1 *sheng*	0.34 market *sheng*
Hsin dynasty	1 *liang*	0.4455 market *liang*	1 *sheng*	0.20 market *sheng*
East Han dynasty	1 *liang*	0.4455 market *liang*	1 *sheng*	0.20 market *sheng*
Wei/Chin dynasty	1 *liang*	0.4455 market *liang*	1 *sheng*	0.21 market *sheng*
North Chou dynasty	1 *liang*	0.5011 market *liang*	1 *sheng*	0.21 market *sheng*
Hsui/Tang dynasty	1 *liang*	1.0075 market *liang*	1 *sheng*	0.58 market *sheng*
Sung dynasty	1 *liang*	1.1936 market *liang*	1 *sheng*	0.66 market *sheng*
Ming dynasty	1 *liang*	1.1936 market *liang*	1 *sheng*	1.07 market *sheng*
Ching dynasty	1 *liang* (*ku ping*)	1.194 market *liang*	1 *sheng* (*ying tsao*)	1.0355 market sheng

Note: The equivalents given above are only approximate values. Today one *liang* is approximately equal to 30.0g.

Scientific Chinese Herb Preparations

Recently the preparation of Chinese medicines has been standardized. Carefully selected by trained pharmacists, the raw materials are condensed by a high-vacuum, reduced-pressure method. The essential oils are then recovered by means of an ultra-high speed, low temperature drying appartus that converts the herbs into granular form or powder. High quality is maintained by tests and chemical analysis. Modern preparation has several distinct advantages over the traditional decoction method. Not only does it facilitate dispensing, it also prevents the loss of active ingredients, rendering the drugs substantially more effective.

Nagakura Onzo of Japan initiated this method of herbal preparation. Twenty years ago the technique was imported to Taiwan. After modification and improvement of Nagakura's process, in 1963 the scientific preparation of Chinese herbal drugs was instituted at the Sun Ten Pharmaceutical Works and the products marketed under the trade name of "Sun Ten's Scientific Chinese Herbal Preparations."

All the formulas now produced scientifically were taken from the *Shang han lun* (傷寒論) and *Chin kuei yao lueh* (金匱要略), written by Chang Chung-ching some 1800 years ago, and from the *I fang chi chieh* (醫方集解) by Wang Ang of the Ching dynasty. The formulas selected were considered to be the more effective ones as attested to by modern scientific studies.

Raw materials for these scientific preparations are carefully selected from the best quality crude drugs by the pharmacognostic specialists using pharmacognostic research methods. Thus the preparations produced from these high-quality raw materials are of a constant high standard. All of them undergo accurate analysis and strict quality control.

The amounts of herbs used are equivalent to those used in the ancient system of the *Shang han lun*. Modern archaeological research has enabled us to calculate and convert the ancient system into modern equivalents. One gram of a formula produced by the scientific method has five to ten times the potency of the original. Moreover, preparations in granular or powder form are much more convenient to use.

All amounts used in this book are expressed in the original form. One can convert them to the equivalent amount of the scientific preparation by multiplying by 6. For example, 6g of raw *Tang-kuei* is equivalent to 1g of refined *Tang-kuei*. However, due to different herbal constituents, the extent of condensation varies. For example, Pueraria and Rehmannia have a richer content of starch and cannot be highly concentrated. Seed drugs, on the other hand, can usually be condensed to one-tenth of their original weight.

For easy and convenient administration, the preparations produced by the Sun Ten Pharmaceutical Works have been so adjusted in their potency that the daily dose falls between 4.5g-6.0g, that is, 1.5g-2.0g taken with water three times daily either between or after meals. If the original formula is bulky, the daily dose may be increased up to 10g.

If more herbs are to be added to a basic formula, the general practice is that the basic formula comprises two-thirds of the dosage and the additional herbs make up one-third of the dosage. For example, when Cnidium and Magnolia flower are added to the formula *Ko-ken-tang* (Pueraria Combination), then a daily dose of 4g of *Ko-ken-tang*, is combined with 1g each of Magnolia flower and Cnidium. The three are then blended together and taken as a single formula.

PART II

DETAILED DISCUSSION OF FORMULA TYPES

Note:

1. The unit of dosages is given in grams, and the dosage indicated for each formula is the maximum daily amount allowed. If there are no directions for administration given after a formula, the formula is decocted in the conventional way, that is, a one-day dosage of the formula is added to 500 ml of water and decocted until 300 ml remains; then the dregs are discarded and the decoction is divided into two or three portions. Each portion is taken warmed one hour before meals, or on an empty stomach. Dosages may vary according to the patient's size and strength, and the severity of the disease.
2. A ~~~ mark given under "Discrimination" means the conformation is the same as the aforementioned formula.
3. An illustration of the human body showing treatment area is placed at the end of each formula monograph.

1.

Chieh Piao Chi

(解表劑, Sudorific Formulas)

Formulas that promote sweating, relieve muscular tension, speed the eruption of measles, and eliminate surface conformations are called *chieh piao chi.* Such formulas are of the "sweating" method, one of eight major therapeutic methods in Chinese medicine.

A sudorific formula expels toxins accumulated on the surface of the body (skin and hair) that have not yet penetrated to the interior. Expulsion of toxins occurs by means of sweating. The *Shang han lun* says, "He who is proficient at treatment always treats the skin and hair." An injury, caused by the six excesses generally manifests itself on the surface; hence it is surface conformation. At this stage, the injurious toxin is still light and shallow can be eliminated by sudorifics which induce sweating, thus dispelling the toxins. The sweating method often precedes other therapeutic methods.

Because most sudorific formulas contain herbs that are acrid, dispersant, light, and evaporative, they should not be overcooked because it causes reduction in effectiveness. At the same time patients treated with a sudorific formula should avoid drafts and the cold and put on more clothes to induce more sweating. Strong sudorifics cause the patient to become soaked with sweat. Note: If there is too little sweating, the toxin is not totally expelled. But excessive sweating may injure normal *ch'i* causing yang to collapse.

Chai-Ko-Chieh-Chi-Tang 柴葛解肌湯

(Bupleurum and Pueraria Combination)

Bupleurum	4.0	Pueraria	4.0	Scute	3.0
Peony	3.0	*Chianghuo*	2.0	Angelica	2.0
Platycodon	2.0	Licorice	2.0	Jujube	2.0
Gypsum	5.0	Ginger	1.0		

Chai-ko-chieh-chi-tang was first mentioned in the *Shang han liu shu* (傷寒六書) by Tao Hua during the Ming dynasty. This formula is used by those with a common cold when both *Kuei-chih-tang* (Cinnamon Combination) and *Ma-huang-tang* (*Ma-huang* Combination) have been ineffective. Further symptoms are high fever, headache, thirst, generalized pain, and epistaxis.

Herbs and Actions

Bupleurum, Scute, Peony, and Gypsum remove "internal heat" from the liver, the chest, and below the heart. Pueraria and Angelica dispel "moist heat" in the body. *Chianghuo* alleviates severe chills, fever, headache, and anhidrosis. Platycodon reinforces the function of the other herbs. Licorice synthesizes the actions of the other herbs.

Indications

Pneumonia, common cold, influenza, and febrile diseases.

Discrimination

Ma-huang-tang (*Ma-huang* Combination): fever; greater yang disease with external fever and firm conformation; floating, tense pulse; no tongue coating, no extreme thirst.

Hsiao-chai-hu-tang (Minor Bupleurum Combination): fever; lesser yang disease with firm fever; thoraco-costal distress; chordal pulse; and bitter taste in the mouth.

Pai-hu-tang (Gypsum Combination): fever; sunlight yang disease with firm fever; sweating and extreme thirst.

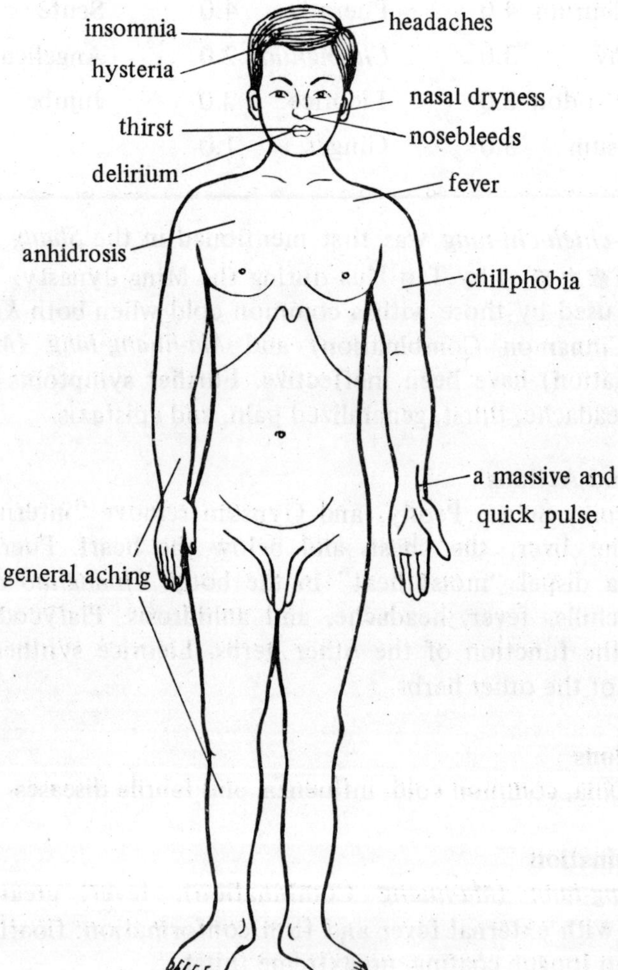
insomnia
headaches
hysteria
nasal dryness
thirst
nosebleeds
delirium
fever
anhidrosis
chillphobia
a massive and
quick pulse
general aching

Ching-Pi-Tang 清鼻湯

(Pueraria Nasal Combination)

Pueraria	6.0	Cnidium	1.5	*Ma-huang*	3.0
Rhubarb	1.5	Cinnamon	2.5	Licorice	1.0
Peony	3.0	Coix	5.0	Ginger	1.5
Platycodon	4.5	Gypsum	2.0	Jujube	2.0
Magnolia flower	4.0				

Ching-pi-tang is good for rhinitis and nasal suppuration. This formula is good to treat nasal drainage, sneezing, shivering due to chills, general fatigue, headache, itching in the nose and throat, viscid nasal mucus, stuffy nose, loss of the sense of smell, and anorexia, snoring, headache due to pus in the nasal cavity, amnesia, lack of vigor, and impatience.

Herbs and Actions

The multiple action of Pueraria, Cnidium, *Ma-huang*, and Cinnamon in combination relieves headache, heaviness in the head, stress, amnesia, poor concentration, and mental instability. Pueraria initiates the discharge of nasal mucus, and in conjunction with Coix, it alleviates stiffness in the shoulders; when added to Platycodon, it can purge pus. The volatile oil of Magnolia flower alleviates stuffy nose. Cnidium and Rhubarb relieve swelling due to mucus accumulation. Gypsum relieves allergies and toxic states.

Indications

Rhinitis and nasal suppuration.

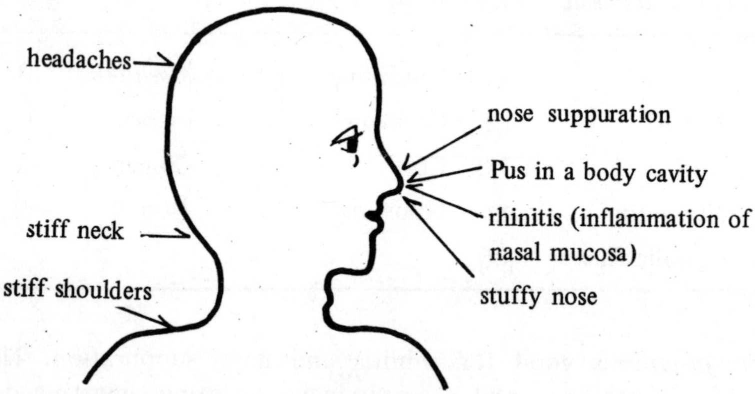

Chiu-Wei-Chiang-Huo-Tang 九味羌活湯

(Chianghuo Combination)

Chianghuo	4.5	Siler	4.5	Jujube	1.0
Atractylodes	4.5	Asarum	1.5	Cnidium	3.0
Angelica	3.0	Rehmannia	3.0	Scute	3.0
Licorice	3.0	Ginger	1.0	Allium	1.0

Chiu-wei-chiang-huo-tang is recorded in *Liu k'o chuen sheng* (六科準繩) by Wang Ken-tang of the Ming dynasty. This formula acts as a diaphoretic, and dispels moisture and internal heat. It is used for treating "wind chill", "moist evil", severe chills, fever, superficial anhidrosis, headache, stiff neck, generalized pain, bitter taste, and thirst.

Herbs and Actions

Chianghuo, Siler, Atractylodes, and Angelica are diaphoretics. dispel "external evil" and internal moisture. Cnidium and Asarum dispel "external evil", remove chills, treat headache and non-specific pain. Rehmannia and Scute are antipyretics. Licorice coordinates the actions of the other herbs. Allium and Ginger act as diaphoretics.

Indications

Influenza, headache with fever, rheumatic neuralgia due to the common cold.

Discrimination

Ko-ken-tang (Pueraria Combination): chillphobia, fever, headaches, body aches, absence of sweat, stiffness and spasms in the neck and back, flushing up, and asthma.
Ma-huang-tang (*Ma-huang* Combination): chillphobia, fever, headaches, body aches, absence of sweat, asthma, chest fullness, and extreme thirst.
Shih-shen-tang (*Ma-huang* and Cimicifuga Combination): chillphobia, fever, headaches, body aches, no sweating, cough, stuffy nose.
Sheng-ma-ko-ken-tang (Cimicifuga and Pueraria Combination): chillphobia, fever, headaches, body aches, no sweating, insomnia, aching eyes, dry nose.

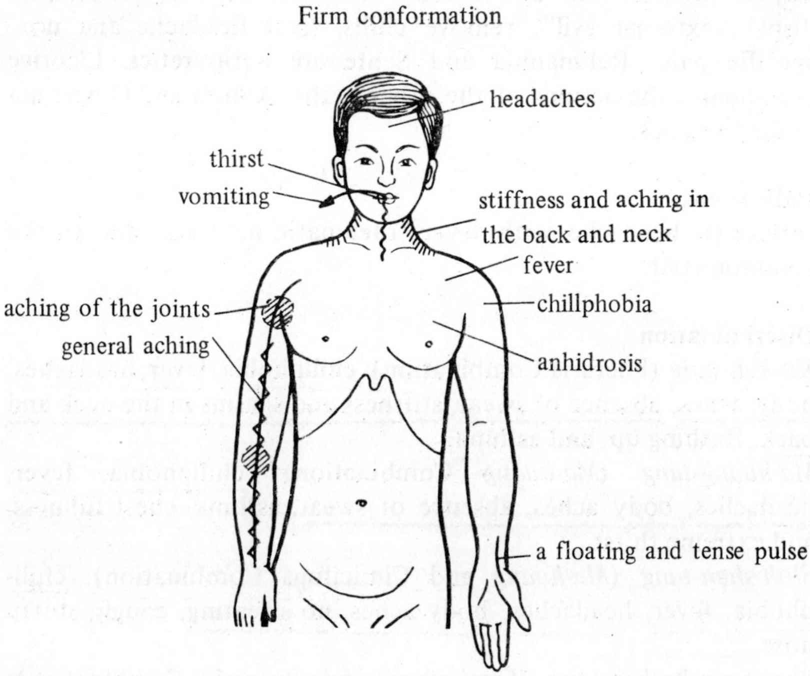

Chuan-Chiung-Cha-Tiao-San 川芎茶調散

(Cnidium and Tea Formula)

Mentha	2.0	Cnidium	3.0	Cyperus	4.0
Schizonepeta	2.0	*Chianghuo*	2.0	Angelica	2.0
Licorice	1.5	Siler	2.0	Tea	1.5

Chuan-chiung-cha-tiao-san is first mentioned in the *Tai ping huei min ho chi chu fang* (太平惠民和劑局方 A.D. 1110) during the Sung dynasty. The formula is a carminative, antipyretic, and analgesic. It is used for treating migraine or other headaches such as those due to a common cold with severe chills, fever, vertigo, stuffy nose, thin-white tongue coating, and a floating pulse.

Herbs and Actions
Cnidium, *Chianghuo,* Angelica, Siler, and Cyperus are carminatives that are effective for headaches. Schizonepeta is also a carminative. Mentha relieves "internal heat". Licorice coordinates the actions of the other herbs. Tea also removes "internal heat".

Indications
Common cold, migraine, nasal congestion, vertigo, and copious sputum.

Hsiang-Su-San 香蘇散

(Cyperus and Perilla Formula)

Cyperus	3.5	Perilla	1.5	Citrus	3.0
Licorice	1.0	Ginger	1.0		

Hsiang-su-san was first recorded in the *Tai ping huei min ho chi chu fang* (太平惠民和劑局方) by Chen Shih-wen during the Sung dynasty. This formula is used for treating common colds due to stagnant *ch'i* and stagnant food. It is also recommended for patients with gastrointestinal weakness who are suffering from a common cold with chest distension even after taking *Kuei-chih-tang* (Cinnamon Combination) or *Ko-ken-tang* (Pueraria Combination). This formula is also suitable for a sinking pulse, subcardiac distension, aching shoulders, headache, vertigo, tinnitus, nausea, and stagnant *ch'i.*

Herbs and Actions
Perilla is a disphoretic that also improves blood circulation. Cyperus dispels stagnant *ch'i.* Citrus is a stomachic and expectorant. Licorice coordinates the actions of the other herbs.

Indications

Common cold, neurasthenia, abdominal pain of emotional origin, blood diseases, amenorrhea, food poisoning caused by eating toxic fish, anosmia, nasal congestion, eructation, and vomiting.

Discrimination

Pan-hsia-hou-pu-tang (Pinellia and Magnolia Combination): mental illness, depressed *ch'i*, and the sensation of broiled meat clinging to the throat.

Kuei-chih-tang (Cinnamon Combination): the common cold and spontaneous sweating, floating and weak pulse.

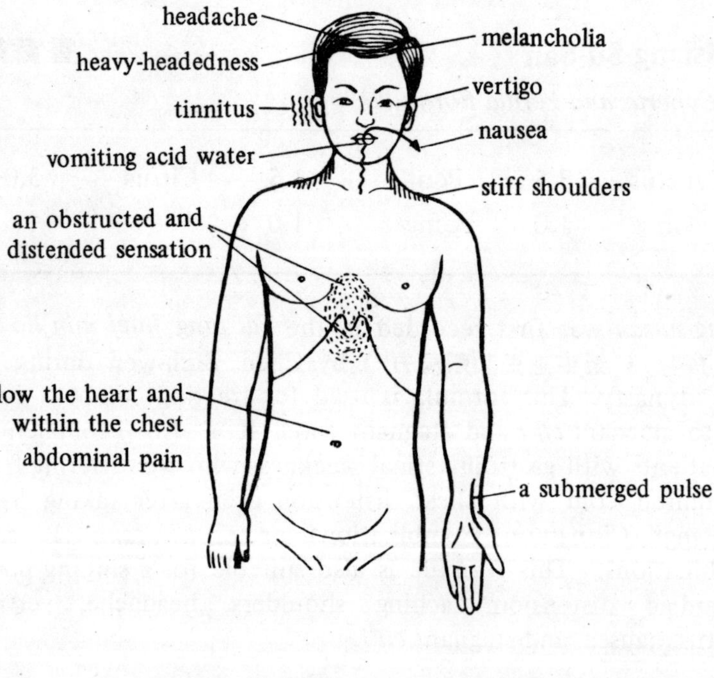

Hsiao-Ching-Lung-Tang 小青龍湯

(Minor Blue Dragon Combination)

Pinellia	6.0	*Ma-huang*	3.0	Peony	3.0
Licorice	3.0	Cinnamon	3.0	Asarum	3.0
Schizandra	3.0	Ginger	3.0		

Hsiao-ching-lung-tang is mentioned early in *Shang han lun* (Treatise on Febrile Diseases) and *Chin kuei yao lueh* (Summaries on Household Drugs) by Chang Chung-ching (A.D. 142-220). This formula is used to treat subcardiac edema, anhidrosis, general aching, dry coughs, fever, asthmatic cough or dyspnea, frothy sputum, decrease of urine, and occasional chills in the back.

Herbs and Actions

Ma-huang and Cinnamon remove surface diseases (severe chills, anhidrosis, general aching, etc.). Cinnamon checks regurgitation. *Ma-huang* cures cough stridor. Asarum, Ginger, and Pinellia relieve ascites. Pinellia alone increases the flow of urine. Schizandra, *Ma-huang*, Asarum, and Peony are antitussive. And Licorice coordinates the actions of the herbs, sedates flushing up, and relieves contraction of tissues.

Indications

1. Cough with fever, stridor, headache, severe chills, flushing up, hiccups, and dizziness.
2. Bronchial or humoral stridor, and watery sputum.
3. Allergic rhinitis.
4. Whooping cough, bronchial dilation, pulmonary asthma.
5. Renal cirrhosis (interstitial inflammation), swelling due to primary nephritis, and colds accompanied by cough and swelling.
6. Conjunctivitis, inflammation of the tear ducts, periorbital edema and lachrymation.
7. Edematous arthritis.

Note: This formula should not be given to patients having weak conformation and night sweats.

Discrimination

Ma-huang-tang (*Ma-huang* Combination): coughing and asthma, fever, external conformation, muscle pain, tense pulse.

Ta-ching-lung-tang (Major Blue Dragon Combination): asthmatic cough, severe symptoms, distress and irritability, a floating and tense pulse.

Mai-men-tung-tang (Ophiopogon Combination): asthmatic cough, coughing and upward congestion of *ch'i*, dry cough, difficulty in expectorating mucus.

Ling-kan-chiang-wei-hsin-hsia-jen-tang (Hoelen and Schizandra Combination): cough, stridor, edema, no fever, weakness and chills, yin conformation.

Hsiao-chai-hu-tang (Minor Bupleurum Combination): asthmatic cough, distressed chest, loss of appetite, chordal pulse.

Ma-hsing-kan-shih-tang (*Ma-huang* and Apricot Combination): asthmatic cough, sweating, and extreme thirst.

Sheng-mi-tang (*Ma-huang* and Magnolia Combination): cough, asthma, mild distressed chest, prolonged labored breathing.

Mu-fang-chi-tang (Stephania and Ginseng Combination): labored breathing, palpitations, hardness beneath the heart, submerged and tense pulse.

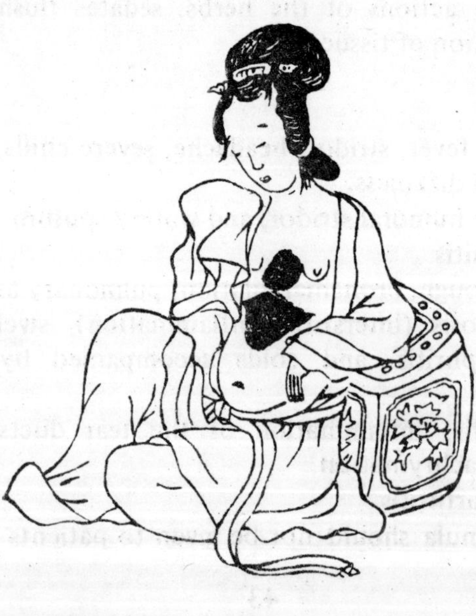

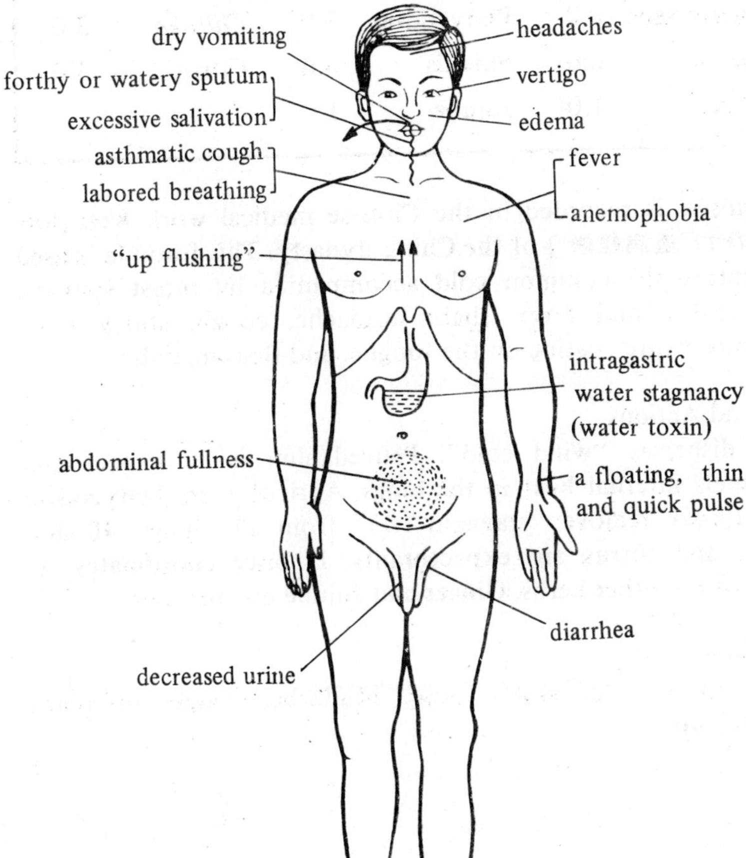
dry vomiting
headaches
forthy or watery sputum
vertigo
excessive salivation
edema
asthmatic cough
labored breathing
fever
anemophobia
"up flushing"
intragastric
water stagnancy
(water toxin)
abdominal fullness
a floating, thin,
and quick pulse
diarrhea
decreased urine

Hsing-Su-San 杏蘇散

(Apricot Seed and Perilla Formula)

Perilla	3.0	Peucedanum	6.0	Licorice	1.5
Apricot seed	6.0	Platycodon	3.0	*Chih-ko*	3.0
Hoelen	6.0	Pinellia	6.0	Citrus	3.0
Ginger	1.0	Jujube	1.0		

Hsing-su-san is recorded in the Chinese medical work *Wen ping tiao pien* (溫病條辨) of the Ching dynasty. This formula is used for treating the common cold accompanied by moist sputum, severe chills, mild fever, slight headache, cough, stuffy nose, anhidrosis, white coating on the tongue, and floating pulse.

Herbs and Actions

Perilla disperses "wind cold". Peucedanum is an expectorant and dispels internal heat in the lungs. Apricot seed, Platycodon, and *Chih-ko* remove "stagnant *ch'i*" from the lungs. Hoelen, Pinellia, and Citrus are expectorants. Licorice coordinates the actions of the other herbs. Ginger and Jujube are nutrients.

Indications

The common cold, stuffy nose, headache, cough, influenza, and bronchitis.

Hua-Kai-San 華蓋散

(Ma-huang and Morus Formula)

Ma-huang	4.0	Citrus	2.0	Hoelen	5.0
Apricot seed	4.0	Morus bark	2.0	Licorice	1.0
Perilla fruit	2.0				

Hua-kai-san was recorded in the Chinese medical work, *Tai ping huei min ho chi chu fang* (太平惠民和劑局方) during the Sung dynasty. This formula is used for treating a common cold, cough, restlessness, distension in the chest, nasal congestion, vertigo, chest congestion, a floating pulse, gastrointestinal weakness, and anorexia.

Herbs and Actions

Hoelen, Citrus, Morus bark, and Perilla fruit are antitussives and expectorants. *Ma-huang* and Apricot seed improve blood circulation, eliminate stagnant water and relieve wheezing and coughing. Licorice coordinates the actions of the other herbs.

Indications

Common cold, cough, wheezing, nasal congestion, bronchitis, and asthma in children.

Discrimination

Hsiao-ching-lung-tang (Minor Blue Dragon Combination): asthmatic cough, thin sputum, stagnant water in the stomach, external fever.

Mai-men-tung-tang (Ophiopogon Combination): asthmatic cough, severe flushing up of *ch'i*, sore throat.

Jen-Sheng-Pai-Tu-San 人參敗毒散

(Ginseng and Mentha Formula)

Ginseng	2.0	*Chianghuo*	2.0	*Tuhuo*	2.0
Bupleurum	2.0	Peucedanum	2.0	Cnidium	2.0
Chih-ko	2.0	Platycodon	2.0	Hoelen	2.0
Licorice	1.0	Mentha	1.0	Ginger	1.0

Jen-sheng-pai-tu-san was recorded in the *I fang chi chieh* (醫方集解) by Wang Jen-an during the Ching dynasty. This formula is used for treating common cold, chills, fever, stiffness in the neck, headache, general pain, anhidrosis, nasal congestion, and productive cough. It is also suitable for treating diarrhea, malaria, and ulcers.

Herbs and Actions

Chianghuo and *Tuhuo* relieve rheumatism and, in combination with Cnidium, relieve headache and neck stiffness. Peucedanum is an expectorant. Bupleurum and Mentha dispel "internal heat". *Chih-ko*, Platycodon, and Hoelen are expectorants that reduce chest distention and nourish the *ch'i*. Licorice coordinates the actions of the other herbs. Ginger dispels chills. Ginseng is a tonic.

Indications

Common cold, cough, nasal congestion, and the early stages of a carbuncle.

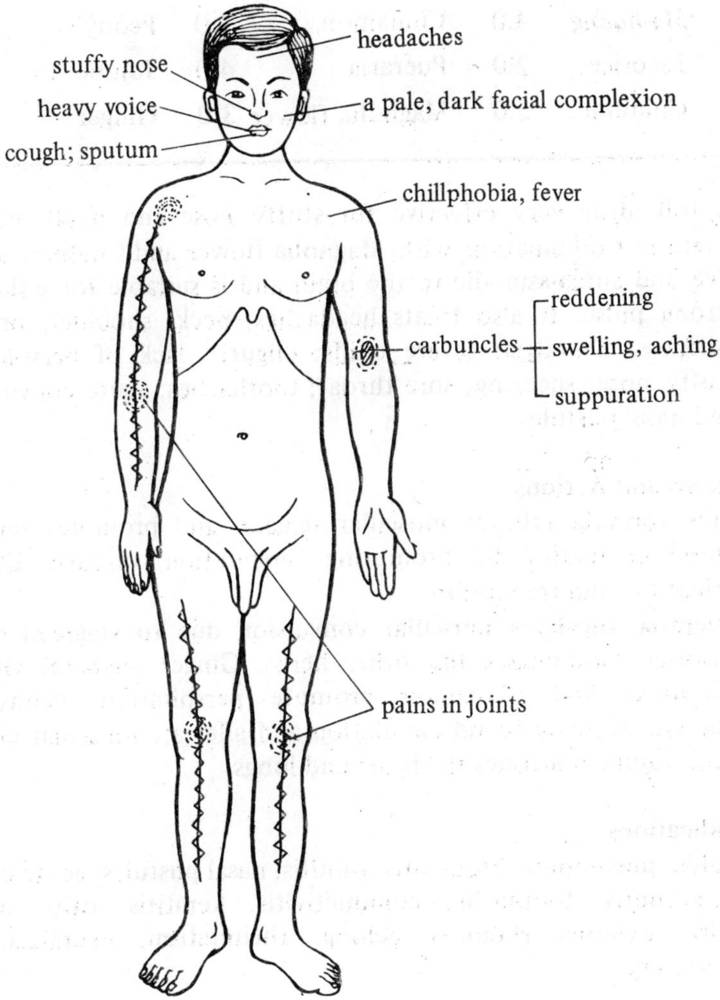
headaches
stuffy nose
heavy voice
a pale, dark facial complexion
cough; sputum
chillphobia, fever
reddening
carbuncles
swelling, aching
suppuration
pains in joints

Ko-Ken-Chia-Hsin-I-Chuan-Chiung 葛根加辛夷川芎

(Pueraria and Magnolia Combination)

Ma-huang	4.0	Cinnamon	2.0	Peony	2.0
Licorice	2.0	Pueraria	4.0	Jujube	3.0
Cnidium	3.0	Magnolia flower	3.0	Ginger	1.0

A folk drug very effective for stuffy nose and nasal pustules. Pueraria Combination with Magnolia flower and Cnidium is sedative and antispasmodic to the brain and is suitable for a floating, strong pulse. It also treats headaches; neck, shoulder, or back stiffness; neuralgia; severe chills; oliguria; lack of perspiration; stuffy nose; sneezing; sore throat; toothaches; acute convulsions; and nasal pustules.

Herbs and Actions

This formula relieves muscular tension and promotes retarded blood circulation by promoting perspiration, vascular dilation, urination, and tranquility.

Pueraria alleviates muscular convulsion due to stagnant blood. Licorice harmonizes the other herbs. Ginger regulates vitality. *Ma-huang* and Cinnamon promote perspiration. Peony and Pueraria regulate blood circulation and alleviate muscular convulsion. Jujube nourishes the heart and lungs.

Indications

Colds, pneumonia, bronchitis, rhinitis, nasal pustules, acute colitis, pararhinitis, toothache, conjunctivitis, keratitis, otitis media, otitis externa, shoulder aching, rheumatism, neuralgia, and dysentery.

Ko-Ken-Tang 葛根湯

(Pueraria Combination)

Pueraria	8.0	*Ma-huang*	4.0	Cinnamon	3.0
Peony	3.0	Jujube	4.0	Licorice	2.0
Ginger	1.0				

Ko-ken-tang is a well-known formula for the common cold. This formula was first recorded in *Shang han lun* (Treatise on Febrile Diseases) and *Chin kuei yao lueh* (A.D. 205, Summaries on Household Drugs), Chinese medical works of the Han dynasty. It is suitable for treating febrile or afebrile common cold with severe chills, floating or strong pulse; stiffness in the neck and back, inflammation, congestion, diarrhea and severe muscle spasms.

Herbs and Actions

Pueraria regulates blood circulation and intestinal function and evacuation. *Ma-huang* and Licorice cure cough and relieve contraction of the skin. *Ma-huang* and Cinnamon promote perspiration. Cinnamon improves blood circulation. Peony strengthens gastrointestinal function. Licorice has a detoxifing action in the liver. Jujube is a nutritive. Ginger promotes blood circulation.

Indications

1. Common cold, influenza, pneumonia, bronchitis, and headache.
2. Shoulder stiffness, 40 years' wrists, 50 years' shoulders, and neuralgia.
3. Skin diseases, eczema, urticaria, rubella, furuncles, and boils.
4. Keratitis, hordeolum, conjunctivitis, and trachoma.
5. Otitis media, rhinitis, stuffy nose, and otitis externa.
6. Meningitis, lymphadenitis, mastitis, and scarlet fever.

Discrimination

Kuei-chih-chia-ko-ken-tang (Cinnamon and Pueraria Combina-

tion): pain in the scapula region, weakness conformation, sweating.
Ma-huang-tang (*Ma-huang* Combination): fever, asthma, tense pulse.

Ma-huang-fu-tzu-hsi-hsin-tang (*Ma-huang*, Aconite, and Asarum Combination): common cold, chill conformation, submerged pulse.

Huang-chin-tang (Scute and Licorice Combination): diarrhea, greater and lesser yang disease, abdominal pain, and diarrhea.
Ko-ken-huang-lien-huang-chin-tang (Pueraria, Coptis, and Scute Combination): fever, internal fever, sweating, obstruction and hardness beneath the heart and the hypochondrium.

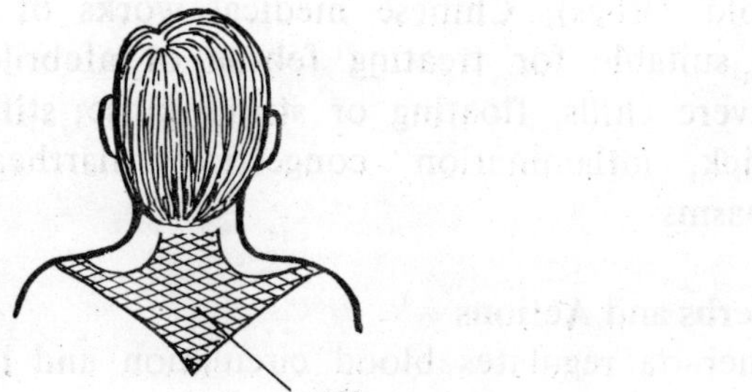

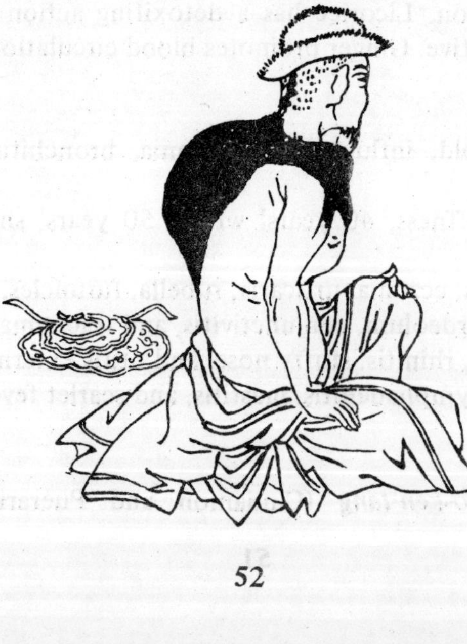

Yang firm conformation

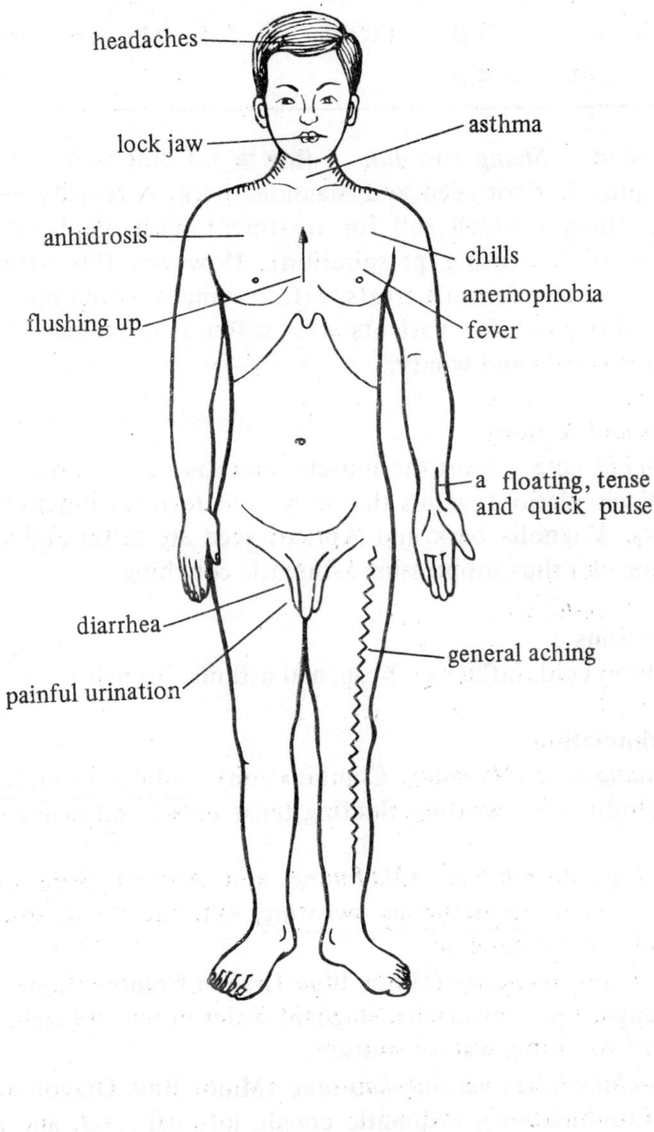

Kuei-Chih-Chia-Hou-Pu-Hsing-Jen-Tang

桂枝加厚朴杏仁湯

(Cinnamon, Magnolia, and Apricot Seed Combination)

Cinnamon	4.0	Peony	4.0	Jujube	4.0
Ginger	4.0	Licorice	2.0	Magnolia bark	1.0
Apricot seed	4.0				

Recorded in *Shang han lun* (傷寒論). Composed of *Kuei-chih-tang* plus Apricot seed and Magnolia bark. A remedy for greater yang diseases which call for treatment with diaphoretics (producing or increasing perspiration). However, this formula is a purgative. The formula treats surface symptoms and mild coughs. It is also good for patients who suffer from coughs or asthma when it is cold and windy.

Herbs and Actions

Kuei-chih-tang relaxes the muscles and causes sweating, stimulates blood circulation, warms the body, and fortifies functions of the viscera. Magnolia bark and Apricot seed are bitter and settle up-rushing *ch'i* thus suppressing asthmatic coughing.

Indications

Common cold, influenza, bronchial asthma, bronchitis.

Discrimination

Ma-huang-tang (*Ma-huang* Combination): asthma, fever, headache, chillphobia, no sweating, floating tense pulse, and firm conformation.

Ma-hsing-kan-shih-tang (*Ma-huang* and Apricot Seed Combination): cough, spontaneous sweating, extreme thirst, discomfort, and adverse flushing up.

Hsiao-ching-lung-tang (Minor Blue Dragon Combination): asthmatic cough, fever, headache, stagnant water in the stomach, flushing up, dry vomiting, watery sputum.

Hsiao-ching-lung-chia-shih-kao-tang (Minor Blue Dragon and Gypsum Combination); asthmatic cough. internal fever, and anxiety.

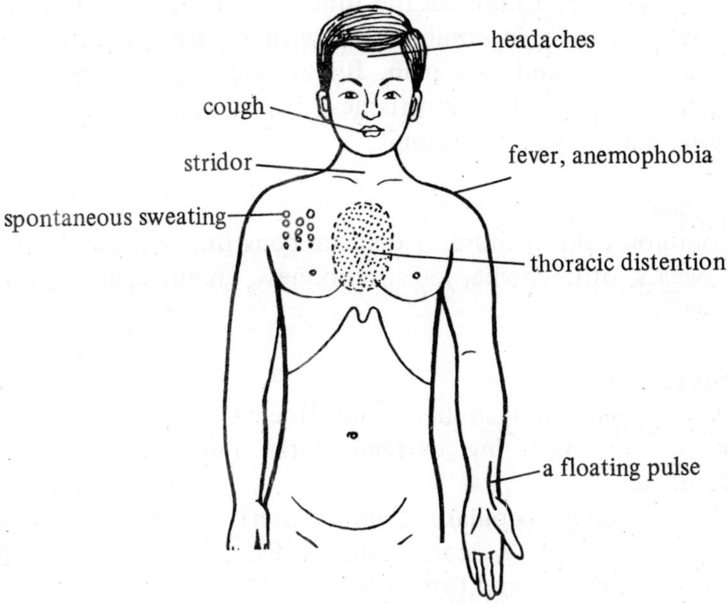

Kuei-Chih-Chia-Huang-Chi-Tang 桂枝加黃耆湯

(Cinnamon and Astragalus Combination)

Cinnamon	4.0	Peony	4.0	Jujube	4.0
Ginger	4.0	Astragalus	3.0	Licorice	2.0

Kuei-chih-chia-huang-chi-tang is recorded in *Chin kuei yao lueh* (金匱要略) of the Han dynasty. This formula is used for treating excessive perspiration on the upper body, pain in the waist and legs, nonspecific pain, stress, dysuria, jaundice, superficial moisture, flaccid skin, night sweats, and numbness.

Herbs and Actions
Cinnamon and Ginger are stimulants, increase blood circulation, warm the body, and improve the functions of the internal organs. Peony is a sedative; in combination with Licorice, it can relieve muscular tension and ease pain. Jujube and Licorice are tonics. Astragalus nourishes the skin tissues, dispels moisture, stops suppuration, and acts as a body tonic.

Indications
The common cold in those of delicate constitution, skin diseases, night sweats, otitis media, facial numbness, jaundice, and "yellow sweating".

Discrimination
Yin-chen-wu-ling-san (Capillaris and Hoelen Formula): jaundice, decreased urine, vomiting, extreme thirst, and stagnant water in the stomach.
Yin-chen-hao-tang (Capillaris Combination): jaundice, decreased urine, head sweating, constipation, distention in the upper abdomen, submerged and firm pulse.
Pu-chung-i-chi-tang (Ginseng and Astragalus Combination): spontaneous sweating, night sweats, fatigability, loss of appetite, thin and weak pulse, and a desire for hot food.
Huang-chi-chien-chung-tang (Astragalus Combination): spontaneous sweating, night sweats, weakness, fatigability, appetite loss, thin and weak pulse, cold arms and legs, abdominal pain.

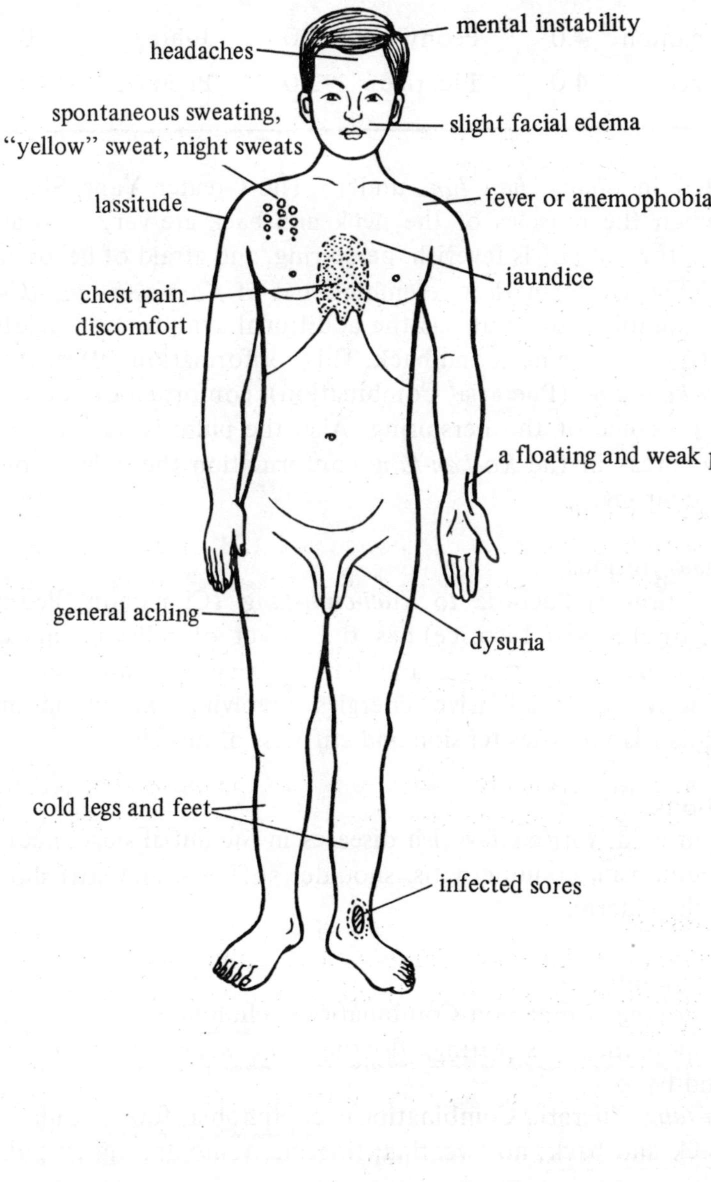
mental instability
headaches
spontaneous sweating,
"yellow" sweat, night sweats
slight facial edema
lassitude
fever or anemophobia
jaundice
chest pain
discomfort
a floating and weak pulse
general aching
dysuria
cold legs and feet
infected sores

Kuei-Chih-Chia-Ko-Ken-Tang 桂枝加葛根湯

(also called *Hsiao-ko-ken-tang*)

(Cinnamon and Pueraria Combination)

Cinnamon	4.0	Peony	4.0	Jujube	4.0
Ginger	4.0	Licorice	2.0	Pueraria	6.0

Recorded in *Shang han lun* under "The Greater Yang Stage." Used when the muscles of the neck and back are very rigid and stiff and the patient is feverish, perspiring, and afraid of becoming chilled. The conformation resembles that of *Kuei-chih-tang* (Cinnamon Combination) but has the additional symptom of rigidity and stiffness of the neck and back. This conformation differs from the *Ko-ken-tang* (Pueraria Combination) conformation because of the presence of the perspiring. Also the pulse is buoyant and weak whereas in the *Ko-ken-tang* conformation the pulse is buoyant and strong.

Herbs and Actions

The addition of Pueraria to *Kuei-chih-tang* (Cinnamon, Peony, Ginger, Jujube, and Licorice) has the effect of relieving muscle tenseness, nullifying toxins, and harmonizing the *jung* and *wei* (constructive and defensive energies involving the blood and *ch'i*). Pueraria mollifies tension and stiffness of muscles.

Indications

Common cold, various feverish diseases in the initial stage, neuralgia, rheumatism, conjunctivitis, shoulder stiffness, and stiff shoulders in the elderly.

Discrimination

Kuei-chih-tang (Cinnamon Combination): chillphobia, fever, headaches, spontaneous sweating, floating and weak pulse, no stiff neck and back.

Ko-ken-tang (Pueraria Combination): chillphobia; fever; headache; stiff neck and back; no sweating; floating, tense and quick pulse.

Hsiao-chai-hu-tang (Minor Bupleurum Combination): headache, stiff neck and back, alternating chills and fever, thoraco-costal distress, bitter taste in the mouth and vomiting.

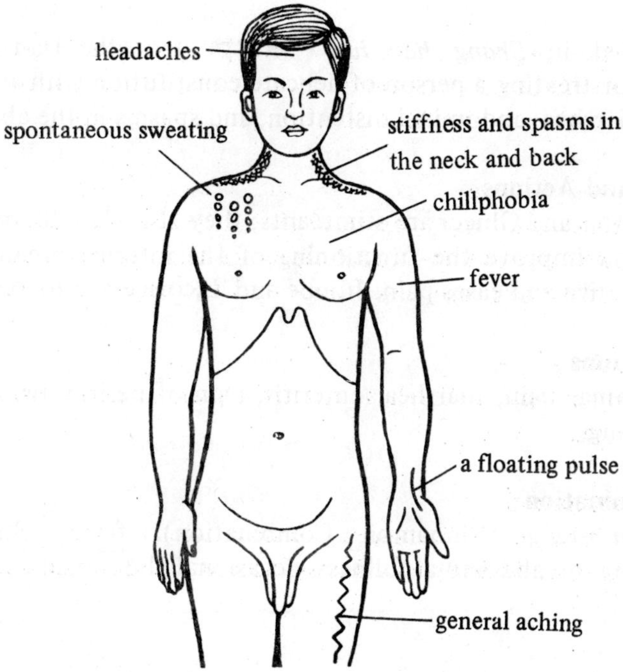

Kuei-Chih-Chia-Shao-Yao-Tang 桂枝加芍藥湯

(Cinnamon and Peony Combination)

Cinnamon	4.0	Peony	6.0	Jujube	4.0
Ginger	4.0	Licorice	2.0		

Recorded in *Shang han lun* (傷寒論) of the Han dynasty. Used for treating a person of delicate constitution with abdominal pain, diarrhea, abdominal distention, and spasms in the abdomen.

Herbs and Actions
Cinnamon and Ginger are stimulants; they stimulate blood circulation and improve the functioning of the internal organs. Peony is a sedative and eases pain. Jujube and Licorice are tonics.

Indications
Abdominal pain, diarrhea, enteritis, pain of peritonitis, and food poisoning.

Discrimination
Kuei-chih-tang (Cinnamon Combination): fever, chillphobia, sweating, no abdominal fullness, occasional abdominal pains.

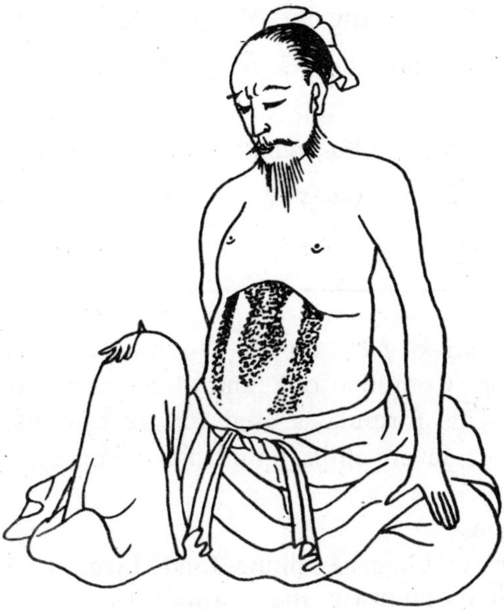

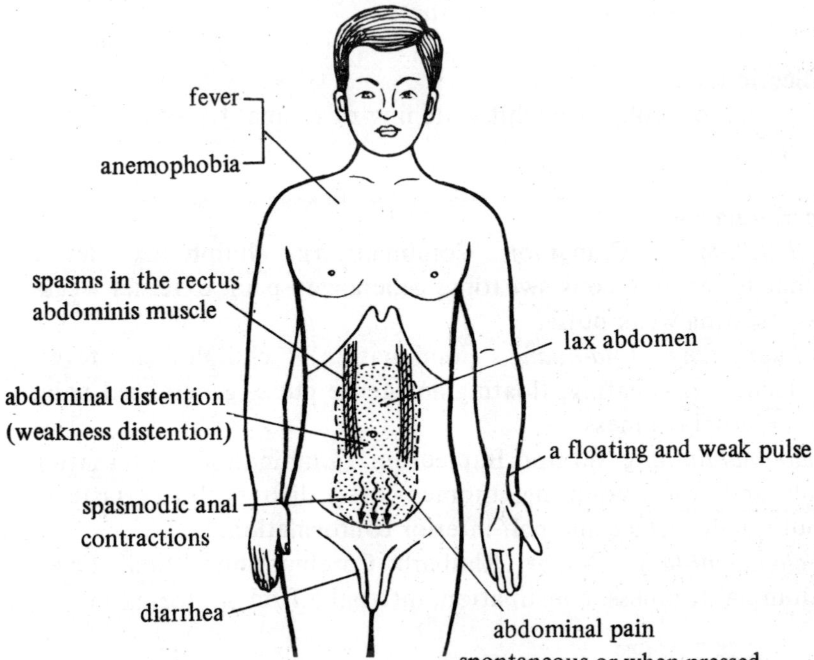
fever
anemophobia
spasms in the rectus abdominis muscle
lax abdomen
abdominal distention (weakness distention)
a floating and weak pulse
spasmodic anal contractions
diarrhea
abdominal pain spontaneous or when pressed

Kuei-Chih-Ma-Huang-Ko-Pan-Tang 桂枝麻黃各半湯

(Cinnamon and Ma-huang Combination)

Cinnamon	3.5	*Ma-huang*	2.0	Peony	2.0
Apricot seed	2.5	Licorice	2.0	Ginger	2.0
Jujube	2.0				

Kuei-chih-ma-huang-ko-pan-tang is a combination of *Kuei-chih-tang* (Cinnamon Combination) and *Ma-huang-tang* (*Ma-huang* Combination). This formula is used for treating ailments due to cold and for fever, severe chills, anhidrosis, and pruritis.

Herbs and Actions
Cinnamon, Peony, Ginger, Jujube, and Licorice of *Kuei-chih-tang* have both diaphoretic and antihidrotic effects. *Ma-huang*, Apricot seed, Licorice, and Cinnamon of *Ma-huang-tang* are diuretics and are used to treat asthma.

Indications
The common cold, bronchitis, itching of dermatitis, eczema, and urticaria.

Discrimination
Kuei-chih-tang (Cinnamon Combination): chillphobia, fever, headache, spontaneous sweating, generalized pain, external weakness, floating weak pulse.
Ma-huang-tang (*Ma-huang* Combination): chillphobia, fever, headache, no sweating, floating and tense pulse, generalized pain, and external firmness.
Hsiao-chai-hu-tang (Minor Bupleurum Combination): alternating chills and fever, vomiting, thoraco-costal distress, bitter taste in mouth, half surface and half interior conformation.
Ta-cheng-chi-tang (Major Rhubarb Combination): tidal fever, abdominal firmness, constipation, internally firm conformation.

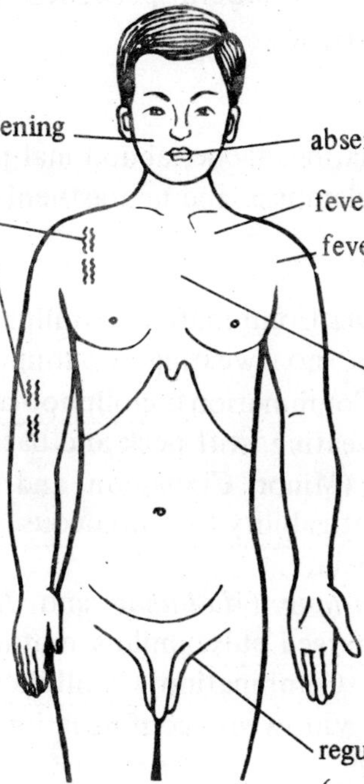

Kuei-Chih-Tang *(Cinnamon Combination)*					**桂枝湯**
Cinnamon	4.0	Peony	4.0	Jujube	4.0
Ginger	4.0	Licorice	2.0		

Kuei-chih-tang was first recorded in the *Shang han lun* (傷寒論) by Chung-ching Chang during the Han dynasty. This formula is used for treating severed chills, fever, headache, and a floating and weak pulse as well as for stimulating the functions of the internal organs.

Herbs and Actions

Cinnamon eliminates flushing up. Peony improves blood circulation and relieves tension in the muscles. Licorice coordinates the action of the other herbs. Jujube dispels chest distension. Ginger and Cinnamon are diuretics.

Indications

Common cold, neuralgia, headache, abdominal pain due to chills, delicate constitution, eclampsia, and neurasthenia.

Discrimination

Ma-huang-tang (*Ma-huang* Combination): chillphobia, fever, headache, external firmness, no sweating, floating and tense pulse.
Ko-ken-tang (Pueraria Combination): chillphobia, fever, headache, external firmness, no sweating, stiff neck and back.
Hsiao-chien-chung-tang (Minor Cinnamon and Peony Combination): weakness and fatigability, spontaneous sweating, internal acute pain, abdominal pain.
Ma-huang-fu-tzu-hsi-hsin-tang (*Ma-huang* and Asarum Combination): chillphobia, submerged pulse, mild sensation of fever.
Chen-wu-tang (Vitality Combination): chillphobia, heavy body, cold hands and feet, yin weak conformation, submerged and minute pulse.
Kuei-chih-chia-huang-chi-tang (Cinnamon and Astragalus Combination): spontaneous and excessive sweating, no fever.
Cheng-chi-tang (Rhubarb Combination): spontaneous sweating, firm conformation, and constipation.
Yueh-pei-chia-chu-tang (Atractylodes Combination): spontaneous sweating, edema, asthmatic cough, and extreme thirst.

Surface, weak conformation

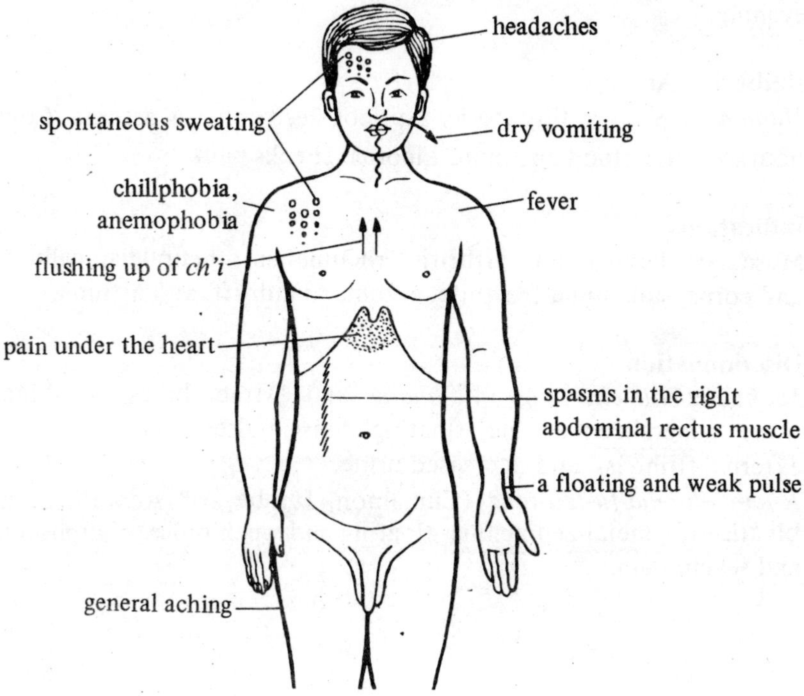

Ma-Hsing-I-Kan-Tang 麻杏薏甘湯

(Ma-huang and Coix Combination)

Ma-huang	4.0	Apricot seed	3.0	Licorice	2.0
Coix	10.0				

Ma-hsing-i-kan-tang was recorded in the *Chin kuei yao lueh* (金匱要略) during the Han dynasty. This formula is used for treating rheumatism with generalized pain and high fever in the evening.

Herbs and Actions

Ma-huang is an antihydrotic. Apricot seed relieves asthma. Coix nourishes the blood and skin. Licorice checks pain.

Indications

Muscular rheumatism, arthritis, rheumatism, neuralgia, calluses and corns, sudamina, frostbite, eczema, dandruff, and asthma.

Discrimination

Ma-huang-chia-chu-tang (*Ma-huang* and Atractylodes Combination): generalized aching; floating, tense pulse; sweating, strong external firmness, and decreased urine.

Kuei-chih-chia-fu-tzu-tang (Cinnamon, Jujube, and Aconite Combination): generalized aching, floating and weak pulse, chillphobia, and severe pain.

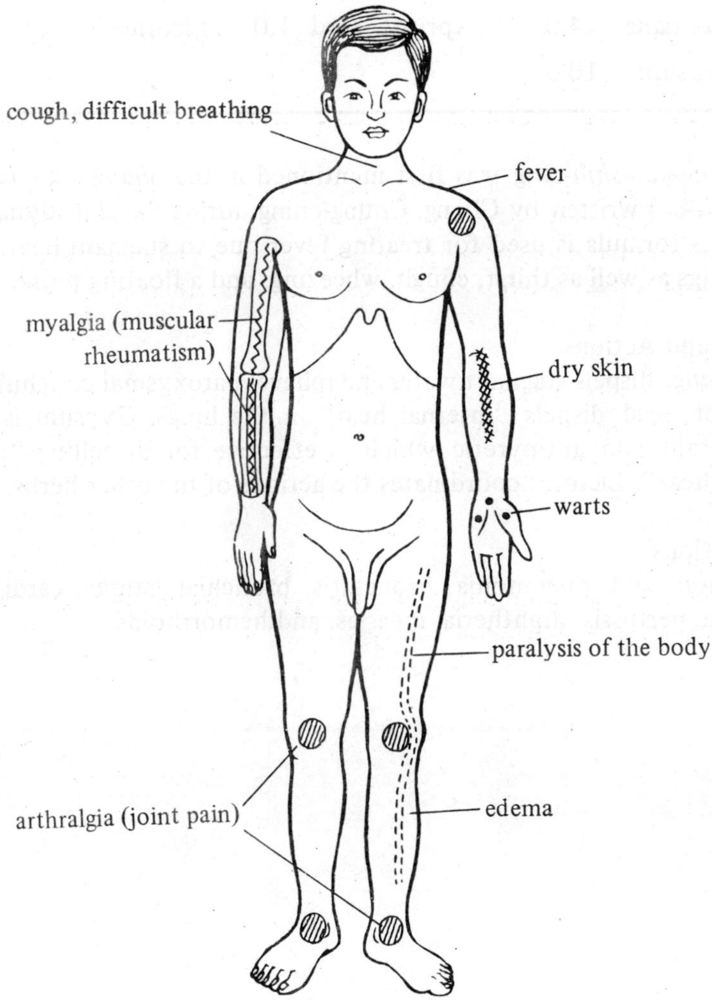
cough, difficult breathing
fever
myalgia (muscular rheumatism)
dry skin
warts
paralysis of the body
arthralgia (joint pain)
edema

Ma-Hsing-Kan-Shih-Tang 麻杏甘石湯

(Ma-huang and Apricot Seed Combination)

Ma-huang	4.0	Apricot seed	1.0	Licorice	2.0
Gypsum	10.0				

Ma-hsing-kan-shih-tang was first mentioned in the *Shang han lun* (傷寒論) written by Chang Chung-ching during the Han dynasty. This formula is used for treating fever due to stagnant heat in the lungs as well as thirst, cough, wheezing, and a floating pulse.

Herbs and Actions

Ma-huang dispels stagnant water and relieves paroxysmal coughing. Apricot seed dispels "internal heat" in the lungs. Gypsum is a refrigerant and antipyretic which is effective for dispelling "internal heat". Licorice coordinates the actions of the other herbs.

Indications

Common cold, pneumonia, bronchitis, bronchial asthma, cardiac asthma, pertussis, diphtheria, measles, and hemorrhoids.

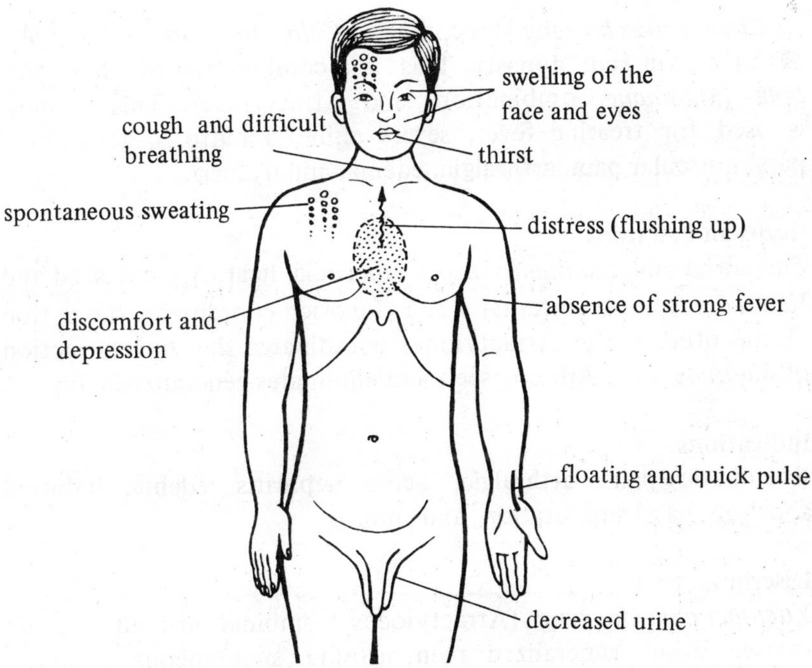
swelling of the
face and eyes
cough and difficult
breathing
thirst
spontaneous sweating
distress (flushing up)
discomfort and
depression
absence of strong fever
floating and quick pulse
decreased urine

Ma-Huang-Chia-Chu-Tang 麻黃加朮湯

(Ma-huang and Atractylodes Combination)

Ma-huang	5.0	Apricot seed	5.0	Licorice	1.5
Cinnamon	4.0	Atractylodes	5.0		

Ma-huang-chia-chu-tang is recorded in *Chin kuei yao lueh* (金匱要略) of the Han dynasty. This is a combination of *Ma-huang-tang* (*Ma-huang* Combination) and Atractylodes. This formula is used for treating fever, severe chills, anhidrosis, generalized pain, muscular pain, arthralgia, edema, and dysuria.

Herbs and Actions

Cinnamon and *Ma-huang* dispel superficial heat. Apricot seed and *Ma-huang* remove internal water. Licorice coordinates the action of the other herbs. Atractylodes coordinates the diuretic action of *Ma-huang* and Apricot seed and eliminates generalized pain.

Indications

Rheumatic pain, arthralgia, acute nephritis, edema, habitual abortion, nasal suppuration, and rhinitis.

Discrimination

Yueh-pei-chia-chu-tang (Atractylodes Combination): edema, decreased urine, generalized pain, asthma, spontaneous sweating, extreme thirst, and hard stools.

Surface-fever-firm conformation

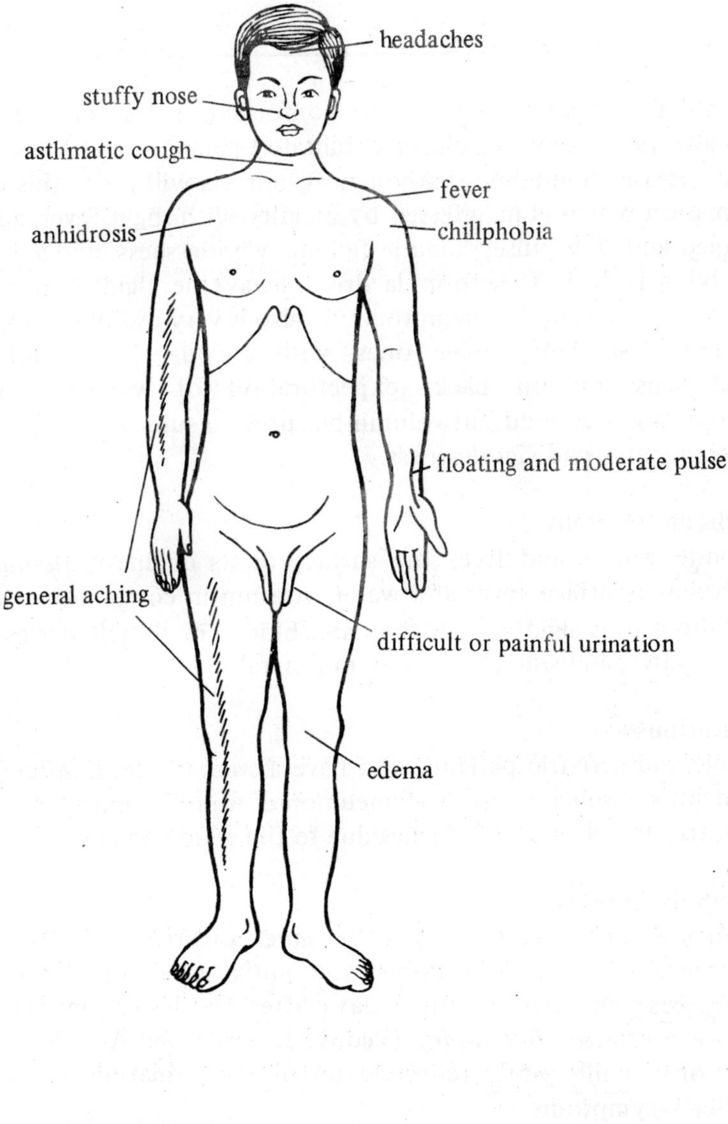

Ma-Huang-Fu-Tzu-Hsi-Hsin-Tang 麻黃附子細辛湯

(Ma-huang and Asarum Combination)

Aconite	0.5~1.0	Asarum	3.0	*Ma-huang*	4.0

Recorded in *Shang han lun.* The conformation for this formula can always be found in old or debilitated persons or at the onset of a disease. Sometimes pathological hidrosis will cause this conformation which is manifested by algidity with slight fever, a submerged and thin pulse, somatic fatigue, vigorlessness, and a desire for lying in bed. This formula drives away the algidity, restores vigor, and alleviates all symptoms. It also is very useful in treating patients, especially feeble ones, with a cough; an occasional algid sensation on back; expectoration of water-like, thin sputum; light colored but voluminous urine; a submerged and thin pulse; anemia; and vigorlessness.

Herbs and Actions

Aconite warms and frees the surface of its coldness. *Ma-huang* disperses a surface fever and water. Asarum in combination with Aconite warms algidity and stimulates blood circulation, drives off chilly water, and warms the body in general.

Indications

Feeble and geriatric patients who have a common cold, influenza, bronchitis, bronchial asthma, pneumonia, rhinitis, sinusitis maxillaris, trigeminalgia, or headaches due to the wind and cold.

Discrimination

Ma-huang-kan-tsao-fu-tzu-tang (*Ma-huang,* Licorice, and Aconite Combination): mild symptoms; the initial stage of the lesser yin disease and two or three days after the lesser yin disease. *Shao-yao-kan-tsao-fu-tzu-tang* (Peony, Licorice, and Aconite Combination): chillphobia, relieve external conformation, no cold "water" symptoms.

Fu-tzu-tang (Aconite Combination): chillphobia, submerged pulse, generalized pain, and aching joints.
Wu-chu-yu-tang (Evodia Combination): headache, chills, dry vomiting, and flushing up.
Szu-ni-tang (Aconite and G. L. Combination): headache, fever, submerged thin pulse, and diarrhea with undigested food.
Ma-hsing-kan-shih-tang (*Ma-huang* and Apricot Seed Combination): cough, yang conformation, extreme thirst, and a forceful pulse.

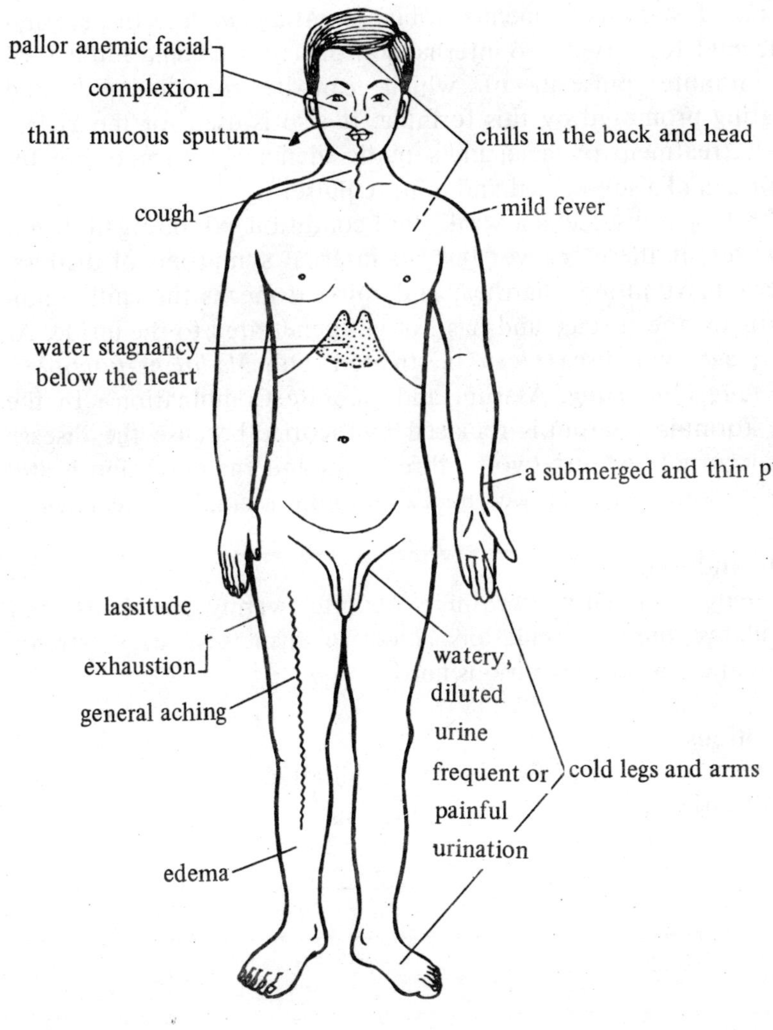

Ma-Huang-Fu-Tzu-Kan-Tsao-Tang 麻黃附子甘草湯
(*Ma-huang, Aconite, and Licorice Combination*)

Ma-huang	3.0	Aconite	0.5~1.0	Licorice	3.0

First recorded in *Shang han lun* (傷寒論). The main indications are lesser yin diseases that have lasted for two or three days with the manifestations of anemophobia, somatic pain, lack of perspiration, mild fever (with no internal conformation), and a submerged and minute pulse-all of which can be corrected by mild sweating promoted by this formula. It also is used for the hydropathic treatment of facial and somatic edema, shortness of breath, dysuria, and a submerged and minute pulse.

Basically yin disease is a weak, chill condition exhibiting no fever. However, if there is fever but no internal symptoms of distress, irritation, vomiting, diarrhea, and thirst it means the chill condition is on the surface and has not yet penetrated to the inside. At this stage, yin disease can be treated with *Ma-huang-fu-tzu-hsi-hsin-tang* (*Ma-huang*, Asarum, and Aconite Combination). In the first formula Asarum, is replaced by Licorice because the disease has occurred for just two to three days and the condition is still mild. Licorice with its sweetness and mildness combats weakness.

Herbs and Actions
Ma-huang stimulates sweating. Aconite warms the body and stimulates blood circulation. Licorice disperses fever, strengthens, and harmonizes various herbs.

Indications
Common cold, influenza in the debilitated, bronchitis, edema, and dysuria.

Yin conformation

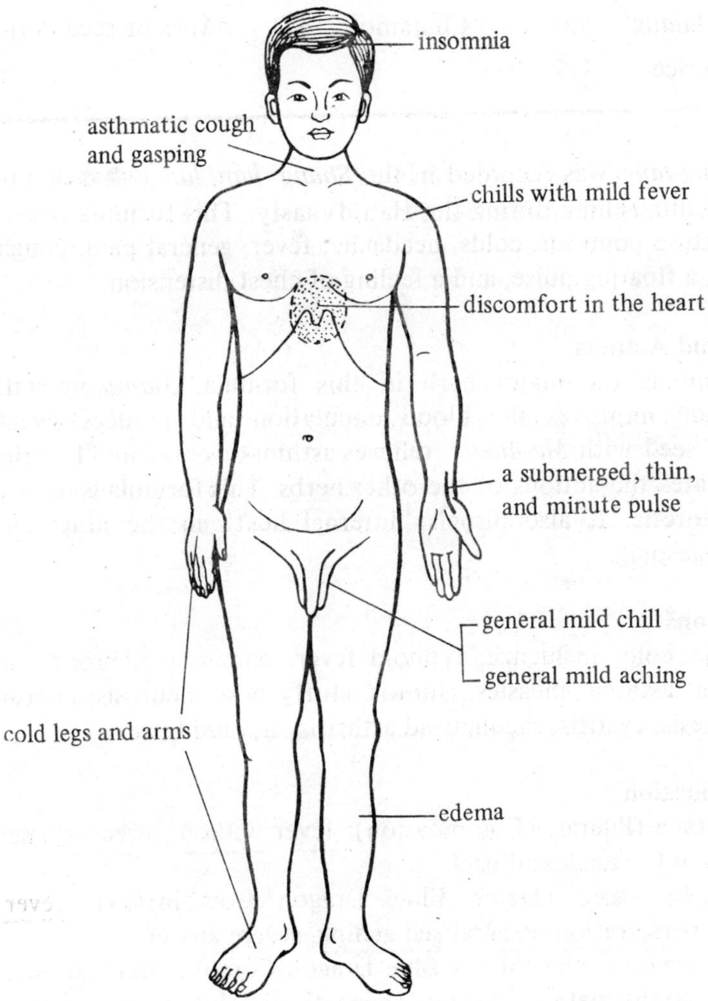

Ma-Huang-Tang 麻黃湯

(Ma-huang Combination)

Ma-huang	5.0	Cinnamon	4.0	Apricot seed	5.0
Licorice	1.5				

Ma-huang-tang was recorded in the *Shang han lun* (傷寒論) by Chang Chung-ching during the Han dynasty. This formula is used for treating common colds, headache, fever, general pain, cough, asthma, a floating pulse, and a feeling of chest distension.

Herbs and Actions

Ma-huang is the major herb in this formula. *Ma-huang* with Cinnamon improves the blood circulation and induces sweat. Apricot seed with *Ma-huang*, relieves asthmatic coughing. Licorice coordinates the actions of the other herbs. This formula is used as a diaphoretic. It also dispels "internal heat" in the lungs and relieves gasping.

Indications

Common cold, influenza, typhoid fever, pneumonia, bronchitis, bronchial asthma, measles, rhinitis, stuffy nose, neurosis, nocturnal enuresis, cystitis, rheumatoid arthritis, and mild pain.

Discrimination

Ko-ken-tang (Pueraria Combination): fever without sweating, and stiffness in the neck and back.

Ta-ching-lung-tang (Major Blue Dragon Combination): fever without perspiration, generalized aching, severe anxiety.

Hsiao-ching-lung-tang (Minor Blue Dragon Combination): asthma, external conformation, "water" beneath the heart, and internal chills.

Kuei-chih-tang (Cinnamon Combination): fever, spontaneous sweating, external conformation, floating and weak pulse.

Ma-hsing-kan-shih-tang (*Ma-huang* and Apricot Seed Combination): asthma, extreme thirst, and spontaneous sweating.

Surface-fever-firm conformation

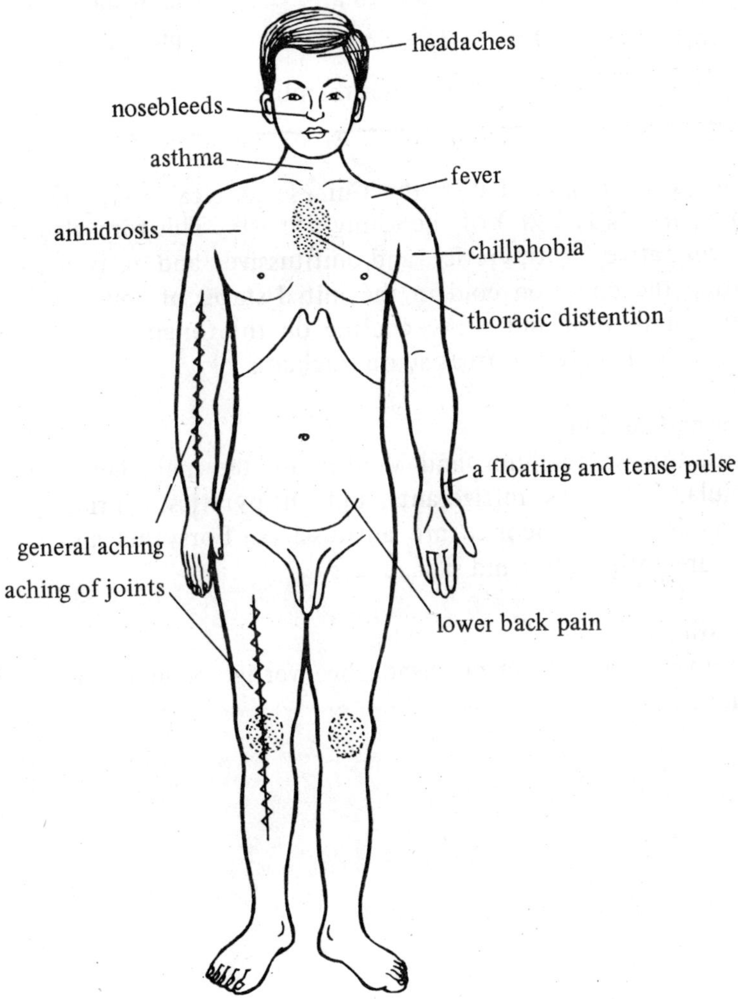

Sang-Chu-Yin 桑菊飲

(Morus and Chrysanthemum Combination)

Morus	12.0	Forsythia	12.0	Mentha	4.5
Apricot seed	9.0	Licorice	4.5	Phragmites	18.0
Platycodon	9.0	Chrysanthemum	9.0		

Sang-chu-yin is recorded in the Chinese medical text, *Wen ping tiao pien* (溫病條辨) of the Ching dynasty. This formula acts as a carminative, antipyretic, and antitussive, and it is used for treating the common cold in the initial stages of coughing, mild fever, thirst, thin and white coating on the tongue, and floating pulse. It is also used to treat acute tracheitis.

Herbs and Actions

Morus, Chrysanthemum, and Mentha are the main herbs in this formula, acting as refrigerants and antipyretics. Apricot seed, Platycodon, and Licorice are antitussives. Forsythia and Phragmites are antipyretics and sialagogues.

Indications

Common cold, influenza, headache, vertigo, cough, and acute tracheitis.

Shih-Shen-Tang 十神湯

(Ma-huang and Cimicifuga Combination)

Cnidium	3.0	Licorice	1.5	*Ma-huang*	3.0
Perilla	3.0	Angelica	1.5	Cimicifuga	1.5
Citrus	3.0	Peony	3.0	Allium	2.0
Pueraria	3.0	Ginger	2.0	Cyperus	3.0

Shih-shen-tang was first recorded in the Chinese governmental medical work of the Sung dynasty, *Tai ping huei min ho chi chu fang* (太平惠民和劑局方 A.D. 1107-1110). This formula is used for treating influenza with headache, chest distension, fever, severe chills, cough, and stuffy nose, but without excessive sweating.

Herbs and Actions

Cnidium, *Ma-huang,* Pueraria, Angelica, Perilla, Citrus, and Cyperus are acrid and aromatic herbs effective for treating a common cold with stuffy nose. Peony is diaphoretic. Licorice synthesizes the actions of other herbs.

Indications

Influenza, headache due to a common cold, fever, severe chills, stuffy nose, cough, and chest distension.

Discrimination

Sheng-ma-ko-ken-tang (Cimicifuga and Pueraria Combination): chillphobia, fever, headaches, anhidrosis, body aches, extreme thirst, insomnia, no cough.

Ko-ken-tang (Pueraria Combination): chillphobia, fever, headache, anhidrosis, body aches, floating and tense pulse, stiffness and spasms in the neck and back.

Ma-huang-tang (*Ma-huang* Combination): chillphobia, fever, headaches, anhidrosis, body aches, asthma, floating and tense pulse, and chest fullness.

Surface firm conformation

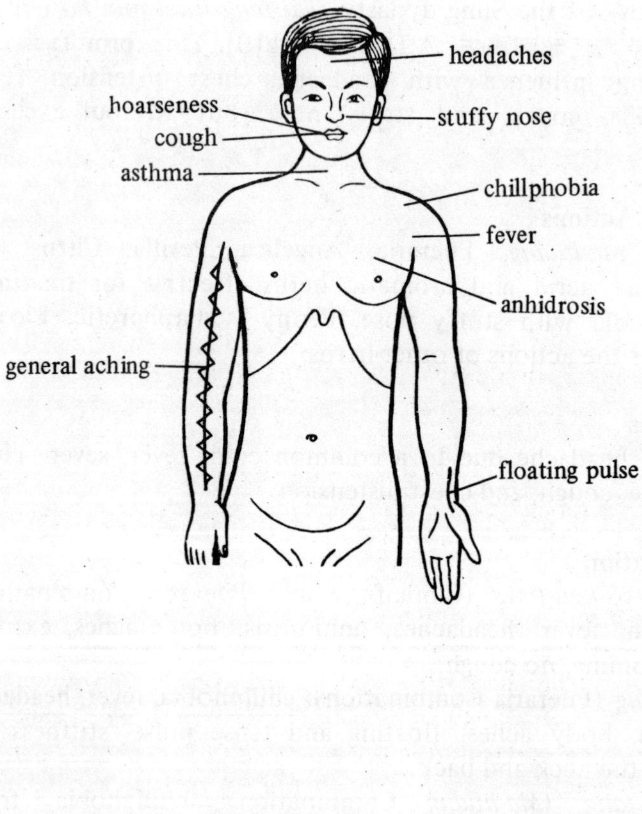

Ta-Ching-Lung-Tang 大靑龍湯

(Major Blue Dragon Combination)

Ma-huang	6.0	Apricot seed	5.0	Cinnamon	3.0
Licorice	2.0	Ginger	3.0	Gypsum	10.0
Jujube	3.0				

Ta-ching-lung-tang is recorded in *Shang han lun* (傷寒論) and *Chin kuei yao lueh* (金匱要略) of the Han dynasty. This formula is used for treating more severe symptoms than those treated by *Ma-huang-tang* (*Ma-huang* Combination) including anhidrosis, tight pulse, stress, edema, and ascites. Those of delicate constitution with sweating and a weak pulse should not take this formula.

Herbs and Actions

Ma-huang is a diaphoretic. Gypsum dispels internal heat and stress. Cinnamon and Apricot seed coordinate with *Ma-huang* to relieve superficial fever and remove "internal water". Licorice, Ginger, and Jujube supply nutrients and help to produce the diaphoretic action of this formula.

Indications

Influenza, acute pneumonia, measles, febrile disease, conjunctivitis, corneal ulcer, hordeolum, acute nephritis, acute edema, acute arthritis, and erysipelas.

Discrimination

Hsiao-ching-lung-tang (Minor Blue Dragon Combination): edema, internal chills, water stagnancy beneath the heart, flushing up of *ch'i*.

Ma-huang-tang (*Ma-huang* Combination): external fever, but no discomfort.

Yueh-pei-tang (*Ma-huang* and Gypsum Combination): edema, spontaneous sweating, no strong fever.

Surface, firm, internal, fever conformation

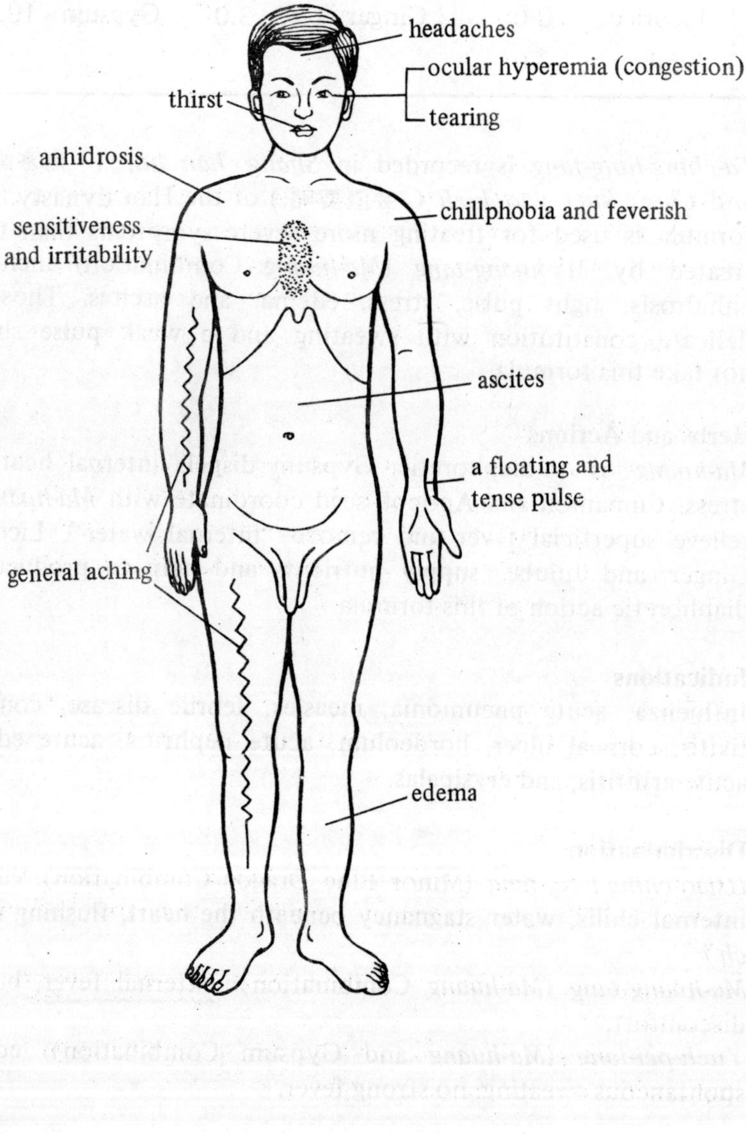

Yin-Chiao-San 銀翹散

(Lonicera and Forsythia Formula)

Lonicera	12.0	Forsythia	12.0	Platycodon	9.0
Arctium	9.0	Mentha	3.0	Licorice	4.5
Bamboo leaves	9.0	Schizonepeta	6.0	Soja	9.0
Phragmites	15.0				

Yin-chiao-san was recorded in the Chinese medical work, *Wen ping tiao pien* (溫病條辨) during the Ching dynasty. This formula acts as a refrigerant, antipyretic and detoxifier; it is used for treating headache, thirst, cough, sore throat, white tongue coating, and a fast and floating pulse.

Herbs and Actions

Lonicera and Forsythia dispel "internal heat". Mentha is a refrigerant. Schizonepeta is a diaphoretic. Bamboo leaves dispel "internal heat". Phragmites removes "internal heat" and increases salivation. Platycodon, Arctium, and Licorice nourish the lungs and dispel sputum.

Indications

Common cold with fever, influenza, acute tonsillitis, initial stages of measles and mumps.

2.

Ho Chieh Chi

(和解劑, Harmonizing Formulas)

Formulas that eliminate toxins by coordinating the liver and spleen or the stomach and intestines are said to "harmonize." The "harmonizing" method is one of the eight major Chinese healing methods. This type of formula is contraindicated when the harmful toxin remains on the surface and the condition has not entered the lesser yang stage, or when the toxin has entered the interior but sunlight yang fever is thriving. Also, harmonizing formulas are not advisable for persons who are fatigued, have internal injuries, irregular diets, weakness in *ch'i* and blood, or fever and chills.

Chai-Hu-Kuei-Chih-Kan-Chiang-Tang
柴胡桂枝乾薑湯

(Bupleurum, Cinnamon,and Ginger Combination)

Bupleurum	6.0	Cinnamon	3.0
Trichosanthes root	3.0	Scute	3.0
Oyster shell	3.0	Ginger	2.0
Licorice	2.0		

Recorded in *Shang han lun* (傷寒論) and *Chin kuei yao lueh* (金匱要略) of the Han dynasty. Used for treating people with a delicate constitution who have a recurrent fever and chills, chest distention, stress, oliguria, thirst, sweating of the head, rapid heart palpitations, cold hands and feet, and soft stools or diarrhea.

Herbs and Actions
Bupleurum eliminates chest distention and recurrent fever and chills, and stimulates liver function. Scute is an antipyretic and sedative. Trichosanthes root relieves dry mouth and thirst. Cinnamon removes flushing and stimulates gastric function.
Oyster shell calms palpitations and stress and relieves sweating of the head and night sweats. Ginger stimulates blood circulation. Licorice coordinates the actions of the other herbs.

Indications
The common cold, pneumonia, bronchitis, tuberculosis, pleurisy, peritonitis, gastric distention, palpitations, insomnia, blood disease, hepatitis, and cholecystitis.

Discrimination
Hsiao-chai-hu-tang (Minor Bupleurum Combination): fever; alternating chills and fever; thoraco-costal distress; mild, firm conformation.
Hsiao-chien-chung-tang (Minor Cinnamon and Peony Combination): spontaneous sweating, night sweats, no abdominal pain, and mild stagnancy bencath the heart.

Chih-kan-tsao-tang (Baked Licorice Combination): palpitations, cardiac palpitations, severe flushing up with a weak fever.
Chen-wu-tang (Vitality Combination): diarrhea, internal fever, abdominal pain, no mild stagnancy beneath the heart.

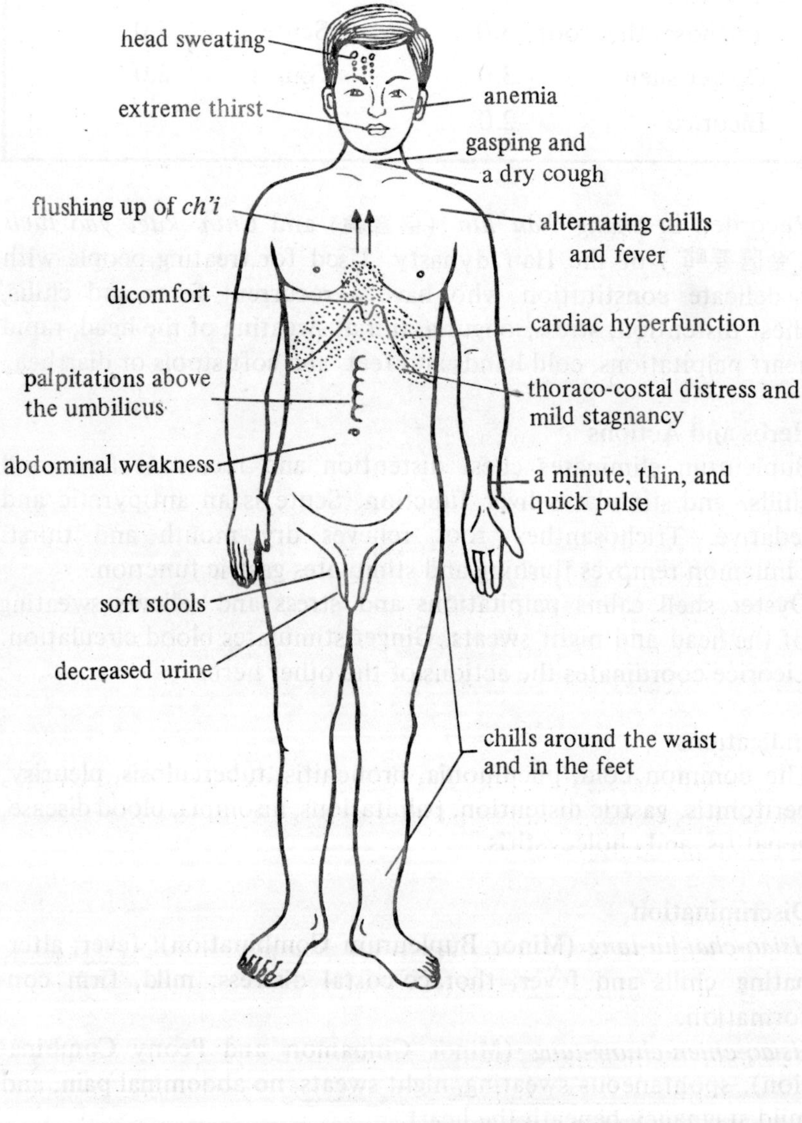

Chia-Wei-Hsiao-Yao-San 加味逍遙散

(Bupleurum and Peony Formula)

Tang-kuei	3.0	Peony	3.0	Gardenia	2.0
Atractylodes	3.0	Hoelen	3.0	Mentha	1.0
Bupleurum	3.0	Moutan	2.0	Ginger	1.0
Licorice	2.0				

Both the medical dictionary of the Sung dynasty, *Tai ping huei min ho chi chu fang* (A.D. 1110) and the *Standards for Treatment* (Cheng Chih Chuen Sheng, A.D. 1602) of the Ming dynasty list *Chia-wei-hsiao-yao-san* for gynecological problems, aching in the arms and legs, dizziness, mental instability, flushing, thirst, night sweating with fever, anorexia, narcolepsy or insomnia, cardiac and limb fever, earache, abdominal distension near the umbilicus, turbid or residual urine, and menstrual irregularity.

The *Japanese Medical News* (醫事新報) No. 1837 also reports that this formula is the best basic remedy for cirrhosis and is very effective for abdominal tenseness, thirst with persistent and bitter taste in the mouth, headache, turbid urine, nosebleed, and odontorrhagia.

Herbs and Actions

The principal herbs of this formula are *Tang-kuei,* Peony, and Bupleurum. *Tang-kuei* has been used as a mild agent for dispeling extravasated blood and as a hematinic. Peony, a mild anticonvulsant and analgesic agent, and *Tang-kuei* have been used to treat blood diseases for 2,000 years. Bupleurum, an antipyretic-stomachic agent for chest distension with resistance and pressing pain and alternating chills and fever, is a principal herb for liver ailments. Gardenia, which is antiphlogistic, analgesic, and hemastatic, is given for depression, glowing sensation, jaundice, anxiety, and insomnia. Moutan is a sedative and anticonvulsive given for headache and lumbago; it also may be used for hypertension, inflammation, bleeding, stagnant blood, and gynecopathy.

Atractylodes and Hoelen are stomachics and diuretics. Mentha is a cooling antidepressive, and stomachic. Ginger warms the body and promotes blood circulation. Licorice synthesizes the actions of all the other herbs.

Indications:
Climacteric disturbance, blood vessel symptoms, infertility, premenstrual tension, menstrual irregularity, stomatitis, leukorrhea, chronic endometritis, chronic hepatitis, cirrhosis, urethritis, cystitis constipation, eczema, hyperkeratosis of the palms, leukoderma, and Basedow's disease.

Discrimination
Hsiao-chai-hu-tang (Minor Bulpeurum Combination): lesser yang disease, firm conformation, distressed chest.
Chai-hu-chiang-kuei-tang (Bupleurum, Cinnamon, and Ginger Combination): lesser yang disease, abdominal palpitations.
Pu-chung-i-chi-tang (Ginseng and Astragalus Combination): weakness fatigability, mild emotional distress.
Tang-kuei-shao-yao-san (*Tang-kuei* and Peony Formula): blood disease, fatigability, absence of muscle tone in the chest and ribs.
I-kan-san-chia-chen-pi-pan-hsia (Bupleurum, Pinellia, and Citrus Formula): blood disease, irritability, insomnia, mental distress, palpitations in the chest to beneath the heart.

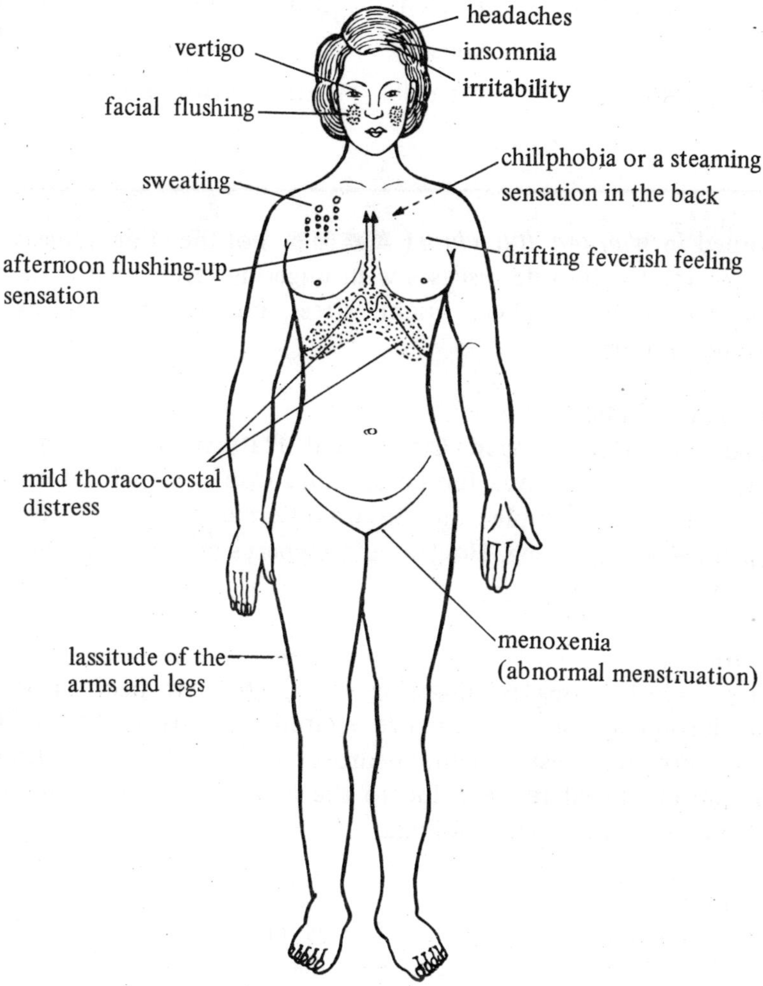
headaches
vertigo
insomnia
irritability
facial flushing
chillphobia or a steaming sensation in the back
sweating
drifting feverish feeling
afternoon flushing-up sensation
mild thoraco-costal distress
menoxenia (abnormal menstruation)
lassitude of the arms and legs

Chu-Ju-Wen-Tan-Tang 竹茹溫膽湯

(Bamboo and Ginseng Combination)

Bamboo	3.0	Licorice	1.0	Coptis	2.0
Bupleurum	5.0	Hoelen	3.0	Ginger	1.0
Pinellia	3.0	Ginseng	2.0	Cyperus	2.0
Platycodon	3.0	Citrus	1.0	*Chih-shih*	1.0

Recorded in *Wan pin hui chun* (萬病回春) of the Ming dynasty. Used for treating febrile diseases with lingering fever, nightmares, stagnant heat in the chest, fright, stress, copious sputum, palpitations, and insomnia.

Herbs and Actions

Pinellia, *Chih-shih*, Ginger, Citrus, and Platycodon are expectorants. Bamboo removes febrile sputum. Coptis dispels internal heat in the heart. Bupleurum dispels internal heat in the liver and gallbladder. Ginseng, Hoelen, and Cyperus nourish the spleen and increase vitality.

Indications

Various febrile diseases, lingering fever, stagnant heat in the chest, insomnia due to excessive sputum and stress. Stagnant sputum in the chest, fright, neurotic palpitation, alcoholism with sputum, facial redness due to the consumption of alcohol, and copious sputum with insomnia.

Discrimination

Chu-yeh-shih-kao-tang (Bamboo Leaves and Gypsum Combination): discomfort in the chest, cough, insomnia, night sweats, dry skin thirst, weak conformation.

Wen-tan-tang (Bamboo and Hoelen Combination): insomnia, nervousness, night sweats, stagnant water in the stomach, weak conformation.

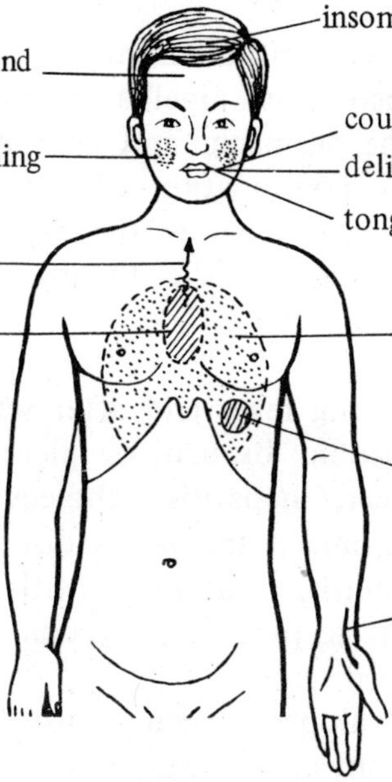

Hsiao-Chai-Hu-Tang 小柴胡湯

(Minor Bupleurum Combination)

Bupleurum	7.0	Scute	3.0	Pinellia	5.0
Ginseng	3.0	Jujube	3.0	Licorice	2.0
Ginger	4.0				

Hsiao-chai-hu-tang has been used mainly as a folk medicine. It was recorded in Chinese medical work *Shang han lun* (Treatise Febrile Diseases) and *Chin kuei yao lueh* (Summaries on Household Drugs, A.D. 205) by Chang Chung-ching of the Han dynasty. This formula is good for the patient of average constitution with chest distension, hardness beneath the heart, pain beneath the ribs when pressure is applied, resistance and pressure pain beneath the liver, loss of appetite, stress, vomiting, bitter taste in the mouth, dry throat, vertigo, abdominal pain, stomachache, white coating on the tongue, and recurrent fever and chills.

Herbs and Actions
Bupleurum and Scute are anti-inflammative and detoxicative and they dispel chest distention. Pinellia and Ginger remove the fluid accumulated in the stomach, and cure nausea, vomiting, and loss of appetite. A combination of Ginseng, Jujube and Licorice is a stomachic and relieves the sensation of fullness beneath the heart. Bupleurum nourishes the liver.

Indication
Common cold with lingering fever and after several days, viscid sputum; acute and chronic bronchitis, pleuritis, pneumonia, disturbance of the liver, hepatitis, cholecystitis, gallstones, jaundice, gastritis, sour stomach and gastric disorder, gastric ulcer, stomachache, lymphadenitis, tonsillitis, otitis media, mumps, mastitis, stiffness in the neck, pyelitis, puerperal fever, severe chills and fever due to uterine diseases, stuttering, epilepsy, impotence in young men, neurosis, alopecia, mental instability in children, and improvement of the physical constitution.

Discrimination
Ta-chai-hu-tang (Major Bupleurum Combination): distressed chest and ribs, alternating chills and fever, vomiting, firmness, acute pain beneath the heart, and constipation.
Chai-hu-chia-lung-ku-mu-li-tang (Bupleurum and Dragon Bone Combination): distressed chest and ribs, palpitations in the chest and abdomen, irritability and mania, decreased urine.
Chai-hu-kuei-chih-tang (Bupleurum and Cinnamon Combination): distressed chest and ribs, external conformation, and non-categorized muscle spasms and abdominal pain.
Chai-hu-chiang-kuei-tang (Bupleurum, Cinnamon, and Ginger Combination): alternating chills and fever, thoraco-costal distress, palpitations beneath the heart, abdominal palpitations, weakness.
Hsiao-hsien-hsiung-tang (Minor Trichosanthes Combination): obstruction and fullness in the chest, pain on pressure beneath the heart, floating and slippery pulse.
Pan-hsia-hsieh-hsin-tang (Pinellia Combination): vomiting, obstruction and hardness beneath the heart, and gas in the abdominal region.

Hsiao-chien-chung-tang (Minor Cinnamon and Peony Combination): abdominal pain, irritability and fever, spasms of abdominal skin, acute abdominal pain.
Huang-lien-tang (Coptis Combination): discomfort and fever in the chest, obstruction and hardness beneath the heart, pain beneath the heart.
Wu-chu-yu-tang (Evodia Combination): vomiting, chest fullness, softness beneath the heart, cold hands and feet, irritability and mania, submerged and slow pulse.
Pu-chung-i-chi-tang (Ginseng and Astragalus Combination): chronic symptoms of mild fever, loss of appetite, deterioration of physical strength, and night sweats.

Half-surface, half-interior conformation

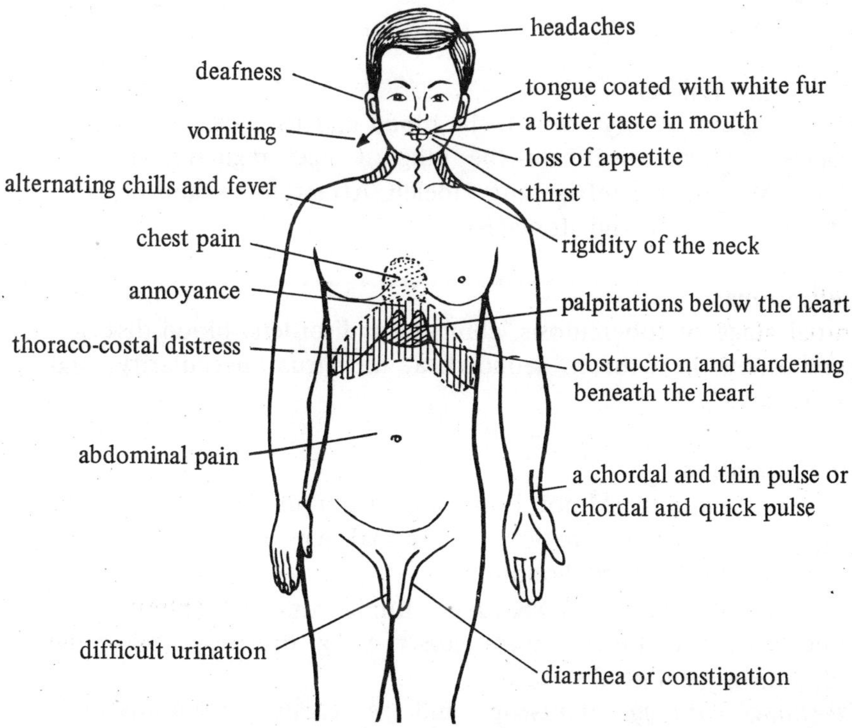

Hsiao-Yao-San 逍遙散

(Bupleurum and Tang-kuei Formula)

Tang-kuei	3.0	Peony	3.0	Mentha	1.0
Bupleurum	3.0	Ginger	2.0	Licorice	1.5
Hoelen	3.0	Atractylodes	3.0		

Hsiao-yao-san was first recorded in the Chinese medical work, *Tai ping huei min ho chi chu fang* (太平惠民和劑局方). This formula is used for treating fever due to stress in the chest cavity and palms due to "internal heat" of the liver; also pain in the arms and legs, heaviness in the head, vertigo, bitter taste in the mouth, dry mouth, anorexia, fever, night sweats, menstrual irregularity, bloating and pain at the umbilicus and in the abdomen, and a weak pulse.

Herbs and Actions

Tang-kuei and Peony nourish the blood and the liver. Bupleurum dispels "internal heat" in the lungs. Ginger regulates *ch'i* and blood. Mentha is a refrigerant. Hoelen, Atractylodes, and Licorice nourish the spleen and stomach.

Indications

Initial stage of tuberculosis, climacteric disorders, blood diseases, nervousness in women, leukorrhea, menstrual irregularity, and insomnia.

Discrimination

Hsiao-chai-hu-tang (Minor Bupleurum Combination): lesser yang diseases, firm conformation, abdominal tension, resistance and pain beneath the hypochondium.

Chai-hu-kuei-chih-kan-chiang-tang (Bupleurum, Cinnamon, and Ginger Combination): treats lesser yang diseases, abdominal palpitations, and head sweating.

Pu-chung-i-chi-tang (Ginseng and Astragalus Combination): fatigability, severe weakness, no neurosis or anxiety.

Tang-kuei-shao-yao-san (*Tang-kuei* and Peony Formula): blood disease, fatigability, no tension in the chest, desire to press the abdomen with warm hands, cold feet.

Huang-Chin-Tang 黃芩湯

(Scute and Licorice Combination)

Scute	4.0	Paeonia	3.0	Licorice	3.0
Jujube	4.0				

Huang-chin-tang is recorded in *Shang han lun* (傷寒論) of the Han dyansty. This formula is used for treating diarrhea, subcardiac distention, abdominal spasms, fever, headache, vomiting, nausea, and thirst. It is suitable for those with abdominal pain and tarry or mucous stools.

Herbs and Actions

Scute is an antiphlogistic and stomachic which improves digestion; in combination with Peony, it relieves abdominal pain and stops diarrhea. Peony coordinates with Licorice to relieve tenesmus. Licorice and Jujube balance the actions of the other herbs in the treatment of abdominal spasms and abdominal pain.

Indications

Acute enteritis, colitis, indigestion, acute appendicitis, annexitis, abdominal pain, and bleeding due to menoplania.

Discrimination

Ko-ken-tang (Pueraria Combination): diarrhea, stiff neck and back, no abdominal pain.

Ta-cheng-chi-tang (Major Rhubarb Combination): diarrhea, firm fever, sunlight yang disease.

Jen-sheng-tang (Ginseng and Ginger Combination): diarrhea and weak chilling.

Association of greater yang and lesser yang conformation

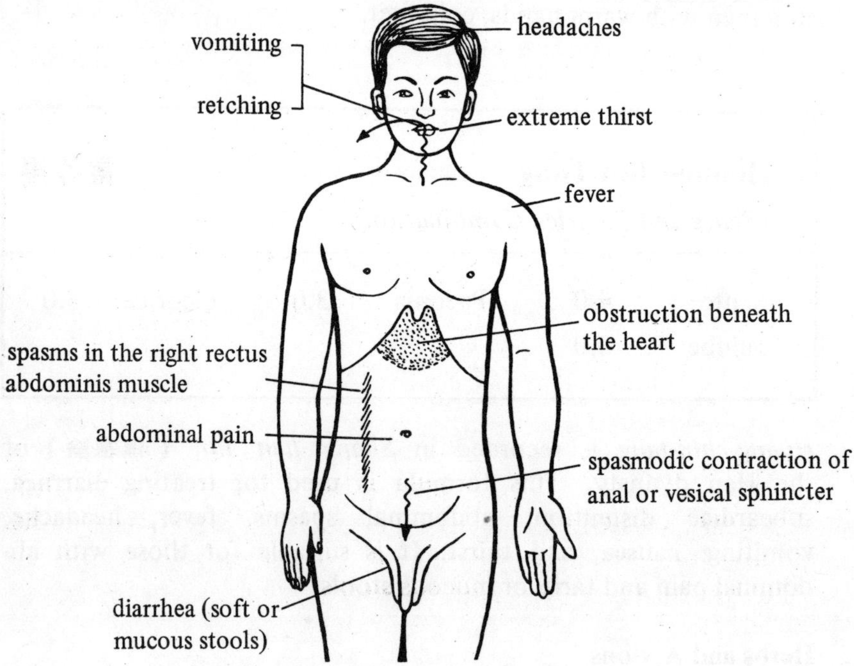

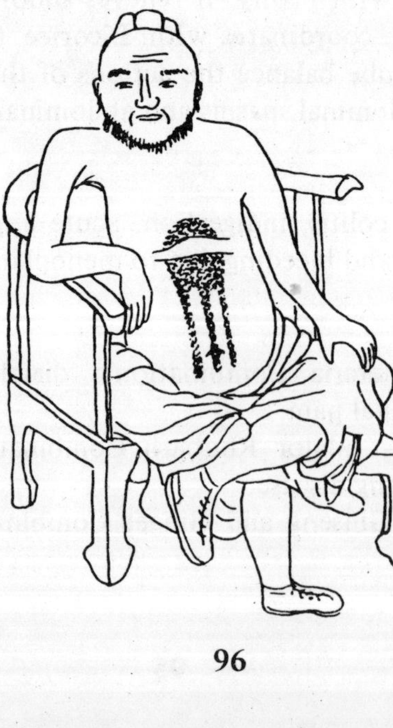

Huang-Lien-Ah-Chiao-Tang 黃連阿膠湯

(Coptis and Gelatin Combination)

Coptis	3.0	Gelatin	3.0	Scute	2.0
Peony	2.5	Egg yolk	1.0		

Huang-lien-ah-chiao-tang is good for treating patients of weak conformation with palpitation, chest distension, insomnia, coarse skin, flushed face, heaviness in the head, and flushing up.

Herbs and Actions
Coptis and Scute are antiphlogistics, antipyretics, sedatives, and hemostatics. Peony, Gelatin, and Egg yolk serve as nutritives, hemostatics, and sedatives. Gelatin and Egg yolk are tonics.

Indications
Insomnia, mental and emotional disorders, bleeding, pneumonia, intestinal fever, scarlet fever, cerebral hemorrhage, and pruritus.

Discrimination
Tao-ho-cheng-chi-tang (Persica and Rhubarb Combination): blood disorders, tense pulse, blood stagnation, firm conformation.
Chai-hu-chia-lung-mu-tang (Bupleurum and Dragon Bone Combination): discomfort, thoraco-costal distress, abdominal movement.
Hsieh-hsin-tang (Coptis and Rhubarb Combination): discomfort, firm conformation.
Ling-kuei-wei-kan-tang (Licorice and Hoelen Combination): discomfort, mild excitability.

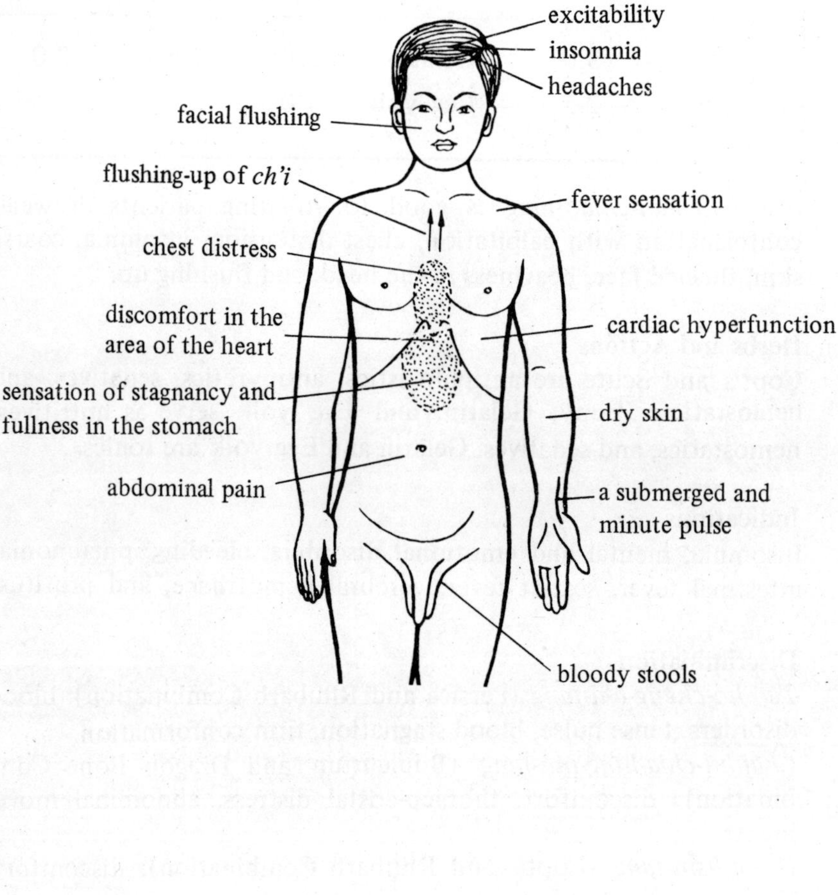
excitability
insomnia
headaches
facial flushing
flushing-up of ch'i
fever sensation
chest distress
discomfort in the area of the heart
cardiac hyperfunction
sensation of stagnancy and fullness in the stomach
dry skin
abdominal pain
a submerged and minute pulse
bloody stools

Huang-Lien-Tang 黃連湯

(Coptis Combination)

Coptis	3.0	Licorice	3.0	Ginger	3.0
Ginseng	3.0	Cinnamon	3.0	Jujube	3.0
Pinellia	6.0				

Huang-lien-tang is recorded in *Shang han lun* (傷寒論) of the Han dynasty. This formula is used for treating "chest heat," abdominal pain, nausea, white and yellow coating on the tongue, gastric ulcer, and duodenal ulcer.

Herbs and Actions

Coptis is chill and bitter in nature and can dispel internal heat in the chest; Ginger and Cinnamon dispel internal chills in the stomach. Pinellia neutralizes the gastric functioning and treats nausea; Ginseng nourishes the *ch'i*. Licorice coordinates the actions of the other herbs. Jujube nourishes the spleen.

Indications

Acute gastroenteritis, indigestion, hangover, stomatitis, cholera, vomiting, diarrhea, abdominal pain, poisoning, and blood disease in women.

Discrimination

Pan-hsia-hsieh-hsin-tang (Pinellia Combination): abdominal pain, obstruction and hardness beneath the heart, and gas. This formula aims at diarrhea and mild abdominal pain.

Ta-chai-hu-tang (Major Bupleurum Combination), *Hsiao-chai-hu-tang* (Minor Bupleurum Combination), and *Chai-hu-kuei-chih-tang* (Bupleurum and Cinnamon Combination): abdominal pain, thoraco-costal distress, acute pain, and distention beneath the heart.

Ta-chien-chung-tang (Major Zanthoxylum Combination) and *Fu-tzu-keng-mi-tang* (Aconite and Oryza Combination): abdominal pain. yin-weakness conformation.

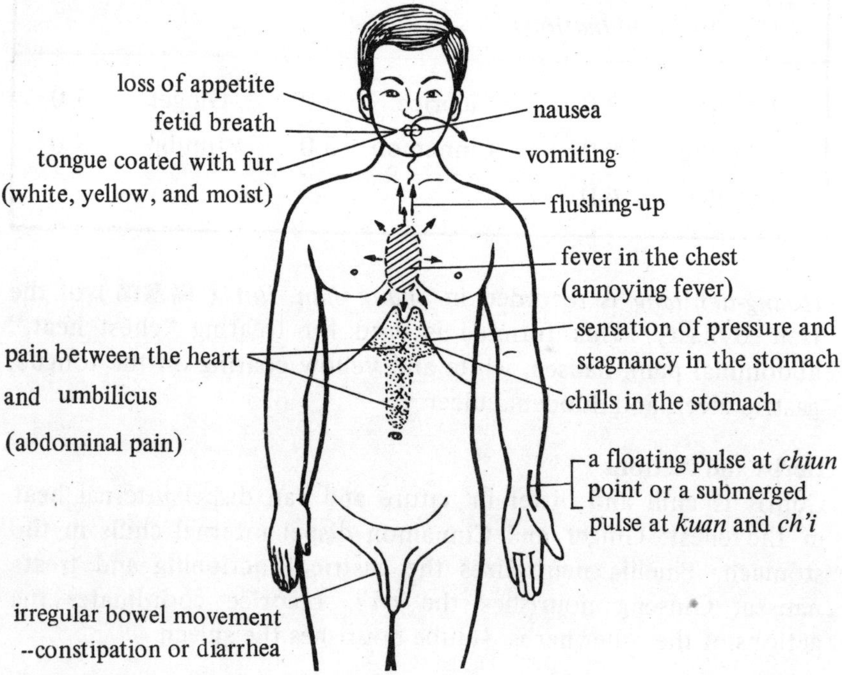

Huo-Hsiang-Cheng-Chi-San 藿香正氣散

(Agastache Formula)

Agastache	1.0	Atractylodes	3.0	Pinellia	3.0
Hoelen	3.0	Magnolia bark	2.0	Citrus	2.0
Platycodon	1.5	Angelica	1.5	Perilla	1.0
Areca	1.0	Jujube	1.0	Ginger	1.0
Licorice	1.0				

Huo-hsiang-cheng-chi-tang was first recorded in the Chinese medical text *Tai ping huei min ho chi chu fang* (太平惠民和劑局

方) of the Sung dynasty. This formula is used for treating gastrointestinal weakness, headache, fever, subcardiac distension, vomiting, diarrhea, abdominal pain, and a strong pulse due to stagnant food and ascites. This formula is also suitable for children with cough, eye ailments, toothache, and sore throat due to stagnant food; it is effective for women with abdominal pain of emotional origin after childbirth.

Herbs and Actions
Agastache, the major herb in this formula, improves gastric function. Perilla and Angelica are carminatives. Hoelen, Pinellia, Citrus, Licorice, Ginger, and Atractylodes dispel ascites and stop vomiting. Magnolia bark, Areca and Platycodon improve gastric function dispel stagnant *ch'i* in the stomach, and relieve abdominal distension.

Indications
Common colds in the summer, acute gastroenteritis, diarrhea in the summer, heatstroke, vomiting, abdominal pain of emotional origin after childbirth, children's cough due to stagnant food, eye disorders, toothache, and sore throat.

Discrimination
Pu-huan-chin-cheng-chi-san (Pinellia, Atractylodes, and Agastache Formula): moisture problems – weak in dispersal activity, however, the formula removes dampness or moisture.
Wu-ling-san (Hoelen Five Herb Formula): sunstroke, moisture problems, water adversity, extreme thirst.

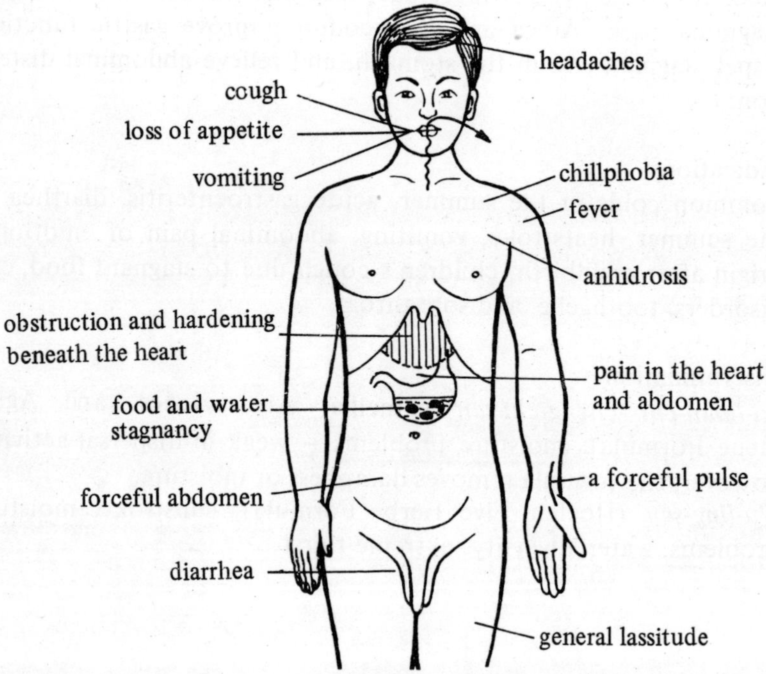
headaches
cough
loss of appetite
vomiting
chillphobia
fever
anhidrosis
obstruction and hardening beneath the heart
pain in the heart and abdomen
food and water stagnancy
a forceful pulse
forceful abdomen
diarrhea
general lassitude

Kan-Tsao-Hsieh-Hsin-Tang 甘草瀉心湯

(Pinellia and Licorice Combination)

Pinellia	5.0	Scute	2.5	Ginger	2.5
Ginseng	2.5	Jujube	2.5	Licorice	3.5
Coptis	1.0				

Kan-tsao-hsieh-hsin-tang is recorded in *Shang han lun* (傷寒論) of the Han dynasty. This formula is used for treating distention beneath the heart, borborygmus, diarrhea, nausea, stress, and mental instability.

Herbs and Actions

The components of this formula are the same as those of *Pan-hsia-hsieh-hsin-tang* (Pinellia Combination) except that here more Licorice is used to reinforce the sedative effect and relieve mental instability.

Indications

Gastroenteritis, hysteria, nervous exhaustion, insomnia, somnambulism, and stomatitis.

Discrimination

Sheng-chiang-hsieh-hsin-tang (Pinellia and Ginger Combination): obstruction and fullness beneath the heart, belching with a fetid odor.

San-huang-hsieh-hsin-tang (Coptis and Rhubarb Combination): obstruction beneath the heart, absence of water vapor, inflammation and congestion, flushing up, and constipation.

Fu-ling-yin (Hoelen Combination): obstruction beneath the heart, water stagnancy in the stomach with a noticeable splashing sound, weak conformation.

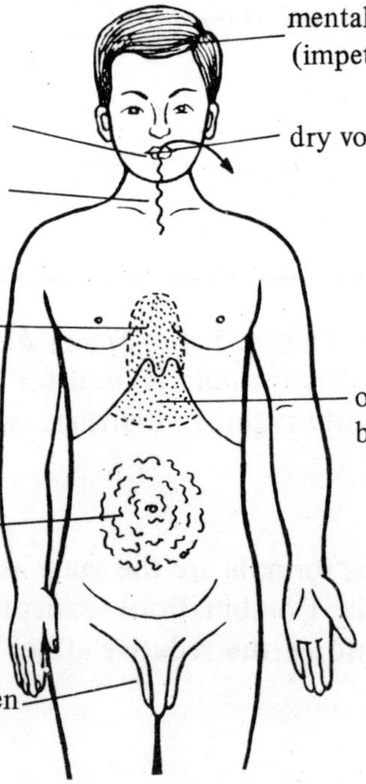

Liu-Ho-Tang 六和湯

(Cardamon Combination)

Cardamon	2.5	Agastache	6.0	Licorice	1.5
Magnolia bark	2.5	Apricot seed	6.0	Pinellia	6.0
Dolichos	6.0	Chaenomeles	4.5	Ginseng	6.0
Atractylodes	6.0	Hoelen	6.0		

Liu-ho-tang was recorded in the *I fang kao* (醫方考) by Wu Kun during the Ming dynasty. This formula is used to treat fatigue, chest distention, gastrosplenic distress due to imbalanced diet, and vomiting and diarrhea due to cholera. It is a commonly used formula during the summer.

Herbs and Actions
Ginseng, Atractylodes, Dolichos, and Licorice nourish the spleen and *ch'i*. Magnolia bark, Cardamon, and Apricot seed increase *ch'i* and stimulate the appetite. Agastache and Pinellia alleviate gastric distress and vomiting. Hoelen and Chaenomeles nourish the spleen and act as diuretics.

Indications
Anorexia, vomiting, diarrhea, thirst, common cold, gastric distress in the summer, hangover, and heatstroke.

Pan-Hsia-Hsieh-Hsin-Tang 半夏瀉心湯

(Pinellia Combination)

Pinellia	6.0	Scute	3.0	Coptis	1.0
Ginseng	3.0	Jujube	3.0	Ginger	3.0
Licorice	3.0				

Pan-hsia-hsieh-hsin-tang is recorded in both the *Shang han lun* (傷寒論) and the *Chin kuei yao lueh* (金匱要略) for treating gastrointestinal disorders. This formula is effective for subcardiac distention, vomiting, nausea, anorexia, resistance below the heart, ascites, borborygmus, diarrhea, and a white tongue coating.

Herbs and Actions
Coptis and Scute are antipyretics that also relieve anxiety due to stress. Pinellia and Ginger cure ascites and vomiting. Ginseng and Licorice improve the gastric function. Licorice and Jujube coordinate the actions of the other herbs.

Indications
Gastritis, enteritis, indigestion, gastromegaly, gastroptosis, gastric ulcer, duodenal ulcer, stomatitis, and motion sickness.

Discrimination

Sheng-chiang-hsieh-hsin-tang (Pinellia and Ginger Combination): obstruction beneath the heart, severe shaking, stagnant water in the stomach, and belching.

Kan-tsao-hsieh-hsin-tang (Pinellia and Licorice Combination): obstruction beneath the heart, severe *ch'i* instability, irritability, emotional and mental instability.

San-huang-hsieh-hsin-tang (Coptis and Rhubarb Combination): obstruction beneath the heart, lack of water in the system, flushing up, and constipation.

Fu-ling-yin (Hoelen Combination): obstruction beneath the heart, severe condition of stagnant water in the stomach, noticeable splashing sound, weak conformation.

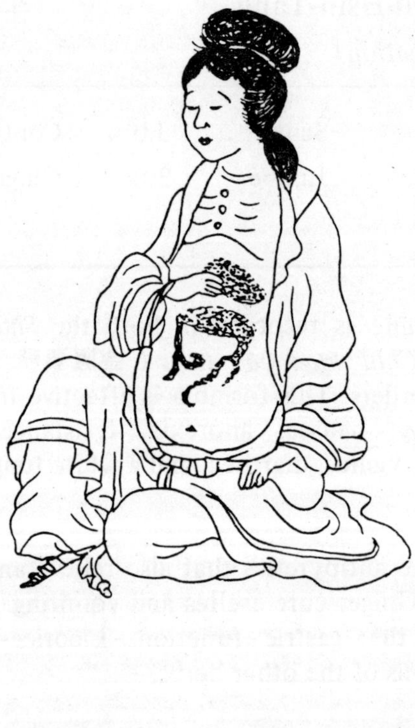

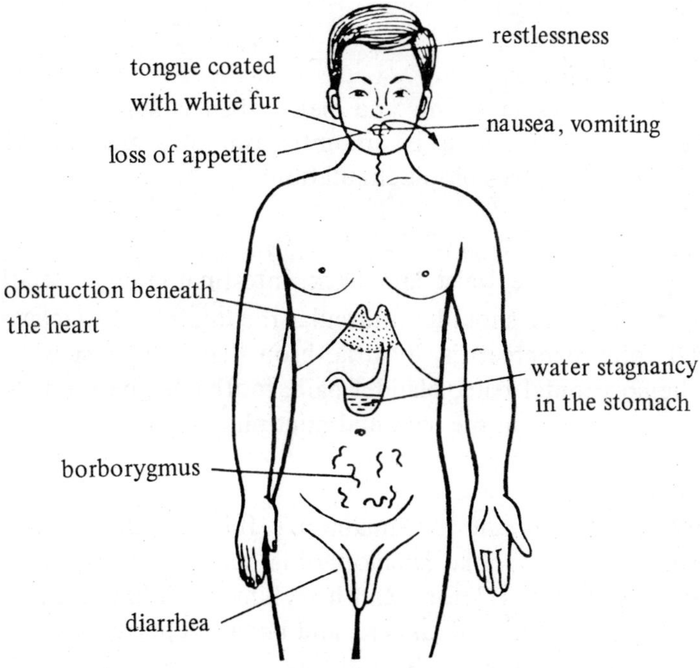
restlessness
tongue coated
with white fur
nausea, vomiting
loss of appetite
obstruction beneath
the heart
water stagnancy
in the stomach
borborygmus
diarrhea

Shao-Yao-Kan-Tsao-Tang 芍藥甘草湯

(Peony and Licorice Combination)

Peony	6.0	Licorice	6.0

Shao-yao-kan-tsao-tang was first recorded in the *Shang han lun* (傷寒論). This formula is used for treating weakness in the legs and severe and painful muscle spasms in the stomach, intestines, bronchi, gallbladder, and ureters.

Herbs and Actions

Peony relieves muscle spasm and palsy, dispels stagnant blood, and checks pain. Licorice is an antispasmodic, analgesic, and detoxifier that improves blood circulation.

Indications

Muscle spasms in the waist and back, intestinal cramps, sciatica, waist pain, 50 years' shoulder, muscular rheumatism, gastrospasm, intestinal colic, pancreatitis, dysuria, bronchial asthma, spasmodic cough, hemorrhoidal pain, bladder pain, toothache, beriberi, palsy in the legs, weakness in the legs, and noctiphobia.

Discrimination

Kuei-chih-chia-fu-tzu-tang (Cinnamon, Jujube, and Aconite Combination): chillphobia, anemophobia, external conformation.
Ta-chien-chung-tang (Major Zanthoxylum Combination): abdominal pain, abdominal weakness, and impaired peristalsis.
Pa-wei-wan (Rehmannia Eight Formula): weakness in the feet, numbness beneath the umbilicus.
Fu-tzu-keng-mi-tang (Aconite and Oryza Combination): abdominal pain, gas, vomiting.

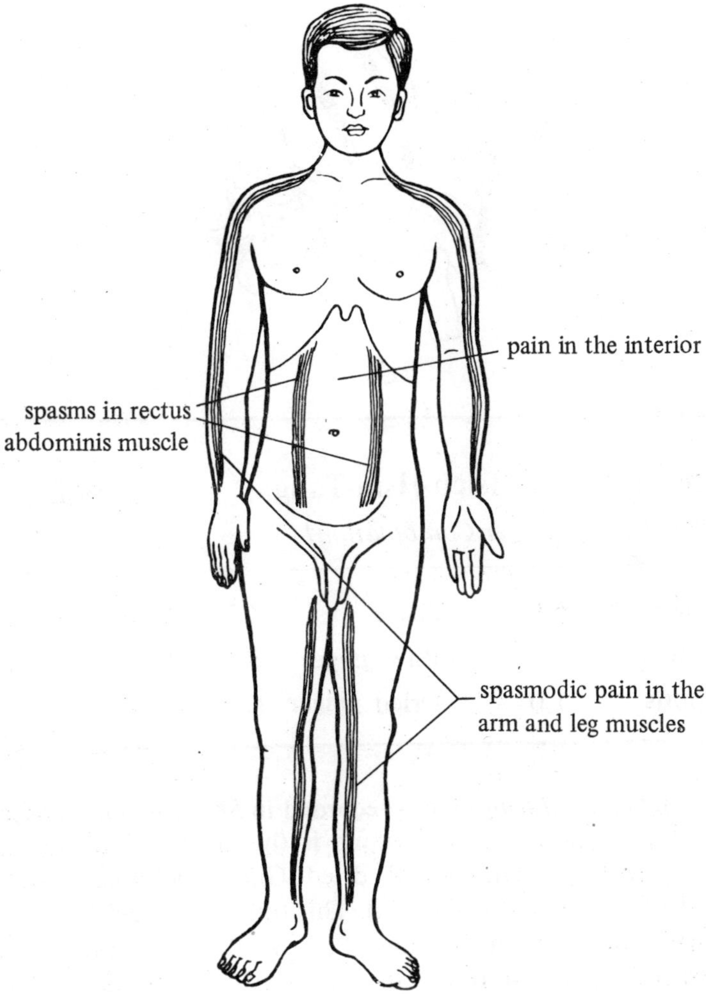
pain in the interior
spasms in rectus abdominis muscle
spasmodic pain in the arm and leg muscles

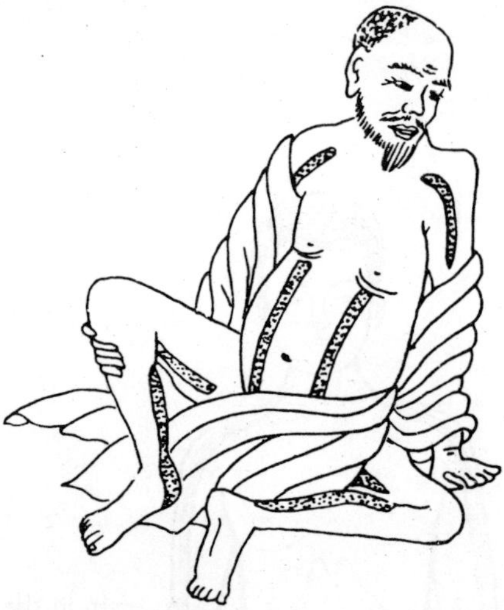

Sheng-Chiang-Hsieh-Hsin-Tang 生薑瀉心湯

(Pinellia and Ginger Combination)

Pinellia	5.0	Scute	2.5	Licorice	2.5
Ginseng	2.5	Raw ginger	2.0	Jujube	2.5
Coptis	1.0	Dried ginger	1.5		

Sheng-chiang-hsieh-hsin-tang is recorded in *Shang han lun* (傷寒論) of the Han dynasty. This formula is the same as *Pan-hsia-hsieh-hsin-tang* with the amount of dried Ginger decreased and the amount of raw Ginger increased. This formula is used for treating eructation, moisture in the chest, "*ch'i* weakness" in the stomach, indigestion, "stagnant food" in the stomach, borborygmus, diarrhea, and moisture in the abdomen.

Herbs and Actions

Pinellia dispels "stagnant water" in the stomach. Pinellia with dried Ginger stops nausea and vomiting. Coptis and Scute are bitter stomachics and can relieve inflammation in the stomach and intestines. Ginseng and raw Ginger improve the blood circulation in the stomach and intestines as well as gastrointestinal functioning. Licorice and Jujube coordinate the actions of the other herbs. Raw Ginger relieves eructation and borborygmus.

Indications
Gastroenteritis, sour stomach, gastric distention, fermentative diarrhea, and gastrectasia.

Discrimination
Kan-tsao-hsieh-hsin-tang (Pinellia and Licorice Combination): obstruction beneath the heart, shaking *ch'i*, irritability, severe mental distress.
San-huang-hsieh-hsin-tang (Coptis and Rhubarb Combination): obstruction beneath the heart, lack of water in the system, flushing up, and constipation.
Fu-ling-yin (Hoelen Combination): obstruction beneath the heart, severe water stagnancy in the stomach, noticeable splashing sound, weak conformation.

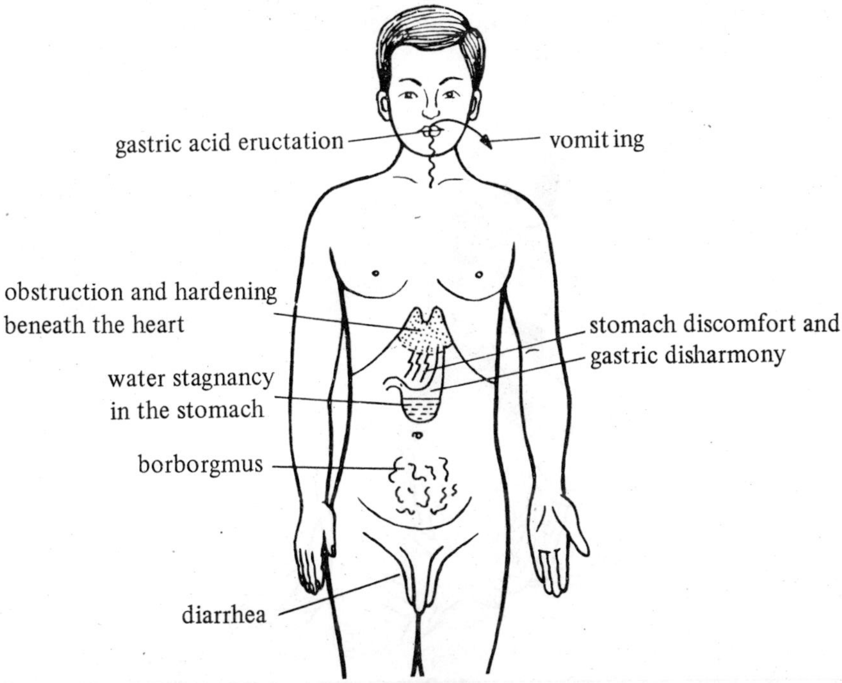

Szu-Ni-San 四逆散

(*Bupleurum and Chih-shih Formula*)

Bupleurum	5.0	Peony	4.0	*Chih-shih*	2.0
Licorice	1.5				

Recorded in the *Shang han lun* (傷寒論) of the Han dynasty. Used for treating chest distention, spasms of the abdomen, cold hands and feet, and irritability caused by nervousness.

Actions of the Herbs

Bupleurum dispels stagnant heat. Peony and Licorice coordinate *ch'i* and blood, relieve spasms, and ease pain. *Chih-shih* gives vitality and increases urine output.

Indications

Cholecystitis (inflammation of the gallbladder), cholelithiasis (gallbladder stones), gastritis, gastric ulcer, pleurisy, rhinitis (inflammation of the nasal mucous membrane), neurosis, epilepsy, and tubercular peritonitis.

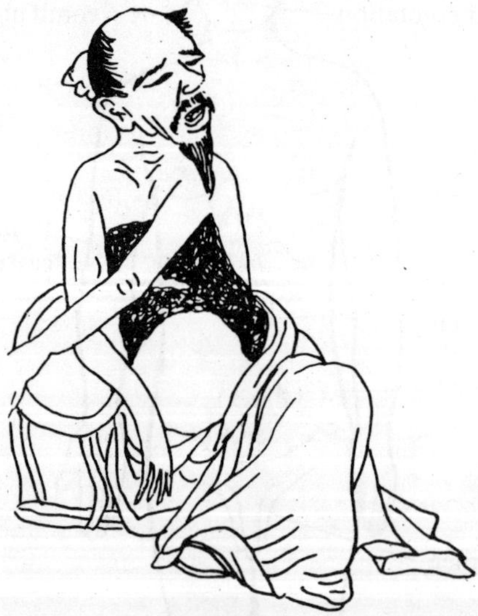

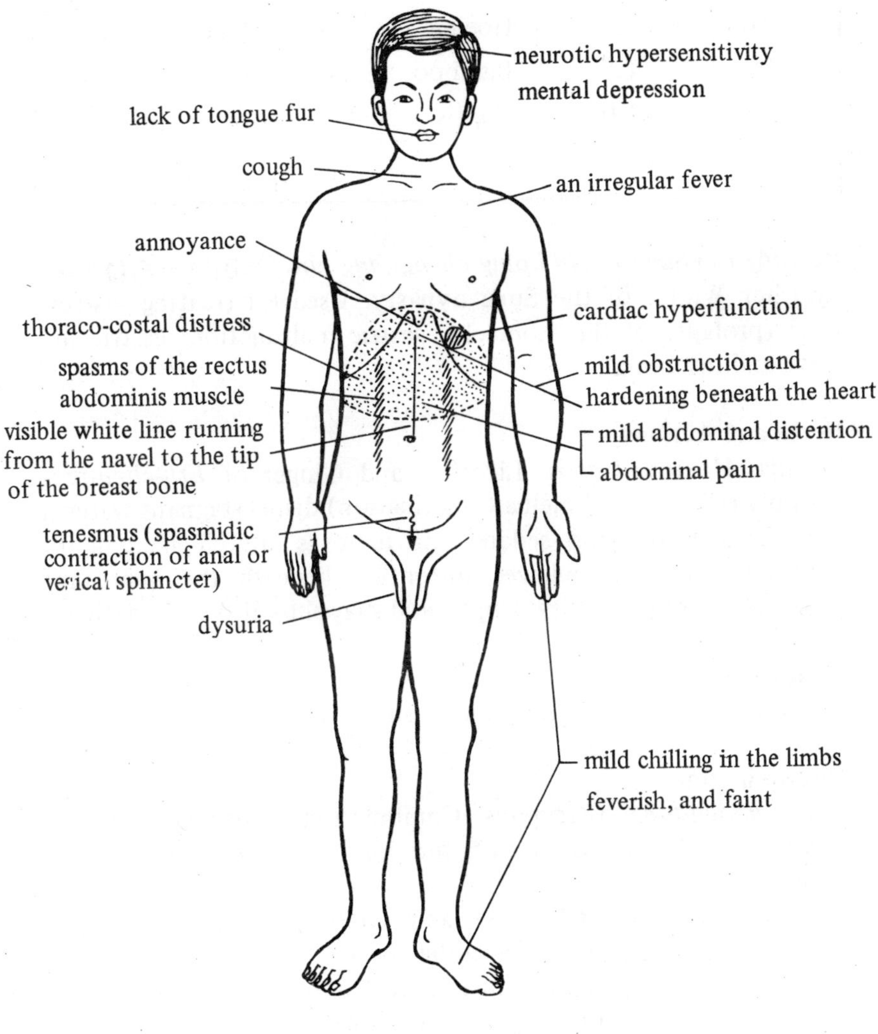
neurotic hypersensitivity
mental depression
lack of tongue fur
cough
an irregular fever
annoyance
cardiac hyperfunction
thoraco-costal distress
spasms of the rectus
abdominis muscle
mild obstruction and
hardening beneath the heart
visible white line running
from the navel to the tip
of the breast bone
mild abdominal distention
abdominal pain
tenesmus (spasmidic
contraction of anal or
vesical sphincter)
dysuria
mild chilling in the limbs
feverish, and faint

Wen-Tan-Tang 溫膽湯

(Bamboo and Hoelen Combination)

Citrus	2.5	Hoelen	6.0	Pinellia	6.0
Chih-shih	1.5	Bamboo	2.0	Ginger	3.0
Licorice	1.0	Coptis	1.0	Zizyphus	3.0

Recorded in *San yin chi i ping cheng fang lun*, (三因極一病證方論) by Chen Wu-tse of the Sung dynasty. Used for treating gastroptosis (prolapse of the stomach), gastric malfunction, gastric distress, and insomnia.

Herbs and Actions

Pinellia, Hoelen, Citrus, Licorice, and Ginger of *Erh-chen-tang* formula (Citrus and Pinellia Combination) dispel stagnant water in the stomach. Bamboo sedates and removes internal heat in the stomach. *Chih-shih* relieves distention beneath the heart and promotes mental stability. Coptis and Zizyphus also are sedatives.

Indications

Insomnia, heart palpitations, and gastric distress.

Discrimination

Suan-tsao-jen-tang (Zizyphus Combination): insomnia, terror, weakness and dryness of *ch'i*, thriving heart fire, weakness and fatigability.

Chu-ju-wen-tan-tang (Bamboo and Ginseng Combination): insomnia, cough, stagnate fever in the chest.

Huang-lien-chieh-tu-tang (Scute and Coptis Combination): insomnia, congestion, flushing up, and uneasiness.

Kuei-pi-tang (Ginseng and Longan Combination): insomnia, mental distress, anemia.

Weak constitution, weakness, and pain after illness

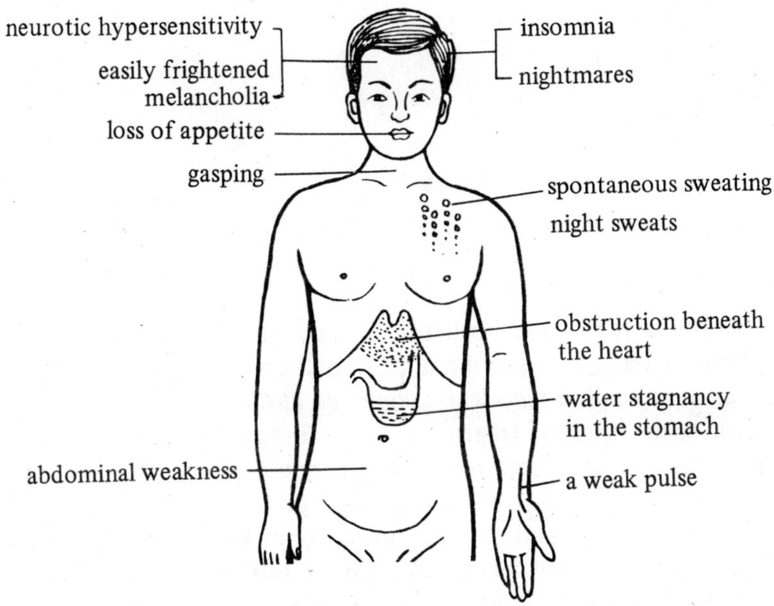

3.

Piao Li Shuang Chieh Chi

(表裏雙解劑, Dual Dissolving Formulas)

Formulas that treat both the surface and the interior at the same time or have a dissolving action in the interior as well as on the exterior are called *piao li shuang chieh chi.*

The basic rules of treatment are to induce sweating for surface diseases and use purgatives or fever-reducing herbs for interior diseases. If the illness is both external and internal, the surface must be treated first and the interior second. However, if the surface condition has not been fully cured but the interior needs immediate treatment, then a dual surface-interior formula is suggested so that the injurious toxin can be dispelled at once. Formulas are prescribed according to whether the conformation is chill or fever, weak or firm. Formulas of this type are classified as a surface-dissolving, interior-attacking; surface-dissolving, interior-cleansing; or surface-dissovling, interior-warming. However, dual formulas are not for all surface-interior diseases. The treatment of disease and selection of a formula depend on the severity of the person's condition and on the priority of treatment. After the severity and priority of the surface and the interior have been determined, dosage proportions between the surface and the internal drugs are then calculated to avoid excessive or inadequate dosing.

Chai-Hu-Kuei-Chih-Tang 柴胡桂枝湯

(Bupleurum and Cinnamon Combination)

Bupleurum	5.0	Pinellia	4.0	Licorice	1.5
Jujube	2.0	Cinnamon	2.5	Scute	2.0
Ginseng	2.0	Peony	2.5	Ginger	1.0

Chai-hu-kuei-chih-tang is recorded in the Chinese medical works *Chin kuei yao lueh* (Summaries on Household Drugs) and *Shang han lun* (Treatise Febrile Diseases, A.D. 205) by Chang Chung-ching of the Han dynasty. This formula is good for those with a somewhat delicate constitution who have a tendency towards fatigue, gastrointestinal weakness, headache, heaviness in the head, neuralgia, fever, moderately severe chills, floating pulse, distention beneath the heart, periumbilical or lower abdominal pain, and tenseness around the public bones.

Herbs and Actions

This is a formula consisting of a combination of *Hsiao-chai-hu-tang* (Minor Bupleurum Combination) and *Kuei-chih-tang* (Cinnamon Combination). Bupleurum promotes blood circulation in the liver and relieves chest distention and moist heat. Scute dispels heat in the chest and may be given for inflammation of the digestive organs. Ginseng improves the functioning of internal organs and increases appetite. Ginger and Pinellia arrest vomiting, decrease expectoration, increase appetite and the flow of urine, and dispel edema in the stomach and chest. Cinnamon cures flushing up and headache. Peony stimulates the action of the digestive organs and is nutritive when in combination with Jujube, Ginger and Licorice.

Indications

1. Common cold, influenza, pneumonia, tuberculosis, and pleuritis.
2. Stomachache, sour stomach, gastric distress, gastric ulcer, duodenal ulcer, acute inflammation of the large intestine,

intestinal ulcer, spleen disorders, gallstones, hepatitis, jaundice, and gallbladder disorders.

3. Chronic appendicitis, peritonitis, abdominal pain, abdominal distension, and constipation.
4. Intercostal neuralgia, headache, arthralgia, nephritis, pyelitis, neurosis, nervous exhaustion, irritability, insomnia, female disorders, hysteria, epilepsy, and cardiac disorders.

Association of greater yang and lesser yang conformations

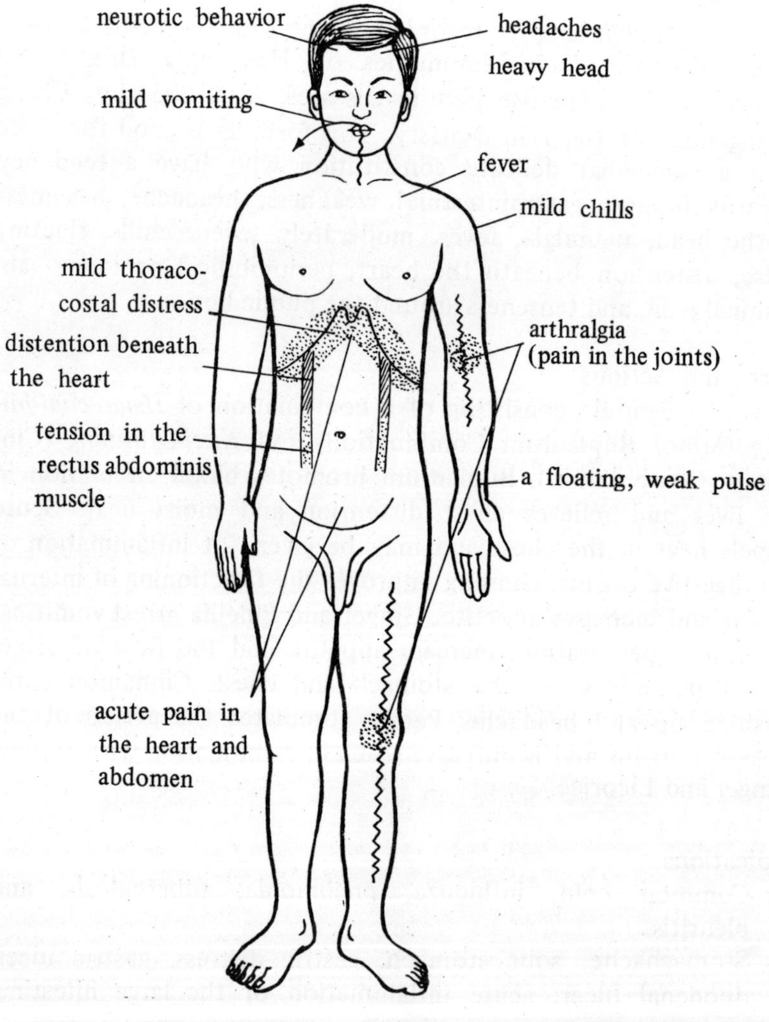

Fang-Feng-Tung-Sheng-San 防風通聖散

(Siler and Platycodon Formula)

Tang-kuei	1.2	Peony	1.2	Gardenia	1.2
Cnidium	1.2	Forsythia	1.2	Ginger	1.2
Schizonepeta	1.2	Siler	1.2	Mentha	1.2
Mirabilitum	1.5	*Ma-huang*	1.2	Licorice	2.0
Rhubarb	1.5	Atractylodes	2.0	Talc	3.0
Platycodon	2.0	Scute	2.0	Gypsum	2.0

Fang-feng-tung-sheng-san is mentioned early in *Hsüan ming lun* by Liu Wan-su (A.D. 1120-1200). This formula is good for those of obese constitution with cardiac disorders, firm muscles, habitual constipation, strong pulse and abdomen, shoulder stiffness, numbness in the hands and feet, fatigue, headache, and heaviness in the head. This formula is also suitable for those not having an obese constitution.

Herbs and Actions

Rhubarb, Mirabilitum, and Licorice remove food poisons from the stomach and intestines. Siler, *Ma-huang*, and Ginger increase skin function. Platycodon, Gardenia, and Forsythia are anti-inflammatives and detoxicants. Schizonepeta and Mentha remove internal heat in the head. Atractylodes and Talcum increase the flow of urine. Scute and Gypsum are anti-inflammatives and sedatives. *Tang-kuei,* Peony, and Cnidium increase blood circulation.

Indications

Obesity, hypertension, apoplexy, arteriosclerosis, diabetes, chronic nephritis, beriberi, asthma, habitual constipation, scabies, red nose, alopecia, skin diseases, hemorrhoids, sciatica, 50 years' shoulder, arthritis, and nasal suppuration.

Discrimination

Ta-chai-hu-tang (Major Bupleurum Combination): hypertension, obstruction and hardness beneath the heart, thoraco-costal distress, and a yang firm conformation in a person with a muscular and obese build.

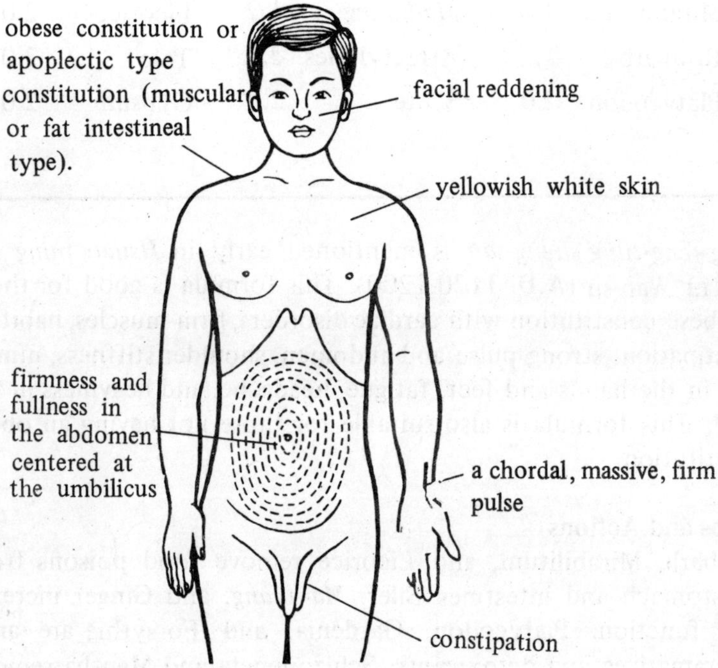

Hou-Pu-Chi-Wu-Tang 厚朴七物湯

(Magnolia Seven Combination)

Magnolia bark	6.0	Rhubarb	2.0	*Chih-shih*	2.5
Cinnamon	1.5	Licorice	2.0	Ginger	3.0
Jujube	2.5				

Hou-pu-chi-wu-tang is recorded in the Chinese medical work *Chin kuei yao lueh* (金匱要略) of the Han dynasty. This formula is used for treating diseases caused by external cold, lingering fever, pain due to abdominal distention, constipation, and floating and fast pulse.

Herbs and Actions
This formula is a combination of *Kuei-chih-chu-shao-yao-tang* and *Hou-pu-san-wu-tang*. Cinnamon, Jujube, Ginger and Licorice dispel "superficial evil" and supply nutrients. Magnolia bark, *Chih-shih,* and Rhubarb improve the "*ch'i*" and dispel internal heat.

Indications
Febrile disease, gastrointestinal disease, peritonitis, and habitual constipation.

Discrimination
Ta-cheng-chi-tang (Major Rhubarb Combination): abdominal distention, firm fever conformation, severe fullness and firmness, submerged and firm pulse.
Tiao-wei-cneng-chi-tang (Rhubarb and Mirabilitum Combination): abdominal fullness, discomfort, pyrophobia instead of chillphobia, vomiting, submerged and firm pulse.

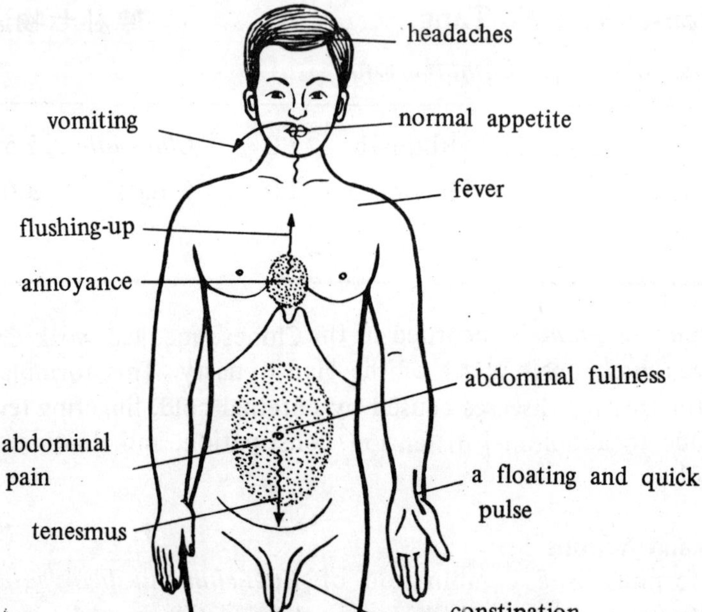

Ko-Ken-Huang-Lien-Huang-Chin-Tang

葛根黃連黃芩湯

(Pueraria, Coptis, and Scute Combination)

Pueraria	6.0	Coptis	3.0	Scute	3.0
Licorice	2.0				

Ko-ken-huang-lien-huang-chin-tang was record in the Chinese medical work *Shang han lun* (傷寒論) during the Han dynasty. This formula is used for treating fever, diarrhea, a feverish sensation in the chest, thirst, gasping, and ephidrosis.

Herbs and Actions

Pueraria relieves muscle tension. Pueraria with Coptis and Scute promotes gastrointestinal functions. Scute and Coptis are antipyretic, antiphlogistics, and stomachics that dispel "moist heat" and check vomiting.

Indications
Dysentery, diarrhea, acute gastroenteritis, influenza, asthma, febrile diseases, erysipelas, measles, ophthalmic disorders, toothache, stomatitis, and hypertension.

Discrimination
Ko-ken-tang (Pueraria Combination): fever, external fever, and stiff neck and back.
Pan-hsia-hsieh-hsin-tang (Pinellia Combination): obstruction beneath the heart, diarrhea, gas, vomiting.
Kuei-chih-jen-sheng-tang (Cinnamon and Ginseng Combination): diarrhea, internal chills and external fever.
Ma-huang-tang (*Ma-huang* Combination): fever, no sweating, asthma.

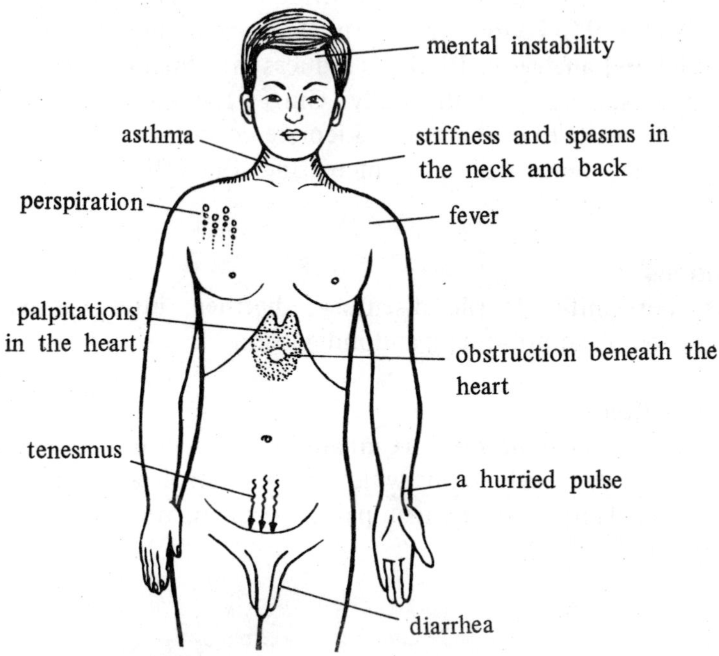

Kuei-Chih-Chia-Shao-Yao-Ta-Huang-Tang
桂枝加芍藥大黃湯

(Cinnamon,Peony, and Rhubarb Combination)

Cinnamon	4.0	Ginger	4.0	Jujube	4.0
Licorice	2.0	Peony	6.0	Rhubarb	1.0

Kuei-chih-chia-shao-yao-ta-huang-tang, also called *Kuei-chih-chia-ta-huang-tang*, is recorded in *Shang han lun* (傷寒論) of the Han dynasty. This formula is a combination of *Kuei-chih-chia-shao-yao-tang* (Cinnamon and Peony Combination) with Rhubarb. It is used for treating conformations that are more firm than *Kuei-chih-chia-shao-yao-tang*. This combination is suitable for "superficial evil", fever with severe chills, abdominal distention, paralytic ileus, and tenesmus due to diarrhea.

Herbs and Actions
Cinnamon is used for relaxing a contracted muscle and dispeling "superficial evil". Peony warms the body and acts as an anti-spasmodic and analgesic. Rhubarb reduces intestinal inflammation and dispels stagnancy in the body. Ginger relieves chills. Jujube can regulate the *ch'i* in the body. Licorice coordinates the actions of the other herbs, thereby increasing the efficiency of the formula.

Indications
Colitis, peritonitis, febrile disentery, diarrhea, intestinal colic, constipation, food poisoning, and indigestion.

Discrimination
Kuei-chih-chia-shao-yao-tang (Cinnamon and Peony Combination): treats external toxin which is not resolved; abdominal fullness and pain; no strong firm pain; no constipation or presence of diarrhea.

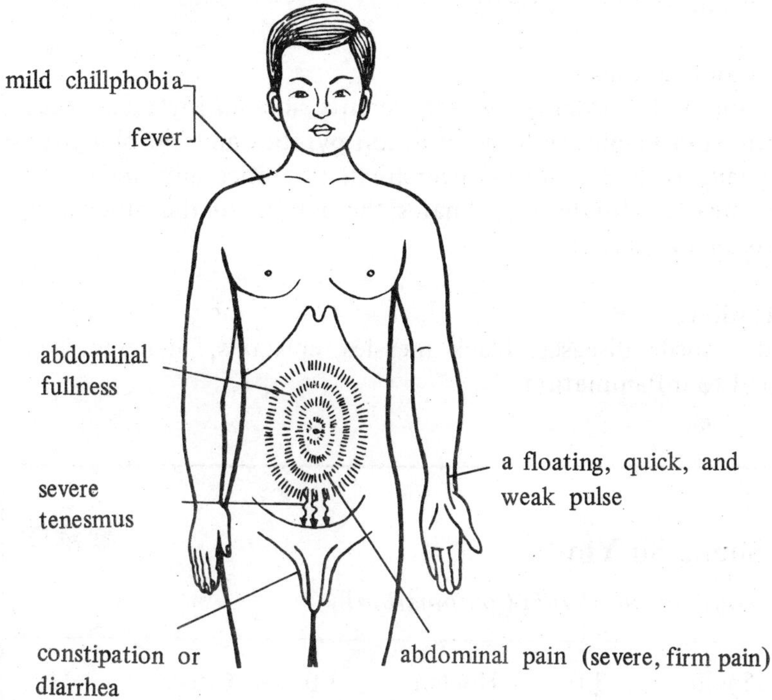

San-Huang-Shih-Kao-Tang 三黃石膏湯

(Gypsum, Coptis, and Scute Combination)

Gypsum	10.0	Scute	3.0	Coptis	1.5
Phellodendron	1.5	Gardenia	2.0	*Ma-huang*	3.0
Soja	2.0	Ginger	1.0	Jujube	1.0
Tea	1.0				

San-huang-shih-kao-tang is recorded in *I fang chi chieh* (醫方集解) of the Ching dynasty. This formula is used for treating warm diseases of heat and firmness conformations; it acts as an antipyretic and antiphlogistic. It is suitable for those with a large and quick pulse, red face, dry mouth, thirst, delirium, measles, epistaxis, and insomnia due to anxiety.

Herbs and Actions

Gypsum and Gardenia are refrigerants and antipyretics. Scute, Coptis, and Phellodendron act as antipyretics and antiphlogistics. *Ma-huang* with Soja and Ginger are diaphoretics and are used to treat measles. Jujube coordinates the actions of the other herbs. Tea is an antipyretic.

Indications

Acute febrile diseases, black measles, epistaxis, all hemorrhages related to inflammation.

Sheng-Su-Yin 參蘇飲

(Ginseng and Perilla Combination)

Pinellia	3.0	Hoelen	3.0	Citrus	2.0
Pueraria	2.0	Platycodon	2.0	Peucedanum	2.0
Perilla	1.0	Ginseng	1.5	*Chih-ko*	1.0
Saussurea	1.0	Jujube	1.5	Licorice	1.0
Ginger	1.5				

Recorded in *Tai ping huei min ho chi chu fang* (太平惠民和劑局方) of the Sung dynasty. Used for treating the common cold, fever, headache, cough, sputum, distention in the stomach, vomiting, nausea, and a delicate constitution. Most effective for common colds with coughing in children, the elderly, and pregnant women.

Herbs and Actions

Perilla, pueraria, and peucedanum are carminatives. Ginseng, Hoelen, and Licorice are tonics. Citrus and Pinellia are expectorants and anti-emetics. *Chih-ko* and Platycodon improve gastric function. Saussurea unblocks stagnant *ch'i.*

Indications
The common cold, bronchitis, pneumonia, stagnant *ch'i*, toxemia during pregnancy, and alcoholic hangovers.

Discrimination
Ma-huang-tang (*Ma-huang* Combination): headache, fever, sweating, asthma, firm conformation, floating and tense pulse, generalized aching.
Ko-ken-tang (Pueraria Combination): headache, fever, no sweating, stiffness in the neck and back, floating and tense pulse.

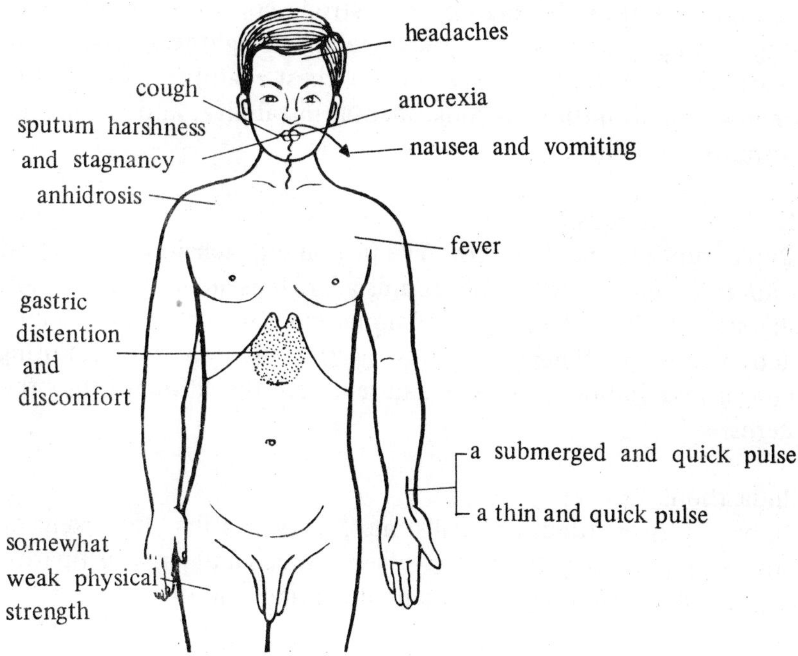

Ta-Chai-Hu-Tang 大柴胡湯

(Major Bupleurum Combination)

Bupleurum	6.0	Scute	3.0	Pinellia	3.0
Ginger	4.0	*Chih-shih*	2.0	Peony	3.0
Rhubarb	1.0	Jujube	3.0		

Ta-chai-hu-tang is recorded in *Shang han lun* and *Chin kuei yao lueh* by Chang Chung-ching (A.D. 142-220) of the Han dynasty. This formula is used for more severe symptoms than those treated by *Hsiao-chai-hu-tang* (Minor Bupleurum Combination). It should be taken by those having obese or strong constitution with good skin, strong and sunken pulse, a feeling of tightness beneath the heart, chest distention, pain in the chest, habitual constipation or diarrhea, vomiting, asthma, mental instability, and a tendency towards irritability.

Herbs and Actions

Bupleurum and Scute remove evil heat and distension in the chest. *Chih-shih* and Peony relieve muscular tenseness, and promote digestion. Rhubarb is anti-inflammative. Ginger relieves nausea and vomiting. Pinellia relieves gastric distress and vomiting. Ginger and Jujube synthesize and reinforce the action of the other herbs.

Indications

Impaired liver function, gallstones, cholecystitis, hypertension, sour stomach, gastritis, gastric ulcer, duodenal ulcer, constipation, asthma, diarrhea, diabetes, impaired hearing, and obesity.

Discrimination

Hsiao-chai-hu-tang (Minor Bupleurum Combination): thoraco-costal distress, pain in the upper abdomen, inclination towards a weak conformation, slight sensation of fullness.

Szu-ni-san (Bupleurum and *Chih-shih* Formula): thoraco-costal distress, a congested condition occurring from below the heart to

the umbilicus.
Chai-hu-chia-lung-ku-mu-li-tang (Bupleurum and Dragon Bone Combination): thoraco-costal distress, palpitations in the abdomen, irritability and fright, emotional upset.
Hsiao-hsien-hsiung-tang (Minor Trichosanthes Combination): tension beneath the heart, floating and slippery pulse, thinness beneath the heart.
Mu-fang-chi-tang (Stephania and Ginseng Combination): obstruction and hardness beneath the heart, dark facial complexion, edema, asthmatic cough, submerged and tense pulse.
Yin-chen-hao-tang (Capillaris Combination): abdominal fullness, internal fever, jaundice, cardiac discomfort, painful urination with red urine.
Shih-tsao-tang (Jujube Combination): obstruction, hardening, and distention beneath the heart; water stagnancy; gasping.

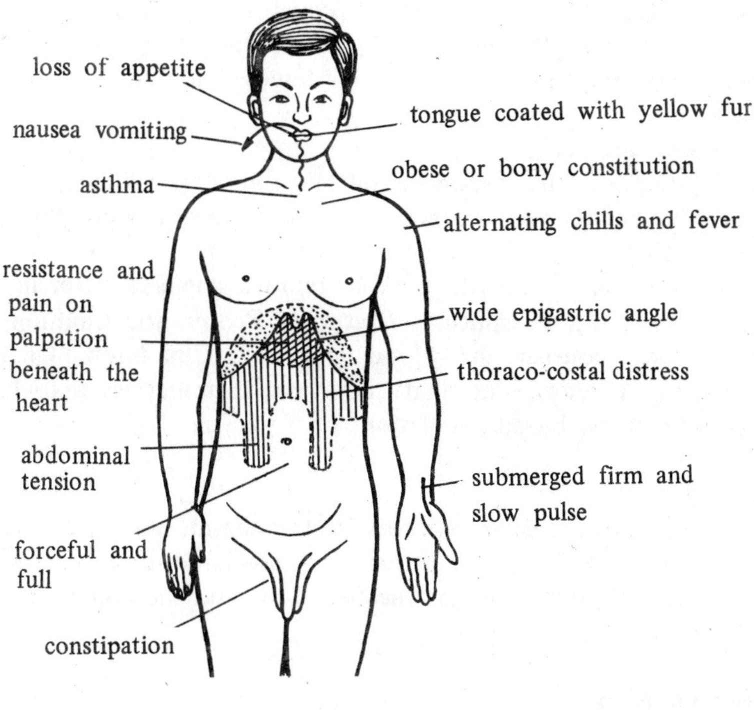

Wu-Chi-San 五積散

(Tang-kuei and Magnolia Formula)

Angelica	1.2	Citrus	2.0	Cinnamon	1.2
Magnolia bark	1.2	*Tang-kuei*	1.2	Cnidium	1.2
Peony	1.2	Hoelen	2.0	Platycodon	1.2
Atractylodes	4.0	*Chih-ko*	1.2	Pinellia	2.0
Ma-huang	1.2	Ginger	1.2	Jujube	1.2
Licorice	1.2	Dry ginger	1.2		

Recorded in *Tai ping huei min ho chi chu fang* (太平惠民和劑局方) of the Sung dynasty. Used for treating stagnant *ch'i*, stagnant blood, stagnant sputum, stagnant cold, and stagnant food. It is best for patients having a delicate constitution, slight anemia, a febrile feeling in the upper body accompanied by chills in the lower body, and pain in the waist and lower abdomen.

Herbs and Actions

Atractylodes, Citrus, Licorice, and Magnolia bark of *Ping-wei-san* (Magnolia and Ginger Formula) remove stagnant food. Pinellia, Hoelen, Citrus, Licorice and Ginger of *Erh-chen-tang* (Citrus and Pinellia Combination) with *Chih-ko* remove stagnant water in the stomach and watery sputum. *Tang-kuei,* Peony, and Cnidium of *Szu-wu-tang* nourish the blood and *ch'i*. Cinnamon, Ginger, *Ma-huang*, Angelica, and Platycodon are carminatives (expelling gas) and increase blood circulation.

Indications

Acute and chronic gastroenteritis, gastric spasm, hernia, aching at the waist, pain during menstruation, valvular disease, neuralgia, rheumatism, beriberi, injury due to falling, and the common cold in the elderly.

Discrimination

Kuei-chih-chia-fu-tzu-tang (Cinnamon, Jujube, and Aconite

Combination): pain, spontaneous sweating, chillphobia, floating pulse.
Ping-wei-san (Magnolia and Ginseng Formula): obstruction and annoyance beneath the heart, overnight indigestion, and congestion.
Tang-kuei-szu-ni-tang (*Tang-kuei* and Jujube Combination): chill conformation, with severe chilling of the arms and legs.

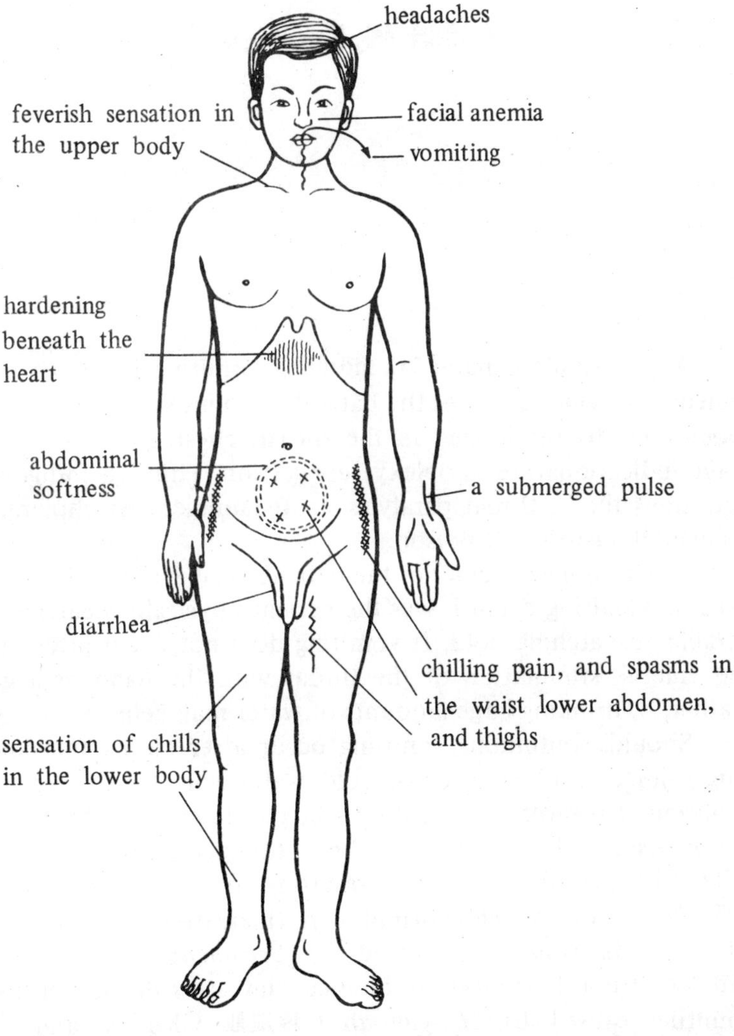

4.
Yung Tu Chi
(涌吐劑, Emetics)

Any formula capable of inducing vomiting is a *yung tu chi* remedy. An emetic causes the patient to vomit sputum, indigested foods, and toxins lodged in the throat, chest, or stomach. The main indications are apoplexy, congestion, fainting, indigestion, poisonous foods, throat paralysis, acute jaundice, dry cholera, and accidental ingestion of poison.

When taking an emetic, the patient must avoid drafty rooms, because vomiting often leaves the patient physically weak and vulnerable to catching cold. If vomiting does not occur after taking the emetic, stimulation of the throat with the hand or a goose feather, or drinking large amounts of water may help.

Should continuous vomiting occur after taking the emetic, ginger juice, cold congee, or cold water will usually arrest the vomiting. However, if vomiting still continues, countermeasures are necessary. For example, 30mg—60mg of musk is an antidote for incessant vomiting resulting from taking *Kua-ti-san* (瓜蒂散 Melon Pedicle Formula). A thick decoction of scullion white treats vomiting induced by *San-sheng-san* (三聖散 Siler and Veratrum Formula). A licorice and aspis decoction arrests vomiting caused by *Hsi-yen-san* (稀涎散 Gleditsia and Alum Formula).

After the vomiting has ceased, stomach upset can be soothed by taking congee to correct inverted *ch'i*. Oily, fried foods or indigestable foodstuffs should be avoided, otherwise the condition may be exacerbated, further injuring the normal *ch'i*.

Although the emetic formula has prompt curative effects for urgent conformations, it can have various harmful effects on the stomach. Therefore, this method of treatment should never be used on weak, debilitated, or elderly patients; it is also prohibited for patients with agitated *ch'i* in the abdomen and inadequacy of *ch'i* and blood; for pregnant women; for persons with amnesia; for patients with hemoptysis (hemorrhage of the larynx, trachea, bronchi or lungs); or for patients with cardiac disease or hypertension.

Kua-Ti-San 瓜蒂散

(Melon Pedicle Formula)

Melon pedicle	1.0	Phaseolus	1.0
Fermented soy bean	5.0		

Kua-ti-san is recorded in *Chin kuei yao lueh* (金匱要略) of the Han dynasty. This formula is an emetic and is used for treating large amounts of phlegm, chest distention, and stagnant food in the stomach.

Herbs and Actions
Melon pedicle is bitter in nature, and acts as an emetic. Phaseolus is sour in nature and reinforces the vomiting function. Fermented soybean removes "stagnant *ch'i*" from the chest.

Indications
Large amounts of phlegm, stagnant food, tonsillitis, jaundice, cholera, and neurotic vomiting.

San-Sheng-San 三聖散

(Siler and Veratrum Formula)

Siler	6.0	Melon pedicle	6.0	Veratrum	3.0

Recorded in *Ju men shih chin* (儒門事親). Used to remove the blockage following hemorrhage. It is indicated in (1) apopletic blockage, loss of voice and "suppressive disorder," distorted eyes and mouth, unconsciousness, lockjaw, a slippery and firm pulse; (2) epilepsy and turbid sputum clogging the chest and generating

pain as it is coughed up; (3) accidental ingestion of poisonous substances. (The remedy can be given only while the patient remains conscious in order that the poisonous substance can be expelled through induced vomiting.)
The action of this formula is comparatively drastic; hence its administration must be carefully attended. It is a common practice to begin with a little dose, increasing the dose until vomiting occurs. It is then withdrawn to prevent injury.

Herbs and Actions
Melon pedicle and Veratrum induce vomiting. Siler is good at expelling, bringing up, and dispersing wind toxin. The three herbs work together to open obstructions of wind sputum.

Indications
Apoplexy, epilepsy, food poisoning.

Sheng-Lu-Yin 蔘蘆飲

(Ginseng Rhizome Combination)

Ginseng rhizome 3.0–6.0

Recorded in *Tan chi's mental ways* (丹溪心法). For debilitated individuals who have profuse saliva and sputum which tend to obstruct passages, a tendency to vomit, and a weak and slippery pulse.
Melon pedicle and Veratrum are emetics, but they are so violent in action and so poisonous that they are suitable only for strong people. If the patient's physical condition is weak and calls for vomiting treatment, then Ginseng rhizome is the proper remedy.

Herbs and Actions
Ginseng rhizome has a bitter taste and warm nature. Its mildness makes it a tonic as well as a dispersing agent; hence it does not deplete vitality.

Indications
Sputum adversity in the debilitated.

Tsou-Ma-Tang *(Croton and Apricot Seed Combination)*			**走馬湯**
Croton	1.0	Apricot seed	1.0

Recorded in *Chin kuei yao lueh* (金匱要略). A strong cathartic agent. It is life giving for some acute cases, and its name *Tsou-ma-tang* means "immediate effect." Given as a single dose drug to stalwart individuals who suddenly contract an acute disease. The disease is generally caused by toxic water or other pathogenic substances and will manifest a feeling of compression and obstruction in the chest, ribs, and throat; acute pain in the heart and abdomen, even acute cardiac paralysis; respiratory paralysis leading to unconsciousness; and other rapidly occurring symptoms. This formula can only be used for patients with a conformation that is cold and firm, and in which severe intoxication is obvious. It is contraindicated for weak individuals.

Herbs and Actions
Croton is acrid and hot in nature, attacks chills, expels toxins, removes thoracic obstructions, and washes and cleans the stomach and intestines, and removes their obstructions. Apricot seed coordinates with Croton. The two herbs collaborate to expel pathogenic toxins. Note: The diarrhea induced by Croton preparations can be alleviated by drinking cold water or cold congee.

Indications
Apoplexy, uremia, convulsions caused by tetanus, contusions and wounds resulting from accidents, acute food poisoning, and cerebral diseases in which the patient has thoracic distress or becomes unconscious. In all of these cases this formula can save the patient from dangerous and acute conditions.

Discrimination

Tzu-yuan (Croton and Hematite Formula) is for cardiac and abdominal distention and pain and gastrointestinal accumulation and blockage when the conditions are mild. It is commonly used for children.

San-wu-pei-chi-wan (Croton, Ginger, and Rhubarb Formula) aims at the toxins in the chest and abdomen with the food poisoning being primary target and water poisoning a secondary target.

Emergent Acute symptoms of the chill-firm conformation

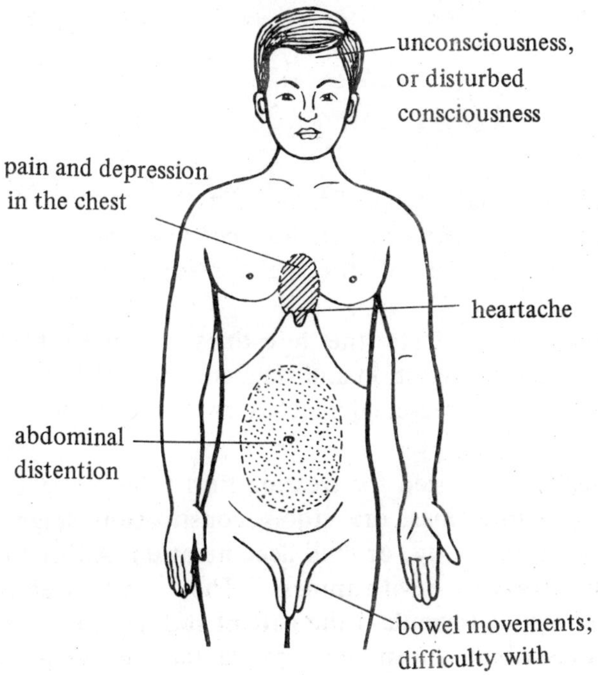

5.
Kung Li Chi
(攻裏劑, Interior Attacking Formulas)

Formulas that attack firmness in the interior of the body are called *kung li chi* or *hsieh hsia chi* (瀉下劑) or purgatives. Purgation is another of the eight major Chinese therapeutic methods.

Purgatives lubricate the intestines, promote bowel movements, eliminate congestion and stagnancy within the stomach and intestines, and decrease edematous swelling of the abdomen or chest.

Purgatives are used for treating firm fever, congestion in the stomach and intestines, dry stools, constipation, stagnated water (fluid) inside the body, or chill accumulation. All of these symptoms are caused by "evil firmness." They can be treated with an interior attacking formula if the patient still has normal vitality.

In prescribing an emetic formula the following precautions need be observed. First, if surface toxin has not been dispelled and the interior is not firm enough, treatment must be carried out according to the rule of surface-first, interior-second. Only after surface toxin has been eliminated and the interior has become firm can a purgative be prescribed. If the surface is not yet cured but the interior has become firm, then, depending on the relative severity of the two, a properly adjusted dual suface-interior attacking formula must be used.

Second, in prescribing purgatives, not only the firmness conformation must be considered but also the weakness conformation. Generally if the patient has a strong tendency toward interior firmness (sound functioning of internal organs), purgation is instituted. If the patient is more inclined to the weakness, then both purgating and supplementing methods are used. Sometimes when constipation is a symptom of the conformation, it should not be treated with a purgative. This prohibition applies especially to physically weak geriatric patients, postpartal women with blood weakness (anemia), recovering patients with inhibited salivation and patients who have lost considerable blood. This type of formula is contraindicated for pregnant women.

Third, most purgatives are injurous and exhaust normal stomach *ch'i* (vitality). Hence their administration should be suspended once they have taken effect, and the patient given a nourishing formula. The patient must be cautioned against eating oily and indigestible foods.

Chieh-Keng-Pai-San 桔梗白散

(Platycodon and Croton Formula)

Platycodon 1.0	Fritillaria 1.0	Croton seed 0.3

Recorded in *Shang han lun*. Has strong expectorant and pus-discharging effects and a purgative action which is contraindicated for people with a feeble physique. If the disease is located above the diaphragm, the formula may encourage vomiting. If the disease is located below the diaphragm, it may encourage purging. The formula treats the following symptoms: distention and bloating in the chest; severe cough; and frequent spitting of fishy, foul-smelling thick sputum or clogging of the throat by a thick mucous sputum which hinders breathing and signifies a dangerous condition. It is suitable for patients with a forceful pulse and a firm fullness beneath the heart. If this formula results in ceaseless diarrhea, one cup of cold water taken all at once will stop the diarrhea.

Herbs and Actions

Croton seed alone has cathartic actions; but in combination with Platycodon and Fritillaria, it has a joint expectorant and pus-discharging action.

Indications

Pulmonary gangrene, acute pneumonia, the initial stage of diphtheria, apoplexy, paroxysms of asthma. To be taken in a one potion regimen.

Hsiao-Cheng-Chi-Tang *(Minor Rhubarb Combination)*		小承氣湯
Rhubarb 2.0	*Chih-shih* 2.0	Magnolia bark 3.0

Hsiao-cheng-chi-tang was recorded in both the *Shang han lun* (傷寒論) and the *Chin kuei yao lueh* (金匱要略) during the Han dynasty. This formula is used for treating symptoms similar to those of the *Ta-cheng-chi-tang* conformation as well as bloating, constipation, moist fever, and a sinking pulse.

Herbs and Actions

Chih-shih and Magnolia bark dispel distention. Rhubarb is an antipyretic.

Indications

Acute febrile diseases, habitual constipation, hypertension, obesity, food poisoning, epilepsy, emotional disorders, food stagnation, tetanus, dysentery, and dysuria.

Discrimination

Ta-cheng-chi-tang (Major Rhubarb Combination): constipation, abdominal fullness, tidal fever, spontaneous sweating, delirium, hiccups, dry tongue with black coat, and gasping.

Tiao-wei-cheng-chi-tang (Rhubarb and Mirabilitum Combination): constipation, fever, abdominal fullness, acute abdominal pain, mild asthma.

Hou-pu-san-wu-tang (Magnolia Three Combination): constipation, abdominal fullness, submerged and firm pulse, abdominal pain.

Sunlight yang conformation

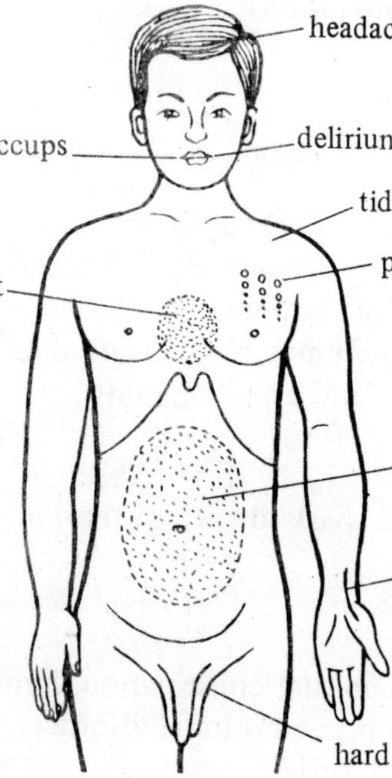

Hsiao-Hsien-Hsiung-Tang *(Minor Trichosanthes Combination)*					小陷胸湯
Trichosanthes seed	3.0	Pinellia	6.0	Coptis	1.5

Hsiao-hsien-hsiung-tang was recorded in the *Shang han lun* (傷寒論) during the Han dynasty. This formula is used for treating sub-cardiac pressure and pain, chest pain on coughing or deep breathing, hyperpnea, viscid sputum, and a floating pulse.

Herbs and Actions

Coptis has bitter and cooling qualities and acts as an antipyretic. Pinellia is an expectorant. The combination of Coptis and Pinellia dispels "internal heat" and serves as a stomachic and expectorant. Trichosanthes seed is an expectorant and antipyretic.

Indications
Pneumonia, bronchitis, pleurisy, gastritis, dyspepsia, intercostal neuralgia, and gallstones.

Discrimination
Ta-hsien-hsiung-tang (Rhubarb and *Kan-sui* Combination): undectable hardness and pain beneath the heart; distention, hardness, and pain occurring from the inferiority of heart to the lower abdomen; submerged and tense pulse.
Sheng-chiang-hsieh-hsin-tang (Pinellia and Ginger Combination): obstruction and hardness beneath the heart; this formula is for swelling and acute pain at the low end of the substernum.

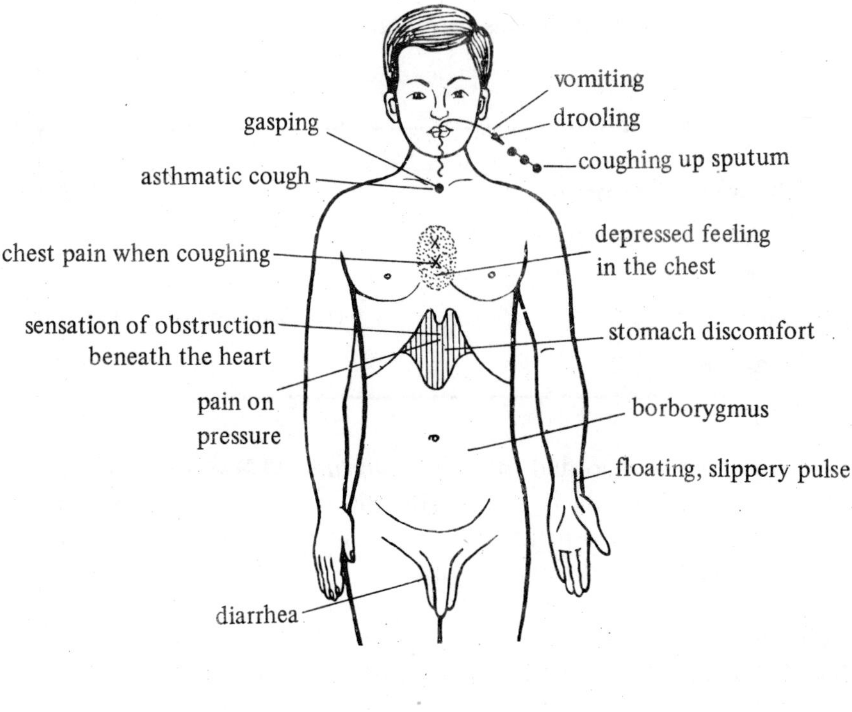

San-Wu-Pei-Chi-Wan 三物備急丸

(Rhubarb, Ginger, and Croton Formula)

Rhubarb	1.0	Ginger	1.0	Croton	1.0

San-wu-pei-chi-wan is recorded in *Chin kuei yao lueh* (金匱要略) of the Han dynasty. This formula is used for treating abdominal distention due to suffering from cold or eating cold foods, with rapid breathing and severe pain.

Herbs and Actions
Croton is a poisonous herb used to treat distention due to chills. Rhubarb is a detoxifier which removes stagnant food. Ginger is warm in nature and treats ailments due to cold. Although not harmful in small doses when processed correctly, great care must be taken when using this formula.

Shih-Tsao-Tang 十棗湯

(Jujube Combination)

Jujube	4.0	*Kansui*	1.0	Euphorbia	1.0
Genkwa	1.0				

Shih-tsao-tang is recorded in *Shang han lun* (傷寒論) of the Han dynasty. This formula is a cathartic and is used for coughs, pain in the chest, hardness in the abdomen, nausea, rapid respirations, headache, vertigo, and sunken pulse.

Herbs and Actions
Kansui, Genkwa, and Euphorbia are cathartics. Jujube is a tonic.

Indications
Pleurisy, cirrhosis, and ascites due to schistosomiasis or nephritis.

Discrimination
Ta-hsien-hsiung-tang (Rhubarb and *Kan-sui* Combination): stagnancy, hardness and fullness beneath the heart, dragging pain at the hypochondrium, constipation, extreme thirst, asthmatic cough, mild sweating of the head, submerged and tense pulse or slow pulse.
Ling-kuei-chu-kan-tang (Atractylodes and Hoelen Combination): stagnant water beneath the heart, gasping, headaches, diminished urine, lack of vitality, weak conformation.
Chih-so-erh-chen-tang (*Chih-shih* and Cardamon Combination): congestive diseases, pain beneath the heart, vomiting, pain radiating toward the waist and lower back, and moving along the chest and the back.

Ta-Cheng-Chi-Tang 大承氣湯

(Major Rhubarb Combination)

Rhubarb	2.0	*Chih-shih*	2.0	Mirabilitum	2.0
Magnolia bark	5.0				

Ta-cheng-chi-tang is recorded in both the *Shang han lun* (傷寒論) and the *Chin kuei yao lueh* (金匱要略) of the Han dynasty. This formula is used for treating patients with a strong abdomen, abdominal distention, a sensation of heaviness in the body, ephidrosis, a sinking-strong pulse, constipation, moist fever, and a dry tongue and mouth. Those with a fast-weak pulse and ascites should not take this formula.

Herbs and Actions
Chih-shih dispels distention and stagnant *ch'i.* Magnolia bark dispels distention and increases vitality. Mirabilitum is a nutritive and laxative. Rhubarb relieves dryness of the stools.

Indications

Acute pneumonia, typhoid, influenza, measles, meningitis, hypertension, tetanus, beriberi, habitual constipation, neurosis, food poisoning, obesity, dysentery, and hemorrhoids.

Discrimination

Hsiao-cheng-chi-tang (Minor Rhubarb Combination): abdominal fullness, hard stools; a *Ta-cheng-chi-tang* conformation is characterized by a hard and full abdomen and dry stools.

Tiao-wei-cheng-chi-tang (Rhubarb and Mirabilitum Combination): abdominal fullness, constipation, irritability, no chillphobia and no sweating.

Hou-pu-chi-wu-tang (Magnolia Seven Combination): abdominal fullness, flushing up, vomiting.

Hou-pu-sheng-chiang-pan-hsia-kan-tsao-jen-sheng-tang (Magnolia Five Combination): abdominal fullness, distention after diarrhea.

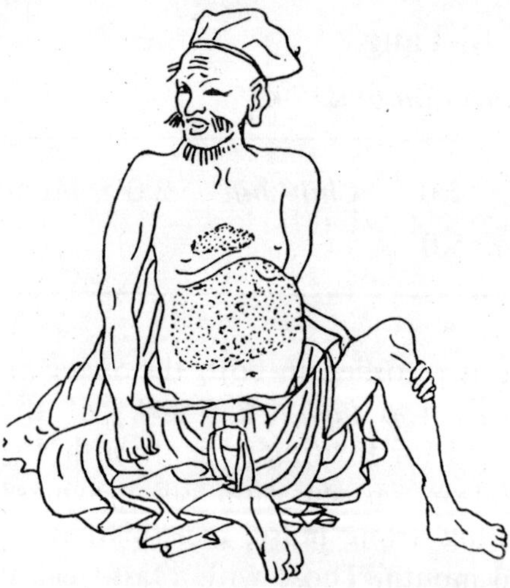

Sunlight yang conformation

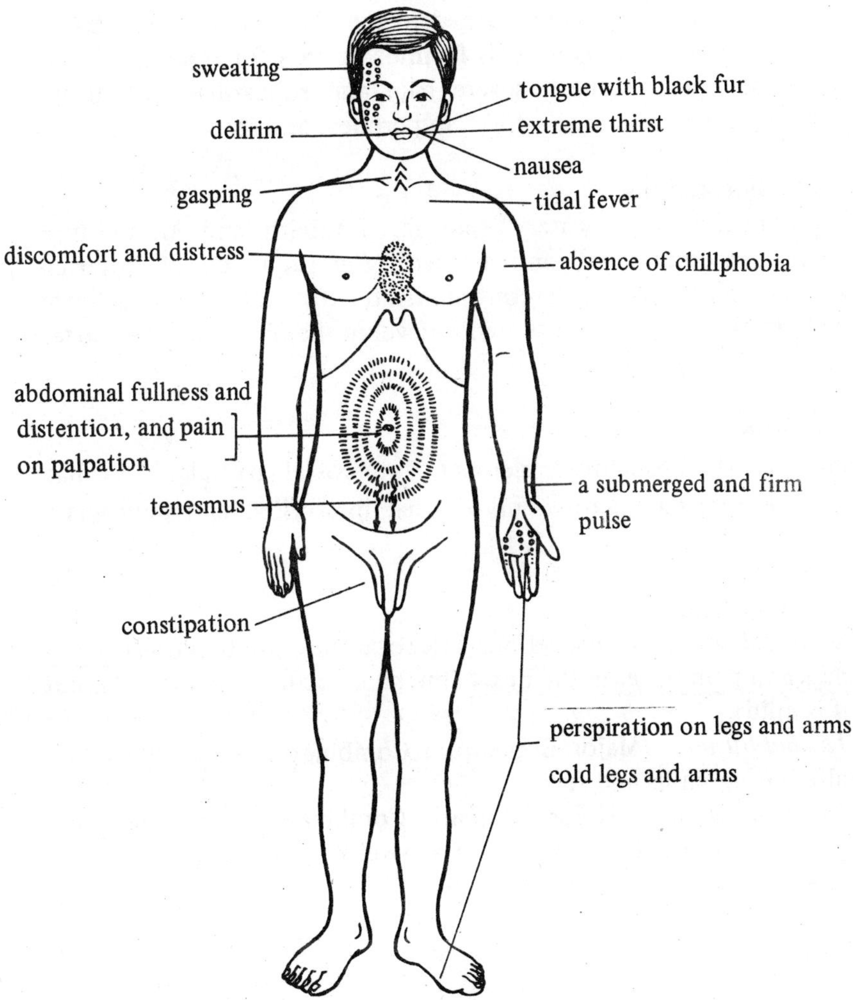

Ta-Hsien-Hsiung-Tang 大陷胸湯

(*Rhubarb and Kan-sui Combination*)

Rhubarb	9.0	Mirabilitum	1.5	*Kan-sui*	1.5

Ta-hsien-hsiung-tang was recorded in the *Shang han lun* (傷寒論) during the Han dynasty. This formula is used for treating "internal heat" in the chest, severe pain and subcardiac distention, constipation, dry mouth, thirst, hyperpnea, and stress.

Herbs and Actions

Kan-sui eliminates watery sputum. Rhubarb and Mirabilitum dispel "internal heat" and act with *Kan-sui* to dispel "internal water". This formula is contraindicated for patients of delicate constitution and patients who develop lienteric diarrhea after taking the formula.

Indications

Pneumonia, bronchitis, pleurisy, intercostal neuralgia, cardiac neuritis, angina pectoris, myocardial infarction, and pulmonary edema.

Discrimination

Hsiao-hsien-hsiung-tang (Minor Trichosanthes Combination): hardness and pain beneath the heart (the pain occurs when pressed, but it is mild).
Ta-chai-hu-tang (Major Bupleurum Combination): internal fever, alternating chills and fever.
Ta-cheng-chi-tang (Major Rhubarb Combination): hardness and fullness, constipation, distention around the umbilicus, and severe tidal fever.

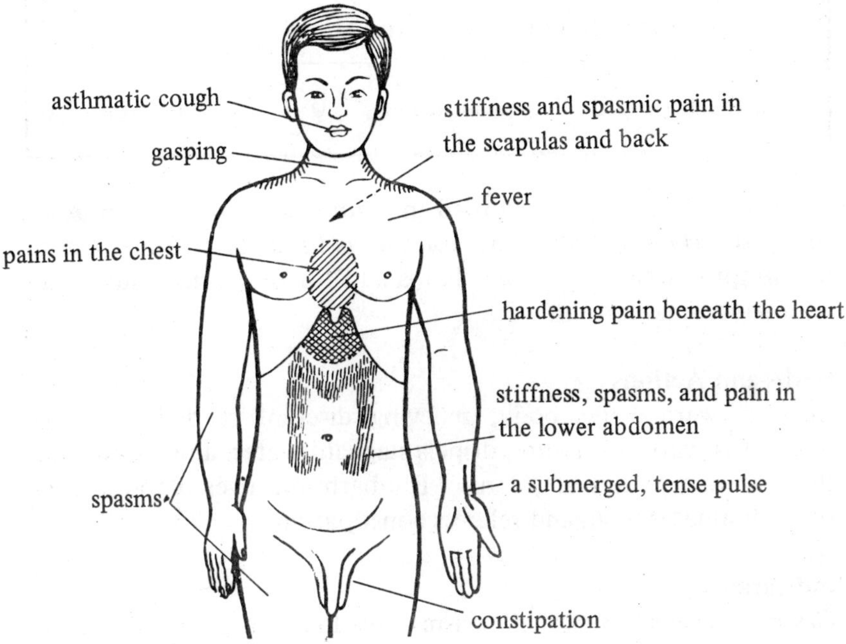
asthmatic cough
gasping
stiffness and spasmic pain in the scapulas and back
fever
pains in the chest
hardening pain beneath the heart
stiffness, spasms, and pain in the lower abdomen
a submerged, tense pulse
spasms
constipation

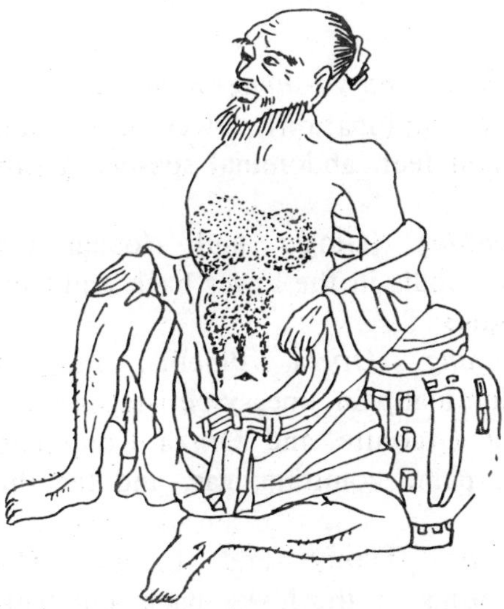

Ta-Huang-Fu-Tzu-Tang 大黃附子湯

(Rhubarb and Aconite Combination)

Rhubarb 1.0	Asarum 2.0	Aconite 0.5–1.0

Ta-huang-fu-tzu-tang is recorded in *Chin kuei yao lueh* (金匱要略)of the Han dynasty. This formula is used for treating pain in the armpits, waist, and lower limbs and for fever, tight pulse, and mild abdominal tension.

Herbs and Actions

Aconite warms the body, relieving discomfort due to chills. Asarum is warm in nature, dispels stagnant water, and coordinates the warming action of Aconite. Rhubarb improves blood circulation, eliminates pain, and relieves constipation.

Indications

Gastric spasms, intestinal spasms, pyelonephritis, renal calculi, gallstones, pancreatitis, intestinal colic, hernia pain, sciatica, intercostal neuralgia, and migraine.

Discrimination

Tang-kuei-szu-ni-chia-wu-chu-yu-sheng-chiang-tang (*Tang-kuei*, Evodia, and Ginger Combination): lower back pain, abdominal pain, cold hands and feet, abdominal spasms, a submerged and thin pulse.

Ling-chiang-chu-kan-tang (Ginger and Hoelen Combination): lower back pain, icy chills in the lower back and feet, diminished urine, submerged pulse.

Chieh-chi-shu-chiao-tang (Oryza, Pinellia, and Zanthoxylum Combination): abdominal pain, uneasy peristalsis, and gas.

Fu-tzu-keng-mi-tang (Aconite and Oryza Combination): abdominal pain, severe pain, vomiting, gas, and the flushing up of *ch'i*.

Shao-yao-kan-tsao-tang (Peony and Licorice Combination): abdominal pain, spasms in the lower back and feet, abdominal spasms–impetuous condition.

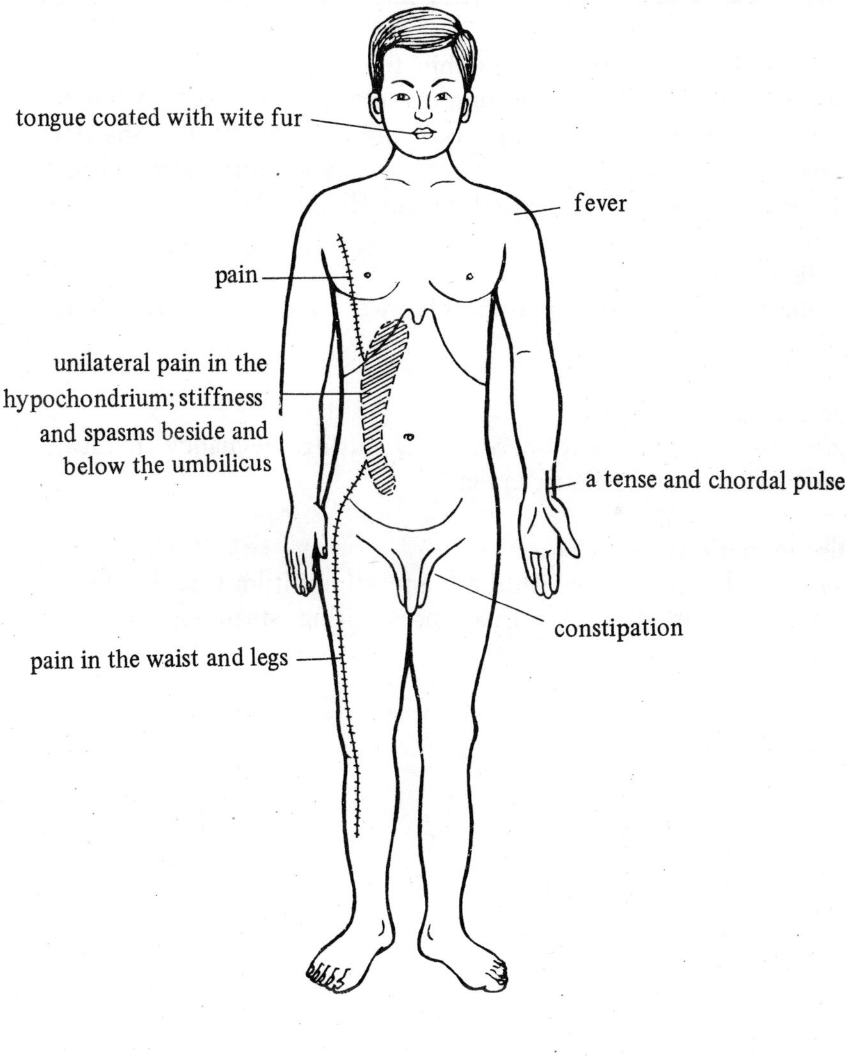
tongue coated with wite fur
fever
pain
unilateral pain in the hypochondrium; stiffness and spasms beside and below the umbilicus
a tense and chordal pulse
constipation
pain in the waist and legs

Ta-Huang-Kan-Tsao-Tang 大黃甘草湯

(Rhubarb and Licorice Combination)

Rhubarb	4.0	Licorice	1.0

Ta-huang-kan-tsao-tang, a combination of *Tiao-wei-cheng-chi-tang* (Rhubarb and Mirabilitum Combination) except Mirabilitum, is recorded in *Chin kuei yao lueh* (金匱要略) of the Han dynasty. This formula is used for treating vomiting after eating, abdominal distention, constipation, and dry stools.

Herbs and Actions
Rhubarb relieves constipation, Licorice stimulates gastric function.

Indications
Gastritis, gastric distention, vomiting during pregnancy, habitual constipation, and pediatric epilepsy.

Discrimination
Tiao-wei-cheng-chi-tang (Rhubarb and Mirabilitum Combination): abdominal distention, constipation, vomiting, steaming fever, dry mouth and tongue.

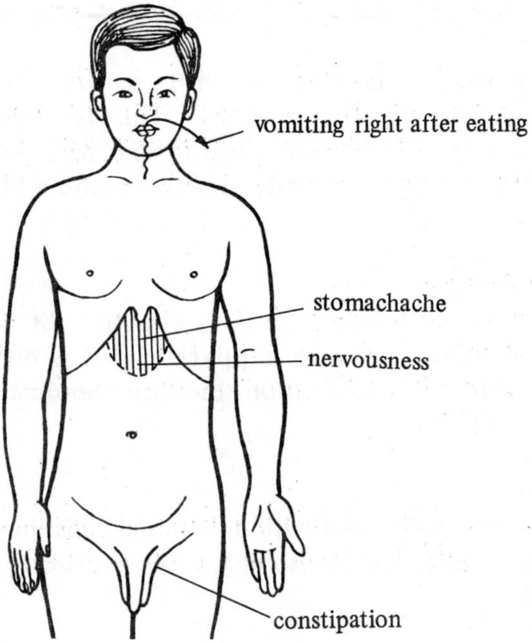
vomiting right after eating
stomachache
nervousness
constipation

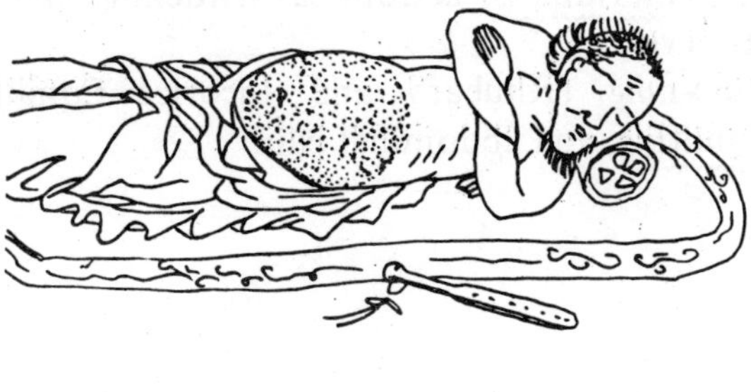

Tiao-Wei-Cheng-Chi-Tang 調胃承氣湯

(Rhubarb and Mirabilitum Combination)

Rhubarb	2.5	Mirabilitum	1.0	Licorice	1.0

Tiao-wei-cheng-chi-tang was recorded in the *Shang han lun* (傷寒論) during the Han dynasty. This formula is used for treating patients of delicate constitution with severe fever, a sinking pulse, a supple abdomen, vomiting, and a dry tongue and mouth.

Herbs and Actions
Rhubarb is an antipyretic which is effective for dryness of the stool. Mirabilitum is also an antipyretic that is effective for dry stools and promoting evacuation. Licorice coordinates the actions of the other herbs.

Indications
Febrile diseases with constipation, habitual constipation, constipation in the elderly, food poisoning, acute gastroenteritis, and food stagnation.

Discrimination
Ta-cheng-chi-tang (Major Rhubarb Combination): constipation, delirium, abdominal fullness, abdominal hardening and fullness, dry stool, severe fever.
Ta-huang-kan-tsao-tang (Rhubarb and Licorice Combination): constipation, vomiting, and abdominal pain.

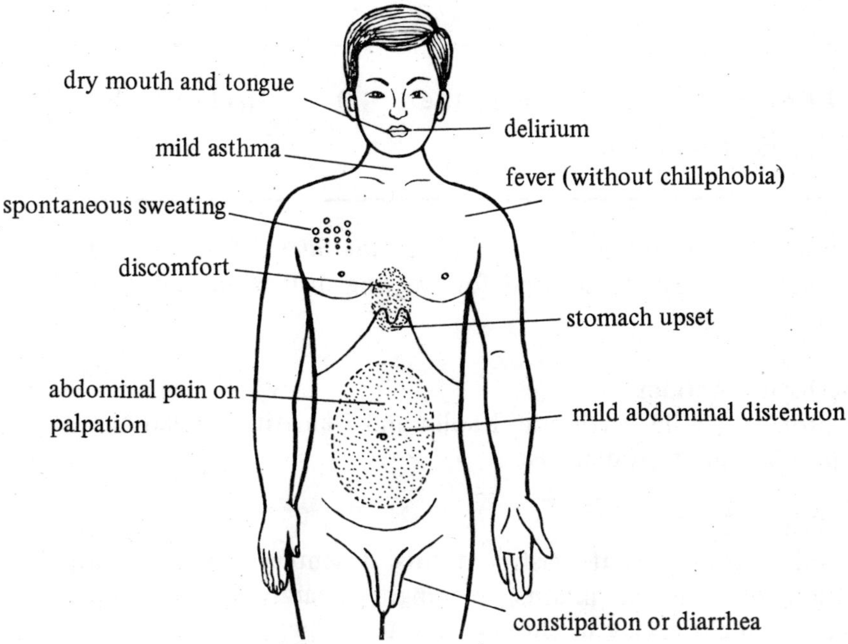
dry mouth and tongue
delirium
mild asthma
fever (without chillphobia)
spontaneous sweating
discomfort
stomach upset
abdominal pain on palpation
mild abdominal distention
constipation or diarrhea

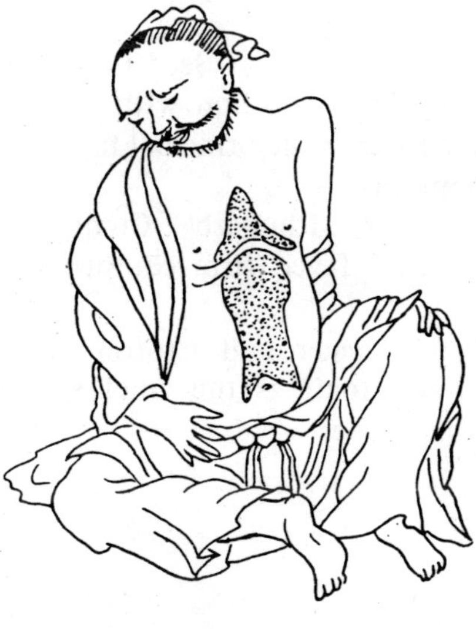

Tzu-Yuan 紫圓

(Croton and Hematite Formula)

Croton	4.0	Hematite	4.0	Kaolin	4.0
Apricot seed	8.0				

Tzu-yuan is recorded in *Chien chin yao fang* (千金要方). This formula is a carthartic used for treating distention in the chest and abdomen.

Herbs and Actions
Croton is a mild carthartic. Kaolin and Hematite are astringests. Apricot seed stops diarrhea.

Indications
Food poisoning, acute gastroenteritis, dysentery, uremia, regurgitation of milk in infants, meningitis, paralytic ileus, cardiac dropsy, night crying in children due to abdominal distention and constipation, beriberi, and external injuries.

Discrimination
Tsou-ma-tang (Croton and Apricot Seed Combination): thoracic-abdominal toxin, an acute condition with severe poisoning, firm conformation. Water toxin is the principal target and food toxin is the subordinate symptom.
Ta-cheng-chi-tang (Major Rhubarb Combination): thoraco-abdominal toxin, internal fever, firm conformation, formula discharges of food toxin.
Pei-chi-wan (Rhubarb, Ginger, and Croton Formula): thoracic-abdominal toxin. Food toxin is the chief symptom and water toxin as the subordinate one.

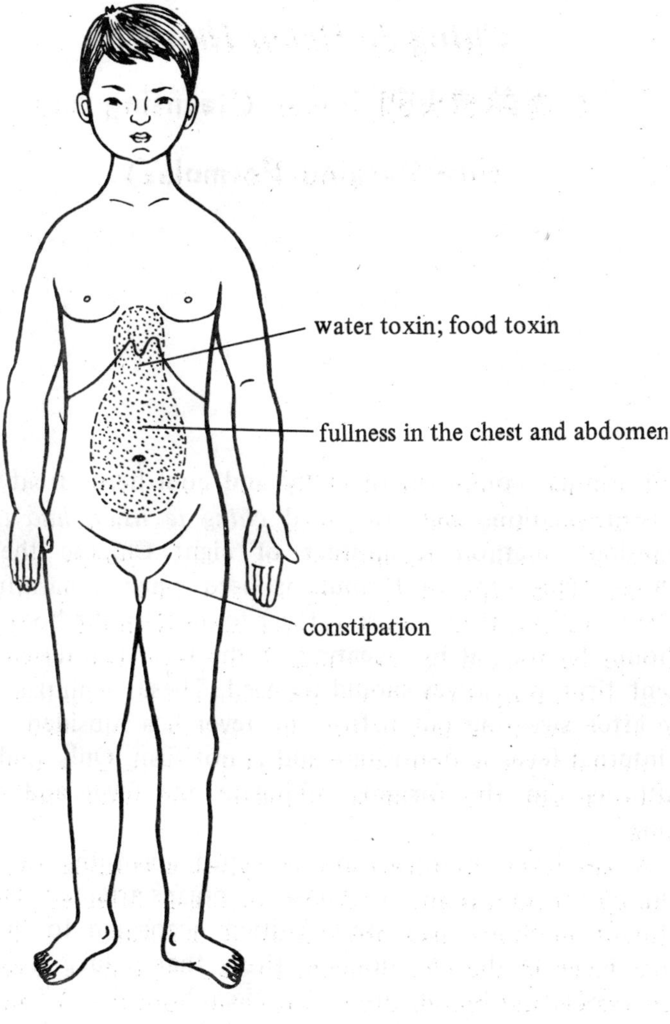
water toxin; food toxin
fullness in the chest and abdomen
constipation

6.
Ching Je Hsieh Huo Chi
(清熱瀉火劑, Fever Cleansing and Fire Purging Formulas)

Formulas composed of chilly and cool herbs treat fever or fire conformations and are called *ching je hsieh huo chi.* This "cleansing" method is another of eight Chinese therapeutic methods. This type of formula is used when a harmful toxin results in a fever. If the injurous fever toxin is on the body surface, it should be treated by sweating; if the fever is internal and the patient firm, purgatives should be used. These formulas are used only after sweating but before the fever has subsided, or when the internal fever is flourishing and is not firm. Only under these conditions can the formula subjugate the fever and result in healing.

A fire-fever conformation is typed according to domain: blood, *ch'i*, firmness and weakness, or organs affected. Therefore, treatment methods also are classified according to those that reduce fever in the *ch'i* domain, those that reduce fever in the blood vessels and blood, those that clean both the *ch'i* and blood, those that purge fire and poisons, and those that reduce visceral and weakness fever.

In prescribing this type of formula certain precautions must be taken. It must be clearly determined whether the fever is genuine or false. A high-grade, short-term fever that expels toxins is termed a real fever whereas a low-grade, persistent fever–such as found in tuberculosis–is deemed a false fever. The same applies to chills. For example, a real-fever, false-chills condition should be treated with a fever-cleansing, fire-purging formula, not with a warming formula, and a false-fever, real-chills condition must be treated with an interior-warming, yang-restoring formula and not with a chill and cool formula.

The dosage must be adjusted to comply with the patient's condition and physical strength. Fever toxin (infection) is liable to reduce or diminish bodily fluids including saliva. Likewise, chilly and cool formulas may cause the harmful toxin to linger and are also delecterious to the stomach and spleen.

If repetitive treatment with fever-cleansing, fire-purging formulas does not bring about a remission of the fever, the condition is considered a conformation which Wang Ping described thusly: "If all efforts fail to lower the fever, it is due to a lack of water (dehydration)." The correct way of treating this kind of conformation is to nourish the yin and augment the water. As the yin is restored, the fever will decrease spontaneously.

Chai-Hu-Ching-Kan-Tang 柴胡清肝湯

(Bupleurum and Rehmannia Combination)

Trichosanthes root	1.5	Cnidium	1.5	Bupleurum	2.0
Phellodendron	1.5	Scute	1.5	Peony	1.5
Platycodon	1.5	Forsythia	1.5	Coptis	1.5
Tang-kuei	1.5	Licorice	1.5	Gardenia	1.5
Rehmannia	1.5	Mentha	1.5	Arctium	1.5

The original prescription was first recorded in *Wai k'o shu yao* (外科樞要) by Hsueh Chi of the Ming dynasty. Later this formula was modified by Itkando and Rohaku Mori. Afterwards the formula became a well-known medication for improving the physical condition. This formula is used for treating internal heat with a darkened skin, and tension and itching in the abdomen.

Herbs and Actions

A combination of *Szu-wu-tang* (*Tang-kuei* Four Combination) and *Huang-lien-chieh-tu-tang* (Coptis and Scute Combination) with Platycodon, Mentha, Arctium, and Trichosanthes root. *Huang-lien-chieh-tu-tang* dispels "strong fire" in the "triple warmers". *Szu-wu-tang* cools "blood heat" and nourishes "blood dryness". Platycodon is an antipyretic. Arctium nourishes the lungs, dispels internal heat, and acts as a detoxifier. Trichosanthes root is salivatory antipyretic, and anti-inflammative. Mentha soothes the *ch'i*.

Indications

Improvement of the physical condition, lymphadenitis, chronic tonsillitis, skin diseases, measles, and pleurisy.

Discrimination

Hsiao-chai-hu-tang (Minor Bupleurum Combination): infantile adenoids and thoraco-costal distress. This formula is also used

for tension in rectus abdominis muscle.
Hsiao-chien-chung-tang (Minor Cinnamon and Peony Combination): infantile adenoids, abdominal muscle tension, weak conformation.

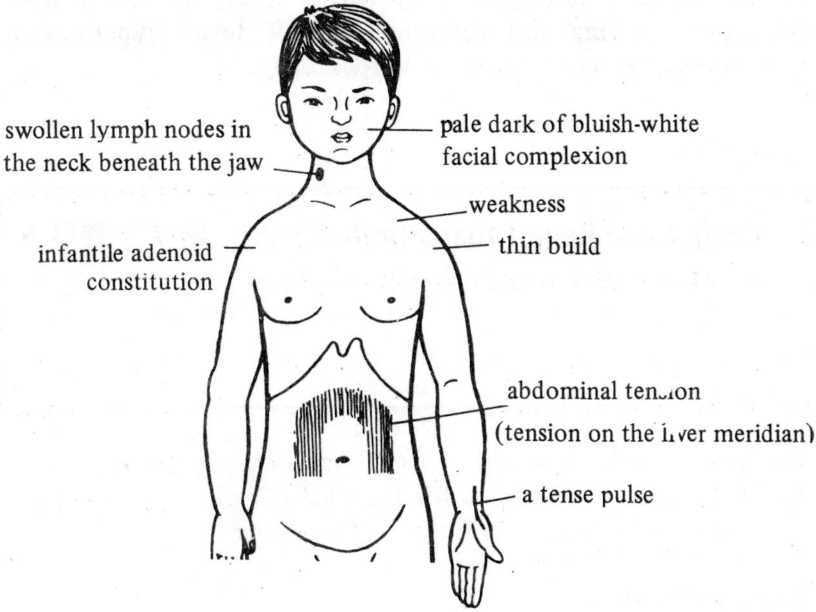

Chih-Tzu-Kan-Tsao-Shih-Tang 梔子甘草豉湯

(Gardenia, Licorice, and Soja Combination)

Gardenia	3.0	Soja	4.0	Licorice	2.0

Incorporates Licorice with *Chih-tzu-shih-tang* (梔子豉湯, Gardenia and Soja Combination). Used for the same conformation except somatic fever is present; also the symptoms, such as superficial respiration or severe pruritus, are more acute.

Herbs and Actions
Gardenia treats intense thoracic fever. Soja liberates thoracic air.

Licorice replenishes the spleen and aids free breathing.

Indications
Esophageal stenosis, insomnia, jaundice, glossitis inflammation of the tongue, laryngitis, pharyngitis, weakness and distress following sweating and vomiting, somatic fever, hypertension, neurasthenia, eczema, dry tinea, herpes, urticaria.

Chih-Tzu-Sheng-Chiang-Shih-Tang 梔子生薑豉湯

(Gardenia, Ginger, and Soja Combination)

Gardenia	3.0	Soja	4.0	Ginger	4.0

Prepared by adding Ginger to *Chih-tzu-shih-tang* (Gardenia and Soja Combination). Suitable for the *Chih-tzu-shih-tang* conformation with the additional symptom of vomiting.

Herbs and Actions
Gardenia has anti-inflammatory, hemostatic, and sedative effects. Soja is a sedative. Ginger is a stomachic and antiemetic.

Indications
See *Chih-tzu-shih-tang.*

Chih-Tzu-Shih-Tang 梔子豉湯

(Gardenia and Soja Combination)

Gardenia	3.0	Soja	4.0

Chih-tzu-shih-tang is recorded in *Shang han lun* (傷寒論) of the Han dynasty. This formula is used for treating stress, insomnia, chest distention, anorexia, sensation of fever, and reddening of the tongue with yellowish fur.

Herbs and Actions
Gardenia treats stress, fever in the chest, and acts as an anti-inflammative and sedative. Soja treats internal *ch'i* in the chest, dispels "weak heat" in the stomach, and also acts as a sedative.

Indications
Catarrhal jaundice, esophageal cancer, esophageal constriction, insomnia, stomatitis, pharyngitis, nervous exhaustion, hemoptysis, and fatigue after sweating or vomiting.

Discrimination
Suan-tsao-jen-tang (Zizyphus Combination): weak discomfort and insomnia, stagnant water in the stomach, flushing up.
Yin-chen-hao-tang (Capillaris Combination): chest discomfort, suppressed fever, jaundice.
San-huang-hsieh-hsin-tang (Coptis and Rhubarb Combination): insomnia, inflammation with severe congestion, firm fever symptoms.

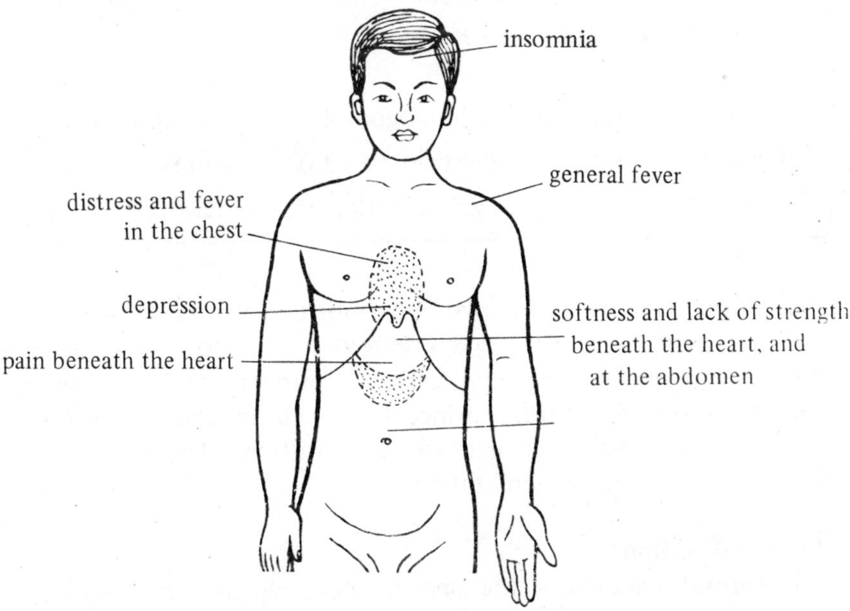

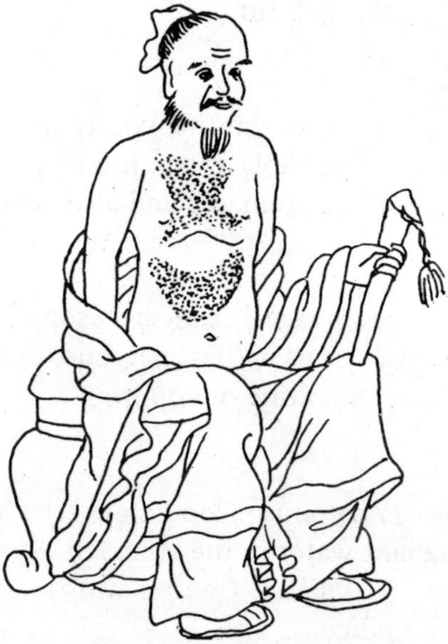

Ching-Hsin-Lien-Tzu-Yin 清心蓮子飲

(Lotus Seed Combination)

Lotus seed	4.0	Ophiopogon	4.0	Hoelen	4.0
Ginseng	3.0	Plantago	3.0	Scute	3.0
Astragalus	2.0	Lycium bark	2.0	Licorice	2.0

Ching-hsin-lien-tzu-yin was first mentioned in *Tai ping huei min ho chi chu fang* (太平惠民和劑局方). This formula is used for treating spleen, lung, and kidney disorders due to excessive drinking; polyuria; turbid urine; nocturnal emission; enuresis; blood-tinged leukorrhea; delicate constitution; diabetic neuropathy; anorexia; and general fatigue.

Herbs and Actions

This formula nourishes the spleen, stomach, and kidneys and

dispels "internal heat" in the heart and the lungs.
Ophiopogon and Lotus seed dispel "internal heat" in the heart and nourish the heart and blood. Plantago and Lycium bark remove "internal heat" from the kidneys and increase the flow of urine. Ginseng, Astragalus, Lycium fruit, Scute, and Ophiopogon remove "internal heat" from the lungs and nourish the kidneys. Ginseng, Hoelen, and Licorice nourish and invigorate the spleen and the stomach.

Indications
Renal calculi, tubercular kidneys, pyelitis, chronic gonorrhea, cystitis, leukorrhea, prostatitis, impotence, urinary retention, diabetes, and stomatitis.

Discrimination
Pa-wei-wan (Rehmannia Eight Formula): the sensation of residual urine, annoying fever in the soles of the feet and hands, no weakness of spleen and stomach.
Chu-ling-tang (Polyporus Combination): frequent urination, firm fever conformation, and red and turbid urine.

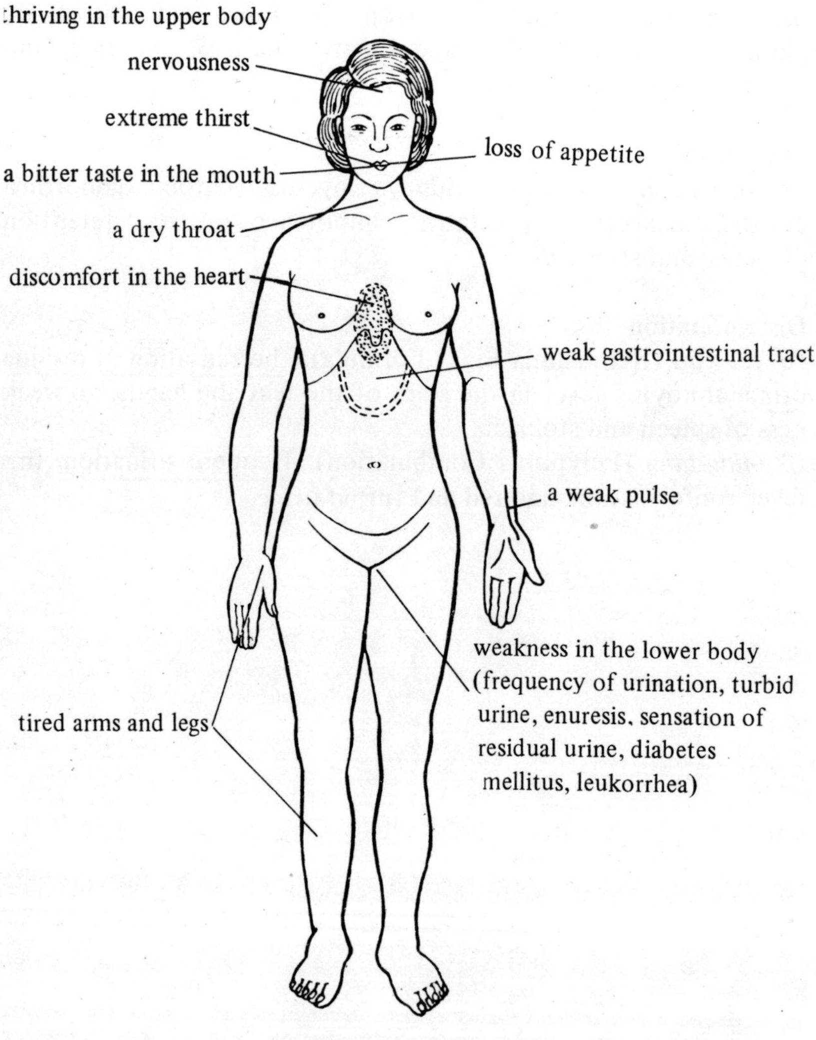
:hriving in the upper body
nervousness
extreme thirst
a bitter taste in the mouth
loss of appetite
a dry throat
discomfort in the heart
weak gastrointestinal tract
a weak pulse
weakness in the lower body (frequency of urination, turbid urine, enuresis, sensation of residual urine, diabetes mellitus, leukorrhea)
tired arms and legs

Ching-Je-Pu-Chi-Tang 清熱補氣湯

(Tang-kuei and Cimicifuga Combination)

Ginseng	3.0	*Tang-kuei*	3.0	Peony	3.0
Ophiopogon	3.0	Atractylodes	3.5	Hoelen	3.5
Figwort	2.0	Cimicifuga	0.5	Schizandra	1.0
Licorice	1.0				

Ching-je-pu-chi-tang is recorded in *Cheng chih chuen sheng* (證治準繩) of the Ming dynasty. This formula is used for treating those of weak conformation with chronic gastritis, lingual ulceration, and absent lingual papilla caused by weakness and fever in the stomach. These patients will also have a numb and aching tongue, weak or soft pulse and abdomen, distention beneath the heart, bitter taste in the mouth, and persistent thirst.

Herbs and Actions
Ginseng, Atractylodes, Hoelen, and Licorice [of *Szu-chun-tzu-tang* (Major Four Herb Combination)] nourish the spleen and stomach. *Tang-kuei* and Peony supplement anemic blood. Schizandra, Ophiopogon, and Figwort have the function of producing saliva and fluid. Cimicifuga can relieve the feeling of heat in the mouth.

Indications
Stomatitis or aphthous stomatitis and reddened tongue after a fever crisis; ulceration of a reddened tongue caused by weak *ch'i*, postpartum hemorrhage, or malignant carcinoma; numbness and loss of the sense of taste due to chronic gastritis.

Discrimination
Jen-sheng-tang (Ginseng and Ginger Combination): spleen weakness. This formula does not contain nourishing or lubricating components.
Pa-wei-wan (Rehmannia Eight Formula): treats stomatitis, no weakness of the spleen and stomach.

Liang-ke-san (Forsythia and Rhubarb Formula): stomatitis with firm fever conformation.

Weak fever of the spleen and stomach

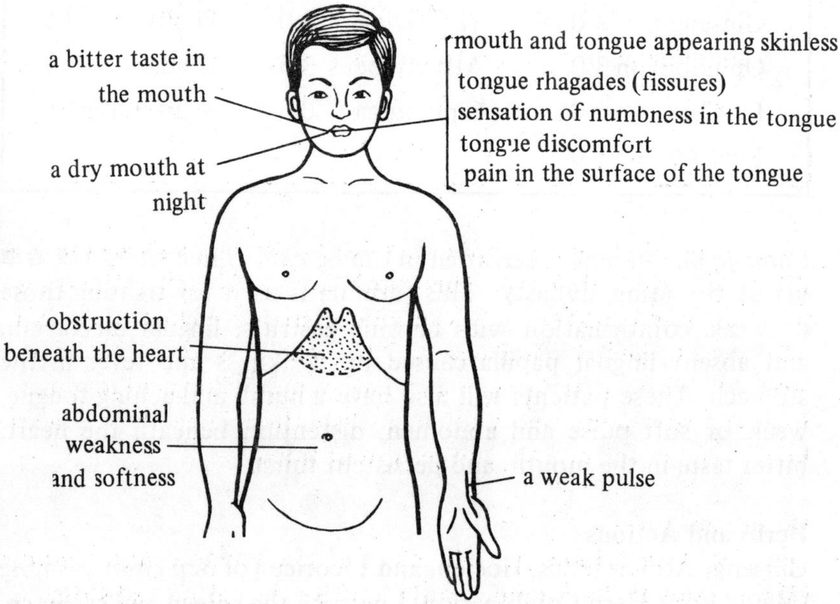

Ching-Wei-San 清胃散

(Coptis and Rehmannia Formula)

Tang-kuei	6.0	Coptis	1.0	Rehmannia	6.0
Moutan	6.0	Cimicifuga	1.0		

Ching-wei-san is recorded in *I fang chi chieh* (醫方集解) by Wang Ang of the Ching dynasty. This formula is used for treating internal heat in the stomach, "moist heat", gingivitis, stomatitis, facial redness with fever, swelling and pain in the gums, and pain in the throat.

Herbs and Actions
Coptis is antiphlogistic and antipyretic. *Tang-kuei* eases ulcerative pain. Gypsum is antipyretic and antiphlogistic. Rehmannia and Moutan dispel internal heat and cool the blood. Cimicifuga is a detoxifier and antipyretic.

Indications
Stomatitis, pain due to swelling in the throat, toothache, and ulceration of the gingiva.

Ching-Yen-Li-Ke-Tang 清咽利膈湯

(Arctium Combination)

Lonicera	3.0	Siler	4.5	Scute	4.5
Gardenia	2.0	Forsythia	2.0	Figwort	2.0
Mirabilitum	2.0	Arctium	2.0	Platycodon	4.5
Schizonepeta	4.5	Coptis	4.5	Rhubarb	2.0
Licorice	2.0	Mentha	4.5		

Ching-yen-li-ke-tang is recorded in *Cheng chih chuen sheng* (證治準繩) of the Ming dynasty. This formula is used for treating laryngeal swelling and pain, chest congestion, distention in the chest, constipation, anxiety, and an insistence on cold foods. It is effective for swelling of the throat and tongue and for excessive sputum and saliva.

Herbs and Actions
Siler, Schizonepeta, Platycodon, and Mentha are detoxifying agents. Coptis, Scute, and Gardenia are bitter and chill in nature, and they can dispel firm fever. Lonicera and Forsythia relieve swelling and disperse pus. Arctium is an antipyretic. Figwort is also an antipyretic. Licorice coordinates the actions of the other herbs. Rhubarb and Mirabilitum reduce fever and facilitate evacuation and micturition.

Indications
Laryngitis and tonsillitis.

Hsi-Chiao-Ti-Huang-Tang 犀角地黃湯

(Rhinoceros and Rehmannia Combination)

Rehmannia	8.0	Peony	3.0	Moutan	2.0
Rhinoceros horn	1.0				

Hsi-chiao-ti-huang-tang was recorded in the *Chien chin yao fang* (千金要方) by Sun Szu-miao during the Tang dynasty. This formula is used for treating "blood heat", hemoptysis, epistaxis, tarry stools, menorrhagia, febrile diseases, sensory disorders, body fever, reddening of the tongue, and a fast pulse. It has refrigerant and hemostatic properties and may be used to dispel "internal heat" and counteract poisons.

Herbs and Actions
Rhinoceros horn, the major component in this formula, is an antipyretic detoxifier, and refrigerant. Rehmannia nourishes the yin and acts as a refrigerant and hemostatic. Peony is an antipyretic. Moutan relieves "internal heat" in the blood, cools the blood, and dispels stagnant blood.

Indications
Hemorrhage due to "blood heat"; febrile infectious diseases with hemorrhage; measles; and mental illness.

Discrimination
San-huang-hsieh-hsin-tang (Coptis and Rhubarb Combination): nosebleeds, flushing up, mental instability, obstruction beneath the heart, constipation, facial flushing.

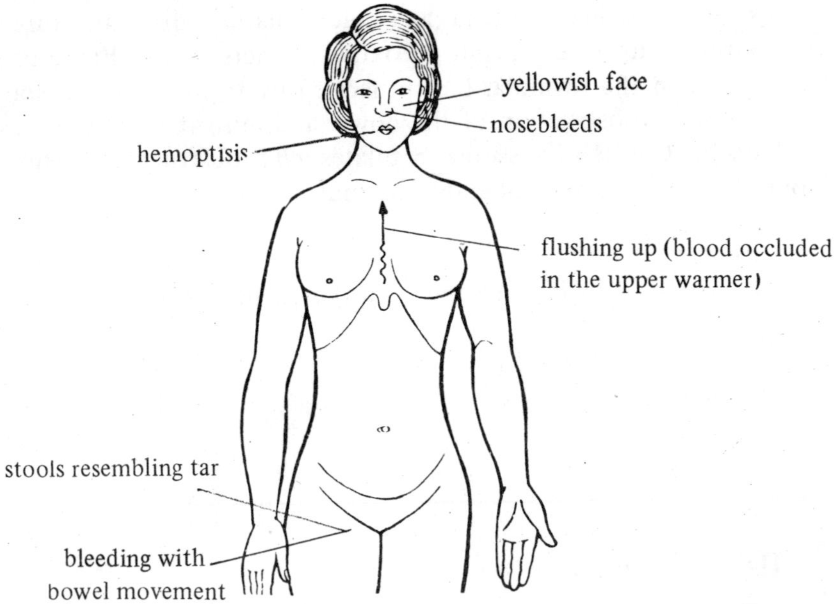

Hsiang-Lien-Wan 香連丸

(Saussurea and Coptis Formula)

Saussurea	3.0	Coptis	12.0

Recorded in *Tai ping huei min ho chi chu fang* (太平惠民和劑局方). Used for feverish diarrhea with the main indications being either red or white diarrhea–more white than red diarrhea–and tenesmus (the persistent desire to urinate or defecate).

Diarrhea generally is caused by irregular and abnormal eating and drinking, cold and heat, and "depressive steaming by moisture and heat." If the blood is harmed, the result is a white diarrhea. The conformation of this formula includes symptoms of simultaneous white and red diarrhea, malfunctioning in *ch'i* and blood, and tenesmus due to obstruction of *ch'i*.

Herbs and Actions

Coptis, which is bitter in taste and cold in nature, dries moisture and warms, purges fever, and detoxifies; it acts as the Emperor component in the formula. It is processed by frying with Evodia which relieves obstruction of the bowel and mitigates the potent coldness of Coptis. Saussurea regulates *ch'i* obstructed in the stomach and intestines and ends tenesmus.

Indications

Dysentery, red and white diarrhea, diarrhea, tenesmus.

Hsieh-Huang-San 瀉黃散

(Siler and Licorice Formula)

Siler	6.0	Licorice	3.0	Gardenia	7.0
Agastache	2.4	Gypsum	6.0		

Hsieh-huang-san is recorded in *Tang tou ko chueh* (湯頭歌訣). This formula is used for treating "moist heat" in the spleen and stomach, halitosis, stomatitis, thirst due to stress, and generalized fever.

Herbs and Actions

Siler is an antipyretic, antiphlogistic, and detoxifier. Agastache treats indigestion and the common cold.

Indications

Halitosis and stomatitis.

Hsieh-Pai-San 瀉白散

(Morus and Lycium Formula)

Morus	4.0	Lycium bark	4.0	Oryza	2.0
Licorice	2.0				

Recorded in *Hsiao erh yao cheng chih chueh* (小兒藥證直訣) by Chieh I of the Sung dynasty. Used for treating internal heat in the lungs, cough, mild asthma, a high fever in the afternoon, thirst, red tongue, and a fast pulse.

Herbs and Actions

Morus, the major herb in this formula, dispels internal heat in the lungs and relieves asthma with coughing. Lycium bark also dispels internal heat in the lungs. Licorice and Oryza nourish the stomach.

Indications

The common cold, a mild asthmatic cough, bronchitis, and the initial stage of tuberculosis.

Hsin-I-Ching-Fei-Tang 辛夷清肺湯

(Magnolia Flower and Gypsum Combination)

Magnolia flower	2.0	Eriobotrya	2.0	Gardenia	3.0
Anemarrhena	3.0	Lily	3.0	Scute	3.0
Cimicifuga	1.0	Ophiopogon	5.0	Gypsum	5.0

Hsin-i-ching-fei-tang was recorded in the *Wai k'o cheng tzung* (外科正宗) by Chen Shih-kung during the Ming dynasty. This formula is used for treating "internal heat" in the lungs, nasal polyps, nasal congestion, rhinitis, and sinusitus.

Herbs and Actions

Magnolia flower relieves nasal congestion. Cimicifuga is an antipyretic and detoxifier. Lily and Ophiopogon act as sialagogues and nourish the lungs. Eriobotrya is a refrigerant and stomachic that removes "internal heat" from the stomach. Scute and Gardenia are antipyretics and antiphlogistics. Gypsum and Anemarrhena are antipyretics and refrigerants which can dispel "strong heat".

Indications

Nasal congestion, rhinitis, and sinusitus.

Hsin-I-San 辛夷散

(Magnolia Flower Formula)

Magnolia flower	3.0	Angelica	3.0	Cimicifuga	3.0
Ko-pun	3.0	Siler	3.0	Cnidium	3.0
Asarum	3.0	Akebia	3.0	Licorice	3.0
Chianghuo	3.0				

Hsin-i-san is recorded in *Cheng chih chuen sheng* (證治準繩) and is effective for nasal disorders. This formula is used for treating nasal congestion, coryza, and anosmia.

Herbs and Actions

Magnolia flower, Cimicifuga, and Angelica increase vitality and nourish the brain. Siler, *Chianghuo, Ko-pun* dispel "internal moisture". Asarum dispels "internal heat" and increases vitality. Cnidium nourishes the liver. Akebia is an adjuvant. Licorice coordinates the actions of the other herbs.

Indications

Nasal congestion, rhinitis, coryza, sinusitis, and polyps.

Huang-Lien-Chieh-Tu-Tang 黃連解毒湯

(Coptis and Scute Combination)

Scute	3.0	Coptis	1.5	Gardenia	2.0
Phellodendron	1.5				

Huang-lien-chieh-tu-tang was recorded in the Chinese text, *Chou hou fang* (肘後方) by Ko Hung during the Chin dynasty(晉朝).

This formula is used for treating congestion, emotional instability, inflammation, anxiety, hematuria, hemorrhage, a sinking-strong pulse, and subcardiac distension and resistance.

Herbs and Actions

Coptis dispels "internal heat" in the heart, spleen, and stomach, and relieves distention beneath the heart and palpitations. Scute dispels "internal heat" in the lungs and intestines and reduces inflammation, congestion, hemoptysis, and bleeding. Phellodendron is a diuretic and astringent effective for "internal heat" in the kidneys and bladder. Gardenia is a sedative, hemostatic, and antiemetic.

Indications

Febrile diseases, hemoptysis, epistaxis, hematuria, blood diseases, anxiety, palpitations, insomnia, neurasthenia, hysteria, urticaria, pruritis, cerebral bleeding, and hypertension.

Discrimination

Hsiao-chai-hu-tang (Minor Bupleurum Combination): fever, alternating chills and fever, thoraco-costal distress.

Pai-hu-tang (Gypsum Combination): fever, generalized fever, burning sensation on the skin, extreme thirst, slippery and quick pulse.

Ta-cheng-chi-tang (Major Rhubarb Combination): fever, dry feces, and abdominal fullness.

Tzu-yin-chiang-huo-tang (Phellodendron Combination): fever, yin-weakness conformation, weak pulse.

San-huang-hsieh-hsin-tang (Coptis and Rhubarb Combination): hemorrhaging, facial flushing, flushing up, mental instability, obstruction beneath the heart, constipation.

Chiung-kuei-chiao-ai-tang (*Tang-kuei* and Gelatin Combination): hemorrhaging, pain in the lower abdomen, vertigo, anemia, abdominal laxity.

Huang-tu-tang (*Fu-lung-kan* Combination): hemorrhaging, anemia, annoying fever in the palms; submerged, thin pulse; weak conformation.

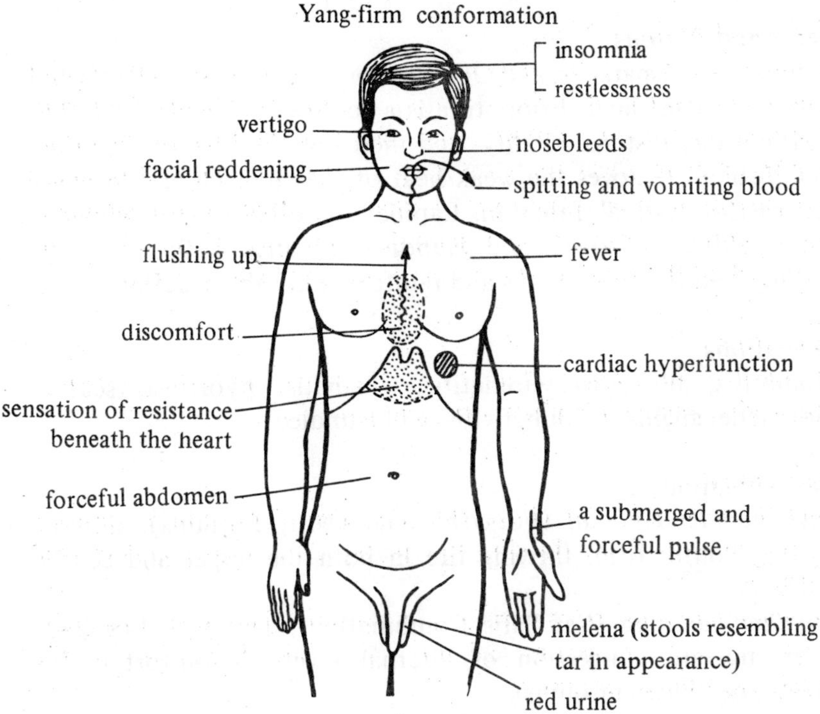

Kan-Lu-Yin *(Sweet Combination)*					甘露飲
Rehmannia	2.5	Ophiopogon	2.5	Asparagus	2.5
Eriobotrya	2.5	*Chih-shih*	2.5	Licorice	2.5
Capillaris	2.5	Dendrobium	2.5	Scute	2.5

Kan-lu-yin was first recorded in the governmental medical dictionary of the Sung dynasty, *Tai ping huei min ho chi chu fang* (A.D. 1107-1110). It has the effects of dispeling heat, moisture, and inflammation, and of purifying the flood. This formula is suitable for moist heat with stagnant blood in the digestive system, for suppuration and swelling in the tongue, gingiva, and throat, and for blepharitis, jaundice, mild edema, fever, constipation, and dysuria.

Herbs and Actions

Rehmannia, Asparagus, and Ophiopogon have nutritive effects and relieve stagnant heat. Eriobotrya is a cooling stomachic. *Chih-shih* is stomachic, restores vitality, and increases the flow of the urine. Dendrobium removes the weak heat of the stomach and balances the gastrointestinal function. Capillaris is effective for jaundice. Scute cures carbuncle and jaundice. Licorice harmonizes the action of all the other herbs and reinforces the above actions.

Indications

Stomatitis, ulcerative stomatitis, gingivitis, pyorrhea, scurvy, toothache, angina, conjunctivitis, and jaundice.

Discrimination

Chia-chien-liang-ke-san (Forsythia and Peony Formula): diseases of the mouth; firm, thriving fire in both the upper and central warmers.

Yin-chen-hao-tang (Capillaris Combination): jaundice, low-grade fever, upward congestion of internal fever, discomfort in the chest, uneasiness, insomnia.

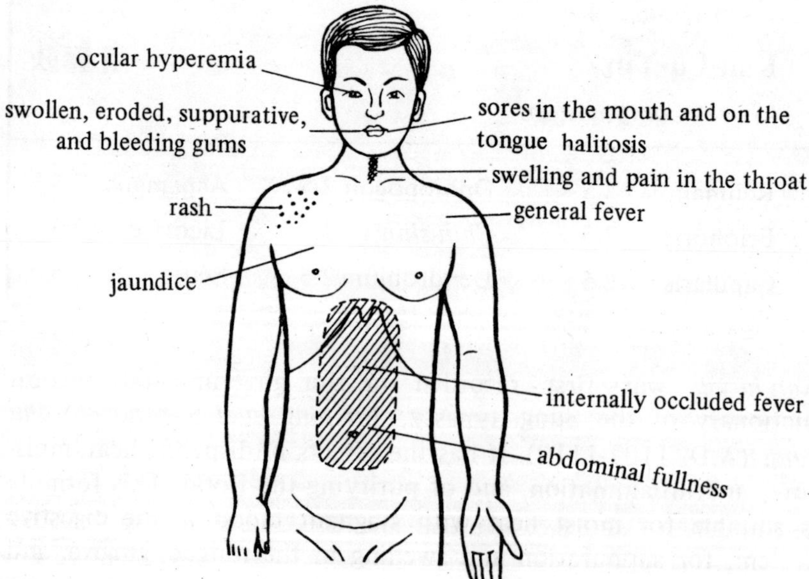

Kuei-Chih-Wu-Wu-Tang 桂枝五物湯

(*Cinnamon Five Herb Combination*)

Cinnamon	4.0	Scute	4.0	Platycodon	3.0
Rehmannia	4.0	Hoelen	8.0		

Kuei-chih-wu-wu-tang was recorded in the Japanese medical text, *Han feng hou shih yao fang chieh so*(漢方後世要方解說). This formula is used for treating toothache, stomatitis, and swelling and pain due to ulcers in the mouth or on the tongue.

Herbs and Actions

Cinnamon is effective for flushing up and improving blood circulation. Platycodon is used to treat suppuration and swelling and to ease pain in the throat and toothache. Scute relieves "moist heat" and heals ulceration. Rehmannia dispels stagnant blood and relieves "internal heat". Hoelen nourishes the spleen, dispels "internal moisture", and removes "water poisoning."

Indications

Toothache, gingivitis, pyorrhea, and stomatitis.

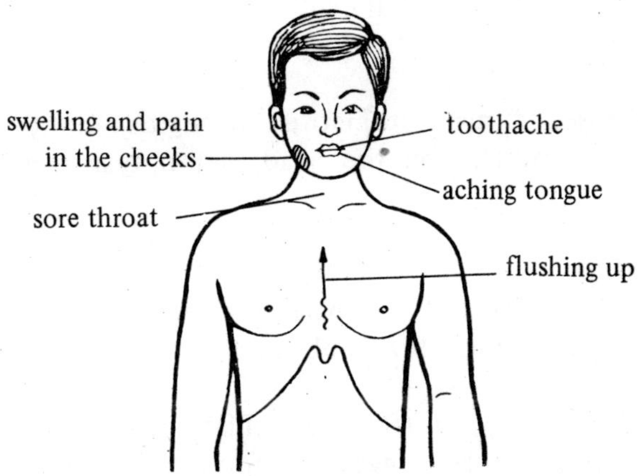

Liang-Ke-San 涼膈散

(Forsythia and Rhubarb Formula)

Forsythia	3.0	Rhubarb	4.5	Scute	3.0
Mirabilitum	3.0	Licorice	2.5	Gardenia	3.0
Bamboo leaves	2.0	Mentha	2.5		

Liang-ke-san is recorded in *Tai ping huei min ho chi chu fang* (太平惠民和劑局方) of the Sung dynasty. This formula is used for treating stagnant heat, stress, thirst, ulceration of the mouth, suppuration of the lips, swelling pain in the throat, ophthalmia, hemoptysis, epistaxis, spasms due to severe heat in the stomach, psychosis, insomnia, and constipation. This formula is effective for treating internal and external heat with constipation, inflammation, and congestion.

Herbs and Actions

Forsythia, Scute, Bamboo leaves, and Mentha dispel internal heat in the upper body. Rhubarb, Mirabilitum, and Gardenia dispel internal heat in the chest. Licorice coordinates the actions of the other herbs, and dispels "heat evil" in the chest.

Indications

Febrile diseases, thrush, stomatitis, laryngitis, diphtheria, tetter on the lips, furuncles on the head, hemoptysis, epistaxis, and gingivitis.

Discrimination

Ta-cheng-chi-tang (Major Rhubarb Combination): constipation, delirium, anxiety, high fever, abdominal hardness and fullness, and dry stools.

Fang-feng-tung-sheng-san (Siler and Platycodon Formula): constipation, inflammatory congestion, food and water toxin, obese and apoplectic constitution.

Lung-Tan-Hsieh-Kan-Tang 龍膽瀉肝湯

(Gentiana Combination)

Gentiana	1.0	Alisma	3.0	Akebia	5.0
Plantago	3.0	*Tang-kuei*	5.0	Rehmannia	5.0
Gardenia	1.0	Scute	3.0	Licorice	1.0

Lung-tan-hsieh-kan-tang is recorded in a Chinese medical work, *Hsùeh-shih i an*, by Hsueh Chi of the Ming dynasty. This formula cures patients with symptoms of pain in the armpits, deafness, swollen ears, blood in the urine, gonorrhea, swelling and itching in the genital areas, leukorrhea, yellow coated tongue, strong pulse, and redness in the mouth, tongue, and eyes.

Herbs and Actions

Gentiana relieves the internal heat of the liver and gallbladder. Bupleurum removes the stagnant internal heat of the liver. Alisma, Akebia, and Plantago increase the flow of urine and reduce inflammation of the urethra and bladder. *Tang-kuei* and Rehmannia nourish the blood and check pain. Gardenia, Scute, and Gentiana are anti-inflammatives and detoxifiers. Licorice coordinates the actions of the other herbs.

Indications

Urethritis, cystitis, endometritis, inflammation of the vagina, leukorrhea, itching and pain in the genital areas, venereal ulcer, groin lymphadenitis, orchitis, and eczema at the genital areas.

Note: This formula should not be given to patients having a delicate constitution and weak conformation.

Discrimination

Ching-hsin-lien-tzu-yin (Lotus Seed Combination): urological diseases, thriving upper body and weak lower body, degenerated vitality.

Chu-ling-tang (Polyporus Combination): occluded fever in the lower warmer, urethritis, stagnant water in the stomach, edema, irritability.

Firm conformation

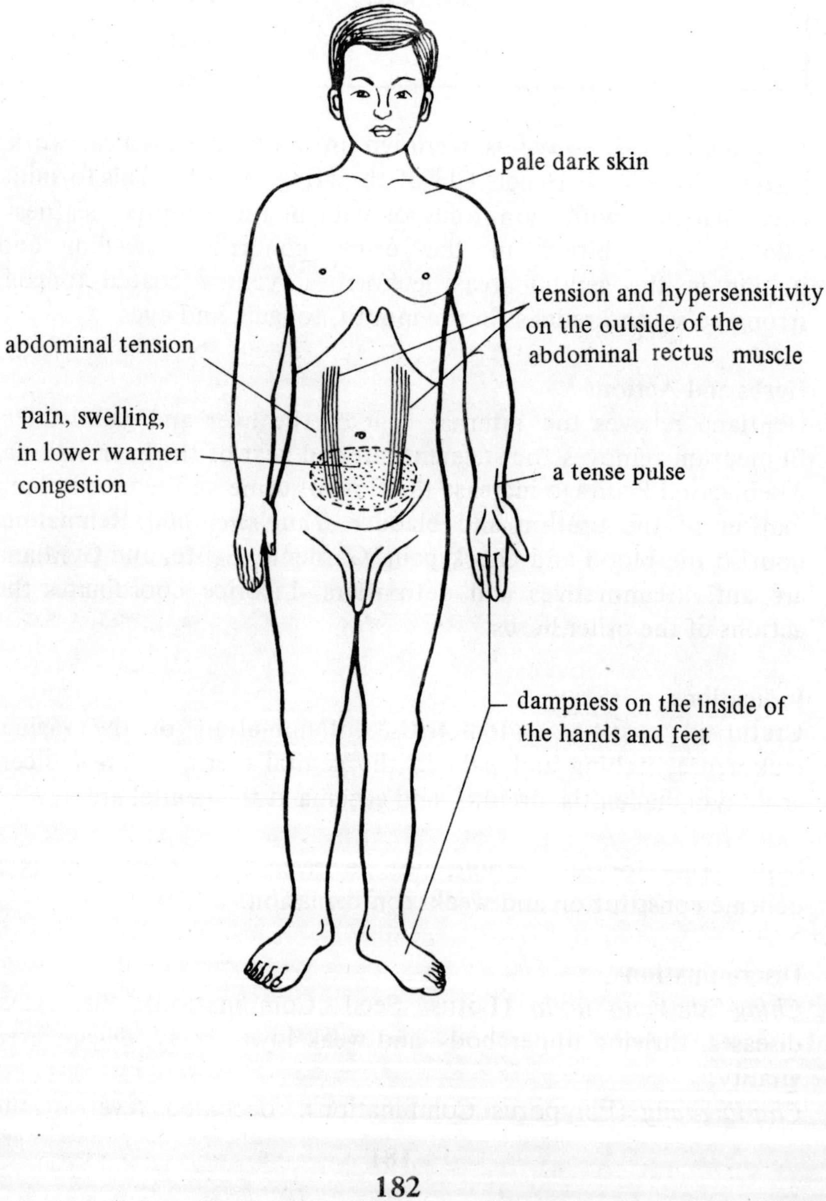

Pai-Hu-Chia-Jen-Sheng-Tang 白虎加人參湯

(Ginseng and Gypsum Combination)

Gypsum	15.0	Anemarrhena	5.0	Oryza	10.0
Licorice	2.0	Ginseng	3.0		

Pai-hu-chia-jen-sheng-tang was recorded in both the *Shang han lun* (傷寒論) and the *Chin kuei yao lueh* (金匱要略) by Chang Chung-ching during the Han dynasty. This formula is used when there is severe thirst, aptyalism, fever, severe chills, and fatigue.

Herbs and Actions

Anemarrhena dispels "internal heat". Gypsum is a sedative which also dispels heat. Oryza is a tonic that relieves chills. Licorice is an adjuvant to Oryza. Ginseng is a tonic.

Indications

Influenza, pneumonia, cerebritis, heatstroke with high fever and thirst, diabetes, cerebral bleeding, Basedow's disease, dermatitis, urticaria, eczema, pruritus, congestion in an area of infection, nephritis, uremia, cholecystitis, and nocturnal enuresis.

Discrimination

Pai-hu-tang (Gypsum Combination): thirst, high fever, and mild fluid deficiency.
Wu-ling-san (Hoelen Five Herb Formula): thirst, decreased urine, adverse congestion of fluid, a splashing sound beneath the heart.
Pa-wei-ti-huang-wan (Rehmannia Eight Formula): thirst, decreased urine or excessive urine, numbness in the lower abdomen, submerged and chordal pulse.

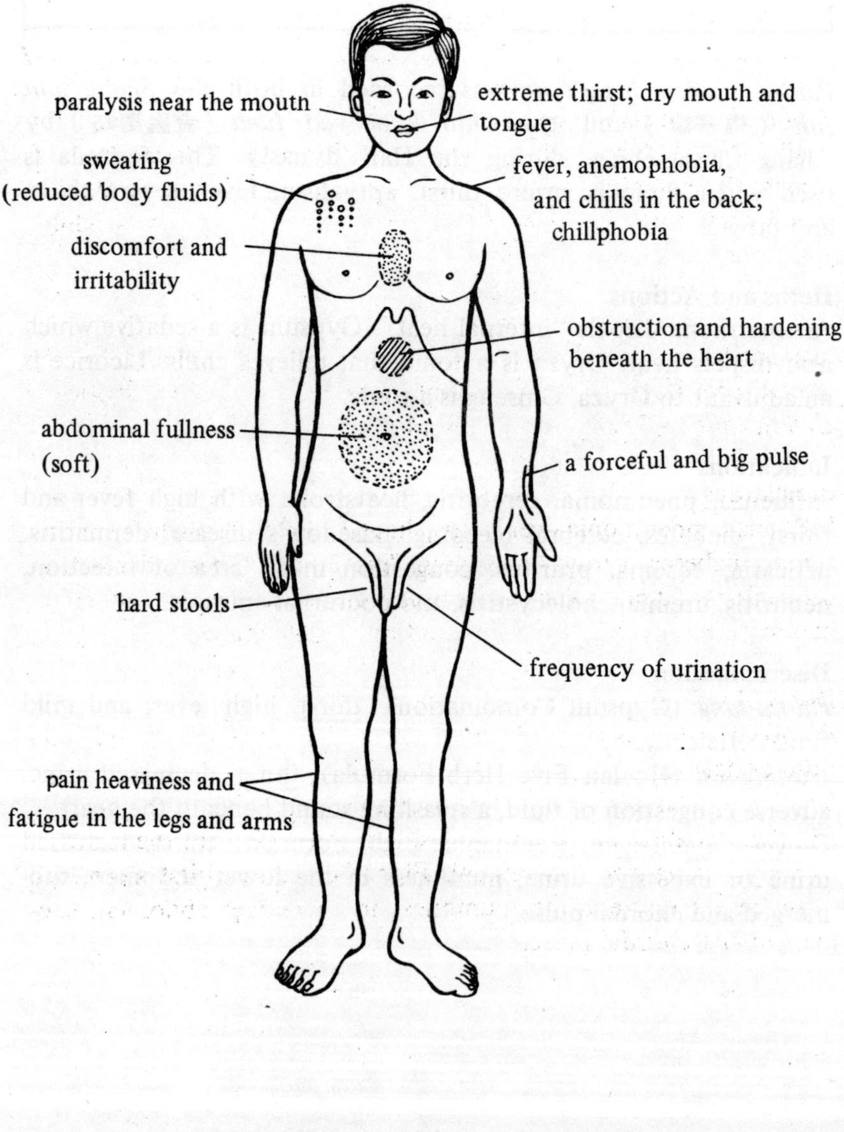
paralysis near the mouth
extreme thirst; dry mouth and tongue
sweating (reduced body fluids)
fever, anemophobia, and chills in the back; chillphobia
discomfort and irritability
obstruction and hardening beneath the heart
abdominal fullness (soft)
a forceful and big pulse
hard stools
frequency of urination
pain heaviness and fatigue in the legs and arms

Pai-Hu-Tang 白虎湯

(Gypsum Combination)

Gypsum	15.0	Anemarrhena	5.0	Licorice	2.0
Oryza	8.0				

Pai-hu-tang was recorded in the *Shang han lun* (傷寒論) during the Han dynasty. This formula is used for treating high fever and sweating with a flushed face, thirst due to stress, white coating on the tongue, and polyuria. Those with severe chills, pallor, and fever, but no sweating or thirst due to stress should not take this formula.

Herbs and Actions
Gypsum and Anemarrhena both are refrigerants and antipyretics used to dispel "internal" and "external heat". Licorice and Oryza coordinate the actions of the other herbs.

Indications
Common cold, influenza, measles, erysipelas, scarlet fever, typhoid fever and meningitis with high fever, thirst, and anxiety, diabetes, emotional disorders, eczema, and pruritus.

Discrimination
Ta-cheng-chi-tang (Major Rhubarb Combination): fever, abdominal fullness, dry stools, submerged and firm pulse.
Ta-ching-lung-tang (Major Blue Dragon Combination): fever, anxiety, no sweating, generalized pain, external firm conformation, floating and tense pulse.
Wu-ling-san (Hoelen Five Herb Formula): extreme thirst, decreased urine, splashing sound beneath the heart, adverse congestion of water.
Pa-wei-wan (Rehmannia Eight Formula): extreme thirst, decreased urine, numbness beneath the umbilicus, submerged and chordal pulse.

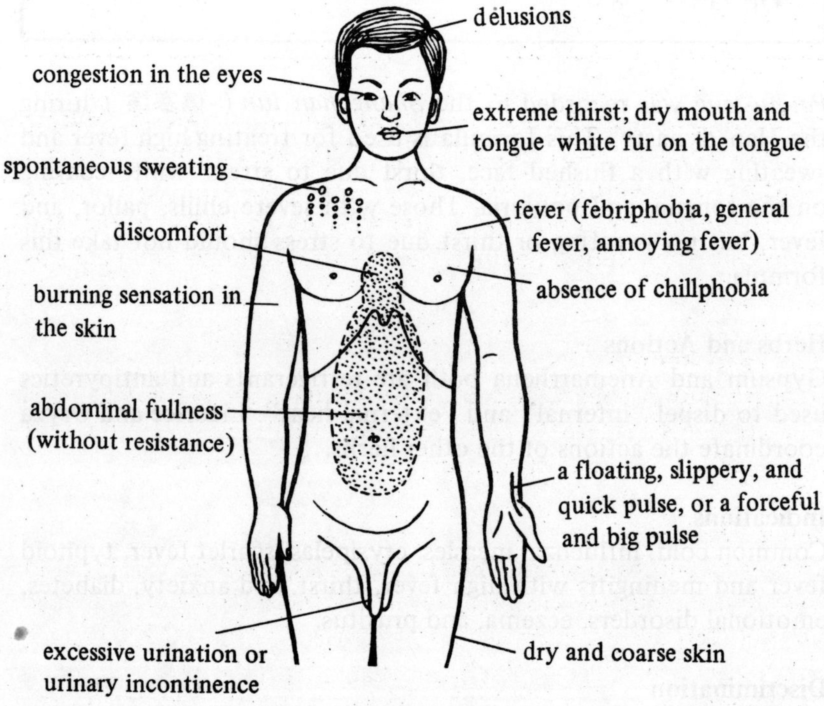
delusions
congestion in the eyes
extreme thirst; dry mouth and tongue white fur on the tongue
spontaneous sweating
fever (febriphobia, general fever, annoying fever)
discomfort
absence of chillphobia
burning sensation in the skin
abdominal fullness (without resistance)
a floating, slippery, and quick pulse, or a forceful and big pulse
excessive urination or urinary incontinence
dry and coarse skin

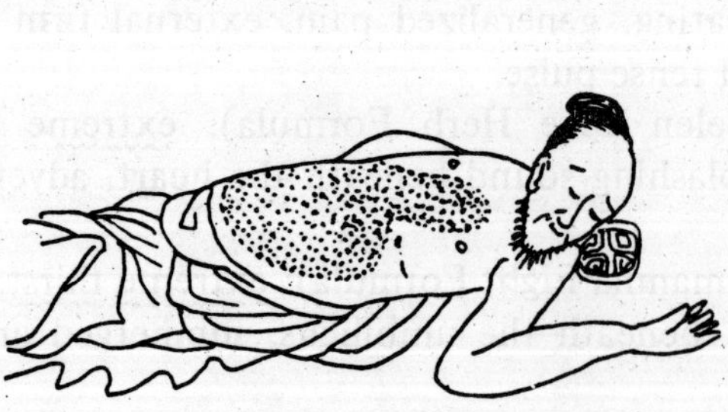

Pai-Tou-Weng-Tang 白頭翁湯

(Anemone Combination)

Anemone	3.0	Coptis	3.0	Fraxinus	3.0
Phellodendron	3.0				

Pai-tou-weng-tang is recorded in *Shang han lun* (傷寒論) of the Han dynasty. This formula is used for treating diarrhea due to internal heat, stools mixed with pus and blood, abdominal pain, thirst, and enteritis.

Herbs and Actions

Anemone dispels "moist heat" in the blood and arrests diarrhea due to "internal heat". Coptis removes "internal heat" and eliminates thirst. Phellodendron also removes "internal heat." Fraxinus is bitter in nature, dispels "moist heat", and arrests diarrhea.

Indications

Febrile diarrhea, acute enteritis, postpartum enteritis, and stools mixed with blood and pus.

Discrimination

Tao-hua-tang (Kaolin and Oryza Combination): diarrhea, abdominal pain, abdominal weakness and fullness, physical weakness, no tenesmus, weak conformation.

Kan-tsao-hsieh-hsin-tang (Pinellia and Licorice Combination): diarrhea, irritability, obstruction and hardness beneath the heart, gas, dry vomiting, and uneasiness.

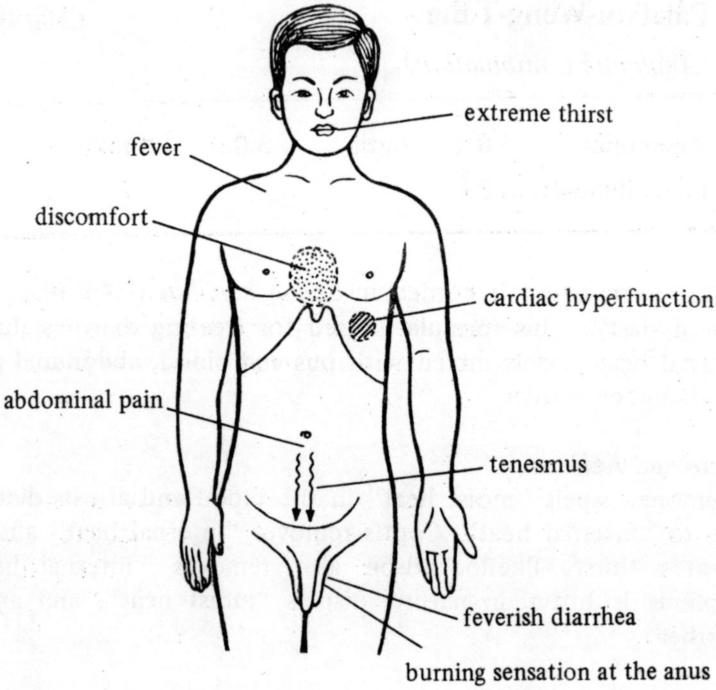

Pai-Tu-San 敗毒散

(Rehmannia and Lonicera Formula)

Rehmannia	4.5	Platycodon	2.5	Forsythia	2.5
Arctium	2.5	Figwort	2.5	Gypsum	3.0
Trichosanthes	2.5	Lonicera	2.5	Moutan	2.0
Bupleurum	2.0	Mentha	1.5	Licorice	1.0
Phellodendron	1.5	Peony	1.5		

Pai-tu-san is recorded in *Yang i ta chuan* (瘍醫大全) of the Ching dynasty. This formula has the function of cooling the lungs and stomach, thereby reducing fever. It is used for treating post-eruption halitosis, stomatitis, perleche, and pain in the throat.

Herbs and Actions

Rehmannia nourishes the body and can lower a resistent fever. Forsythia, Platycodon, Trichosanthes, Peony, and Lonicera are antiphlogistics which purify the blood and reduce swelling. Figwort dispels the feverish feeling in the mouth or throat. Bupleurum eliminates liver fever. Moutan clears the blood fever. Arctium and Mentha dispel wind and fever on the upper torso. Phellodendron is an antiphlogistic, bactericide, and stomachic. Gypsum can expel internal fever. Licorice coordinates the actions of the other herbs.

Indications

Stomatitis, ulcerative stomatitis, halitosis, glossitis, and laryngitis.

Pu-Chi-Hsiao-Tu-Yin 普濟消毒飲

(Scute and Cimicifuga Combination)

Scute	9.0	Coptis	6.0	Isatis	12.0
Forsythia	12.0	Arctium	9.0	Figwort	9.0
Licorice	3.0	Platycodon	3.0	Cimicifuga	2.4
Bupleurum	6.0	Lasiosphaera	3.0	Citrus	3.0
Mentha	4.5	Silkworm	6.0		

Pu-chi-hsiao-tu-yin was recorded in the *I fang chi chieh* (醫方集解) during the Ching dynasty. This formula is used for treating severe chills, fever, facial edema, thirst, restlessness, swelling and pain in the throat, and a floating-strong pulse.

Herbs and Actions

Coptis, Scute, Isatis, Cimicifuga, Forsythia, Licorice, and Lasiosphaera are antipyretics, antiphlogistics, and detoxifiers. Mentha, Arctium, Silkworm, and Bupleurum alleviate discomforts due to cold. Figwort nourishes the yin and dispels "internal heat". Citrus dispels stagnant *ch'i*. Platycodon dispels "internal heat in the triple warmers".

Indications
Erysipelas, mumps, and carbuncles.

San-Huang-Hsieh-Hsin-Tang 三黃瀉心湯

(Coptis and Rhubarb Combination)

Rhubarb	1.0	Scute	1.0	Coptis	1.0

San-huang-hsieh-hsin-tang has been an important decoction highly recommended by Chinese physicians since it was first recorded in an ancient Chinese medical work *Chin kuei yao lueh* (Summaries of Household Drugs, A.D. 205) of the Han dynasty.

Herbs and Actions
All three herbs of this formula are bitter antiphlogistics and laxatives. Rhubarb contains various anthraquinone derivatives and emodins and a special tannin. Scute contains wogonin, baicalin, etc. Coptis contains berberine, worenine, coptisine, etc. Their combined pharmacology facilitates bile secretion and bowel evacuation, produces sedation, and is anti-inflammative. When used clinically, it produces nearly miraculous effects due to the synergy of the Chinese formula, a concept that is difficult to explain in modern pharmacological terms.

Indications
Congestion, regurgitation, anxiety, shoulder stiffness, stomach distention, and constipation.
In modern medicine, the formula may be used for:
1. Habitual constipation . . . improvement of bile secretion will promote smooth defecation.
2. Gastritis, peptic ulcer, and gastrorrhagia.
3. Flushed faces, white-coated tongue, anxiety, mental instability, insomnia, shoulder stiffness, ophthalmia, and tinnitus aurium.

4. Prevention of and recuperation from hypertension, arteriosclerosis, liver disorders, and apoplexy.
5. Hemorrhoids, hemorrhoidal bleeding, and flushed faces.

Discrimination

Ta-huang-huang-lien-hsieh-hsin-tang (Rhubarb Combination): palpitations of the heart; this formula is for mild inflammation and congestion.
Huang-tu-tang (*Fu-lung-kan* Combination): hemorrhaging, irritability, weak conformation, anemia.
Chih-tzu-shih-tang (Gardenia and Soja Combination): discomfort and fever in the heart, insomnia, yang and weak conformation, mild irritability.
Chih-kan-tsao-tang (Baked Licorice Combination): irritability and insomnia, yang and weak conformation, lax and dry abdomen.
Suan-tsao-jen-tang (Zizyphus Combination): irritation and discomfort in the chest, insomnia, weak conformation, lassitude.

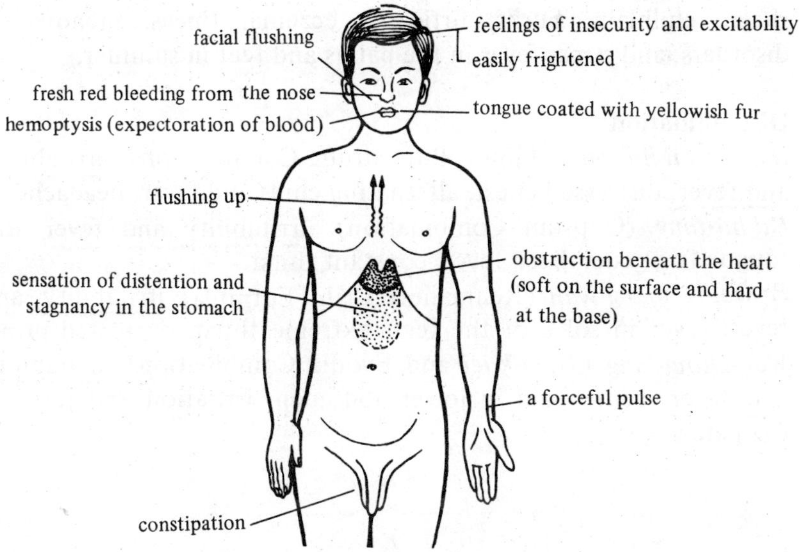

San-Wu-Huang-Chin-Tang 三物黃芩湯

(Scute Three Herb Combination)

Scute	3.0	Sophora	3.0	Rehmannia	6.0

San-wu-huang-chin-tang is recorded in *Chin kuei yao lueh* (金匱要略) of the Han dynasty. This formula is used for treating postpartum fever, stress fever, fatigue, dry tongue, and stress heat in the palms and feet.

Herbs and Actions

Scute is an antipyretic, antiphlogistic, and stomachic. Sophora is a diuretic, antipyretic, and vermifuge. Rehmannia nourishes the blood and removes "blood heat".

Indications

Postpartum fever, tuberculosis, insomnia, autonomic nerve disorders, stomatitis, hemorrhage during childbirth, hemoptysis, hemorrhage, chilblain, burns, urticaria, eczema, tineas, menopausal disorders, and stress fever in the palms and feet in summer.

Discrimination

Hsiao-chai-hu-tang (Minor Bupleurum Combination): irritability and fever, distressed chest, alternating chills and fever, headache.
Pai-hu-tang (Gypsum Combination): irritability and fever, dry tougue fur, generalized fever, constant thirst.
Pa-wei-ti-huang-wan (Rehmannia Eight Formula): irritability and fever; fever in soles of the feet, extreme thirst, decreased urine.
Wen-ching-tang (*Tang-kuei* and Evodia Combination): irritability and fever, acute pain in lower abdomen, irritation and fever in the palms.

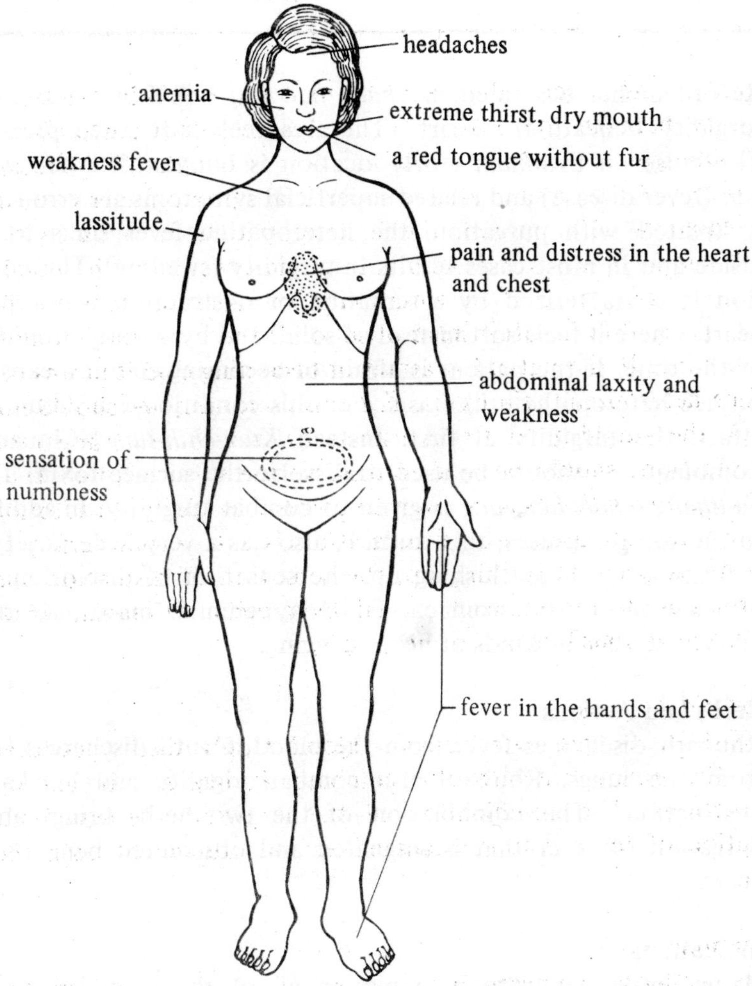
headaches
anemia
extreme thirst, dry mouth
a red tongue without fur
weakness fever
lassitude
pain and distress in the heart and chest
abdominal laxity and weakness
sensation of numbness
fever in the hands and feet

Ta-Huang-Huang-Lien-Hsieh-Hsin-Tang
大黃黃連瀉心湯

(Rhubarb Combination)

Rhubarb	2.0	Coptis	1.0

Recorded and described in *Shang han lun* (傷寒論): "It treats turgidity beneath the heart. (The area feels soft when pressed.) The pulse on the *kuan* (fort) location is buoyant." When *shang han* (fever disease) and related superficial symptoms are erroneously treated with purgation, the heteropathic fever sinks to the inside and in most cases results in turgidity (swelling). This condition is characterized by a sensation of obstruction beneath the heart, where it feels soft instead of solid, and by constipation most of the time. If the patient is afraid of becoming cold it means the surface heteropathy still exists. For this condition one should not attack the turgidity at first. Instead *Kuei-chih-tang* (Cinnamon Combination) should be used to dissolve the surface toxin. Then *Ta-huang-huang-lien-tang* is given to combat turgidity. In addition to the foregoing uses, this formula also has a very wide variety of indications such as flushing up, the sensation of distention and obstruction in the stomach, facial hyperemia, insomnia, irritability, and various kinds of hemorrhaging.

Herbs and Actions

Rhubarb discharges fever from the blood; Coptis discharges fever from the lungs. Rhubarb also combats rigidity and breaks up obstructions. The combination of the two herbs brings about purgation of fever that is stagnated and obstructed beneath the heart.

Indications

Mania, epilepsy, amnesia, coma; in all of these conditions the patient has a ruddy face and subcardiac obstruction and turgidity. Subcardiac turgidity with nosebleeds, the coughing up of blood, vomiting of blood, and bloody stools. Apopletic coma, unconsciousness, palpitations, and cardiac hyperfunction.

Discrimination

Hsieh-hsin-tang (Coptis and Rhubarb Combination) is for most bleeding conditions with a firm conformation, subcardiac tension, and flushing up.

Huang-tu-tang (*Fu-lung-kan* Combination) is for heart problems, hemorrhage, and anemia in a person with a weak conformation.

Chih-tzu-shih-tang (Gardenia and Soja Combination) is for fever in the heart, insomnia, a yang-weakness conformation, and distressing weakness.

Chih-kan-tsao-tang (Baked Licorice Combination) is for cardiac problems, insomnia, yang-weakness conformations, and soft and dry abdomens.

Suan-tsao-jen-tang (Zizyphus Combination) is for discomfort and irritation in the chest, insomnia, a weak conformation, and fatigue.

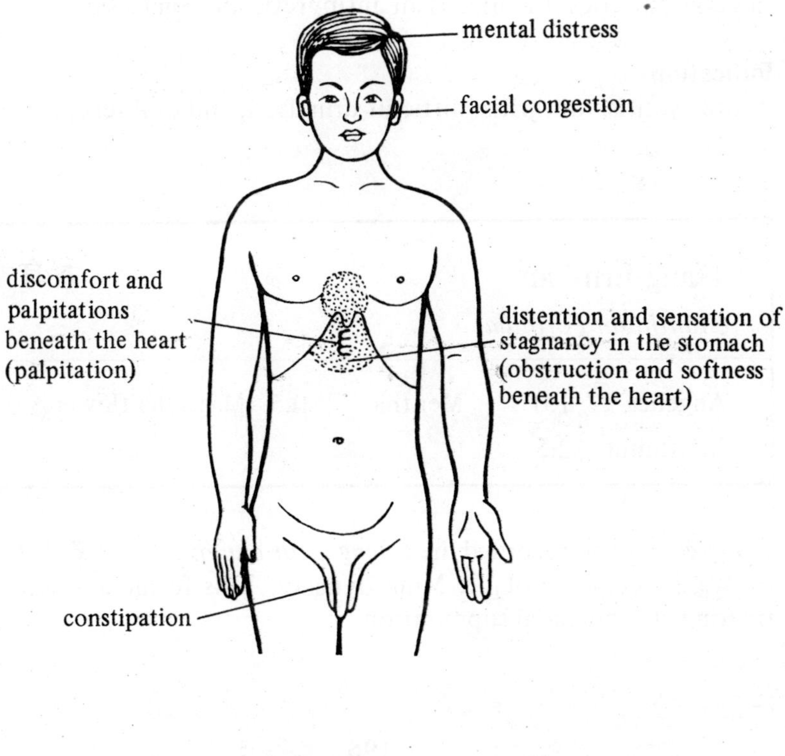

Tao-Chih-San 導赤散

(Rehmannia and Akebia Formula)

Rehmannia	15.0	Akebia	3.0	Lophatherum	3.0
Licorice	3.0				

Tao-chih-san, a good formula for relieving heat in the small intestine and heart, is recorded in *Hsiao erh yao cheng chih chueh* (小兒藥證直訣) of the Sung dynasty. This formula is suitable for fatigue, flushed face, thirst, yellowish urine, ardor urine, and tetters on the tongue or in the mouth.

Herbs and Actions
Rehmannia, the main drug, acts as an antipyretic and nourishes the blood and the kidneys. Lophatherum and Akebia are antipyretics and diuretics. Licorice is an antipyretic and analgesic.

Indications
Acute cystitis, urethritis, difficult urination, and oral tetters.

Tsang-Erh-San 蒼耳散

(Xanthium Formula)

Angelica	1.0	Mentha	0.5	Magnolia flower	5.0
Xanthium	2.5				

Tsang-erh-san is recorded in *Cheng chih chuen sheng* (證治準繩) by Wang Ken-tang of the Ming dynasty. This formula is used for treating chronic nasal suppuration.

Herbs and Actions:
Angelica can relieve the discomfort of rheumatism. Magnolia flower removes internal stomach heat. Xanthium removes internal moisture. Mentha dispels internal heat in the liver and lungs.

Indications
Nasal suppuration and chronic rhinitis.

Tsing-Fu-Tang 淨腑湯

(Bupleurum and Pinellia Combination)

Bupleurum	3.0	Pinellia	2.0	Hoelen	3.0
Alisma	1.5	Atractylodes	2.0	Scirpus	1.5
Zedoaria	1.5	Crataegus	1.5	Ginseng	1.5
Coptis	1.0	Polyporus	1.5	Scute	1.5
Ginger	1.0	Jujube	1.0	Licorice	1.0

Tsing-fu-tang, a modified combination of *Chai-ling-tang* (Bupleurum and Hoelen Combination), is recorded in *Wan ping hui chun* (萬病回春) of the Ming dynasty. This formula is used for treating hard tumors in children who also exhibit abdominal tension. Typically, these occur in the initial stage of tubercular peritonitis when the rigid, firm, and tight subcardiac and abdominal tenseness appears to coalesce into a hard mass (a combination of the intestines and the abdominal wall). It is suitable for children's tabes mesentericus (the initial stage of the mesenteric tubercles of tuberculous origin), abdominal distention, recurrent chills and fever, retained hematuria, and thirst. This formula is also suitable for adults.

Herbs and Actions
Tsing-fu-tang is a combination of *Hsiao-chai-hu-tang* (Minor Bupleurum Combination), *Wu-ling-san* (Hoelen Five Herb Formula), *po-ch'i-chi* (Carminatives), and *chien-wei-hsiao-hua-ch*

(Stomachic and Digestive Agents). *Hsiao-chai-hu-tang* treats chest distress, subcardiac distention, and recurrent chills and fever. *Wu-ling-san* treats thirst, retained hematuria, and watery stool. Scirpus and Zedoaria disintegrate tumors and relieve hardness and coalescence in the abdomen. Hawthorn and Coptis are digestives and antiphlogistics which move the stagnant foods and reduce the fever.

Indications
Tuberculous peritonitis, mesenteric tubercles of tuberculous origin, indigestion, tabes mesenteria, epilepsy, adenopathic physique, and high fever of unknown origin in children.

Discrimination
Hsiao-chai-hu-tang (Minor Bupleurum Combination): thoraco-costal distress, bitter taste in mouth, white fur, and vomiting.
Chai-hu-chiang-kuei-tang (Bupleurum, Cinnamon, and Ginger Combination): treats thoraco-costal distress, extreme thirst, cardiac hyperfunction, head sweating, a weak conformation.

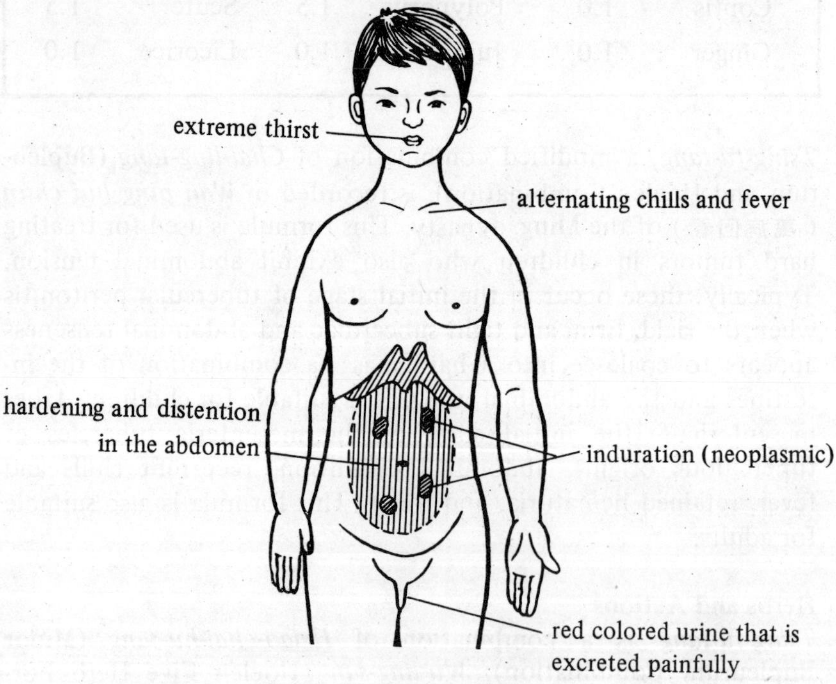

Tzu-Yin-Chiang-Huo-Tang 滋陰降火湯
(Phellodendron Combination)

Tang-kuei	2.5	Peony	2.5	Rehmannia	2.5
Asparagus	2.5	Ophiopogon	2.5	Citrus	2.5
Atractylodes	3.0	Anemarrhena	1.5	Licorice	1.5
Phellodendron	1.5				

Recorded in *Wan ping hui chun* (萬病回春). Used for treating fevers, coughing, viscid sputum, asthma, night sweats, dry mouth, darkened skin, dry stools, and a weak pulse. Patients with a pallor, sweating, coughing with profuse sputum, gastrointestinal weakness, and a tendency towards diarrhea should not take this formula.

Herbs and Actions
Tang-kuei, Peony, and Rehmannia nourish the liver. Ophiopogon and Asparagus nourish the lungs. Rehmannia, Anemarrhena, and Phellodendron dispel internal heat in the kidneys. Atractylodes, Citrus, and Licorice nourish the spleen and stomach.

Indications
Tuberculosis, acute and chronic bronchitis, acute and chronic pyelitis (inflammation of the pelvis of a kidney), tuberculosis of the kidneys, diabetes, pleurisy, and nocturnal emission.

Discrimination
Chai-hu-kuei-chih-kan-chiang-tang (Bupleurum, Cinnamon, and Ginger Combination): fever, cough, thoraco-abdominal pain, alternating chills and fever, irritability, flushing up.
Mai-men-tung-tang (Ophiopogon Combination): persistent congestion, dry throat, severe flushing up of *ch'i*, cough, facial flushing.
Ching-fei-tang (Platycodon and Fritillary Combination): pulmonary fever, cough, sticky sputum, flushing up of *ch'i*.
Chih-kan-tsao-tang (Baked Licorice Combination): weakness and

fatigability, hiccups, cardiac hyperfunction, knotty and alternate pulse.
Huang-chi-pieh-chia-tang (Astragalus and Tortoise Shell Combination): fatigue with a cough, steaming fever in the bones, spontaneous sweating, fatigability.

Yin weakness and fire agitation

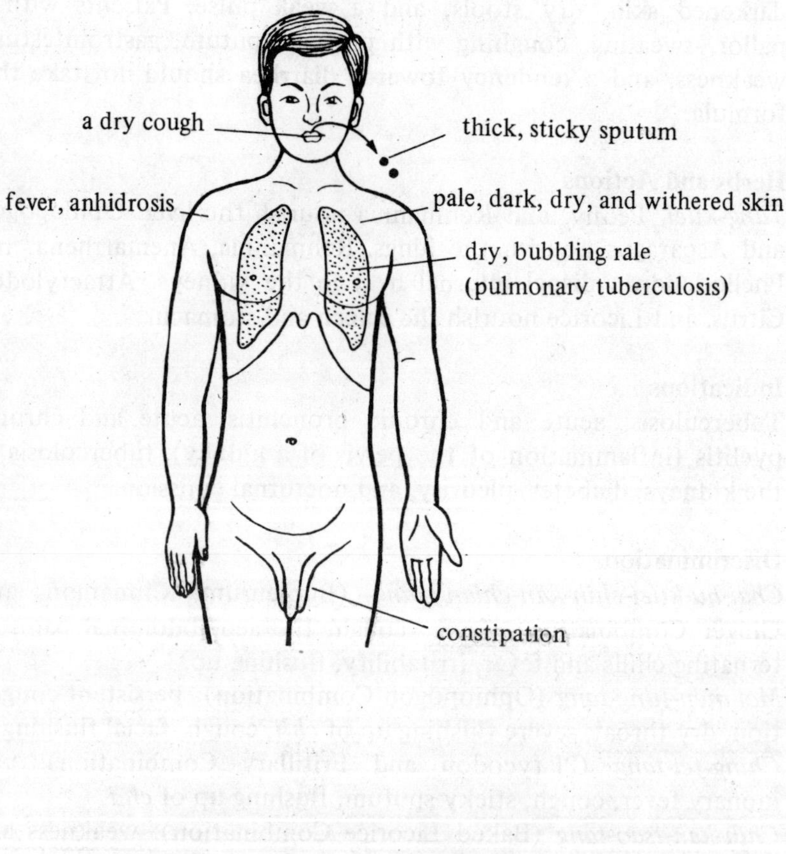

Yu-Nu-Chien 玉女煎

(Rehmannia and Gypsum Combination)

Gypsum	9.0	Rehmannia	9.0	Ophiopogon	6.0
Anemarrhena	4.5	Achyranthes	4.5		

Recorded in *Ching yueh fa hui* (景岳發揮) by Yao Chiu of the Ching dynasty. Used for treating internal heat in the stomach, fever caused by stress, thirst, headache, toothache, nosebleed, hemoptysis (spitting of blood), red tongue with white or dry yellow coating, and fast pulse.

Herbs and Actions

Rehmannia nourishes yin and Gypsum is an antipyretic; both are the major components in this formula. Anemarrhena and Gypsum dispel internal heat in the stomach. Ophiopogon and Rehmannia nourish yin. Achyranthes removes internal heat.

Indications

Swelling pain in the gingiva (tissue surrounding a tooth), internal heat in the stomach, nosebleed, and thirst.

7.
Hsiao Tao Chi
(消導劑, Digestive Formulas)

Formulas that aid digestion and dissolve congestion are called *hsiao tao chi* or *hsiao tao hua chi chi*. The "digestion" method is another of eight Chinese therapeutic methods.

Drinks and foods may injure the stomach, causing nausea, distention, belching with an acidic and fetid odor, and diarrhea. Treatment stimulates digestion and channels the accumulation of undigested food. If there is a conflict between chills, fever, sputum and food and congestion of *ch'i* and blood have resulted in the formation of a hard mass, palpable or non-palpable, treatment focuses on dissolving the hardening and accumulation. Hence, this type of formula is used for conditions due to malfunctioning of the spleen and stomach, for impeded circulation of *ch'i* that results in obstruction and distention, and for movable or non-movable tumors which have developed from the accumulation of moisture, phlegm, food, and blood. Digestive formulas stimulate circulation of *ch'i* and blood and restore normal functioning of the organs.

Both the digestive and the purgative formulas are used to eliminate tangible harmful toxins. However, clinically they are used differently. A purgative formula is indicated for urgent, tangible, harmful toxins whereas a digestive formula is indicated for obstruction, distention, and tumors. A digestive treats by means of slowing digestion and moderately dispersing.

Although a digestive formula is milder in action than a purgative, it can be useless or even destructive and is prohibited in weak conformations. Severe accumulation or large growths need to be treated by more potent formulas. A digestive formula might prove too weak and may delay and even hinder recovery. Hence, the practitioner must first weigh the weakness and firmness, consider the harmful toxin and *ch'i*, and recognize the acuteness or chronicity and the mildness or severity of the disease before diagnosing the conformation and prescribing the appropriate formula.

Chi-Pi-Tang 啓脾湯

(Lotus and Citrus Combination)

Atractylodes	4.0	Hoelen	4.0	Ginseng	3.0
Lotus seed	3.0	Dioscorea	3.0	Hawthorn	2.0
Citrus	2.0	Alisma	2.0	Licorice	1.0

Chi-pi-tang is recorded in *Wan ping hui chun* (萬病回春) of the Ming dynasty. This formula is used for treating watery diarrhea due to gastrosplenic weakness, indigestion in children, anorexia, persistent diarrhea, frequent abdominal pain, frequent vomiting, and jaundice.

Herbs and Actions

Ginseng, Atractylodes, Hoelen, and Licorice of *Szu-chun-tzu-tang* (Four Major Herb Combination) nourish the spleen and stomach, and with Citrus are stomachics and improve digestion. Lotus seed nourished the spleen and stops diarrhea. Alisma is a diuretic and treats thirst. Dioscorea treats thirst and diarrhea and has nutrient value.

Indications

Indigestion, chronic gastroenteritis, intestinal tuberculosis, watery diarrhea, chronic diarrhea, and loss of appetite during sickness.

Discrimination

Sheng-ling-pai-chu-san (Ginseng and Atractylodes Formula): watery diarrhea, proneness to *ch'i* stagnancy, and gas.
Jen-sheng-tang (Ginseng and Ginger Combination): watery diarrhea, copious saliva, and excessive urination.
Kuei-chih-jen-sheng-tang (Cinnamon and Ginseng Combination): diarrhea, obstruction beneath the heart, fever symptoms, floating pulse.
Chen-wu-tang (Vitality Combination): diarrhea, weakness, vomiting, abdominal pain, and chill conformation.
Wei-feng-tang (Atractylodes and Setaria Combination): diarrhea, and profuse toxic *ch'i* in the rectum.

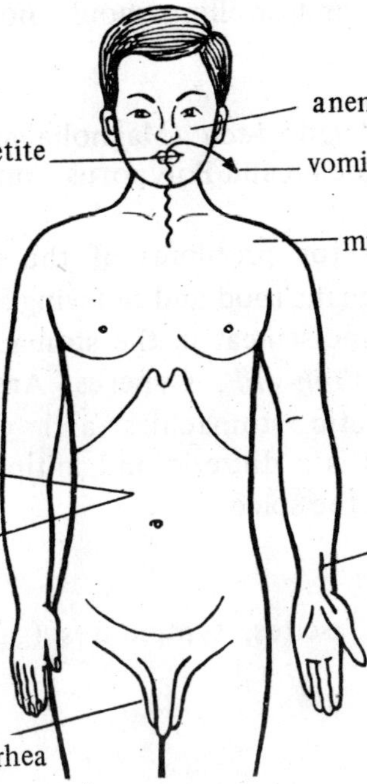

Fen-Hsiao-Tang 分消湯
(Hoelen and Alisma Combination)

Atractylodes	2.5	Hoelen	2.5	Citrus	2.0
Magnolia bark	2.0	Cyperus	2.0	Polyporus	2.0
Alisma	2.0	*Chih-shih*	1.0	Areca	1.0
Cardamon	1.0	Saussurea	1.0	Ginger	1.0
Juncus	1.0				

Recorded in *Wan ping hui chun* (萬病回春) of the Ming dynasty. Used for treating stagnant *ch'i*, stagnant food, edema, the initial stage of ascites (a kind of edema), distention beneath the heart, insufficient stools, severe constipation, gas in the intestines, sour stomach, and loss of appetite. Persons with a delicate constitution and swelling should not take this formula.

Herbs and Actions

A combination of *Ping-wei-san* (Magnolia and Ginger Formula) with *Szu-ling-tang* (Hoelen and Polyporus Combination) and other herbs.

Ping-wei-san is good for problems of the stomach and spleen and for dispelling stagnant food and relieving ascites.

Szu-ling-tang dispels moist heat in the stomach and treats dysuria (painful urination). *Chih-shih*, Cyperus, Areca, Cardamon, and Saussurea are aromatic stomachics and good for dispelling stagnant *ch'i*. Juncus is a diuretic and antipyretic that increases vitality and nourishes the spleen.

Indications

Peritonitis, nephritis, ascites, tympanites (gas in the intestines), and cirrhosis.

Discrimination

Pu-chi-chien-chung-tang (Atractylodes and Citrus Combination): distention and swelling of the abdomen; the abdomen lacks elasticity and recovers slowly after pressing; degenerated vitality and weak conformation.

Pa-wei-ti-huang-wan (Rehmannia Eight Formula); edema, yin conformation and weak swelling, numbness beneath the umbilicus.

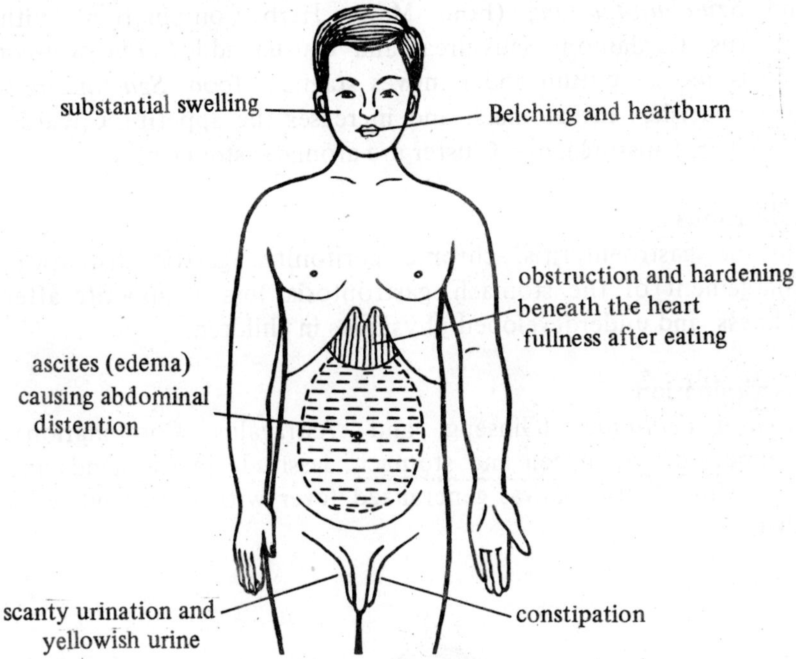

Hsiang-Sha-Yang-Wei-Tang 香砂養胃湯

(Cyperus and Cluster Combination)

Atractylodes	3.0	Hoelen	3.0	Ginseng	2.0
Magnolia bark	2.0	Citrus	2.0	Cyperus	2.0
Cluster	2.0	Saussurea	1.5	Cardamon	1.5
Licorice	1.5	Jujube	1.5	Ginger	1.5

Recorded in *Wan ping hui chun* (萬病回春) of the Ming dynasty. Treats gastrointestinal weakness with loss of appetite and chest distention, nourishes the stomach, dispels stagnant water poisoning and food poisoning, and stimulates digestive functions. When taken regularly it builds physical stamina in children.

Herbs and Actions

A combination of *Ping-wei-san* (Magnolia and Ginger Formula) and *Szu-chun-tzu-tang* (Four Major Herb Combination) with Cyperus, Cardamon, Saussurea, and Cluster added. *Ping-wei-san* dispels moist sputum and removes stagnant food; *Szu-chun-tzu-tang* nourishes the stomach and increases the appetite. Cpyerus, Cinnabar, Saussurea, and Cluster are aromatic stomachics.

Indications

Chronic gastroenteritis, chronic peritonitis, gastric distention, enlargement of the stomach, gastroptosis, loss of appetite after sickness, and underdeveloped physiques in children.

Discrimination

Pu-chung-i-chi-tang (Ginseng and Astragalus Combination): weakness of the spleen and stomach, lassitude in the hands and feet, white frothy saliva, generalized fever with a big and weak pulse.

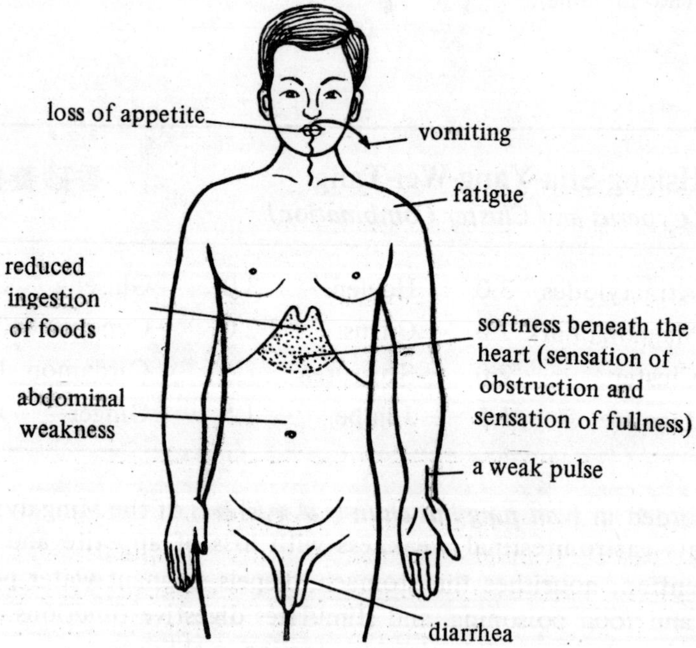

Jen-Sheng-Yang-Wei-Tang 人參養胃湯

(Ginseng Stomach Combination)

Atractylodes	4.0	Pinellia	4.0	Hoelen	4.0
Magnolia bark	2.0	Citrus	2.0	Agastache	1.5
Tsao-kuo	1.5	Ginseng	1.5	Mume	1.5
Ginger	1.5	Jujube	1.5	Licorice	1.0

Recorded in *Ho chi chu fang* (和劑局方). As implied by its name, the formula is used to nourish the stomach. It mainly warms and supplements the stomach and spleen. The combination of *Liu-chun-tzu-tang* (Six Major Herb Combination) and *Ping-wei-san* (Magnolia and Ginger Formula), is given to people who have weak stomachs and intestines or obstructed and impeded stomach functioning due to the wind and cold or ingestion of raw and cold food. It is also prescribed for the onset of diseases with malaria-like symptoms–fever and chills; headaches, heavy headedness, and dizziness; and spasms of arms and legs. Other uses are for geriatric patients with a low fever and inability to eat caused by stagnant water in the stomach and for children with parasitic worms who have alternating fever and chills.

Herbs and Actions

Ginseng, Hoelen and Licorice are sweet tasting. They supplement a deficiency of the stomach; Citrus, Atractylodes, and Magnolia bark have an acrid taste, and dissipate internal moist turbidity, thus drying and strengthening the spleen; Pinellia awakens the spleen; Agastache increases the appetite; and *Tsao-kuo* elminiates obstructions. Because of the ingenious incorporation of these herbs with Ginger, Jujube and Mume, the formula promotes digestion, moves the *ch'i*, and expels toxins.

Indications

Weakened stomach and intestines resulting from cold; alimentary disorders occurring when acclimatizing to a new environment; malaria; parasitic worms; and dyspepsia.

Discrimination

Tsing-fu-tang (Bupleurum and Pinellia Combination): food stagnancy; hard mass; high fever; extreme thirst; painful urination with red urine, firm fever conformation.

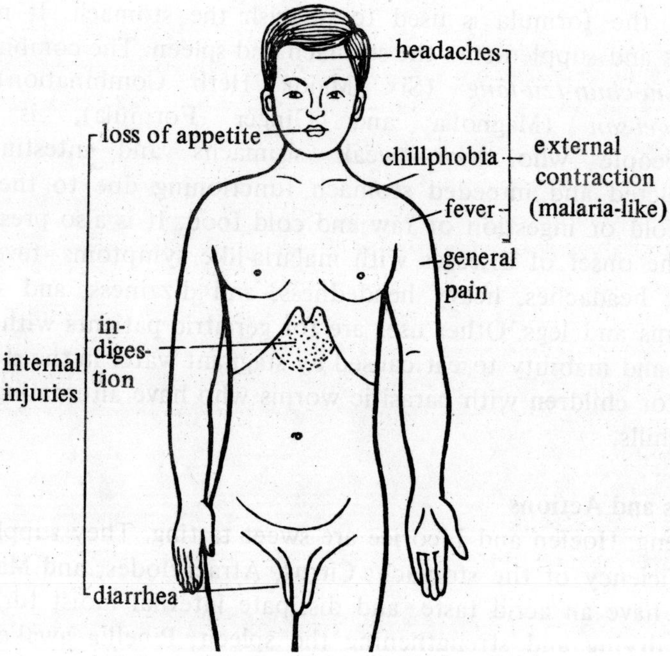

Ko-Hua-Chieh-Hsing-Tang 葛花解醒湯

(Pueraria Flower Combination)

Saussurea	0.6	Ginseng	1.5	Polyporus	1.5
Hoelen	3.0	Citrus	1.5	Atractylodes	1.5
Blue citrus peel	1.5	Ginger	1.5	*Shen-chu*	1.5
Alisma	1.5	Cardamon	3.0	Cluster	3.0
Pueraria flower	3.0				

Ko-hua-chieh-hsing-tang was recorded in the *Lan shih mi tsang* (蘭室秘藏) by Li Kao during the Yuan dynasty. This formula is used for treating hangover, "internal moisture" in the spleen and stomach, vertigo, vomiting, chest distension, anorexia, fatigue, and dysuria.

Herbs and Actions

Pueraria flower eases discomfort of a hangover. As diuretics, Hoelen, Polyporus, and Alisma dispel "moist heat". Cluster and Cardamon also help hangover discomfort. *Shen-chu* is a hangover remedy which also removes stagnant food. Saussurea and Ginger regulate the *ch'i*. Blue citrus peel and Citrus are expectorants. Ginseng and Atractylodes nourish the *ch'i*.

Indications

Intoxication and hangover.

Pao-Ho-Wan 保和丸

(Citrus and Crataegus Formula)

Crataegus	12.0	*Shen-chu*	4.0	Raphanus	2.0
Pinellia	6.0	Citrus	2.0	Forsythia	2.0
Hoelen	6.0				

Pao-ho-wan is recorded in *Tan hsi hsin fa* (丹溪心法). This formula is used for treating stagnant food, indigestion, abdominal distention, abdominal pain, eructation, diarrhea, and thick coating on the tongue.

Herbs and Actions
Crataegus, *Shen-chu*, and Raphanus remove stagnant food and distention, and regulate the *ch'i*. Pinellia, Hoelen, and Citrus are diuretics and improve gastric functioning. Forsythia dispels "internal heat".

Indications
Gastric distress, eructation, indigestion, diarrhea, and abdominal pain.

Ping-Wei-San 平胃散

(Magnolia and Ginger Formula)

Atractylodes	4.0	Magnolia bark	3.0	Citrus	3.0
Jujube	2.0	Licorice	1.0	Ginger	1.0

Ping-wei-san was recorded in the Chinese medical dictionaries of the Sung dynasty: *Chien yao chi chung fang* (A.D. 1051) and *Tai ping huei min ho chi chu fang* (A.D. 1107-1110), as a drug to be used for increasing digestive absorption and removing stagnant water in the stomach. This formula is suitable for detoxification and as treatment for cough with sputum, gastrointestinal weakness, poor digestion, persistent bitter taste, loss of appetite, abdominal distention, borborygmus and diarrhea after eating, chest distention, and pallor. However, those of weak conformation with anemia and severe relaxation around the pubic bones should not use this formula.

Herbs and Actions
Atractylodes removes fluid accumulated in the stomach. Citrus and Magnolia bark improve gastric function and digestion. Licorice harmonizes all the other herbs and improves gastric function. Ginger and Jujube increase vitality.

Indications
Acute and chronic gastritis, gastric relaxation, gastrectasis, gastric ulcer, peptic ulcer, indigestion, obesity, chlorosis, parasitic diseases, and gastrointestinal weakness.

Discrimination
Pan-hsia-hsieh-hsin-tang (Pinellia Combination): pain beneath the heart, obstruction and hardness beneath the heart, firm fever conformation.
Chai-hu-kuei-chih-tang (Bupleurum and Cinnamon Combination): pain beneath the heart; obstruction and hardness beneath the heart; rectus abdominis muscle tension; mild, firm conformation.
Chien-chung-tang (Hoelen and Jujube Combination): pain beneath the heart, mild obstruction and hardness beneath the heart, mild tension in the abdominal muscle, mild weak conformation.
An-chung-san (Cardamon and Fennel Formula): delicate constitution with a stomachache, vomiting of gastric acid, indigestion, stagnant food in the chest, and tense and hard abdomen.

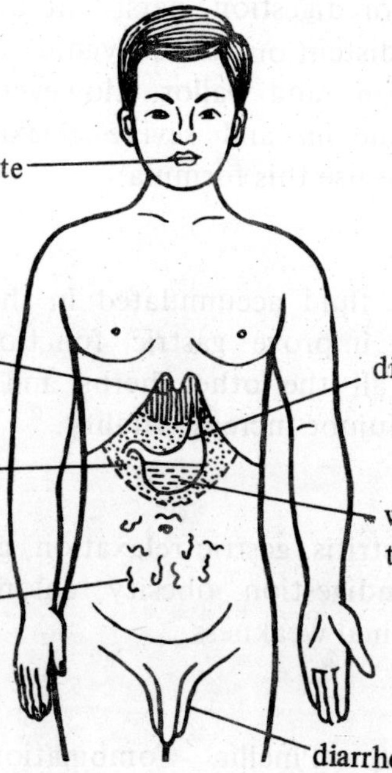

Pu-Huan-Chin-Cheng-Chi-San 不換金正氣散

(Pinellia, Atractylodes, and Agastache Formula)

Atractylodes	4.0	Citrus	3.0	Pinellia	6.0
Magnolia bark	3.0	Agastache	1.0	Licorice	1.0
Ginger	3.0	Jujube	3.0		

Pu-huan-chin-cheng-chi-san was recorded in the *Tai ping huei min ho chi chu fang* (太平惠民和劑局方) during the Sung dynasty. This formula is used for treating the common cold, plague, recurrent fever and chills, cholera, vomiting, diarrhea, dysentery, and acclimation fever.

Herbs and Actions

This formula is a combination of *Ping-wei-san* (Magnolia and Ginger Formula) with Pinellia and Agastache. *Ping-wei-san* regulates the function of the spleen and stomach and is effective for digestive disorders. Pinellia relieves flushing up and "internal moisture". Agastache is an appetizer and antiemetic.

Indications

Acute gastroenteritis, poisoning due to contaminated drinking water, cholera, and acclimation fever.

Discrimination

Huo-hsiang-cheng-chi-san (Agastache Formula): plagues and epidemics chiefly of a dispersal action; *Pu-huan-chin-cheng-chi-san* eliminates moisture.

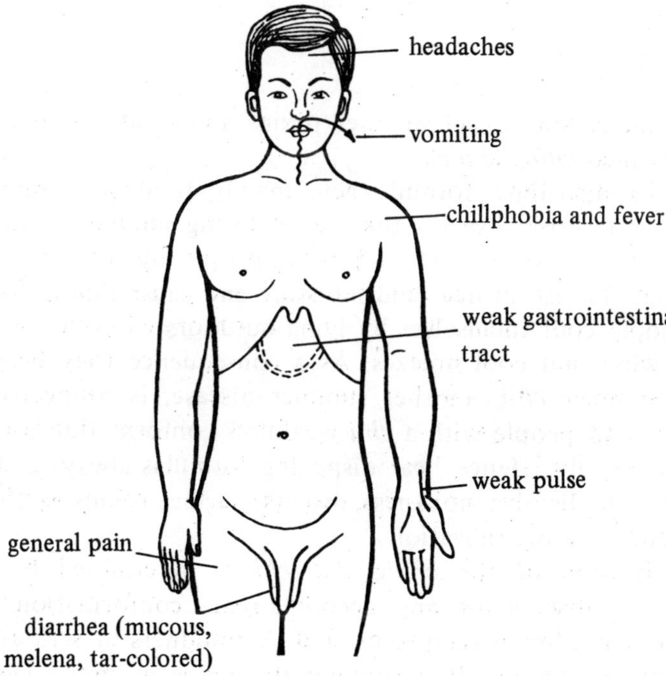

8.
Ching Shu Chi
(清暑劑, Heat Dispelling Formulas)

Formulas that expel summer toxins and treat summer diseases are called *ching shu chi.*

A heat-dispelling formula acts mainly to dispel "summer toxins," or feverish diseases that occur during summer when the earth is humid and hot. At such times people are subject to the toxins that flourish in heat and moisture and cause illness. Sometimes people cool themselves by lying outdoors without concern for the wind and cool breezes. As a consequence they become chilled. Summer *ch'i,* another summer disease, is connected to the heart, and people with a *ch'i* weakness conformation usually sweat excessively. Hence heat dispelling formulas always include herbs that can dissolve moistness, disperse surface toxins, strengthen *ch'i*, and promote salivation.

Application of the *ching shu chi* is determined by the presence or absence of any accompanying conformation, the chief and subordinate symptoms, and the mildness or seriousness of a summer disease. If a summer disease is accompanied by a "moist condition" such that the disease is serious but fluid retention mild, the "moisture condition" often turns to fever. Thus the formula prescribed should not be too warm and dry or it will dry up the saliva and body fluids. If the fluid retention is more severe and the summer fever mild, the fever often will be masked by the accumulated moisture. If this condition prevails, a sweet and chilly formula should be prescribed.

Ching-Shu-I-Chi-Tang 清暑益氣湯

(Astragalus and Atractylodes Combination)

Ginseng	3.0	Astragalus	3.0	Atractylodes	3.0
Shen-chu	1.0	Blue citrus peel	2.0	Citrus	3.0
Licorice	1.0	Ophiopogon	3.0	Schizandra	1.0
Tang-kuei	3.0	Phellodendron	1.0	Alisma	2.0
Cimicifuga	0.5	Pueraria	2.0		

Ching-shu-i-chi-tang is a formula originated by Li Kao (李杲, A.D. 1180-1251) of the Yuan dynasty. This formula is used for treating weakness in the arms and legs, hematuria, frequent watery stools, thirst, anorexia, sweating, and a weak pulse.

Herbs and Actions

Ginseng and Astragalus nourish *ch'i*. Atractylodes dispels moisture and nourishes the spleen. Ophiopogon and Schizandra nourish the lungs and severe as sialagogues. Phellodendron dispels moisture and "internal heat". Blue citrus peel nourishes the liver and dispels stagnant blood. *Tang-kuei* nourishes the blood and neutralizes yin. *Shen-chu* initiates elimination of stagnant food. Cimicifuga and Pueraria dispel "muscular heat". Alisma dispels "moist heat". Citrus increases vitality. Licorice regulates the action of the other herbs.

Indications

Heatstroke, autonomic nerve disorders, thirst, weakness in the arms and legs, and anorexia.

Weak conformation

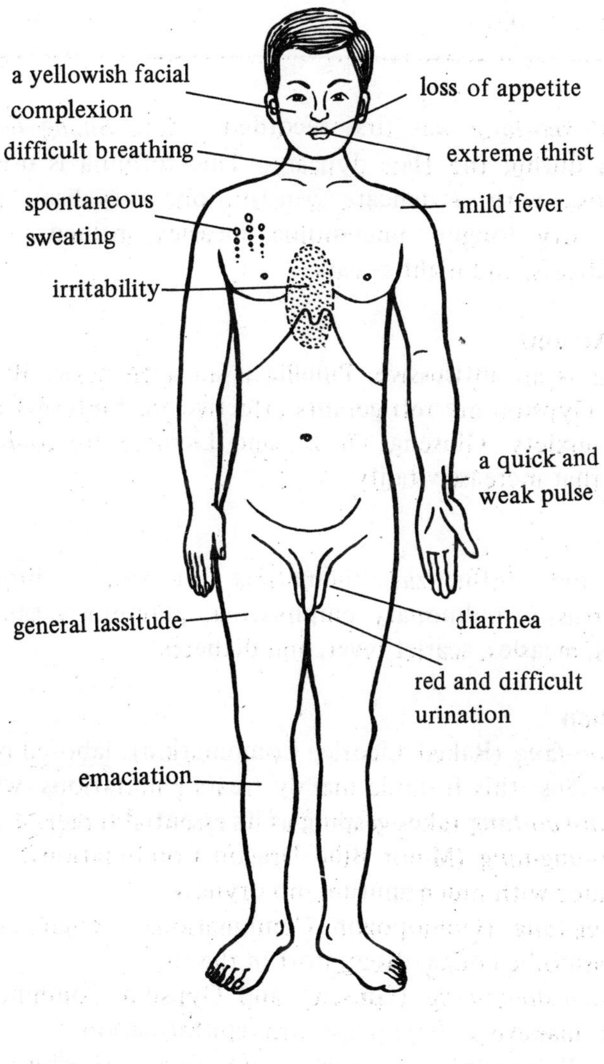

Chu-Yeh-Shih-Kao-Tang 竹葉石膏湯

(Bamboo Leaves and Gypsum Combination)

Ophiopogon	6.0	Oryza	6.0	Pinellia	4.0
Ginseng	3.0	Bamboo leaves	2.0	Licorice	2.0
Gypsum	10.0				

Chu-yeh-shih-kao-tang was first recorded in the *Shang han lun* (傷寒論) during the Han dynasty. This formula is used for treating those with a delicate constitution, aptyalism, coarse skin, thirst, dry tongue, pneumonia, measles, influenza, fever, cough, ephidrosis, and night sweats.

Herbs and Actions

Ophiopogon is an antitussive. Pinellia is an antiemetic. Bamboo leaves and Gypsum are refrigerants effective for "internal heat", thirst, and anxiety. Ginseng, Oryza, and Licorice are tonics and sialagogues that increase vitality.

Indications

Common cold, influenza, pneumonia, bronchitis, bronchial asthma, pertussis, pulmonary emphysema, pulmonary gangrene, tuberculosis, measles, scarlet fever, and diabetes.

Discrimination

Chih-kan-tsao-tang (Baked Licorice Combination): labored breathing, palpitations; this formula mainly treats palpitations, whereas *Chu-yeh-shih-kao-tang* takes gasping as its essential target.
Hsiao-ching-lung-tang (Minor Blue Dragon Combination): cough, asthma, stridor with much sputum, no dryness.
Mai-men-tung-tang (Ophiopogon Combination): cough, asthma, dryness, spasmodic cough, discomfort in the throat.
Pai-hu-chia-jen-sheng-tang (Ginseng and Gypsum Combination): fever, thirst, massive and big pulse, firm conformation.
Pa-wei-wan (Rehmannia Eight Formula): thirst, excessive urine, and numbness in the lower abdomen.

Chih-tzu-kan-tsao-shih-tang (Gardenia, Licorice, and Soja Combination): gasping, and chest depression and distress.

Yang, weak conformation

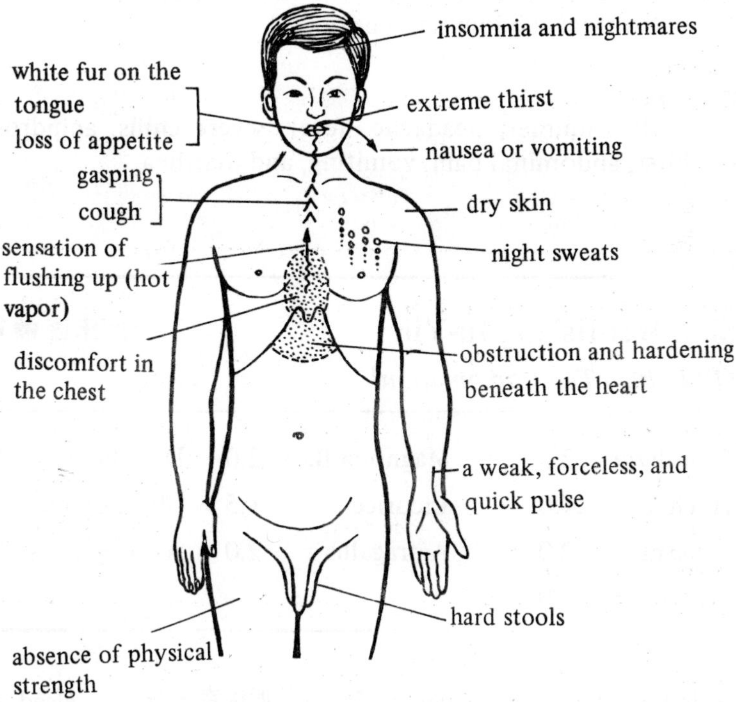

Hsiang-Ju-Yin 香薷飲

(Elsholtzia Combination)

Elsholtzia	6.0	Dolichos	6.0	Magnolia bark	3.0

Hsiang-ju-yin is recorded in *Tai ping huei min ho chi chu fang* (太平惠民和劑局方) of the Sung dynasty. This formula is used for treating nutritional imbalance, headache due to summer heat, fever, severe chills, stress, thirst, abdominal disorders, pain in the abdomen and heart, vomiting, and diarrhea. This formula acts as a diaphoretic and antipyretic.

Herbs and Actions
Elsholtzia is a diuretic and diaphoretic; in combination with Magnolia bark it is a stomachic. Dolichos dispels heat, stops diarrhea, and treats abdominal tension.

Indications
Chills in the summer, headache, fever, severe chills, anhidrosis, stress, thirst, abdominal pain, vomiting, and diarrhea.

Shih-Wei-Hsiang-Ju-Yin 十味香薷飲
(Elsholtzia Ten Combination)

Elsholtzia	2.5	Magnolia Bark	2.0	Dolichos	2.0
Hoelen	4.0	Licorice	1.5	Chaenomeles	2.0
Ginseng	2.0	Astragalus	2.0	Atractylodes	3.0
Citrus	2.0				

Recorded in *Tsou hou pai i fang* (肘後百一方). Used for patients with a weak constitution who suffer from common colds in the summer and experience giddiness, heavy headedness, general lassitude, vomiting or diarrhea, profuse sweating, and a weak pulse.

Herbs and Actions
Elsholtzia is acrid and warm and capable of acting as a carminative and diuretic. Magnolia bark evaporates dampness and harmonizes the stomach. Dolichos lessens heat and harmonizes the spleen. Hoelen is a diuretic. Ginseng is a tonic as well as an excitant. Astragalus eases respiration and solidifies the surface. Atractylodes and Citrus strengthen the stomach. Chaenomeles is a stimulant

and an analgesic. Licorice mollifies the actions of the various herbs.

Indications
Summer heat (heatstroke), weak stomach, common colds contracted in the summer by debilitated individuals.

9.

Pu I Chi

(補益劑, Supplementing Formulas or Tonics)

Formulas that nourish and supplement inadequacy of *ch'i,* blood, yin, and yang are called *pu i chi.* "Supplementing" is one of the eight Chinese therapeutic methods. When the human body is healthy, Chinese physicians say there is a "balance of yin and yang." If either yin or yang is excessive or insufficient, the body is in an abnormal state. A *pu i chi* formula functions to supplement or enrich inadequacy of *ch'i* and blood, to adjust an abundance of yin and yang, and to restore the proper balance. [An ancient saying is, inadequacy is supplemented and surplus is deducted (by these formulas).]

Precautions must be taken in prescribing tonics. Attention must be paid to the phenomenon "strong firmness with weak manifestation" which is a pseudo-weak conformation. This conformation may appear quite similar to a weak and chilly surface conformation, when in fact it is a firm fever accumulated in the interior. If this condition is treated with a tonic formula, it will be aggravated. Cases in which a surface conformation is accompanied by internal weakness or a weak conformation by firmness must be treated with great care. If they are treated with a tonic, a condition likened to "confine the burglar inside the door" may suddenly develop.

Chai-Shao-Liu-Chun-Tzu-Tang 柴芍六君子湯

(B. P. and Six Major Herb Combination)

Ginseng	4.0	Atractylodes	4.0	Hoelen	4.0
Pinellia	4.0	Bupleurum	3.0	Peony	3.0
Citrus	2.0	Jujube	2.0	Ginger	2.0
Licorice	1.0				

Chai-shao-liu-chun-tzu-tang, a combination of *Liu-chun-tzu-tang* (Six Major Herb Combination) with Bupleurum and Peony, is an experimental formula from Japan. This formula is used for the *Liu-chun-tzu-tang* conformation, i.e. distention beneath the heart, loss of appetite, anemia, weak conformation with chilled limbs, and a tendency towards fatigue. It is suitable for abdominal cramps and chest distention.

Herbs and Actions

Ginseng, Atractylodes, Hoelen, Pinellia, Licorice, and Citrus can nourish the spleen and stomach and act as dessicants and expectorants. Bupleurum treats distention in the chest and ribs. Peony is a sedative and analgesic.

Indications

Gastrointestinal weakness, gastritis, gastroptosis, peptic ulcer, indigestion, peritonitis, anorexia, and vomiting.

Chi-Wei-Tu-Chi-Wan 七味都氣丸

(Rehmannia and Schizandra Formula)

Rehmannia	6.0	Cornus	3.0	Dioscorea	3.0
Alisma	3.0	Hoelen	3.0	Moutan	3.0
Schizandra	1.0				

Recorded in *Tang tou ko chueh* (湯頭歌訣). Composed of *Liu-wei-ti-huang-wan* (Rehmannia Six Formula) and schizandra. Primarily this formula is for yin disease symptoms such as weakness, cough, and abundance of water which turns to sputum. Additionally the formula is efficacious for drying up saliva, for severe coughs which prevent the patient from sleeping, and for sore throat and hoarseness. Experience has shown this formula to be quite effective for coughs.

Herbs and Actions

Rehmannia, Cornus and Dioscorea are all nutritive and hemopoeitic (blood building) agents. Alisma and Hoelen are diuretics, which by the removal of fluid harmonize the stomach. Moutan cortex purges fever and cools the blood while Schizandra is an astringent that suppresses asthma and coughs.

Indications

Coughs, bronchial asthma, pulmonary emphysema, and pulmonary tuberculosis.

Chia-Wei-Pa-Hsien-Tang 加味八仙湯

(Siler and Chianghuo Combination)

Tang-kuei	2.5	Peony	2.5	Cnidium	2.5
Rehmannia	2.5	Citrus	2.5	Pinellia	2.5
Atractylodes	6.0	Hoelen	5.0	Ginseng	1.5
Achyranthes	1.5	Siler	1.5	*Chianghuo*	1.5
Chin-chiu	1.5	Bupleurum	1.0	Cinnamon	1.0
Licorice	1.0	Jujube	1.0	Ginger	1.0

Chia-wei-pa-hsien-tang is recorded in *Wan ping hui chun* (萬病回春) of the Ming dynasty. This formula is used for treating numbness or pain in the limbs, and facial spasms and numbness.

Herbs and Actions

Tang-kuei, Peony, Cnidium, and Rehmannia are tonics which nourish the blood. Ginseng, Atractylodes, Hoelen, Licorice, Citrus, and Pinellia of *Liu-chun-tzu-tang* (Six Major Herb Combination) can strengthen the spleen and stomach and act as dessicants and expectorants. Siler and *Chianghuo* treat numbness of the joints. Achyranthes is an analgesic which can strengthen the muscles and bones of the flanks and feet. Cinnamon coordinates the actions of the other herbs, warms the meridians, and regulates the pulses. Bupleurum is an analgesic which also nourishes the liver and relieves anxiety. Gentiana nourishes muscle and acts as an antirheumatic and analgesic. Ginger and Jujube treat paralysis.

Indications

Numbness of the limbs, palsy and pain due to cerebral hemorrhage, facial numbness, and facial spasms.

Chien-Shih-Pai-Chu-San 錢氏白朮散

(Atractylodes and Pueraria Formula)

Atractylodes	4.0	Hoelen	4.0	Pueraria	4.0
Ginseng	3.0	Saussurea	1.0	Agastache	1.0
Licorice	1.0				

Chien-shih-pai-chu-san is recorded in *I fang kao* (醫方考) by Wu Kun of the Ming dynasty. This formula is a combination of *Szu-chun-tzu-tang* (Four Major Herb Combination) with Pueraria, Agastache, and Saussurea. It is to be taken by children with gastrointestinal weakness and by those with fever, thirst, and decreased salivation due to vomiting and diarrhea.

Herbs and Actions

Ginseng, Atractylodes, Hoelen, and Licorice of *Szu-chun-tzu-tang* nourish the spleen. Pueraria relieves muscular heat. Agastache and Saussurea are aromatic stomachics.

Indications

Indigestion in children, the common cold with vomiting and diarrhea, and diabetes with anorexia.

Discrimination

Wu-ling-san (Hoelen Five Herb Formula): vomiting, diarrhea, extreme thirst, stagnant water in the stomach, decreased urine but no dryness or excessive fluids.

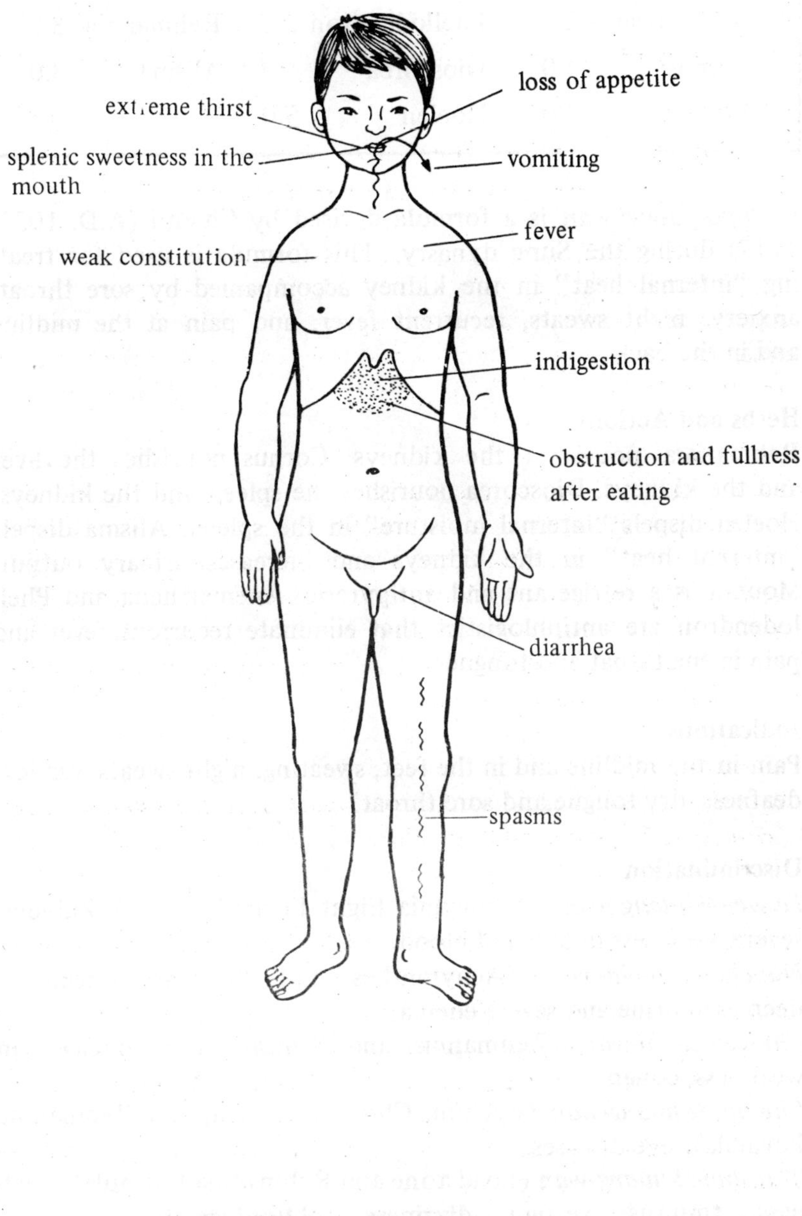
loss of appetite
extreme thirst
splenic sweetness in the mouth
vomiting
fever
weak constitution
indigestion
obstruction and fullness after eating
diarrhea
spasms

Chih-Po-Pa-Wei-Wan 知蘗八味丸

(Anemarrhena, Phellodendron, and Rehmannia Formula)

Anemarrhena	2.0	Phellodendron	2.0	Rehmannia	8.0
Cornus	4.0	Dioscorea	4.0	Alisma	3.0
Moutan	3.0	Hoelen	3.0		

Chih-po-pa-wei-wan is a formula devised by Chien I (A.D. 1035-1117) during the Sung dynasty. This formula is used for treating "internal heat" in the kidney accompanied by sore throat, anxiety, night sweats, recurrent fever, and pain at the midline and in the back

Herbs and Actions
Rehmannia nourishes the kidneys. Cornus nourishes the liver and the kidneys. Dioscorea nourishes the spleen and the kidneys. Hoelen dispels "internal moisture" in the spleen. Alisma dispels "internal heat" in the kidneys and increases urinary output. Moutan is a refrigerant and antipyretic. Anemarrhena and Phellodendron are antiphlogistics that eliminate recurrent fever and pain in the throat and tongue.

Indications
Pain in the midline and in the feet, sweating, night sweats, vertigo, deafness, dry tongue,and sore throat.

Discrimination
Pa-wei-ti-huang-wan (Rehmannia Eight Formula): weak kidneys, severe weakness in *ch'i* and blood.
Niu-che-shen-chi-wan (Achyranthes and Plantago Formula): decreased urine and severe edema.
Chi-wei-tu-chi-wan (Rehmannia and Schizandra Formula): yin weakness; cough.
Chi-chu-ti-huang-wan (Lycium, Chrysanthemum, and Rehmannia Formula): eye diseases.
Tzu-shih-ti-huang-wan (Loadstone and Rehmannia Formula): deafness, tinnitus, vertigo, dizziness, blurred vision.

Chin-Chiu-Fu-Lei-Tang 秦艽扶羸湯

(Chin-Chiu and Bupleurum Combination)

Chin-chiu	3.0	Bupleurum	3.0	Tortoise shell	3.0
Aster	2.0	Lycium bark	2.0	Ginseng	2.0
Tang-kuei	5.0	Pinellia	5.0	Licorice	1.0
Mume	2.5	Jujube	1.5	Ginger	1.5

Used to treat tidal fever and coughs from pulmonary tuberculosis. It is definitely effective for tidal fever but indicated principally for pulmonary adynia and the "bone-steaming" fever resulting in a phthiatic cough, chills, fever, hoarseness or laryngitis, somatic weakness with spontaneous perspiration, and weakness in the arms and legs.

Herbs and Actions

Chin-chiu, Tortoise shell, Lycium bark and Bupleurum diminish pulmonary phthiasis and the accompanying wasting fever. Pinellia dries moisture and expels sputum. Aster and Mume suppress coughs and stimulate expectoration. Ginseng and Licorice restore normal breathing. *Tang-kuei* supplements the blood.

Indications

Pulmonary tuberculosis, residual symptoms of pneumonia, pleuritis, a constant mild fever from chronic influenza that persists.

Chin-Chiu-Pieh-Chia-San 秦艽鼈甲散

(Chin-chiu and Tortoise Shell Formula)

Chin-chiu	2.0	*Ching-hao*	2.0	Mume	2.0
Anemarrhena	2.0	*Tang-kuei*	3.0	Tortoise Shell	3.0
Bupleurum	3.0	Lycium bark	3.0	Ginger	1.5

Chin-chiu-pieh-chia-tang is recorded in *Wei sheng pao chien* (衛生寶鑑). This formula is used for treating hyperplastic tuberculosis. This form of the disease has some standard tubercular chest symptoms, but lacks the cough, sputum, and high fever. Rales can be clearly detected by stethoscope, but a cough is almost never present. The patient has fatigue, flushed cheeks, night sweats, and progressive emaciation. Recovery is very difficult in this type of tuberculosis. Today, antibiotic therapy is widely used. If the symptoms are mild, this formula may be administered even though there are lesions.

Herbs and Actions

Chin-chiu is an antipyretic and can relieve the distressing symptoms of tuberculosis. Tortoise shell and Anemarrhena nourish the yin and rid the body of internal heat. Lycium bark and *Ching-hao* remove hidden fever and weak fever, and they cool the blood. *Tang-kuei* is a hematinic and carminative. Bupleurum acts as an antipyretic and muscle relaxant. Mume is an astrigent which checks sweating.

Indications

Pneumonia, hyperplastic tuberculosis, and pleurisy.

Discrimination

Hsiao-chai-hu-tang (Minor Bupleurum Combination): mild fevers, thoraco-costal distress, mild firm fever conformation.

Chai-hu-chiang-kuei-tang (Bupleurum, Aconite, and Ginger Combination): mild fevers and abdominal palpitations.

Huang-chi-chien-chung-tang (Astragalus and Peony Combination): weakness and fatigability, and dryness.

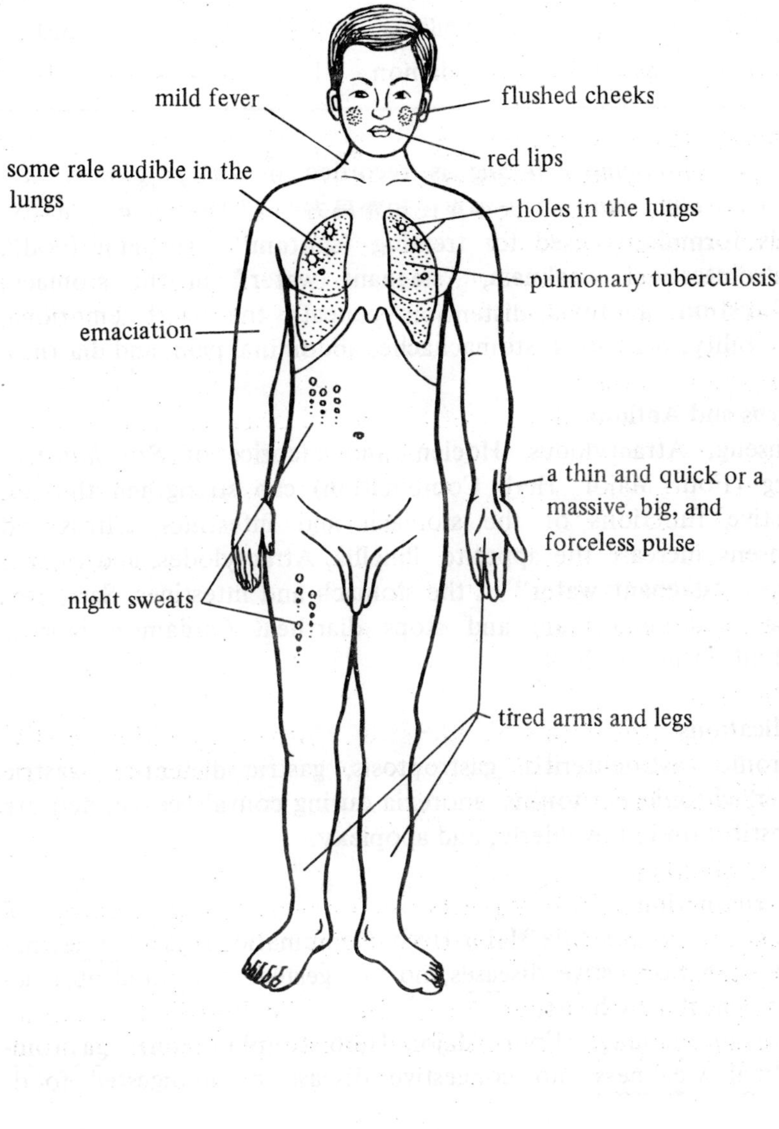
mild fever
flushed cheeks
red lips
some rale audible in the lungs
holes in the lungs
pulmonary tuberculosis
emaciation
a thin and quick or a massive, big, and forceless pulse
night sweats
tired arms and legs

Hsiang-Sha-Liu-Chun-Tzu-Tang 香砂六君子湯

(*Saussurea and Cardamon Combination*)

Ginseng	6.0	Atractylodes	6.0	Hoelen	6.0
Licorice	3.0	Pinellia	6.0	Citrus	3.0
Saussurea	1.5	Cardamon	1.5		

Hsiang-sha-liu-chun-tzu-tang is recorded in *Tai ping huei min ho chi chu fang* (太平惠民和劑局方) of the Sung dynasty. This formula is used for treating "sputum", "stagnant food", gastrointestinal weakness, "stagnant water" in the stomach, indigestion, anorexia, distention beneath the heart, emotional instability, occasional stomachache, abdominal pain, and diarrhea.

Herbs and Actions

Ginseng, Atractylodes, Hoelen, and Licorice of *Szu-chun-tzu-tang* (Four Major Herb Combination) can strengthen the respective functions of the stomach and intestines. Citrus and Ginseng increase the appetite. Pinellia, Atractylodes, and Hoelen dispel "stagnant water" in the stomach and intestines. Saussurea eases abdominal pain and stops diarrhea. Cardamon relieves distention in the chest.

Indications

Chronic gastroenteritis, gastroptosis, gastric distention, gastric ulcer, chronic peritonitis, anorexia during convalescence, delicate constitution in the elderly, and apoplexy.

Discrimination

Liu-chun-tzu-tang (Six Major Herb Combination): gastrointestinal weakness, congestive diseases, no undigested food, mild obstruction beneath the heart.

Szu-chun-tzu-tang (Four Major Herb Combination): gastrointestinal weakness, no congestive disease or undigested food.

Huang-Chi-Kuei-Chih-Wu-Wu-Tang 黃耆桂枝五物湯

(Astragalus and Cinnamon Five Herb Combination)

Astragalus	3.0	Peony	3.0	Cinnamon	3.0
Jujube	3.0	Ginger	3.0		

Huang-chi-kuei-chih-wu-wu-tang is recorded in *Chin kuei yao lueh* (金匱要略) of the Han dynasty. This is a variation of *Hsiao-chien-chung-tang* (Minor Cinnamon and Peony Combination) in which Licorice is omitted and Astragalus is added. This formula is used for treating paralysis in the legs and arms, generalized pain, and weak pulse.

Herbs and Actions

Astragalus is an antihidrotic. Cinnamon and Ginger improve blood circulation, warms the body, and reinforces the functioning of the internal organs. Peony is a sedative. Jujube and Ginger increase the *ch'i*.

Indications

Beriberi, monoplegia, Bell's palsy, and neurosis.

Discrimination

Pu-chung-i-chi-tang (Ginseng and Astragalus Combination): numbness in the hands and feet, weakness in the digestive function, weakness and desire for hot food.

Huang-chi-chien-chung-tang (Astragalus Combination): difficulty walking due to nervous lesion, pain, and cramps of the rectus abdominis muscle.

Pa-wei-ti-huang-wan (Rehmannia Eight Formula): neuroparalysis, cold loins and feet, and excessive urine at night.

Huang-Chi-Pieh-Chia-San 黃耆鱉甲散

(Astragalus and Tortoise Shell Formula)

Bupleurum	2.0	Astragalus	2.0	Tortoise shell	2.0
Peony	2.0	Rehmannia	2.0	Ophiopogon	3.0
Hoelen	3.0	Ginseng	1.0	Morus	1.0
Pinellia	1.0	Platycodon	1.0	Cinnamon	1.0
Lycium bark	1.5	Anemarrhena	1.5	*Chin-chiu*	1.5
Aster	1.5	Licorice	1.0		

Huang-chi-pieh-chia-san is recorded in *Tai ping huei min ho chi chu fang* (太平惠民和劑局方) of the Ming dynasty. This formula is used for treating fatigue, chronic cough, sensation of heat in the chest, and mild lingering fever due to the common cold.

Herbs and Actions

Rehmannia and Anemarrhena are antipyretics, refrigerants, and renal nutritives. Ophiopogon is a nutrient tonic which also nourishes the lungs. Bupleurum, Tortoise shell, and Peony dispel internal heat in the liver. Astragalus, Ginseng, Cinnamon, Hoelen, and Licorice nourish the skin, spleen, and lungs. Aster is an antitussive and sedative which also nourishes the lungs. *Chin-chiu* and Lycium bark are refrigerants and antipyretics. Morus, Pinellia, and Platycodon are expectorants and antitussives.

Indications

Tuberculosis, chronic bronchitis, pneumonia, and chronic malaria.

Discrimination

Chin-chiu-fu-lei-tang (*Chin-chiu* and Bupleurum Combination): treats tubercular fever, even when symptoms of the chest change. Usually with no coughing and only rarely a fever.

Chin-chiu-pieh-chia-san (*Chin-chiu* and Tortoise Shell Formula):

tubercular fever, fever, and coughing.
Chai-hu-chiang-kuei-tang (Bupleurum, Cinnamon, and Ginger Combination): tubercular fever, diarrhea, and extreme thirst.
Mai-men-tung-tang (Ophiopogon Combination): tubercular fever, and spasmodic cough.

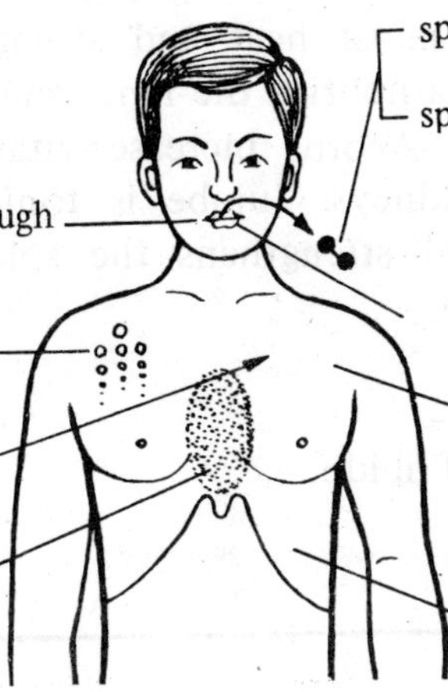

Huan-Shao-Tan *(Lycium Formula)*					還少丹
Acorus	1.2	Dioscorea	1.2	Achyranthes	1.2
Cornus	1.2	Polygala	1.2	Morinda	1.2
Schizandra	1.2	Cistanche	1.2	Broussonetia	1.2
Hoelen	1.2	Lycium	1.2	Rehmannia	1.2
Fennel	1.2	Eucommia	1.2	Jujube	4.0

Huan-shao-tan is a folk drug recorded in *Yung shih fang*. This is a tonic formula for improving the functions of the heart, kidneys, spleen, and stomach. It is good to increase vigor and to treat nocturnal emmission, loss of appetite, fever, night sweats, toothache, weakness, pain at the waist, fatigue, and uterine diseases.

Herbs and Actions
This formula is a nutritive. Cistanche, Morinda, and Fennel are good for the kidneys and spleen. Rehmannia and Lycium nourish the kidneys and increase vigor. Eucommia and Achyranthes help the waist and knees and strengthen the kidneys. Hoelen and Dioscorea remove moist heat and strengthen the spleen. Dioscorea and Schizandra nourish the lungs and correct nocturnal emission. Polygala and Acorus increase vitality and improve the function of the kidneys. Jujube is tonic and hematinic, nourishes the lungs and strengthens the spleen. Broussonetia is a nutritive.

Indications
Weakness and decrease of libido.

I-Chi-Chung-Ming-Tang 益氣聰明湯

(Ginseng, Astragalus and Pueraria Combination)

Astragalus	3.0	Ginseng	3.0	Pueraria	1.5
Vitex	1.5	Peony	1.0	Cimicifuga	1.0
Licorice	1.5	Phellodendron	1.0		

I-chi-chung-ming-tang, one of the ophthalmics, is recorded in *I fang chi chieh* (醫方集解) of the Ching dynasty. This formula is used for treating deafness, tinnitus, and dimness of vision in the initial stage of cataract. It is suitable for restoring visual and aural acuity, but is not effective in treating acute inflammation of ears and eyes.

Herbs and Actions
Ginseng and Astragalus are stimulants and tonics. Vitex, Cimicifuga, Pueraria, and Peony are effective for tic douloureux and act as antipyretics and sedatives. Phellodendron is an antiphlogistic

and detoxifying agent. Licorice nourishes the spleen and stomach.

Indications
Tinnitus, poor cerebral circulation, tic douloureux, and the primary stage of cataract.

Jen-Sheng-Yang-Yung-Tang 人參養榮湯

(Ginseng Nutritive Combination)

Ginseng	3.0	*Tang-kuei*	4.0	Peony	4.0
Rehmannia	4.0	Atractylodes	4.0	Hoelen	4.0
Cinnamon	2.5	Astragalus	2.5	Citrus	2.5
Polygala	1.5	Schizandra	1.5	Licorice	1.5

A basic principle of Chinese medicine is: "The superior physician prevents disease." Maintaining balanced activities of bodily functions is of prime importance in preventing disease and maintaining health. When bodily functions are weak, disease occurs. Nutritives should be given "to supplement the weak and to nourish the impaired." *Jen-sheng-yang-yung-tang* is a nutritive for weak vitality, anemia, and impaired viscera.
According to *Tai ping huei min ho chi chu fang*, the governmental dictionary of the Sung dynasty (1107-1110 A.D.), this formula may be used in treating chronic weakness, impaired viscera, thinness and paleness, fever and severe chills, general debility, marked tiredness, anorexia, mental instability, coughing and gasping, insomnia, night sweats, amnesia, diarrhea, and turbid urine.

Herbs and Actions
Ginseng, Astragalus, Atractylodes, Hoelen, Licorice and Citrus enhance vitality. *Tang-kuei* nourishes the liver; Rehmannia, the kidneys; Schizandra, the lungs; and Polygala, the heart. Cinnamon assists in the synergism of the herbs.

Indications

Various postpartum and post-illness weaknesses, (dry) tuberculosis, pleurisy, amnesia, nocturnal emission, impotence, constipation, and baldness.

Discrimination

Shih-chuan-ta-pu-tang (Ginseng and *Tang-kuei* Ten Combination); weakness of *ch'i* and blood, covert dryness and exhaustion of fluids.

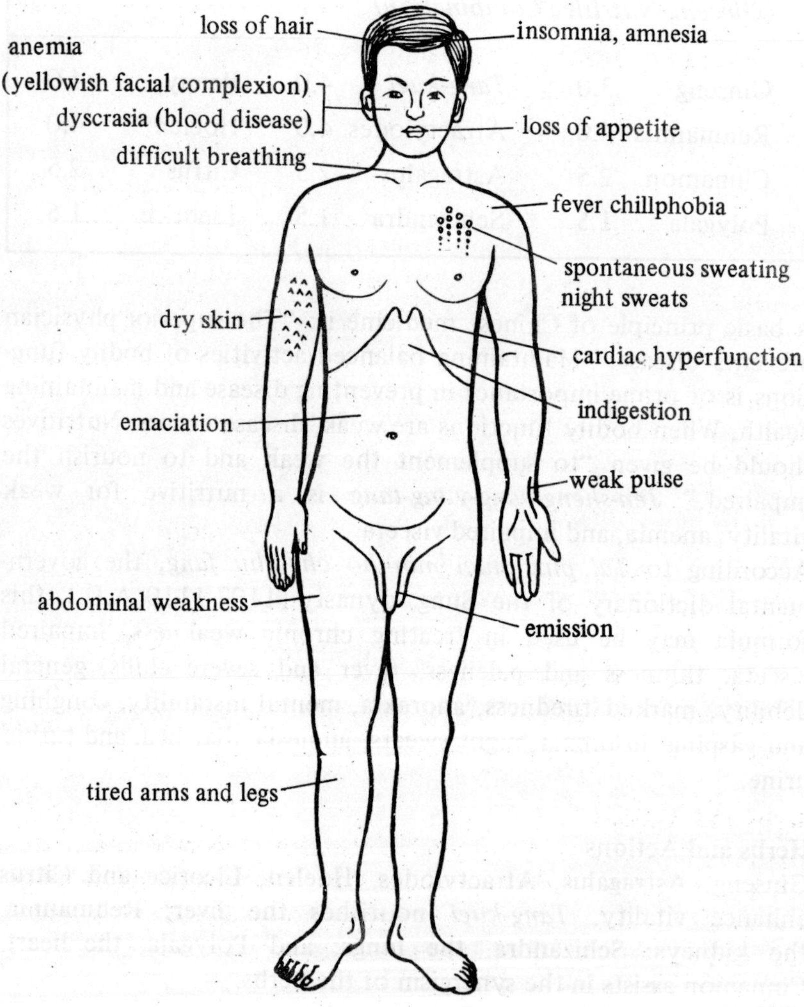

Jen-Sheng-Tang-Shao-San 人參當芍散

(Ginseng and Tang-kuei Formula)

Tang-kuei	3.0	Peony	3.0	Hoelen	3.0
Atractylodes	3.0	Alisma	3.0	Cnidium	2.5
Ginseng	3.0	Licorice	1.0	Cinnamon	1.5

Jen-sheng-tang-shao-san is a combination of *Tang-kuei-shao-yao-san* (*Tang-kuei* and Peony Formula) with Ginseng, Licorice, and Cinnamon. It is used for treating anemia. flushing up, vertigo, heaviness in the head, dizziness, aching shoulders, menstrual irregularity, and chills in the lower abdomen, waist, and feet.

Herbs and Actions

Tang-kuei is a hematinic, nutritive, and antianemic. Peony nourishes the blood and eases pain. Atractylodes dispels stagnant water. Cnidium nourishes the blood and regulates the *ch'i.* Hoelen and Alisma are diuretics. Cinnamon is effective for flushing up. Ginseng nourishes the spleen and stomach. Licorice is a tonic and stomachic.

Indications

Anemia, menstrual irregularity, infertility, leukorrhea, uteritis, neurasthenia, hysteria, gastroptosis, gastrospasm, edema, nephritis, renal atrophy, neuralgia, rheumatic pain, hemorrhoids, rectal prolapse, frostbite, acne, headache, vertigo, opthalmologic disorders, and ear disorders.

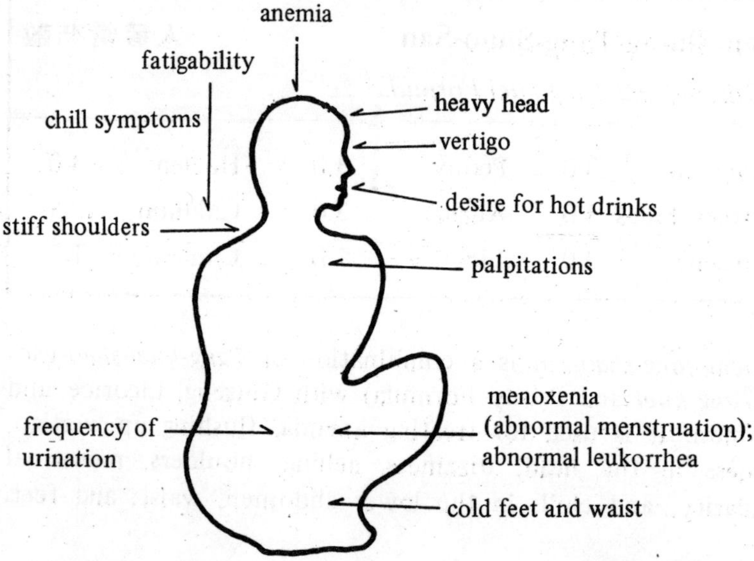

Liu-Chun-Tzu-Tang 六君子湯

(Six Major Herb Combination)

Ginseng	4.0	Atractylodes	4.0	Hoelen	4.0
Pinellia	4.0	Citrus	2.0	Ginger	2.0
Jujube	2.0	Licorice	1.0		

Recorded in the Chinese governmental medical dictionary of the Sung dynasty, *Tai ping huei min ho chi chu fang* (太平惠民和劑局方 1107-1110 A.D.). Treats gastrointestinal weakness with stagnant water in the stomach, indigestion, distention beneath the heart, loss of appetite, a tendency towards fatigue, loss of weight, anemia, a weak abdomen, a weak pulse, and cold hands and feet.

Herbs and Actions

Ginseng, Atractylodes, Licorice, and Hoelen nourish the stomach and intestines and improve the digestive functions. Citrus and

Ginseng increase the appetitie and dispel internal moisture in the stomach. Pinellia, Atractylodes, and Hoelen remove stagnant water from the stomach and increase gastrointestinal functioning.

Indications

Chronic gastritis, gastroptosis, gastric distention, gastric ulcer, gastric cancer, chronic peritonitis, indigestion, loss of appetite, rickets, neurotic vomiting, vomiting, toxemia of pregnancy, and nervous exhaustion.

Discrimination

Szu-chun-tzu-tang (Four Major Herb Combination): weak *ch'i* and sputum diseases; this formula aims at *ch'i* weakness as its main target.

Pan-hsia-hsieh-hsin-tang (Pinellia Combination): weakness of spleen and stomach, obstruction and hardness beneath the heart, firm conformation.

Weak conformation

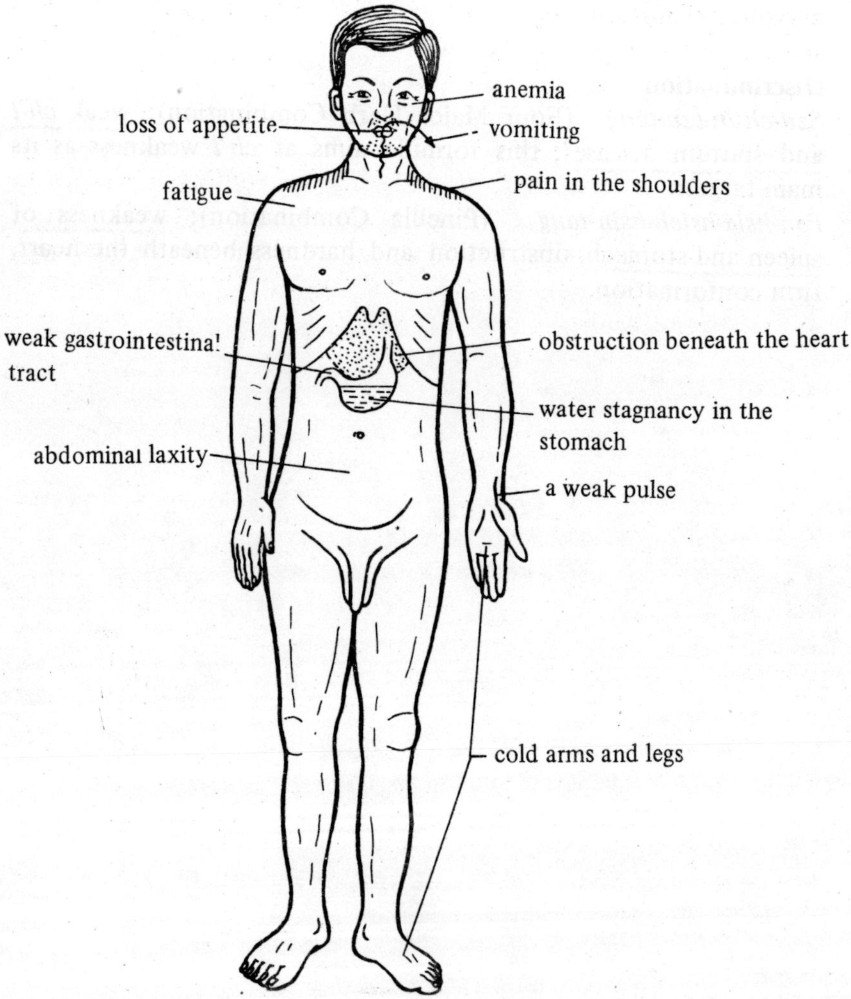

Liu-Wei-Ti-Huang-Wan 六味地黃丸

(Rehmannia Six Formula)

Cornus	3.0	Dioscorea	3.0	Alisma	3.0
Hoelen	3.0	Moutan	3.0	Rehmannia	6.0

In the Sung dynasty, Chein I (A.D. 1035-1117) removed Cinnamon and Aconite from *Pa-wei-ti-huang-wan* (Rehmannia Eight Formula) and formulated *Liu-wei-ti-huang-wan* for milder cases than those for which *Pa-wei-ti-huang-wan* was suitable. It is mainly for symptoms caused by weak kidneys such as flushing up of inner heart, dizziness, dry tongue and sore throat, diminshed hearing capacity, numbness and weakness at the waist and kness, pain in the heels, sweating and night sweats, nocturnal emission, and urinary incontinence.

Herbs and Actions

This formula is mainly for a yin deficiency. Rehmannia is a tonic for the kidneys and increases their blood volume. Cornus warms the liver and strengthens the kidneys. Moutan cools the blood and relieves heat. Dioscorea nourishes the spleen and strengthens the kidneys. Hoelen increases the flow of urine, reduces swelling, and removes moist heat of the spleen. Alisma is both a diuretic and a tonic for the ears and eyes.

Indications

Impotence, nocturnal emission, senility, diabetes, chronic nephritis, nephroatrophy, nocturia and muscular weakness.

Discrimination

Pa-*wei-ti-huang-wan* (Rehmannia Eight Formula): weakness of the kidneys, severe weakness of *ch'i* and blood.

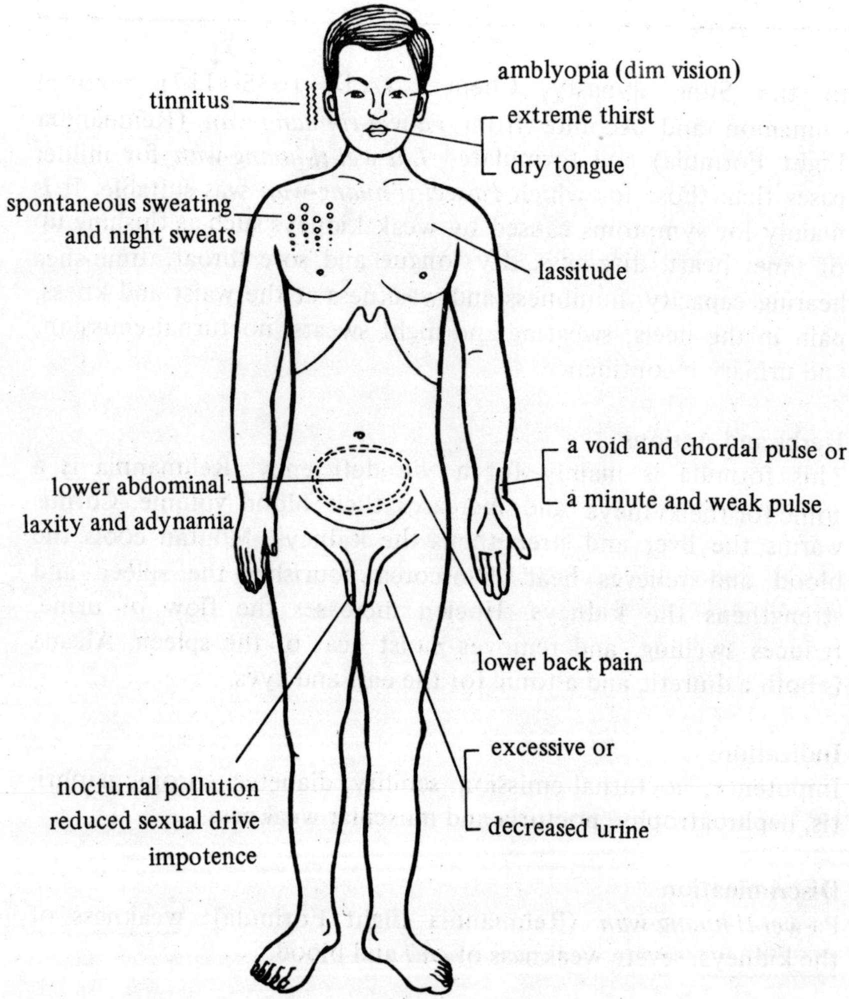
amblyopia (dim vision)
tinnitus
extreme thirst
dry tongue
spontaneous sweating
and night sweats
lassitude
a void and chordal pulse or
a minute and weak pulse
lower abdominal
laxity and adynamia
lower back pain
excessive or
decreased urine
nocturnal pollution
reduced sexual drive
impotence

Niu-Che-Shen-Chi-Wan 牛車腎氣丸

(Achyranthes and Plantago Formula)

Rehmannia	5.0	Cornus	3.0	Dioscorea	3.0
Alisma	3.0	Hoelen	3.0	Moutan	3.0
Cinnamon	1.0	Aconite	0.5	Achyranthes	3.0
Plantago	3.0				

Niu-che-shen-chi-wan is recorded in *Chi sheng fang* (濟生方) by Yen Yung-ho of the Sung dynasty. This formula is a combination of *Pa-wei-ti-huang-wan* (Rehmannia Eight Formula) with Achyranthes and Plantago. It is used for treating symptoms which are similar to those of *Pa-wei-ti-huang-wan* with edema, marked dysuria, weakness of the spleen and kidneys, abdominal distention, edema in the arms and legs, asthma, copious sputum, urine of deep color, and thirst.

Herbs and Actions

Rehmannia is a tonic, nourishes the kidneys, removes internal heat, nourishes the blood, and relieves dryness. Cornus is an aphrodisiac, and it strengthens the waist and knees. Dioscorea increases the "*ch'i*", removes "weak heat", and nourishes the skin. Hoelen dispels "stagnant water" in the stomach and, in combination with Alisma, it can increase the flow of urine. Moutan dispels stagnant blood in the Lower Warmer and improves metabolism. Cinnamon coordinates with Rehmannia to improve blood circulation, and with Hoelen to increase the flow of urine and arrest flushing up. Aconite increases vitality. Achyranthes and Plantago are diuretics and tonics.

Indications

Nephritis, renal calculi, nephrotuberculosis, albuminuria, anuria, enuresis, arteriosclerosis, hypertension, hypotension, prostatomegaly, diabetes, sciatica, beriberi, cerebral hemorrhage, nervous exhaustion, amnesia, nocturnal emission, skin disease, eye ailments, and ear disorders.

Discrimination
Please refer to the section on *Pa-wei-ti-huang-wan*

Pa-Chen-Tang 八珍湯
(Tang-kuei and Ginseng Eight Combination)

Tang-kuei	3.0	Rehmannia	3.0	Cnidium	3.0
Hoelen	3.0	Atractylodes	3.0	Licorice	1.5
Peony	3.0	Ginseng	3.0	Jujube	1.5
Ginger	3.0				

According to the medical dictionaries of the Ming dynasty (1368-1628), *Wan ping hui chun* and *Cheng chih chuen sheng, Pa-chen-tang* is used to treat anemia and lack of vitality, liver and spleen weakness, underweight, severe chills and fever, thirst or dizziness, coarseness of the skin, general weakness during convalescence, anorexia, lower abdominal distention, degeneration of the circulatory and digestive organs and metrorrhagia during childbirth.

Herbs and Actions
This formula is a combination of *Szu-wu-tang* (*Tang-kuei* Four Combination) and *Szu-chun-tzu-tang* (Four Major Herb Combination).
The *Tang-kuei,* Rehmannia, Peony, and Cnidium in *Szu-wu-tang* are hematinics. *Tang-kuei* and Rehmannia increase the amount of hemoglobin and the number of red corpuscles in the blood and have calmative and nutritive effects. Peony and Cnidium dispel extravasated blood and promote blood circulation. The Ginseng, Atracytlodes, Hoelen, and Licorice in *Szu-chun-tzu-tang* are moderate tonics. Ginseng and Atractylodes are stomachics, while Hoelen and Licorice are splenotonics; the four together promote sound digestive functions.

Indications
Weakness during convalescence, anemia, midline pain in women,

menstrual irregularity, and circulatory ailments.

Discrimination
Shih-chuan-ta-pu-tang (Ginseng and *Tang-kuei* Ten Combination): anemia, generalized weakness, gastrointestinal weakness, loss of appetite, coarse skin, no fever.
Pa-wei-ti-huang-wan (Rehmannia Eight Formula): annoyance and thirst, "blood fever", "blood weakness", and weakness and insufficiency of *ch'i*.

Weakness in both the vitality and the blood

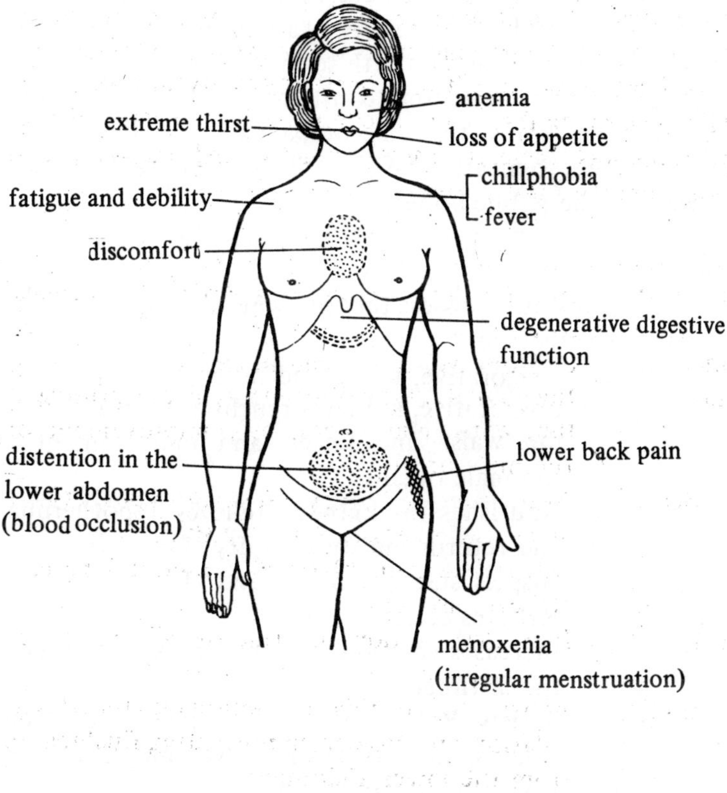

Pa-Wei-Ti-Huang-Wan 八味地黃丸

(Rehmannia Eight Formula)

Rehmannia	5.0	Cinnamon	1.0	Aconite	1.0
Hoelen	3.0	Dioscorea	3.0	Alisma	3.0
Moutan	3.0	Cornus	3.0		

Chin kuei yao lueh (A.D. 205), an old Chinese medical dictionary of the Han dynasty, records that *Pa-wei-ti-huang-wan* may be used for numbness, beriberi, stagnant water in the stomach, diabetes, and gynecological diseases. This formula actually reactivates the functions of degenerated kidneys, adrenals, and reproductive organs, and it is effective as a preventive and remedy for senility. It is given to patients with severe fatigue and lassitude, sluggish gastrointestinal funciton, constipation, dysuria or polyuria, cold or warm limbs, thirst accompanied by a dry tongue, lumbago, weakness beneath the umbilicus, and hardness and tenseness around the public bones.

Herbs and Actions

The herbs in this formula possess the following astringent, hematinic, and nutritive activities:

Rehmannia . . . Invigorative, tonic, and nutritive.

Cornus . . . . . . Invigorative, kidney-strenghtening, warming at the waist and knees, and improvement of the male organ.

Dioscorea . . . . Nourishes the kidneys, relieves hypothermia, and returns moisture to dry skin.

Moutan . . . . . . Dispels stagnant blood and alleviates pain.

Hoelen . . . . . . Relieves ascites.

Alisma . . . . Increases the flow of urine and alleviates continual thirst.

Cinnamon . . . . Assists Rehmannia in improving blood circulation and Hoelen in preventing flushing up from the lower abdomen.

Aconite . . . . . . Increases body temperature, reactivates the functions of degenerated organs, and is diuretic when combined with Hoelen and Cinnamon.

Indications

1. Nephritis, (nephrosclerosis, nephrolithiasis, nephrotuberculosis), pyelitis, (nephro-atrophy), albuminuria, and edema.
2. Cystitis, cystolithiases, cysto-tuberculosis, senile cysto-atrophy, prostatomegaly, dysuria, urinary incontinence, and nocturia.
3. Diabetes and urinary incontinence.
4. Cerebral hemorrhage, arteriosclerosis, hypertension, and hypotension.
5. Neurasthenia, amnesia, nocturnal emmission, uncontrolled emission, impotence, and inappropriate erection of penis.
6. Lumbago, sciatica, deformed vertebra, numbness of the legs, and beriberi.
7. Cataract, glaucoma, decrease of eyesight, and keratitis.
8. Eczema, tinea, senile itching, vaginal itching, dry skin, and urticaria.
9. Chronic gonorrhea, rectoptosis, climacteric disturbance, and related disorders.

Note: Patients having chronic gastrointestinal weakness, frequent diarrhea, marked ascites, and facial flushing with fever should not take this formula.

Discrimination

Hsiao-chien-chung-tang (Minor Cinnamon and Peony Combination): fatigability, excessive urine, and tension in the rectus abdominis muscle of the upper abdomen.
Kuei-chih-chia-lung-ku-mu-li-tang (Cinnamon and Dragon Bone Combination): lower torso weakness, excessive urine, abdominal *ch'i*, chordal pulsation.
San-wu-huang-chin-tang (Scute Three Herb Combination): distress and fever, annoying fever in the arms and legs and the soles of the feet.
Wen-ching-tang (*Tang-kuei* and Evodia Combination): distress and fever, irritating fever in the palms, dry mouth and lips.
Chu-ling-tang (Polyporus Combination): extreme thirst, frequent urination, pain after urinating.

Chu-yeh-shih-kao-tang (Bamboo Leaf and Gypsum Combination): annoying thirst, massive and big pulse, normal urination.
Shih-chuan-ta-pu-tang (Ginseng and *Tang-kuei* Ten Combination): irritation and fever in the palms and feet, fatigability, weakness, absence of abdominal muscle tone.
Chih-kan-tsao-tang (Baked Licorice Combination): similar to a *Hsiao-chien-chung-tang* conformation; irritation and fever in the palms and feet, dry mouth, gasping, knotty and irregular pulse or disorderly pulse, and constipation.

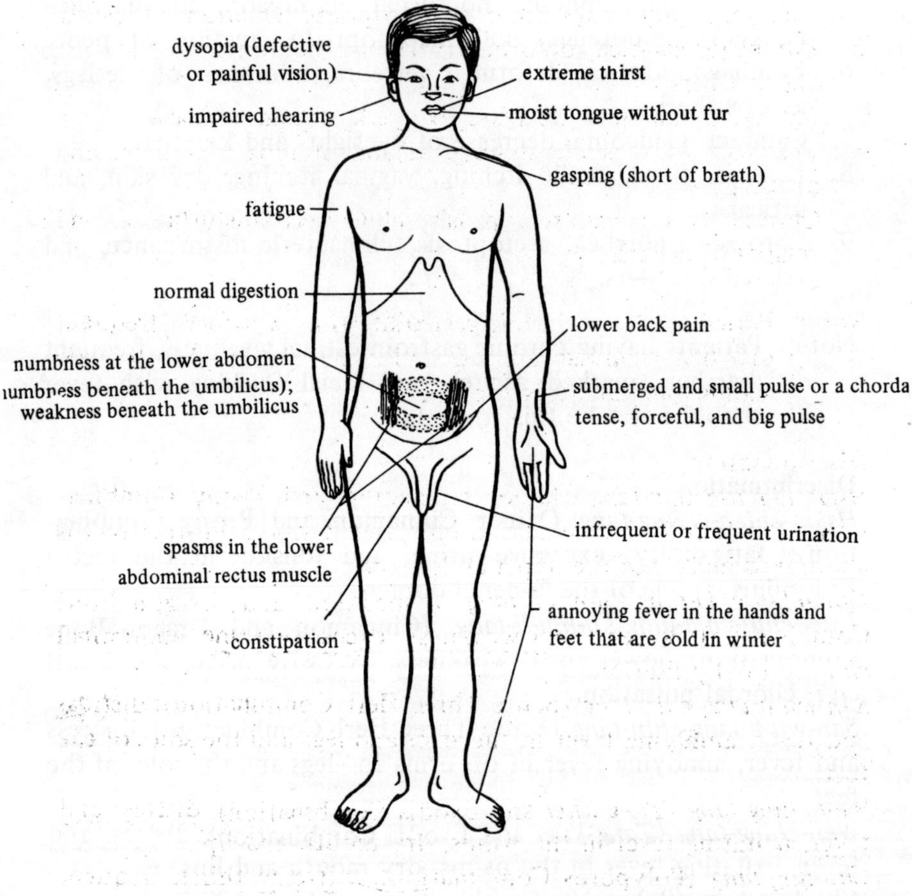

Pai-Ho-Ku-Chin-Tang 百合固金湯

(Lily Combi

Lily	4.0	Peony	3.0	*Tang-kuei*	4.0
Fritillaria	3.0	Licorice	0.5	Rehmannia	4.0
Ophiopogon	6.0	Figwort	3.0	Platycodon	2.0

Pai-ho-ku-chin-tang is a formula created by Chao Chi-an and recorded in the *I fang chi chieh* (醫方集解) during the Ching dynasty. This formula is a tonic, antipyretic, and expectorant which also nourishes the lungs and kidneys. It is used to alleviate pain in the throat, coughing, hemoptysis, stress fever in the hands and feet, red tongue with little coating, and a rapid pulse.

Herbs and Actions
Lily nourishes the lungs and restores mental stability. Ophiopogon is an antipyretic. Figwort and Rehmannia nourish the blood. Fritillaria dispels "internal heat" in the lungs and is used as an expectorant. *Tang-kuei* and Peony nourish the blood and lungs. Licorice and Platycodon remove "internal heat" in the lungs and dispel sputum.

Indications
Pharyngitis, hoarseness, hemoptysis, coughing, and wheezing.

Pan-Hsieh-Liu-Chun-Tzu-Tang 半瀉六君子湯

(Pinellia and Ginseng Six Combination)

Ginseng	3.0	Atractylodes	3.0	Hoelen	3.0
Licorice	2.0	Pinellia	3.0	Citrus	3.0
Ginger	3.0	Scute	3.0	Coptis	3.0
Oyster shell	3.0				

Pan-hsieh-liu-chun-tzu-tang is a combination of *Pan-hsia-hsieh-hsin-tang* (Pinellia Combination) and *Liu-chun-tzu-tang* (Six Major Herb Combination), and is used for general gastrointestinal disorders. Most lingering gastrointestinal disorders become chronic and may be aggravated by overwork, insufficient sleep, and an imbalanced diet.

Herbs and Actions

Pinellia, Scute, Coptis, Ginger, Ginseng, and Licorice of the *Pan-hsia-hsieh-hsin-tang* formula are effective for subcardiac distention, vomiting, anorexia, borborygmus, diarrhea, and ascites. Ginseng, Atractylodes, Hoelen, Licorice, Pinellia, and Citrus in the *Liu-chun-tzu-tang* formula are effective for gastrointestinal weakness, ascites, subcardiac distention, anorexia, chills, anemia, and a tendency to become fatigued.

Indications

Acute and chronic gastroenteritis, gastric ulcer, duodenal ulcer, gastroptosis, ptosis of the internal organs, abdominal distention, dyspepsia, and diarrhea.

Pu-Chung-I-Chi-Tang 補中益氣湯

(Ginseng and Astragalus Combination)

Astragalus	4.0	Ginseng	4.0	Licorice	1.5
Atractylodes	4.0	Citrus	2.0	*Tang-kuei*	3.0
Cimicifuga	1.0	Bupleurum	2.0	Ginger	2.0
Jujube	2.0				

Pu-chung-i-chi-tang is recorded in the *Nei wai shang pien huo Lun* (內外傷辨惑論) by Li Kao of the Yuan dynasty. This formula is used for treating a weak pulse, general fatigue, mild fever, anorexia, headache, night sweats, decreased gastrointestinal function, and palpitation at the umbilicus.

Herbs and Actions

Ginseng and Astragalus nourish the lungs and act as antihydrotics. Ginseng and Licorice nourish the spleen and the stomach and increase vitality. Atractylodes and Citrus improve the functioning of the spleen and stomach. *Tang-kuei* nourishes the blood and, in combination with Astragalus, nourishes the skin. Bupleurum and Cimicifuga are antipyretics. Ginger and Jujube coordinate the actions of the other herbs.

Indications

Improvement of a delicate constitution, common cold in those with a delicate constitution, peritonitis, tuberculosis, gastroptosis, anorexia, abdominal distention, loss of weight during the summer, neurasthenia, impotence, uterine prolapse, hemorrhoids, rectal prolapse, monoplegia, ephidrosis, hernia, chronic,gonorrhea, diarrhea, persistent malaria, suppuration, and hemorrhage.

Discrimination

Hsiao-chai-hu-tang (Minor Bupleurum Combination): mild fever, thoraco-costal distress, alternating chills and fever, mild firmness conformation, and chordal pulse.

Chai-hu-chiang-kuei-tang (Bupleurum, Cinnamon, and Ginger Combination): mild fever, mild distress, abdominal palpitations, night sweats, mild weakness conformation, thin pulse.
Chia-wei-hsiao-yao-san (Bupleurum and Peony Formula): mild fever, mild distress, swelling in the abdomen, blood and mild weakness conformation.
Shih-chuan-ta-pu-tang (Ginseng and *Tang-kuei* Ten Combination): generalized weakness, dry skin, discharge of semen, anemia.
Tzu-yin-chiang-huo-tang (Phellodendron Combination): yin-weakness conformation, poor complexion, hoarse voice, thin and quick pulse.
Chen-wu-tang (Vitality Combination): cold hands and feet, generalized weakness, diarrhea.

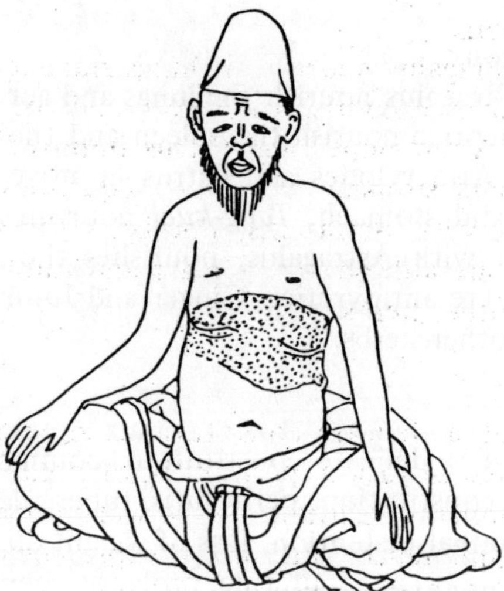

Weak conformation

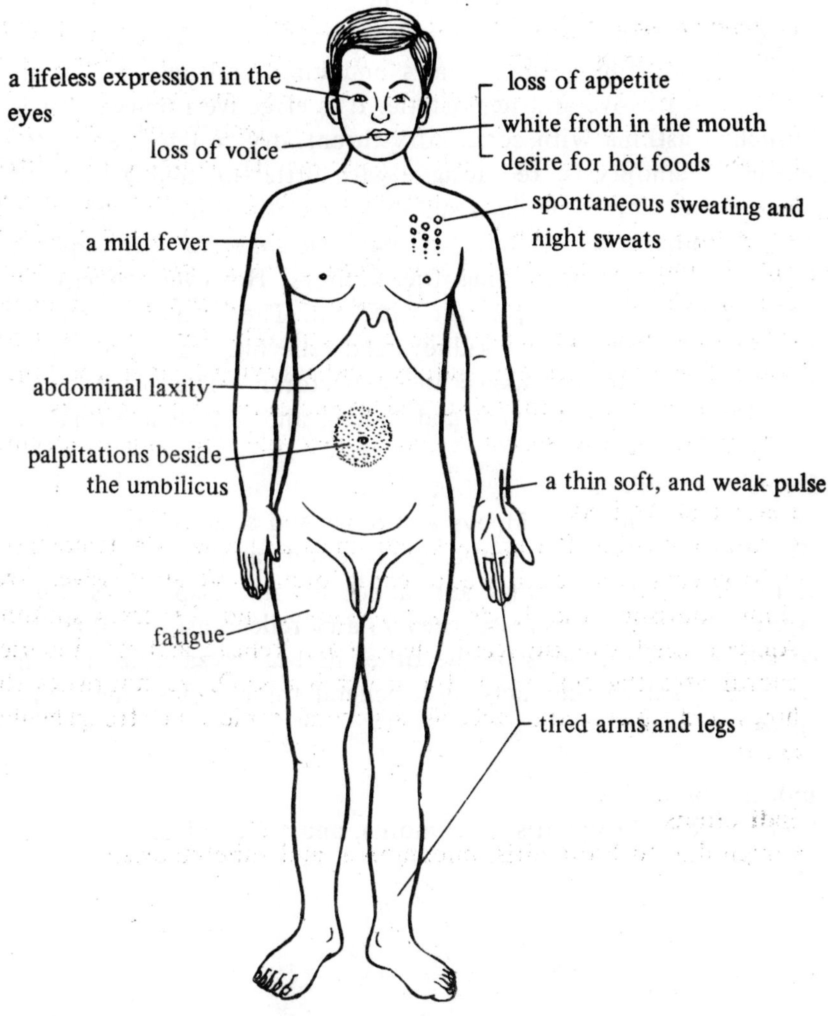

Pu-Fei-Ah-Chiao-Tang 補肺阿膠湯

(Gelatin and Aristolochia Combination)

Gelatin	9.0	Aristolochia	9.0	Arctium	9.0
Licorice	6.0	Apricot seed	6.0	Oryza	15.0

Pu-fei-ah-chiao-tang is recorded in *Hsiao erh yao cheng chih chueh* (小兒藥證直訣) of the Sung dynasty. This formula is used for nourishing the kidneys and lungs and acts as an antipyretic, antitussive and hemostatic. It is effective for weak lungs, bronchial asthma with cough, dry throat, dry cough due to little sputum, hemoptysis, red tongue with little fur, and a thin and quick pulse. This formula is suitable for both adults and children. This formula is as effective as *Mai-men-tung-tang* (Ophiopogon Combination) in nourishing the kidneys. However, therapeutically, their basic principles are different. The former is used for nourishing the lungs and kidneys and relieving heat in the lungs; it also acts as an antitussive and expectorant. The latter is used for nourishing the stomach and kidney and acts as a stomachic.

Herbs and Actions

Gelatin nourishes the kidneys and lungs and acts as a hemostatic. Aristolochia is an antipyretic, expectorant, and antitussive. Arctium nourishes the lungs and abdomen and disperses sputum. Apricot seed can decrease the *ch'i* and relieve asthma. Licorice coordinates the actions of the other herbs. Oryza nourishes the lungs and spleen and acts as a general tonic and strengthening agent.

Indications

Cough due to bronchitis, pneumonia, and tuberculosis.

Pu-Yin-Tang 補陰湯

(Tang-kuei and Rehmannia Combination)

Ginseng	2.0	Peony	2.0	Citrus	2.0
Achyranthes	2.0	Psoralea	2.0	Eucommia	2.0
Tang-kuei	3.0	Hoelen	3.0	Fennel	1.0
Anemarrhena	1.0	Raw rehmannia	1.0	Licorice	1.0
Phellodendron	1.0	Cured rehmannia	1.0		

Pu-yin-tang is recorded in *Wan ping hui chun* (萬病回春) of the Ming dynasty. This formula is used for treating low back pain. It is suitable for slack constitution, dry skin, low back pain when arising from a sitting position, weak pulse and abdomen, and renal weakness.

Herbs and Actions

Tang-kuei, Peony, and Rehmannia nourish the kidneys and improve the blood circulation. Ginseng and Hoelen increase the vitality and strengthen the heart. Anemarrhena and Phellodendron both nourish and dispel inflammation in the kidneys Achyranthes nourishes the kidneys and relieves low back pain. Psoralea is an aphrodisiac and treats lumbago. Fennel with Eucommia is an analgesic. Citrus regulates the *ch'i.* Licorice coordinates the actions of the other herbs.

Indications

Lumbago, sciatica, spinal cord inflammation, chronic nephritis, hernia, and ephidrosis.

Discrimination

Pa-wei-wan (Rehmannia Eight Formula): lower back pain, numbness beneath the umbilicus, annoying fever in the hands and feet, and extreme thirst.
Ling-chiang-chu-kan-tang (Ginger and Hoelen Combination): lower back pain, chilling pain, palpitations beneath the heart.

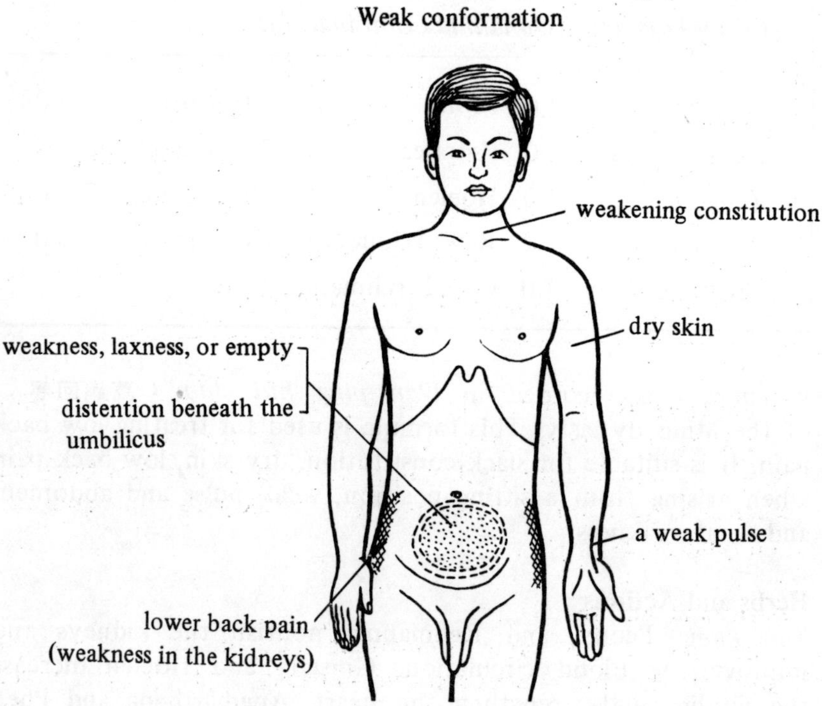

Sheng-Ling-Pai-Chu-San 參苓白朮散

(Ginseng and Atractylodes Formula)

Ginseng	3.0	Dolichos	4.0	Atractylodes	3.0
Hoelen	3.0	Dioscorea	1.5	Lotus seed	4.0
Coix	5.0	Cardamon	2.0	Platycodon	2.0
Licorice	1.5				

Sheng-ling-pai-chu-san is listed as a nutritive in a Chinese governmental medical dictionary of Sung dynasty, *Tai ping huei ming ho chi chu fang* (A.D. 1107-1110). This formula is used to treat gastrointestinal weakness, loss of appetite, watery diarrhea, weak pulse and abdomen, anemia, tendencies towards fatigue and chills, abdominal distention, borborygmus, and severe fatigue during convalescence.

Herbs and Actions

Ginseng, Atractylodes, Licorice, and Hoelen of *Szu-chun-tzu-tang* (Four Major Herb Combination) nourish the spleen. Dolichos, Hoelen, Dioscorea, Lotus seed, and Coix nourish the spleen and stomach. Cardamon acts as a diuretic and improves stomach function. Platycodon nourishes the stomach and cures diarrhea.

Indications

Chronic gastroenteritis, chronic diarrhea, intestinal tuberculosis, indigestion, gastroptosis, anorexia during convalescence, leukorrhea, and uterine bleeding.

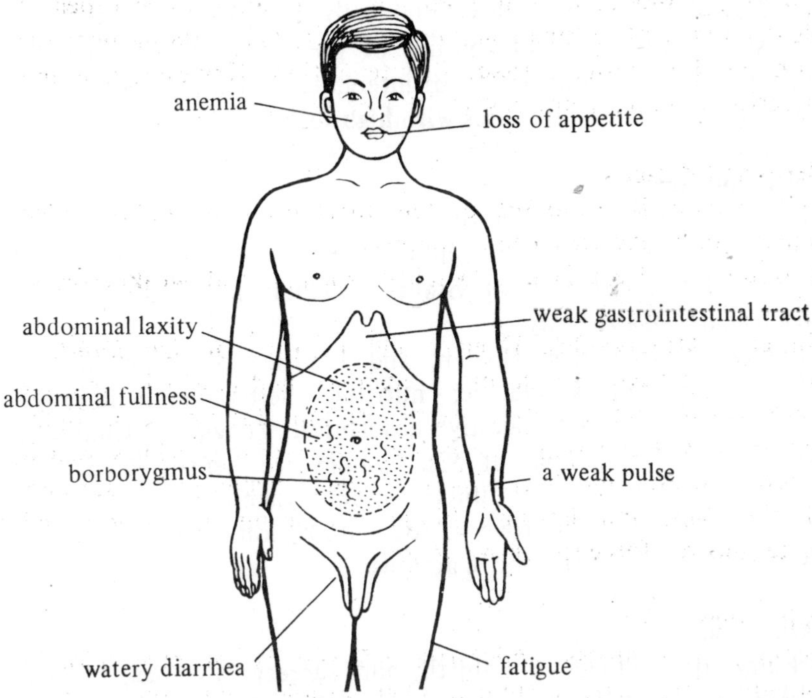

Shih-Chuan-Ta-Pu-Tang 十全大補湯

(Ginseng and Tang-kuei Ten Combination)

Ginseng	3.0	Astragalus	3.0	Atractylodes	3.0
Peony	3.0	Hoelen	3.0	Rehmannia	3.0
Tang-kuei	3.0	Cnidium	3.0	Cinnamon	3.0
Licorice	1.0				

This formula was first recorded in the revised *Tai ping huei min ho chi chu fang,* medical dictionary of the Sung dynasty, (A.D. 1107-1110) by Chen Shih-wen and Pei Chung-yuan. It can cure men as well as women with debilities due to various causes, anorexia, decreased gastrointestinal function, underweight, weakness due to prolonged disease, remittent fever, muscle spasm, coarse skin, nocturnal emission, pallor, weak knees, anxiety, and loss of blood. It is also suitable for treating three types of ulcers: (1) with a small amount of pus; (2) without pus; (3) with pus but without tissue disintergration. However, it is not effective in severe, acute cases with high fever.

Herbs and Actions

This formula is composed of ten different herbs and is called Ginseng and *Tang-kuei* Ten Combination.

It is used to treat lack of vitality, anemia, and weaknesses in various parts of the body.

Ginseng, Atractylodes, Hoelen, and Licorice of *Szu-chun-tzu-tang* are potent stomachic, nutritive herbs which improve anorexia and increase digestive absorption. *Tang-kuei*, Cnidium, Peony, and Rehmannia of *Szu-wu-tang* are hematinics which improve cardiac and liver functions, cure anemia and coarseness of the skin, and improve blood circulation. Cinnamon and Astragalus reinforce the above actions.

Indications

Debility after illness, childbirth, and surgery; anemias, bloody dysentery, malaria, carbuncle, hemorrhoidal bleeding, caries, scrofula, leukemia, nocturnal emission and rectocele; nephrophthisis, osteophthisis, decreased eyesight, chilblain, uterine carcinoma, menopause, postpartum beriberi, poliomyelitis, skin diseases, and auricular ailments.

Discrimination

Kuei-chi-chien-chung-tang (*Tang-kuei,* Astragalus, and Peony Combination): fatigability, anemia and mild dryness. This formula was known as *Shih-chuan-ta-pu-tang* in ancient times.

Pa-chen-tang (*Tang-kuei* and Ginseng Eight Combination): weakness in both *ch'i* and blood. Given to patients with a relatively higher temperature than *Shih-chuan-ta-pu-tang.*

Pu-chung-i-chi-tang (Ginseng and Astragalus Combination): fatigability, severe *ch'i* weakness, mild blood weakness.

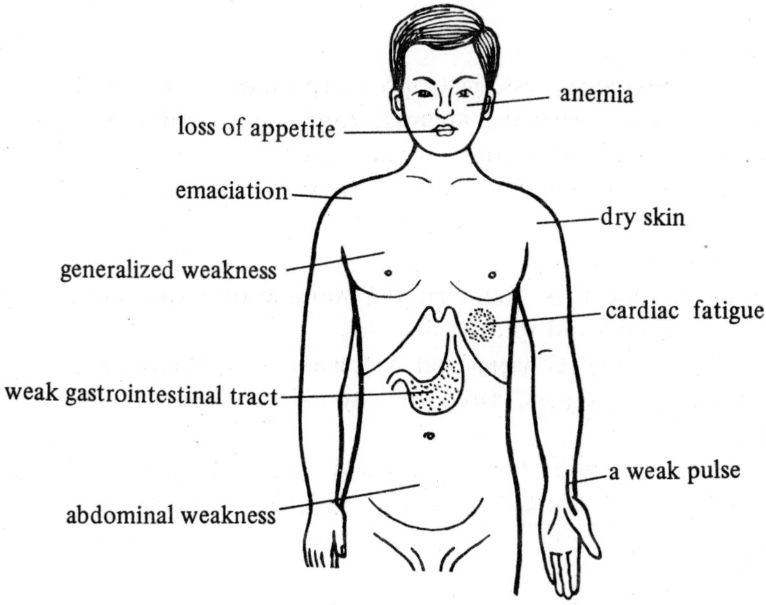

Szu-Chun-Tzu-Tang 四君子湯

(Four Major Herb Combination)

Ginseng	4.0	Atractylodes	4.0	Hoelen	4.0
Licorice	1.5				

Recorded in *Tai ping huei min ho chi chu fang* (太平惠民和劑局方) of the Sung dynasty. Used for treating gastrointestinal weakness, loss of appetite, vomiting, borborygmus (gas), diarrhea, weak abdomen, pallid complexion, and weakness of the arms and legs.

Herbs and Actions

Ginseng nourishes the spleen and stomach. Atractylodes removes stagnant water collected in the stomach. Hoelen also dispels stagnant water in the stomach. Licorice coordinates the actions of the other herbs.

Indications

Gastrointestinal weakness, gastroptosis (prolapse of the stomach), gastric flaccidity, gastritis, anemia, vomiting, diarrhea, bleeding, weak conformation bleeding, weak hands and feet, monoplegia (partial paralysis), and enuresis (involuntary urination).

Discrimination

Liu-chun-tzu-tang (Six Major Herb Combination): the spleen and stomach weakness and sputum diseases.

Pu-chung-i-chi-tang (Ginseng and Astragalus Combination): spleen and stomach weakness, tired and weak hands and feet, generalized fever.

Hsiang-sha-liu-chun-tzu-tang (Saussurea and Cardamon Combination): spleeen and stomach weakness, indigestion, and congestion.

Weak conformation

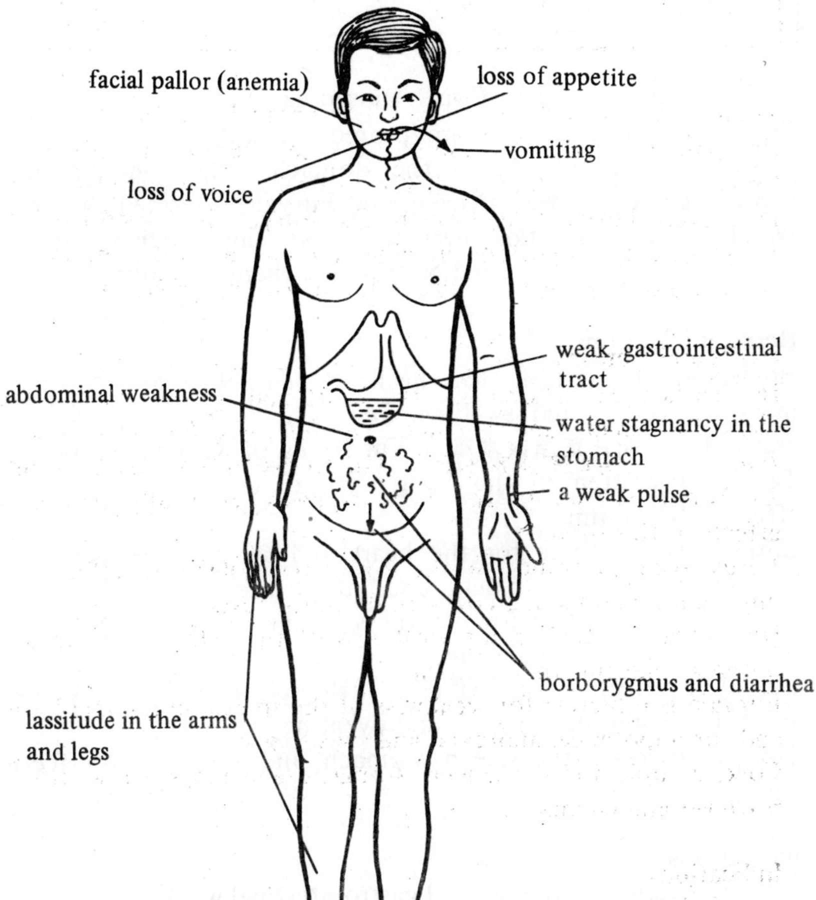

Szu-Shen-Tang 四神湯

(Dioscorea Combination)

Dioscorea	2-4	Lotus seed	2-4	Hoelen	2-4
Euryale	2-4	Coix	2-4		

Chinese herbs such as Coix, Dioscorea, Lotus seed, Euryale, Rehmannia, and dendrobium promote vitality and are used as tonics for the spleen and the stomach. The combination of Dioscorea, Lotus seed, Hoelen, and Euryale is termed the "Four Wonders", an important nervine known since ancient times. It is especially effective for indigestion in asthenic children.

Herbs and Actions

Hoelen is used as tonic for the heart and spleen and as a treatment for edema and swelling. *Ta ming jih hua chu chia pen tsao* (大明日華諸家本草 , On Herbs of Various Schools by Ta Ming) written in the Sung dynasty especially stresses the effects of this tonic.

Lotus seed, a tonic for the heart and spleen, is effective for impotence, anorexia, anxiety, and "moist fever".

Dioscorea is effective for weakness of the spleen and lungs, impotence, phlegm, and diarrhea.

Euryale is effective for weakness of the spleen, lungs, and kidneys and for impotence, anorexia, and sweating.

Coix, a tonic for the spleen, stomach, and lungs is also effective for fever and edema.

Indications

Indigestion, anorexia, and gastrointestinal weakness.

Tang-Kuei-Pu-Hsieh-Tang 當歸補血湯

(Tang-kuei and Astragalus Combination)

Astragalus 30.0 *Tang-kuei* 6.0

Recorded in *I fang chi chieh* (醫方集解 A Collection and Explanation of Medical Formulas). Indications are weakness of both blood and *ch'i*, flushed face and red eyes, dry and feverish skin, distress, and thirst. It is also effective for symptoms occurring after delivery or rupture of an abscess, such as blood weakness with a fever and a large but weak pulse that becomes minute when heavily pressed.

The body is cool when the blood is firm and healthy and becomes feverish when the blood is weak and empty. This formula treats yin blood that has been injured by starvation, continual overeating, or the weariness from over working. Manifestations are muscular fever, the distress and thirst of *Pai-hu-tang* (Gypsum Combination). *Tang-kuei-pu-hsieh-tang's* conformation is similar to that of *Pai-hu-tang. Pai-hu-tang* conformation is contracted externally and has an internal, thriving firm fever causing a large and forceful pulse. The conformation for this formula, however, is an internal injury that has blood weakness with fever and a large but forceless pulse. The distinction can only be done clinically.

Herbs and Actions

Tang-kuei is sweet in taste, strong in odor, and capable of nourishing the yin and stimulating the production of blood. Astragalus is sweet in taste, mild in odor, and capable of supplementing and benefiting the yang *ch'i* (outward vitality). This formula contains five times as much Astragalus as *Tang-kuei* and is said to have the same hemapoeitic quality, which is the main function of *Tang-kuei.* Blood cannot reproduce itself. It requires the warmth of yang *ch'i*, like sunshine, for nourishment. Thus it is said, "The yin grows as long as the yang grows."

Indications

Nourishing the *ch'i* (vitality) and stimulating the production of blood.

Weak conformation

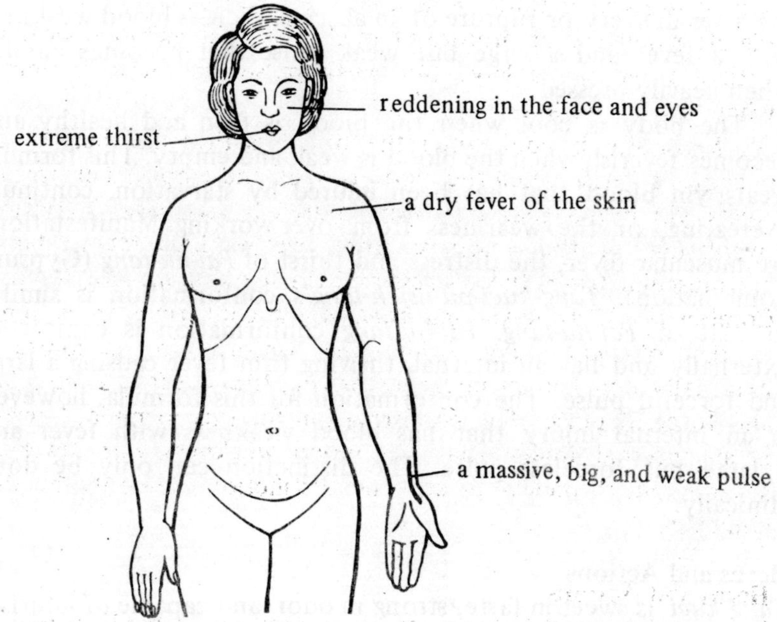

Tang-Kuei-Sheng-Chiang-Yang-Zou-Tang 當歸生薑羊肉湯

(Tnag-kuei, Ginger, and Mutton Combination)

Tang-kuei	18	Ginger	30	Mutton	240

Recorded in *Chin kuei yao lueh* (金匱要略). Alleviates abdominal pain resulting from blood weakness with chills. The main symptom is abdominal cramping with continuous aching in the abdomen. The patient desires warmth and pressure (with his hands) on his stomach. This formula also treats chill hernia, wasting diseases, and general weakness.

Herbs and Actions

Tang-kuei enriches the blood and kills pain. Mixed with Ginger it warms the insides and disperses chills. Used in large quantities mutton warms the insides and supplements weakness. The combination of these components warms the insides, enriches the blood, disperses chills, and kills pain.

Indications

All blood weaknesses with chill symptoms, symptoms exhibiting "chill hernia" with abdominal pain, postpartum abdominal pain, phthisis with insufficiency.

Tien-Wang-Pu-Hsin-Tan 天王補心丹

(Ginseng and Zizyphus Formula)

Rehmannia	1.2	Ginseng	1.2	Scrophularia	1.2
Salvia	1.2	Hoelen	1.2	Platycodon	1.2
Polygala	1.2	Biota	1.2	Asparagus	1.2
Ophiopogon	1.2	*Tang-kuei*	1.2	Schizandra	1.2
Acorus	1.2	Cinnabar	1.2	Zizyphus	1.2
Coptis	1.2				

Tien-wang-pu-hsin-tan was recorded in the *Shih i te hsiao* (世醫得效) by Wei I-lin of the Yuan dynasty. This formula is used for treating anemia, congestion emotional instability, palpitation, amnesia, ephidrosis, constipation, stomatitis, insufficient tongue-coating, and a rapid pulse.

Herbs and Actions
Rehmannia and Scrophularia, the major herbs in this formula, act as antipyretics. Salvia and *Tang-kuei* nourish the blood. Ginseng and Hoelen nourish the heart. Schizandra nourishes the heart. Asparagus dispels "internal heat". Ophiopogon improves metabolism. Biota dispels stagnant *ch'i.* Zizyphus nourishes the blood. Polygala improves mental disposition. Platycodon dispels "internal heat" of the liver. Cinnabar is an antipyretic and sedative. Acorus is an expectorant.

Indications
Neurasthenia, palpitation, insomnia, nocturnal emission, night sweats, amnesia, and emotional instability.
Note: Those having gastrointestinal weakness with moist, tenacious sputum should avoid taking this formula.

Tzu-Sheng-Tung-Erh-Tang 滋腎通耳湯

(Scute Combination)

Tang-kuei	3.0	Cnidium	3.0	Peony	3.0
Anemarrhena	3.0	Rehmannia	3.0	Scute	3.0
Phellodendron	3.0	Bupleurum	3.0	Angelica	3.0
Cyperus	3.0				

Tzu-sheng-tung-erh-tang was recorded in the *Wan ping hui chun* (萬病回春) during the Ming dynasty. This formula is used for treating tinnitus and hearing difficulty due to nephrasthenia. It is suitable for elderly patients.

Herbs and Actions

Tang-kuei, Cnidium, Peony, and Rehmannia are in the *Szu-wu-tang* (四物湯) formula (*Tang-kuei* Four Combination). They nourish the yin and improve blood circulation. Anemarrhena and Phellodendron supply nutrients for yin and dispel "internal heat" in the kidneys. Angelica coordinates the actions of the other herbs in the upper body. Cyperus and Bupleurum dispel "internal heat" in the liver. Scute is an antipyretic and antiphlogistic.

Indications

Deafness, otitis media, deafness in the elderly, and the initial stages of drug-induced deafness.

Tsu-Shih-Ti-Huang-Wan 磁石地黃丸

(Loadstone and Rehmannia Formula)

Rehmannia	6.0	Cornus	3.0	Dioscorea	3.0
Moutan	3.0	Hoelen	3.0	Alisma	3.0
Loadstone	1.0				

Recorded in *Tang tou ko chueh* (湯頭歌訣). Combines *Liu-wei-ti-huang-wan* (Rehmannia Six Formula) and magnetic iron. Used chiefly for renal fire (renal insufficiency) and its resultant deafness, tinnitus, dizziness, and "clouded eyes." If the deafness is accompanied by swelling and pain or dizziness and "sparkling eyes," this formula is not suitable.

Herbs and Actions

Rehmannia nourishes yin and replenishes the kidney; it generates the production of blood and sperm. Cornus warms the insides and prevents involuntary loss of sperm. Moutan cortex cools the blood and fevers. Dioscorea enriches the spleen and firms the kidneys. Hoelen drains moist fever of the spleen. Alisma discharges water toxin from the bladder, and sharpens hearing and vision. Loadstone ore contains iron; hence it calms nervous excitement and enriches the blood.

Indications

Deafness, tinnitus, dizziness, blurred vision.

Tzu-Wan-Tang 紫菀湯

(Aster Combination)

Aster	3.0	Anemarrhena	3.0	Fritillaria	3.0
Gelatin	3.0	Licorice	1.5	Ginseng	1.5
Hoelen	1.5	Platycodon	1.5	Schizandra	1.5

Tzu-wan-tang is recorded in *I fang chi chieh* (醫方集解) of the Ching dynasty. This formula is mainly used for treating pulmonary tuberculosis. It is effective for reducing fever, prolonged cough, caseous necrosis, and hemoptysis of tuberculosis.

Herbs and Actions

Gelatin is an effective treatment for hemoptysis. Anemarrhena is an antipyretic and antiphlogistic. Aster can reduce prolonged coughing, dry cough, tubercular cough, and hemoptysis. Platycodon and Fritillaria dispel sputum and pus, act as antiphlogistics, and ease the cough. Schizandra and Licorice are astrigents and demulcents. Ginseng nourishes the lungs and increases vitality. Hoelen nourishes the whole body, particularly the spleen.

Indications

Caseous necrosis, hemoptysis, weak lungs, fever, and prolonged coughing episodes of tuberculosis.

Wei-Cheng-Fang 痿症方

(Eucommia and Achyranthes Formula)

Tang-kuei	5.0	Peony	2.0	Eucommia	1.0
Achyranthes	3.0	Astragalus	2.0	Rehmannia	4.0
Atractylodes	3.0	Phellodendron	1.0	Anemarrhea	3.0

Wei-cheng-fang is a widely used formula developed by Hukui Futei of Japan. It is used mainly for treating the primary state of weakness near the waist and in the feet. Patients with anorexia or diarrhea after taking this formula should stop taking it.

Herbs and Actions

Rehmannia is a blood tonic. *Tang-kuei* and Peony nourish the blood. Achyranthes and Eucommia nourish the feet and the area near the waist. Anemarrhena and Phellodendron are antipyretics, and they nourish the kidneys. Astragalus nourishes the muscle. Atractylodes is a stomachic which also nourishes the spleen.

Indications

Weakness of the feet during convalescence, weak knees after childbirth, myelophthisis, myelitis, paralysis of the lower limbs due to beriberi, and polio.

Yang-Hsin-Tang 養心湯

(*Astragalus and Zizyphus Combination*)

Astragalus	4.0	Hoelen	4.0	Cnidium	4.0
Tang-kuei	4.0	Pinellia	4.0	Ginseng	1.0
Biota	1.0	Cinnamon	1.0	Schizandra	1.0
Polygala	1.0	Licorice	0.5	Zizyphus	1.0
Fu-shen	4.0				

Yang-hsin-tang is recorded in *I fang chi chieh* (醫方集解) of the Ching dynasty. This formula is used for treating heart weakness, anemia, palpitations, insomnia with night sweats, fever, and anxiety. It is a tonic and is effective for neuralgia.

Herbs and Actions

Ginseng, Astragalus, and Licorice supplement the *ch'i*. Hoelen, Polygala, Biota, and Zizyphus disperse the heat in the heart and act as tranquilizers. *Tang-kuei* regulates the *ch'i* and nourishes the blood. Cnidium promotes blood circulation. Pinellia is an expectorant. Schizandra nourishes the lungs. Cinnamon channels the actions of the other herbs into the *hsin-ching* (heart veins).

Indications

Anemia, amnesia, insomnia, neurasthenia, and neurogenous palpitations.

10.
Chu Han Chi
(祛寒劑, Chill Dispelling Formulas)

Formulas composed chiefly of warm- or hot-natured herbs intended to dispel "stale chills" residing in the viscera are called *chu han chi*.

The *chu han chi* treat a degenerated yang *ch'i* when yin chills are thriving internally. Ancient proverbs say to "heat chills," or "treat chills with hot herbs." Thus the rule of treatment for dispelling chills.

Interior chills are due to a yang deficiency, or to external chills that have invaded the interior, or to an injury of yang *ch'i* as a consequence of taking the wrong medication. Therefore, formulas recorded in this section are divided into two types: interior-warming, chill-dispelling formulas and yang-restoring, chill-curing formulas.

A fever lying dormant internally causes chills and the stronger the fever, the more severe the chills. This condition is one of internal real fever and external pseudochills. The doctor after carefully analyzing and diagnosing this condition should not prescribe a warm or hot formula. Dosages must vary according to the individual's condition. For persons with a thriving fever or an injured yin from loss of blood, the dose should be kept small even if the patient has a chill conformation that calls for a warm formula. As soon as the formula has taken effect, it should be suspended so that it will not affect the patient's physique and induce unnecessary changes.

Chen-Wu-Tang 眞武湯

(Vitality Combination)

Hoelen	5.0	Peony	3.0	Atractylodes	3.0
Ginger	3.0	Aconite	0.5–1.0		

Chen-wu-tang is recorded in the *Shang han lun* (傷寒論) during the Han dynasty. This formula is used for treating metabolic disorders, dysuria due to stagnant water, abdominal pain, diarrhea, vertigo, palpitation, abdominal weakness, severe fatigue, cold hands and feet, and pain in the arms and legs.

Herbs and Actions

Hoelen and Atractylodes dispel ascites and promote gastrointestinal function. Peony relieves the muscle tension, spasm, and pain. Aconite and Ginger improve metabolism and increase vitality.

Indications

Common cold, influenza, pneumonia, pleurisy, tuberculosis, neurasthenia, cerebral bleeding, hypertension, valvular diseases, gastrointestinal weakness, chronic enteritis, indigestion, intestinal tuberculosis, gastroptosis, peritonitis, ascites, cyclic vomiting, nephritis, renal atrophy, monoplegia, rheumatic pain, and pruritus in the elderly.

Discrimination

Jen-sheng-tang (Ginseng and Ginger Combination): diarrhea, weakness and chills, excessive urine, no flushing up of *ch'i*.

Hsiao-chien-chung-tang (Minor Cinnamon and Peony Combination): lassitude, internal weakness (no edema or diarrhea), excessive urine, and palpitations.

Szu-ni-tang (Aconite and G. L. Combination): diarrhea, no splashing sound beneath the heart and diarrhea with indigested food.

Ling-kuei-chu-kan-tang (Atractylodes and Hoelen Combination):

vertigo, submerged tense pulse, and orthostatic vertigo.

Weak yin conformation

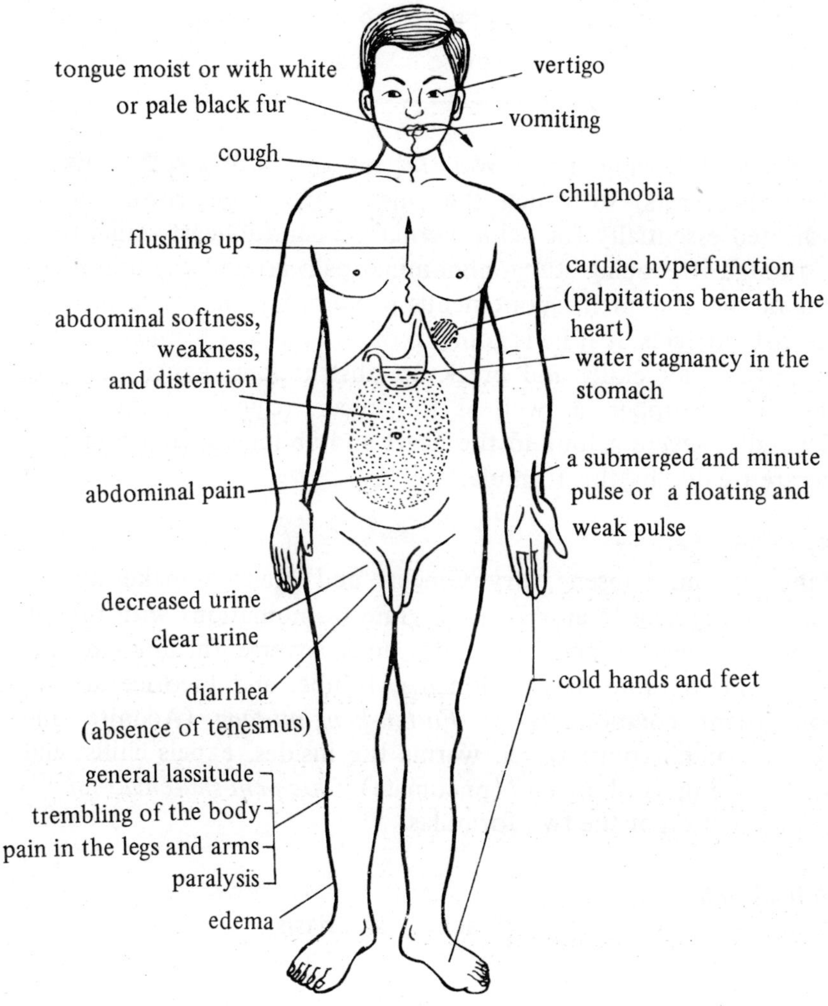

Chieh-Chi-Shu-Chiao-Tang 解急蜀椒湯

(Zanthoxylum Combination)

Dry ginger	1.5	Ginseng	3.0	Aconite	0.5
Zanthoxylum	2.0	Oryza	8.0	Pinellia	5.0
Jujube	3.0	Licorice	1.5	Maltose	2.0

Recorded in Wang Tau's *Wai tai mi yao* (外臺秘要 Extra Medical Secrets) in which the chief usage is described: "It is indicated essentially for "chill hernia", a painful heart which feels as though it is being stung, abdominal pain around the umbilicus and in the abdomen, spontaneous perspiration that is so profuse the patient feels as if he is going to die." Thus this formula is used to drive away chills and break up obstructions, hence relieving pain in the upper, as well as the lower, regions of the body. Generally, severe aching in the heart and abdomen, vomiting, and gas are treated by this formula.

Herbs and Actions

Zanthoxylum Ginseng, dry Ginger, and Maltose make up *Ta-chien-chung-tang* (Major Zanthoxylum Combination) with replenishes weakness, expels chills, descends adverse flushing-up, and kills pain. Aconite, Oryza, Pinellia, Jujube, and Licorice are the constituent components of *Fu-tzu-keng-mi-tang* (Aconite and Oryza Combination) which warms the insides, expels chills, and settles the up-flushing *ch'i* (pneumata). *Chieh-chi-shu-chiao-tang* is a combination of the two formulas.

Indications

"Chill hernia", abdominal aches, ascariasis.

Chien-Chin-Tang-Kuei-Tang 千金當歸湯

(Tang-kuei Combination)

Tang-kuei	5.0	Pinellia	5.0	Peony	3.0
Magnolia bark	3.0	Cinnamon	3.0	Ginseng	3.0
Ginger	1.5	Astragalus	1.5	Licorice	1.0
Zanthoxylum	1.5				

Recorded in *Chien chin fang* (千金方) for the treatment of "... colic in the abdomen and the heart, various chills and weaknesses, and aches due to gas distention." Therefore, it is used for a somewhat weak conformation with slight chills and for subcardiac colic that penetrates to the back; or for chronic abdominal hernia and the so-called *pi nang ping* (a collective term for prolapse of the stomach, loose-bowels, and stomach distention—all of which share the common symptom of gastric water stagnancy).

Herbs and Actions

Tang-kuei nourishes the blood and disperses internal chill. Pinellia decreases the rate of respiration and eliminates distention. Magnolia bark dissolves occlusion, settles the stomach, and eases abdominal pain. Ginseng restores respiration and calms the spirit. Astragalus enriches the spleen and aids respiration. Peony eliminates paralysis and removes extravasation. Cinnamon, Zanthoxylum, Ginger, and Licorice all collaborate to harmonize the exterior with the interior, to warm the interior, and to drive away chills. The synergism of the various components causes the actions of warming the interior, breaking up stagnation, expelling chills, and alleviating pain.

Indications

Angina pectoris, colic of the heart and abdomen owing to arteriosclerosis, chill conformation abdominal pain, gastric ulcers, prolapse and distention of the stomach.

Discrimination

Hsiao-chien-chung-tang (Minor Cinnamon and Peony Combination) is used for abdominal pain, aches and fever in the limbs, cardiac palpitation, dry throat and mouth, and pains that are mild and not so severe as to spread to the back.

Chih-so-erh-chen-tang (*Chih-shih* and Cardamon Combination): pain beneath the heart, chest pain, vomiting, water stagnancy in the stomach.

Chai-hu-kuei-chih-tang (Bupleurum and Cinnamon Combination): resistance and pain beneath the heart when palpated, distention beneath the heart, excessive acid in the stomach, heartburn, mildly distressed chest.

Weak conformation and chill conformation

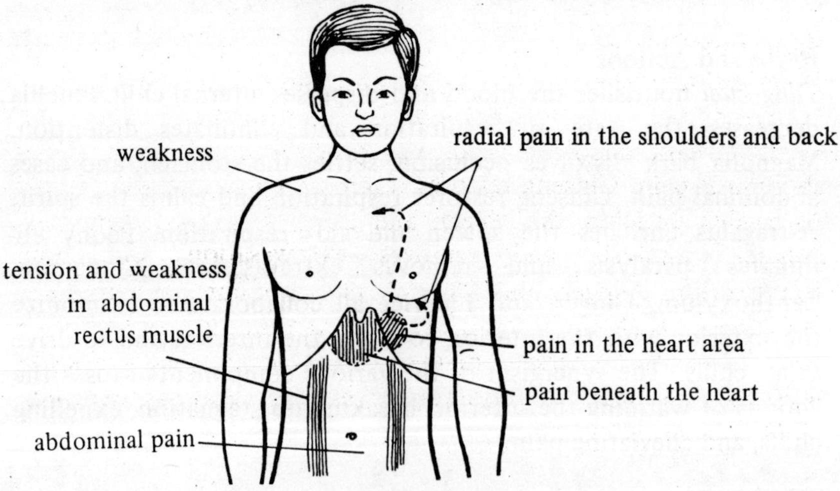

Fu-Ling-Szu-Ni-Tang 茯苓四逆湯

(Hoelen, G. L. and Aconite Combination)

Aconite	0.5–1.0	Ginger	2.0	Licorice	2.0
Ginseng	2.0	Hoelen	4.0		

Fu-ling-szu-ni-tang, a combination of *Szu-ni-tang* (Aconite and G. L. Combination) with Ginseng and Hoelen, is recorded in *Shang han lun* (傷寒論) of the Han dynasty. This formula is used for treating chills, diarrhea, vomiting, abdominal distention, chills in the hands and feet, anemia, palpitations, anxiety due to stress, and edema.

Herbs and Actions
Aconite relieves chills. Ginger is warm in nature, and treats local anemia. Licorice is a tonic, and reinforces the functioning of the internal organs. Ginseng and Hoelen act as sedatives, salivants, and diuretics; they also nourish the *ch'i* and treat anxiety due to stress.

Indications
Influenza; intestinal fever; cholera; diarrhea; neurotic vomiting; gastroenteritis; indigestion; jaundice; ephidrosis; and hemorrhage due to external injuries, surgery, or childbirth.

Discrimination
Kan-tsao-kan-chiang-tang (Licorice and Ginger Combination): vomiting, cold hands and feet, anxiety, and dry throat.
Wu-chu-yu-tang (Evodia Combination): cold hands and feet, vomiting, diarrhea, anxiety, severe shaking of *ch'i*, headache, and slobbering.
Tao-hua-tang (Kaolin and Oryza Combination): diarrhea containing mucus, blood and pus; abdominal pain; and diminished urine.
Chen-wu-tang (Vitality Combination): diarrhea, degenerating metabolism, cardiac hyperfunction, diminished urine, abdominal pain, and vertigo.

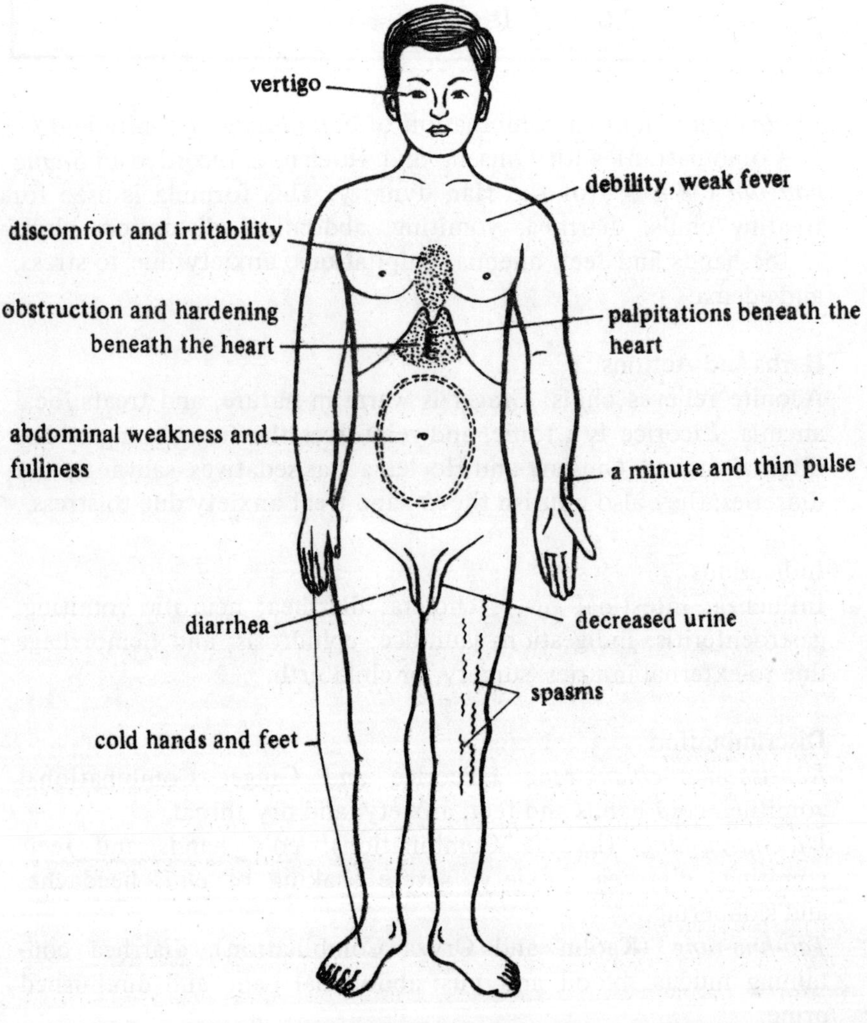
vertigo
debility, weak fever
discomfort and irritability
obstruction and hardening beneath the heart
palpitations beneath the heart
abdominal weakness and fullness
a minute and thin pulse
diarrhea
decreased urine
spasms
cold hands and feet

Fu-Tzu-Keng-Mi-Tang 附子粳米湯

(Aconite and Oryza Combination)

Aconite	0.5–1.0	Oryza	7.0	Pinellia	5.0
Jujube	3.0	Licorice	1.5		

Fu-tzu-keng-mi-tang is recorded in *Chin kuei yao lueh* (金匱要略) of the Han dynasty. This formula is used for treating those of delicate constitution with metabolic disorders, a chilled feeling in the abdomen, borborygmus, severe recurrent pain, flushing up, chest distention, nausea, and vomiting.

Herbs and Actions

Aconite is warm in nature and improves the metabolic functions. Pinellia and Oryza treat vomiting. Licorice and Jujube treat acute symptoms and in combination with Aconite can eliminate pain.

Indications

Intestinal colic, gastric spasms, gastric ulcer, peritonitis, gallstones, pancreatitis, and pylorospasm.

Discrimination

Shao-yao-kan-tsao-tang (Peony and Licorice Combination): abdominal pain, no vomiting, and severe gas.
Wu-tou-kuei-chih-tang (*Wu-tou* and Cinnamon Combination): abdominal pain, no vomiting, and gas.
Ta-wu-tou-chien (Major *Wu-tou* Combination): abdominal pain, no vomiting, and gas.
Ta-chien-chung-tang (Major Zanthoxylum Combination): abdominal pain and excessive peristalsis.

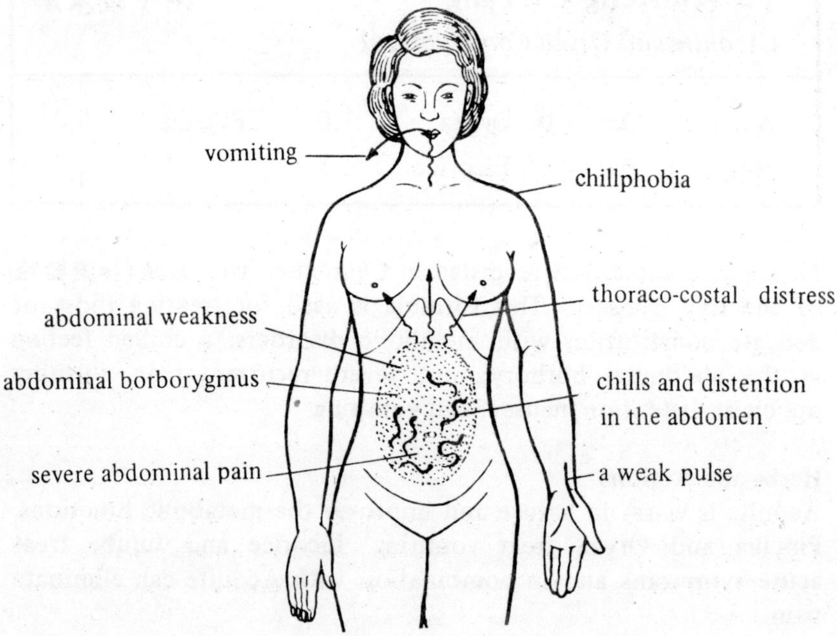
vomiting
chillphobia
thoraco-costal distress
abdominal weakness
abdominal borborygmus
chills and distention
in the abdomen
severe abdominal pain
a weak pulse

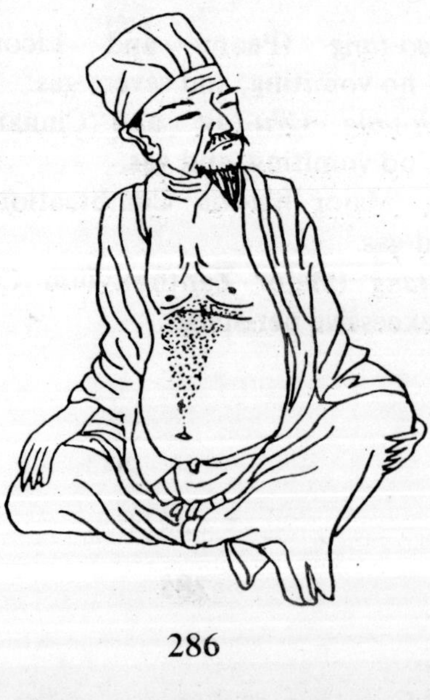

Fu-Tzu-Li-Chung-Tang 附子理中湯

(Aconite, Ginseng, and Ginger Combination)

Ginseng	3.0	Ginger	3.0	Licorice	3.0
Atractylodes	3.0	Aconite	0.5–1.0		

Fu-tzu-li-chung-tang is recorded in *Shang han lun* (傷寒論) of the Han dynasty. This is a combination of *Jen-sheng-tang* (Ginseng and Ginger Combination) with Aconite. This formula is used for treating severe diarrhea, severe abdominal pain, chills in the hands and feet, severe chills, weakness of the spleen and stomach, and weak pulse.

Herbs and Actions
Ginseng, Ginger, Licorice, and Atractylodes of *Jen-sheng-tang* can nourish the *ch'i* and spleen and dispel chills. Aconite warms the body and improves metabolic functioning.

Indications
Gastroenteritis, gastric distention, gastroptosis, toxemia during pregnancy, nervous vomiting in children, bleeding, and indigestion.

Discrimination
See *Jen-sheng-tang* (Ginseng and Ginger Combination).

Fu-Tzu-Tang 附子湯

(Aconite Combination)

Aconite	0.5–1.0	Hoelen	4.0	Peony	4.0
Atractylodes	5.0	Ginseng	3.0		

Fu-tzu-tang is recorded in *Shang han lun* of the Han dynasty. This formula is used for treating generalized pain, arthralgia, severe chills in the back, chills in the hands and feet, white coating on the tongue, sunken and weak pulse, and severe anemia.

Herbs and Actions

Aconite is warm in nature and relieves severe chills and pain. Atractylodes and Hoelen dispel "water poisoning". Ginseng is a tonic and can adjust metabolic disorders. Peony is also a tonic, and it relieves severe chills and pain.

Indications

The common cold, influenza, neuralgia, rheumatism, arthritis, abdominal pain due to chills, peritonitis, edema, ascites, stomatitis, abdominal pain during pregnancy, apoplexy, facial paralysis, monoplegia, dermatitis, eczema, and urticaria.

Discrimination

Chen-wu-tang (Vitality Combination): abdominal pain; aims chiefly at the internal symptoms and secondarily at the surface symptoms; diarrhea; submerged and weak pulse.

Kuei-chih-fu-tzu-tang (Cinnamon and Aconite Combination): chillphobia, generalized pain, external feverish symptoms.

Shao-yao-kan-tsao-fu-tzu-tang (Peony, Licorice, and Aconite Combination): chillphobia; abdominal pain; spasms in the abdomen, lower back and feet; a minute, harsh pulse.

Kan-tsao-fu-tzu-tang (Licorice and Aconite Combination): chillphobia, pain; external fever; arthritis; floating, weak, and quick pulse.

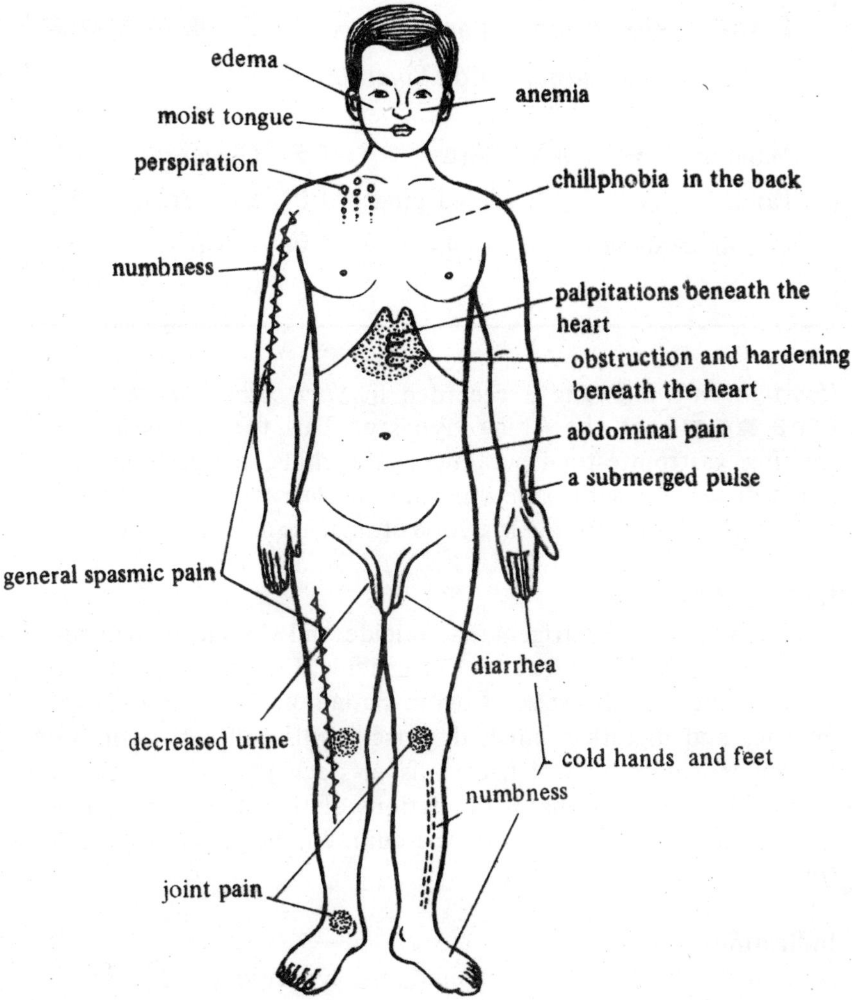
edema
moist tongue
perspiration
numbness
anemia
chillphobia in the back
palpitations beneath the heart
obstruction and hardening beneath the heart
abdominal pain
a submerged pulse
general spasmic pain
diarrhea
decreased urine
cold hands and feet
numbness
joint pain

Hou-Pu-Wen-Chung-Tang 厚朴溫中湯

(Magnolia and Saussurea Combination)

Magnolia bark	4.5	Citrus	4.5	Ginger	1.0
Hoelen	2.0	Dried ginger	1.0	Saussurea	1.5
Cochin cardamon	2.0	Jujube	1.0	Licorice	1.5

Hou-pu-wen-chung-tang is recorded in *Shen shih tsun sheng shu* (沈氏尊生書) of the Ching dynasty. This formula is used for treating gastrointestinal weakness and chills, indigestion, abdominal distention with pain, vomiting of clear water, and diarrhea. Each herb of this formula is a good stomachic and analgesic.

Herbs and Actions

Magnolia bark is an astrigent, bactericide, and stomachic. Saussurea can improve the *ch'i* and act as a stomachic. Citrus can decrease the *ch'i* and act as a digestive. Cochin cardamon is an aromatic, stomachic, and digestive which disperses chills and stops vomiting. Hoelen is a diuretic which can dispel stagnant water in the stomach. Licorice coordinates the actions of the other herbs. Ginger warms the body and disperses the chill. Jujube is a stomachic and tonic.

Indications

Abdominal pain, lumbago, appendicitis, gynecological diseases.

Hsiao-Chien-Chung-Tang 小建中湯

(Minor Cinnamon and Peony Combination)

Cinnamon	4.0	Ginger	4.0	Peony	6.0
Jujube	4.0	Licorice	2.0	Maltose	20.0

Both the medical works of the Han dynasty, *Shang han lun* and *Chin kuei yao lueh* (Summaries on Household Drugs) by Chang Chung-ching (A.D. 142-220), list *Hsiao-chien-chung-tang* as a general tonic. This formula is to be taken by those of delicate constitution with a tendency towards fatigue. It is also used for improving the vitality of children with a delicate constitution, lack of vigor, abdominal pain, palpitations, nose-bleed, night sweats, hot palms and feet, tired limbs, nocturnal emission, dry mouth, and frequent urination.

Herbs and Actions

Maltose and Jujube have nutritive effects. Licorice relieves the prominent symptoms; in combination with Peony, its analgesic effects are improved. Cinnamon with Licorice stops palpitations. Ginger is stomachic and promotes absorption of the herbs.

Indications

For improving the vitality of children with delicate constitution and as treatment for bed-wetting, frequent urination, night crying, gastritis, diarrhea in children, constipation in children, necrosis, arthritis, rickets, neurosis, hernias in children, asthma, purpura, habitual headache in children, tonsillitis, neurasthenia and neuro-palpitation.

Discrimination

Ta-chien-chung-tang (Major Zanthoxylum Combination): abdominal pain, hyperfunctioning of intestinal peristalsis, acute pain, submerged weak pulse.

Jen-sheng-tang (Ginseng and Ginger Combination): abdominal pain, chronic but mild symptoms, diarrhea, abdominal laxity.

Hsiao-chai-hu-tang (Minor Bupleurum Combination): abdominal pain, firm fever conformation, distressed chest and ribs.
Kuei-chih-chia-lung-ku-mu-li-tang (Cinnamon and Dragon Bone Combination): fatigability, palpitations, weakness in the lower body, nocturnal emissions, mental and emotional instability.

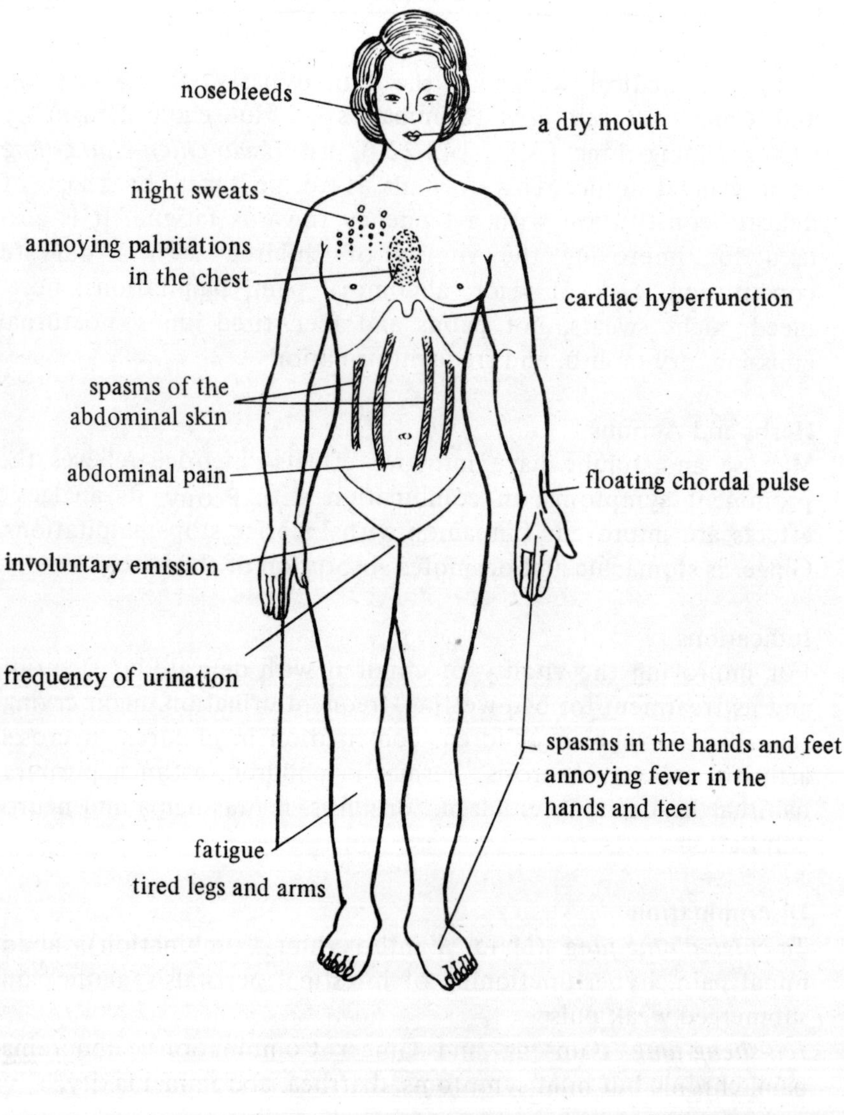

Huang-Chi-Chien-Chung-Tang 黃耆建中湯

(Astragalus Combination)

Peony	6.0	Cinnamon	3.0	Ginger	3.0
Jujube	3.0	Licorice	3.0	Astragalus	1.5
Maltose	20.0				

Huang-chi-chien-chung-tang is recorded in *Chin kuei yao lueh* (金匱要略) of the Han dynasty. This formula is a combination of *Hsiao-chien-chung-tang* (Minor Cinnamon and Peony Combination) with Astragalus. This formula is used for symptoms treated by *Hsiao-chien-chung-tang* in patients of delicate constitution who also have ephidrosis, night sweats, abdominal spasms, abdominal pain, palpitations, fatigue, dry skin, and suppurative swelling.

Herbs and Actions

Maltose nourishes the spleen and stomach. Cinnamon and Ginger relieve internal chills. Licorice and Jujube coordinate with Maltose to nourish the spleen and stomach. Peony eases pain. Astragalus nourishes the skin and relieves suppuration.

Indications

Weakness during convalescence, night sweats, delicate constitution in children, chronic otitis media, suppuration, chronic ulceration, hemorrhoids, carbuncle, and gangrene.

Discrimination

Hsiao-chien-chung-tang (Minor Cinnamon and Peony Combination): weakness and fatigability in the absence of severe weakness.
Tang-kuei-chien-chung-tang (*Tang-kuei,* Cinnamon, and Peony Combination): weakness and fatigability, severe anemia, and drastic pain in the lower abdomen of women.

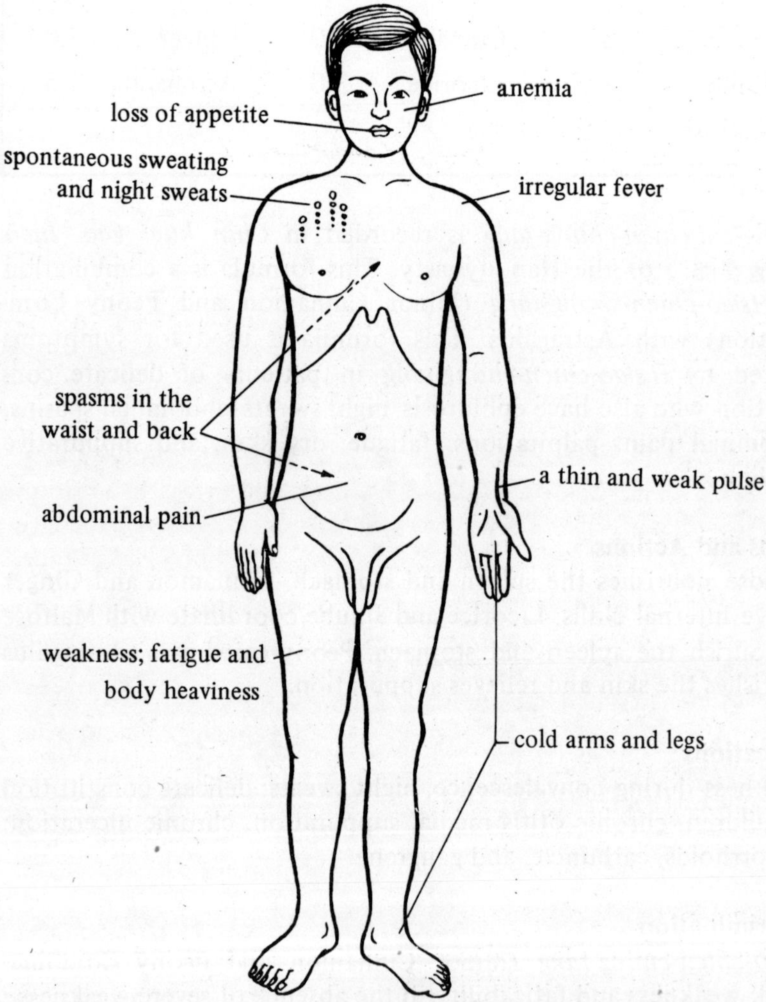
anemia
loss of appetite
spontaneous sweating
and night sweats
irregular fever
spasms in the
waist and back
a thin and weak pulse
abdominal pain
weakness; fatigue and
body heaviness
cold arms and legs

Jen-Sheng-Tang 人參湯

(Ginseng and Ginger Combination)

Ginseng	3.0	Licorice	3.0	Atractylodes	3.0
Ginger	3.0				

Ginseng, a favorite herb of the Chinese since ancient times, is considered to be a longevity elixir. With Ginseng as the principal herb, *Jen-sheng-tang* is an efficacious hematinic and stomachic. Chang Chung-ching's *Shang han lun* and *Chin kuei yao lueh* (Summaries on Household Drugs), compiled in the Han dynasty, contain detailed descriptions of this formula. It is used for gastrointestinal weakness, pallor, moist tongue without coating, polyuria, and tendencies toward fatigue and cold limbs, loose stools, frequent vomiting, headache with fever, body aches, edema, insomnia, hemoptysis, and intestinal bleeding. In addition *Jen-sheng-tang* is effective as a demulcent when treating excessive salivation and chills in the chest occurring during convalescence.

Herbs and Actions

This formula is called *Jen-sheng-tang* in the *Chin kuei yao lueh*. In the *Shang han lun,* it is called *li* (to regulate) *chung* (the middle) *tang* (tea) or "to regulate the middle burning place" i.e., (spleen and stomach). Ginseng, the principal herb, nourishes and warms the spleen and stomach, strengthens the gastrointestinal function, promotes metabolism, improves physical strength, and has sedative, diuretic, and antifatigue properties. Ginger assists Ginseng in warming the spleen and stomach. Atractylodes dispels stagnant water in the stomach. Licorice relieves pain. In short, this formula is excellent for weak digestion, malabsorption, and poor metabolism.

Indications

Acute and chronic gastroenteritis, gastric weakness, gastroptosis, gastrectasia, pernicious vomiting, excessive salivation, peptic ulcer, diarrhea, tapeworm, dyspepsia, mild labor pains, ~~birth control,~~ intoxication, diabetes, shoulder ache, cholera, hemoptysis, chilled feet, intestinal bleeding, hemorrhoidal bleeding, uterine bleeding, leukorrhea, and sneezing of a common cold.

Discrimination

Hsiao-chien-chung-tang (Minor Cinnamon and Peony Combination): abdominal pain, weakness without *ch'i* conformation, tension in the rectus abdominis muscle, warm hands and feet.
Ta-chien-chung-tang (Major Zanthoxylum Combination): abdominal pain, flatulence, and disturbed peristalsis.
Fu-ling-yin (Hoelen Combination): sensation of stagnancy beneath the heart, no diarrhea, mild illness.
Pan-hsia-hou-pu-tang (Pinellia and Magnolia Combination): fatigability, splashing sound under the heart, obstruction in the throat.
Chen-wu-tang (Vitality Combination): abdominal pain, diarrhea, coldness, decreased urine, shivering.
Ling-kuei-chu-kan-tang (Atractylodes and Hoelen Combination): anemia; cardiac palpitations; submerged and tense pulse; decreased urine, water, and *ch'i*.
Kan-tsao-hsieh-hsin-tang (Pinellia and Licorice Combination): obstruction beneath the heart, diarrhea, cold conformation, obstruction and hardness beneath the heart, flatulence.

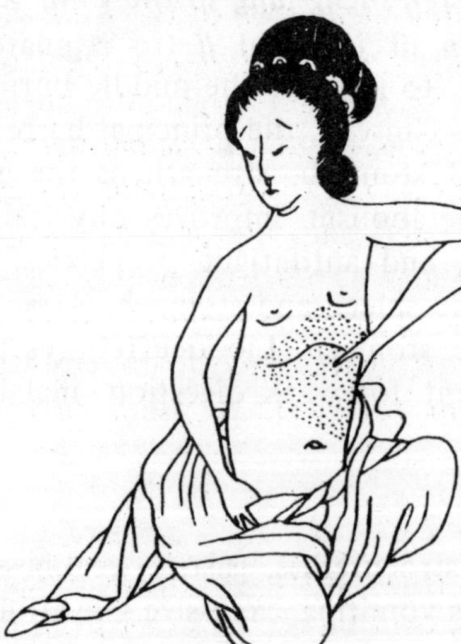

The weak chill conformation of greater yin disease

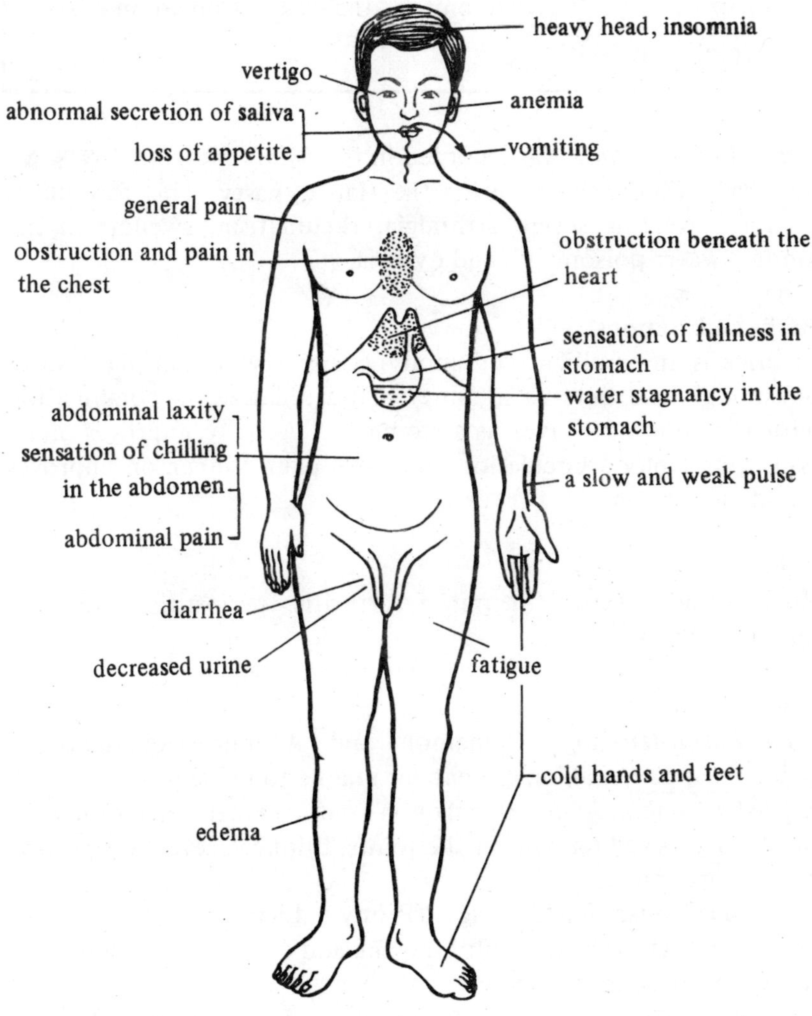

Kan-Tsao-Fu-Tzu-Tang 甘草附子湯

(Licorice and Aconite Combination)

Licorice	2.0	Aconite	0.5–1.0	Cinnamon	3.5
Atractylodes	4.0				

Kan-tsao-fu-tzu-tang was recorded in the *Shang han lun* (傷寒論) by Chang Chung-ching during the Han dynasty. This formula is used for treating severe arthralgia, rheumatism, swelling in the joints, "water poisoning", and dysuria.

Herbs and Actions

Licorice is an emollient and anodyne. Atractylodes dispels "water poisoning" and acts as a diuretic and sedative; in combination with Cinnamon it serves as a stomachic. Aconite improves metabolism and blood circulation and eases pain. Cinnamon improves blood circulation.

Indications

Rheumatoid arthritis, neuralgia, arthritis, periostitis, influenza, lumbago, and tenalgia.

Discrimination

Kuei-chih-fu-tzu-tang (Cinnamon and Aconite Combination): generalized pain making the patient unable to move.
Kuei-shao-chih-mu-tang (Cinnamon and Anemarrhena Combination): pain, swelling pain in the joints, thinness, severe congestion of *ch'i*, firm pulse.
Shao-yao-kan-tsao-fu-tzu-tang (Peony, Licorice, and Aconite Combination): pain, difficulty moving and extending the limbs, no fever, upward congestion.
Kuei-chih-chia-fu-tzu-tang (Cinnamon, Jujube, and Aconite Combination): pains of the soft tissue.

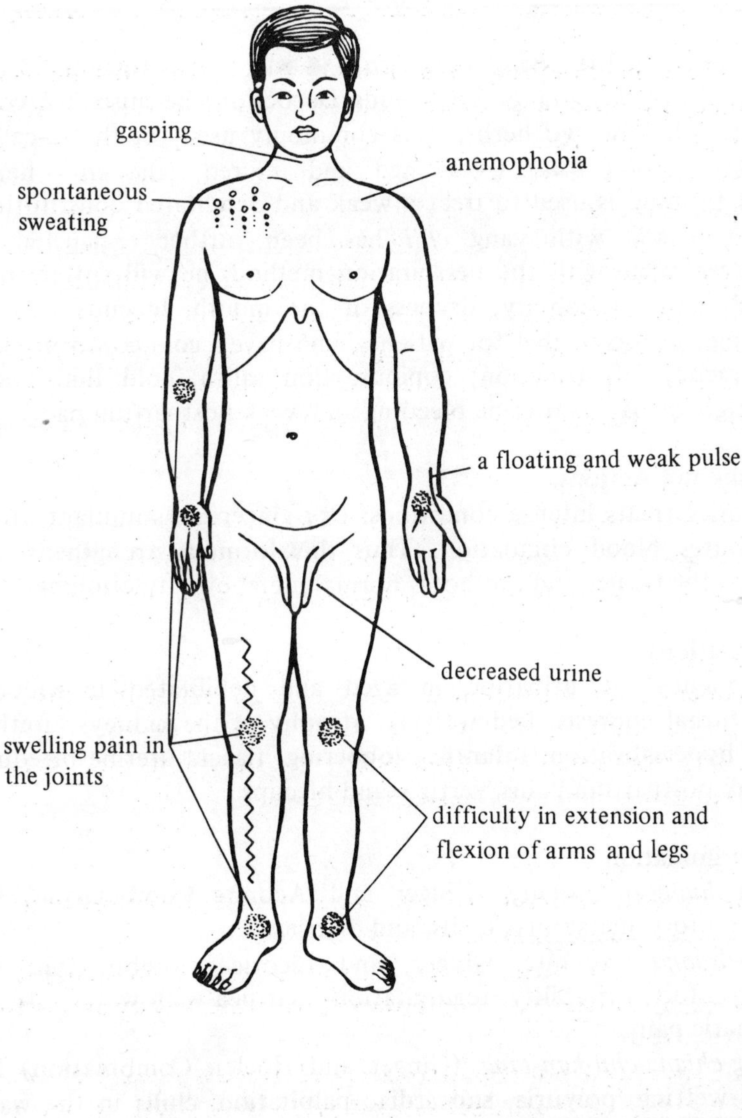
gasping
anemophobia
spontaneous sweating
a floating and weak pulse
decreased urine
swelling pain in the joints
difficulty in extension and flexion of arms and legs

Kan-tsao-Kan-Chiang-Tang 甘草乾薑湯

(Licorice and Ginger Combination)

Licorice	4.0	Ginger	2.0

Recorded in the *Shang han lun* (傷寒論). This formula is also named *Erh-sheng-tang* (Two Gods Decoction) because it is composed of only two herbs. It is commonly used for the so-called *yang chi shu hsun* (weakened and injured yang *ch'i*) hence this formula is used to treat a weak and debilitated constitution. If a person with yang *ch'i* has been further exhausted by mistreatment with the perspiration method, he will suffer from cold limbs, irritability, dryness of the mouth, hiccups and vomiting. It also is used for patients who have a cold conformation; frequency of urination; copious, thin saliva; cold limbs; and vertigo; or flaccid uterine bleeding and weak postpartum pains.

Herbs and Actions

Licorice treats intense conditions. Dry ginger is a stimulant which activates blood circulation. Thus this formula strengthens and tones the tissues and promotes normal metabolic functioning.

Indications

Frequency of urination in aged and debilitated individuals, nocturnal enuresis, bed wetting, atrophy of the kidneys, urethritis, hypersalivation, infantile slobbering, flaccid uterine bleeding, weak postpartum pains, vertigo, and hiccups.

Discrimination

Kan-chiang-fu-tzu-tang (Ginger and Aconite Combination) for discomfort, irritability, chills, and diarrhea.

Szu-ni-tang (Aconite, Ginger, and Licorice Combination) for discomfort, irritability, regurgitation, diarrhea with watery stools, somatic pain.

Ling-chiang-chu-kan-tang (Ginger and Hoelen Combination) for bed wetting, polyuria, subcardiac palpitation, chills in the waist area.

Pai-hu-tang (Gypsum Combination) for bed wetting, polyuria, feverish symptoms, thirst.

Jen-sheng-tang (Ginseng and Ginger Combination) for slobbering, subcardiac distention and rigidity, dysuria.

Hsiao-ching-lung-tang (Minor Blue Dragon Combination) for slobbering, subcardiac water stagnancy, buoyant and quick pulse.

Wu-chu-yu-tang (Evodia Combination) for slobbering, discomfort, irritability, headache, dysuria.

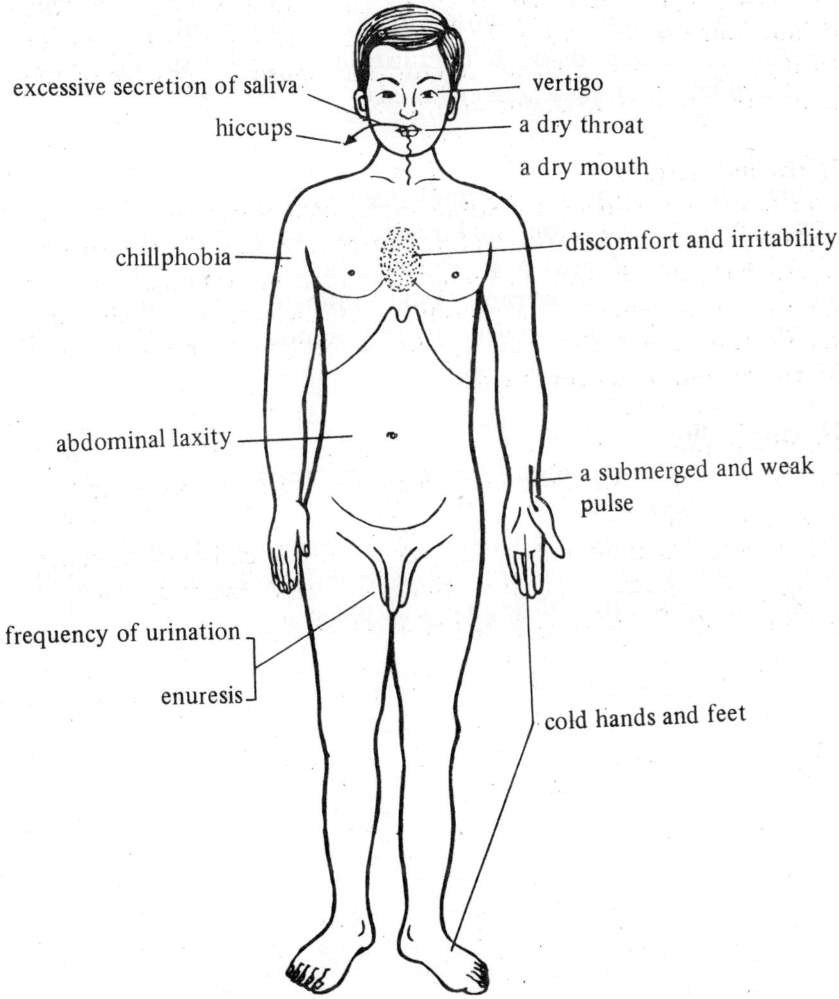

Kuei-Chih-Chia-Fu-Tzu-Tang 桂枝加附子湯

(Cinnamon and Aconite Combination)

Cinnamon	4.0	Peony	4.0	Licorice	2.0
Ginger	4.0	Jujube	4.0	Aconite	0.5–1.0

Kuei-chih-chia-fu-tzu-tang, which was recorded in *Shang han lun* (傷寒論) of the Han dynasty, is a combination of *Kuei-chih-tang* (Cinnamon Combination) with Aconite. This formula is used for treating ephidrosis, difficult micturition, muscular spasms of the arms and legs, neuralgia, and arthralgia.

Herbs and Actions

Cinnamon and Ginger are stimulants which warm the body, increase blood circulation, and reinforce the functioning of the internal organs. Peony is a sedative which in combination with Licorice can relieve tension and eliminate pain. Jujube and Licorice are tonics that relieve acute symptoms. Aconite is warm in nature, and treats ephidrosis.

Discrimination

Kuei-chih-tang (Cinnamon Combination): fever, sweating, and no lesser yin symptoms.

Szu-ni-tang (Aconite and G. L. Combination): chillphobia, generalized fever; body pain; true chills and false fever; submerged, weak pulse or floating, slow and weak pulse.

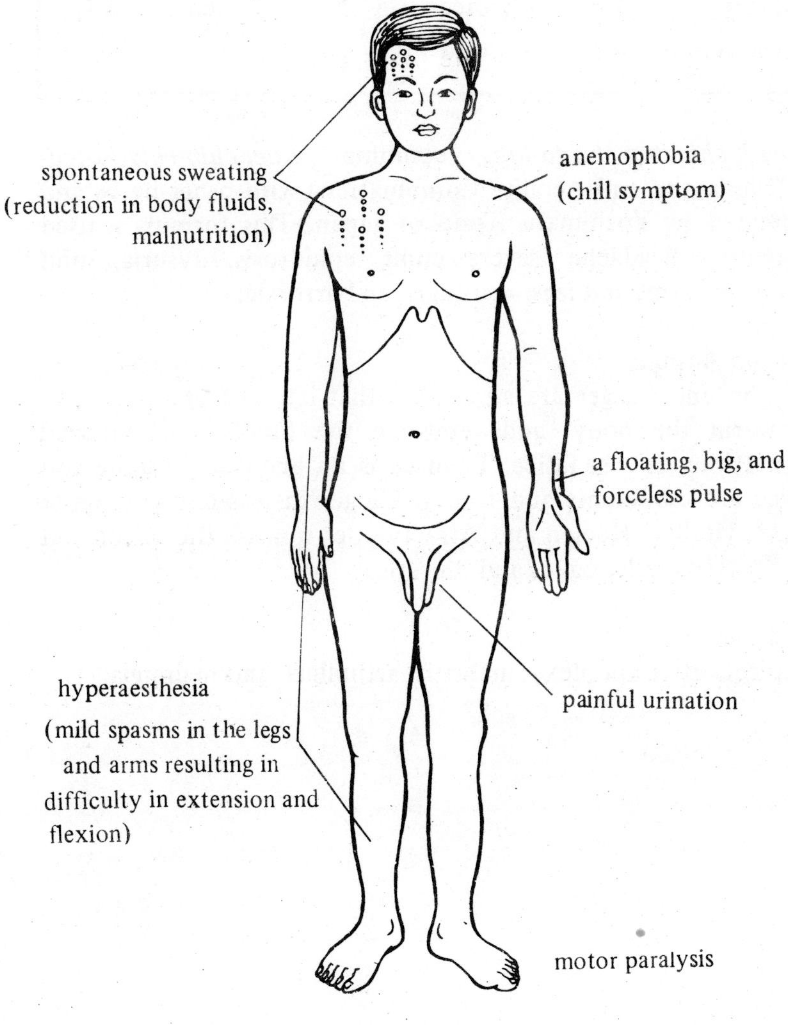
spontaneous sweating
(reduction in body fluids,
malnutrition)
anemophobia
(chill symptom)
a floating, big, and
forceless pulse
hyperaesthesia
(mild spasms in the legs
and arms resulting in
difficulty in extension and
flexion)
painful urination
motor paralysis

Kuei-Chih-Chia-Ling-Chu-Fu-Tang 桂枝加苓朮附湯

(Cinnamon and Atractylodes Combination)

Cinnamon	4.0	Peony	3.0	Jujube	3.0
Ginger	3.0	Licorice	1.5	Hoelen	5.0
Atractylodes	5.0	Aconite	0.5–1.0		

Kuei-chih-chia-ling-chu-fu-tang combines *Kuei-chih-chia-fu-tzu-tang* (Cinnamon and Aconite Combination) with other herbs and was created by Yoshimasu Todo of Japan. This formula is used for treating headache, severe chills, ephidrosis, dysuria, mild spasm in the arms and legs, neuralgia, and arthralgia.

Herbs and Actions

Cinnamon and Ginger are stimulants that improve blood circulation, warm the body, and reinforce the function of internal organs. Peony is a sedative. Licorice is an anodyne. Jujube and Licorice are emollients and tonics. Ginger dispels chills. Aconite increases vitality. Hoelen and Atractylodes nourish the spleen and *ch'i,* and act as sialogogues and diuretics.

Indications

Monoplegia after apoplexy, arthritis, arthralgia, and neuralgia.

Kuei-Chih-Fu-Tzu-Tang 桂枝附子湯

(Cinnamon, Aconite, and Ginger Combination)

Cinnamon	4.0	Aconite	0.5–1.0	Ginger	3.0
Jujube	3.0	Licorice	2.0		

For rheumatism and *shang han* conditions (chills and fever) that have lasted for eight or nine days in which wind toxin is in conflict with water toxin. The somatic pain and irritation make it virtually impossible for the afflicted to turn over. The patient exhibits no thirst or vomiting but his pulse is buoyant, weak, and harsh, denoting a surface yang weakness of a severe nature.

If after taking this formula, the stools become firm and urination normal, it means that yang has become mobile once again and free, and the excess fluid in the system has lessened through vaporization. At this point the Cinnamon is omitted and Atractylodes added to strengthen the spleen and remove any further excess fluids. The formula so adjusted becomes *Pai-chu-fu-tzu-tang*, also a treatment for *shang han* conditions.

Herbs and Actions

Cinnamon channels yang and cures surface symptoms. In combination with Aconite it warms yang and vaporizes moisture. Licorice mollifies impetuous conditions.

Indications

Muscular rheumatism, gout, and arthritis.

Discrimination

Pai-chu-fu-tzu-tang (Atractylodes and Aconite Combination) is for conflicts between the wind and the water toxins in which the inner yang is weakened and the symptoms are comparatively mild.

Kan-tsao-fu-tzu-tang (Licorice and Aconite Combination) is also used for a conflict between the wind and water, but yang is weakened both inside and outside.

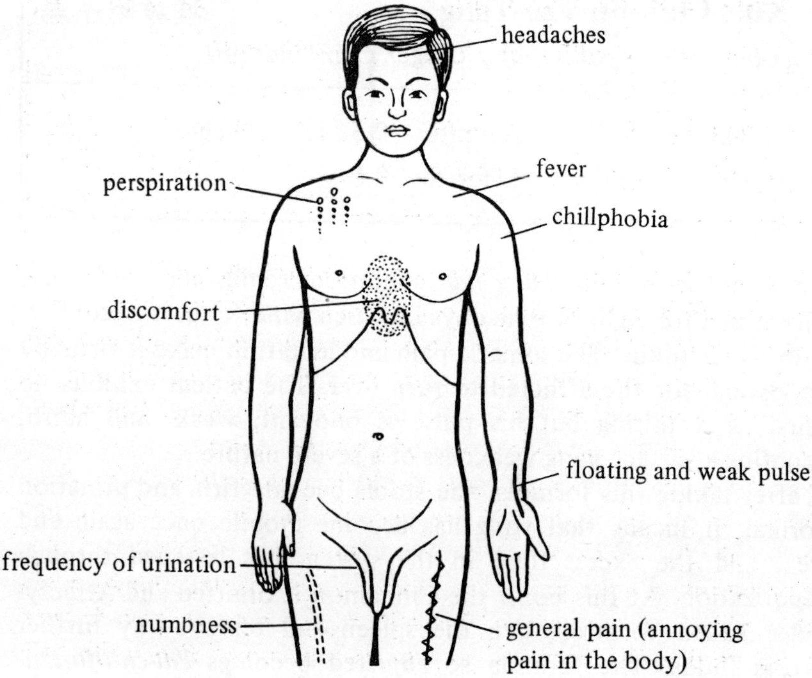

Kuei-Chih-Jen-Sheng-Tang 桂枝人參湯

(Cinnamon and Ginseng Combination)

Cinnamon	4.0	Ginseng	3.0	Licorice	3.0
Atractylodes	3.0	Ginger	2.0		

Kuei-chih-jen-sheng-tang was recorded in the *Shang han lun* (傷寒論) during the Han dynasty. This formula is a combination of *Jen-sheng-tang* (Ginseng and Ginger Combination) plus Cinnamon. It is used for treating headache, fever, ephidrosis, diarrhea, subcardiac distention, abdominal pain, palpitation beneath the heart, weakness of the arms and legs, cold feet, and dysuria.

Herbs and Actions
Cinnamon relieves muscle tension. Ginseng nourishes the *ch'i* and alleviates subcardiac distention. Atractylodes and Ginger dispel "internal chill". Licorice coordinates the actions of the other herbs and eases pain.

Indications
Acute gastroenteritis, nervous palpitations, heart disorders, repeated headache, common cold, and influenza.

Discrimination
Jen-sheng-tang (Ginseng and Ginger Combination): diarrhea with an internal chill conformation and mild external fever.
Ko-ken-tang (Pueraria Combination): diarrhea, firm conformation, floating and tense pulse.
Ko-ken-huang-lien-huang-chin-tang (Pueraria, Coptis, and Scute Combination): diarrhea, external or internal firm fever conformation, and hurried pulse.
Szu-ni-tang (Aconite and G. L. Combination): diarrhea, slow and submerged pulse.
Chen-wu-tang (Vitality Combination): diarrhea, vertigo, and shivering.
Wu-ling-san (Hoelen Five Herb Formula): diarrhea, extreme thirst, scanty urine, and vomiting.
Pan-hsia-hsieh-hsin-tang (Pinellia Combination): diarrhea, firm fever, obstruction and hardness beneath the heart.

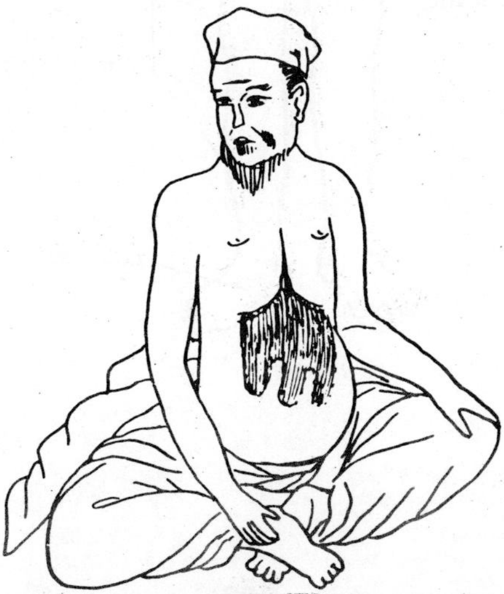

Surface fever and interior chill conformation

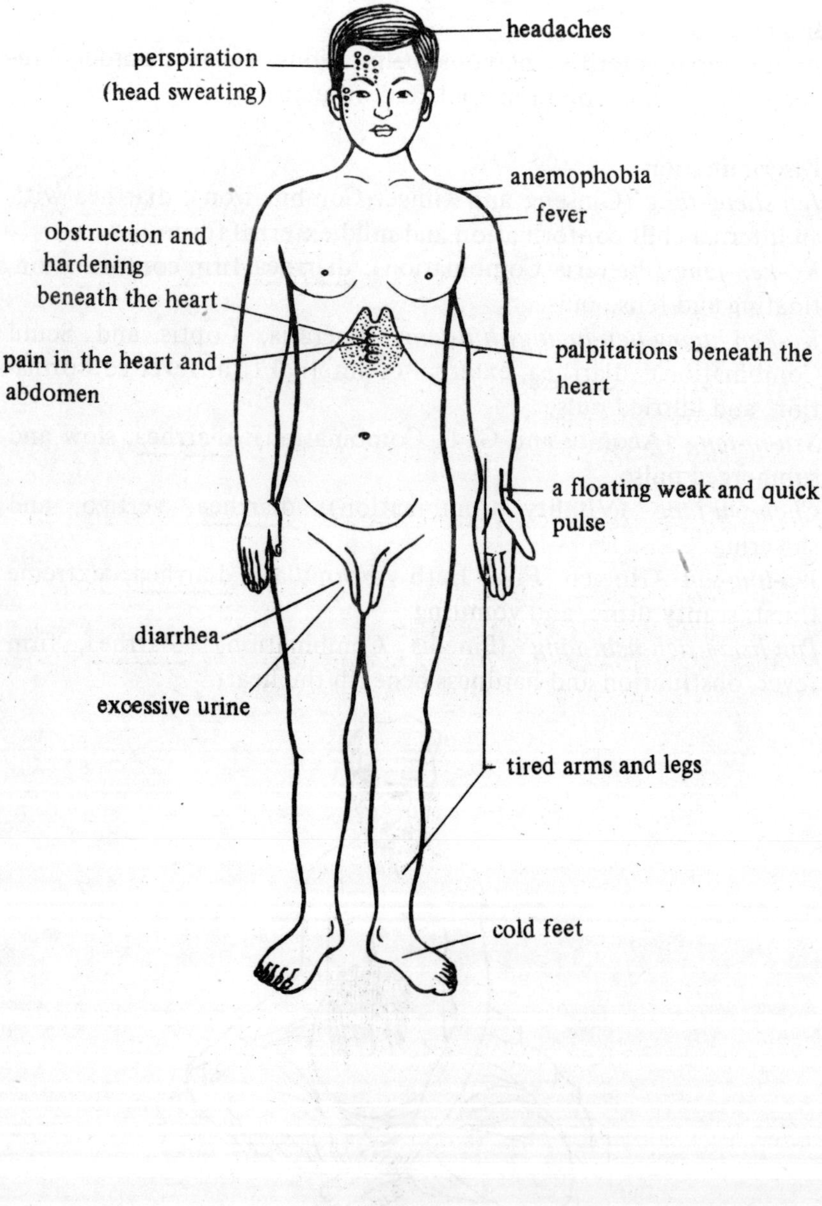

Pai-Chu-Fu-Tzu-Tang 白朮附子湯

(Atractylodes and Aconite Combination)

Atractylodes	3.0	Ginger	3.0	Jujube	3.0
Licorice	2.0	Aconite	1.0		

Recorded in *Chin kuei yao lueh* (金匱要略). This formula is made by omitting Cinnamon from *Kuei-chih-fu-tzu-tang* (Cinnamon and Aconite Combination) and adding Atractylodes in its place. Hence it is also named *Kuei-chih-fu-tzu-chu-kuei-chia-chu-tang* (Atractylodes and Aconite Combination) and is suitable for a *Kuei-chih-fu-tzu-tang* conformation and, in addition, for somatic discomfort and pain, inability to turn over by oneself, hard stools, urinary incontinence, heaviness in the head, vertigo, and loss of taste.

Herbs and Actions

Atractylodes strengthens the spleen and removes moistness and when combined with aconite, it vaporizes moistness. Licorice mollifies intense symptoms.

Indications

Neuralgia, myalgia (muscular pain), myositis (inflammation of muscles), sinusitis maxillaris (inflammation of the sinus) with heavy headedness, and paralysis of facial nerves.

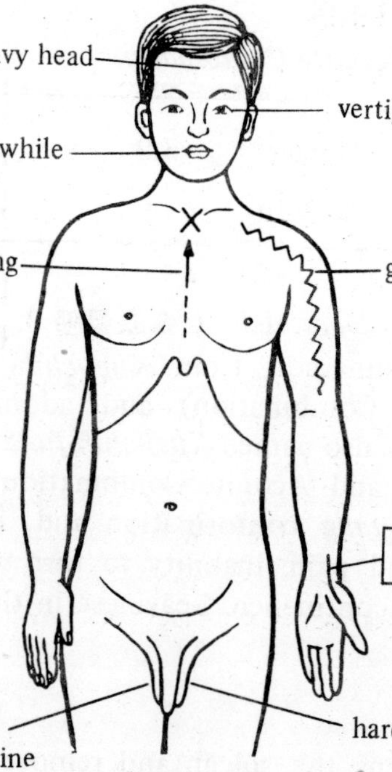

Shao-Yao-Kan-Tsao-Fu-Tzu-Tang 芍藥甘草附子湯

(Peony, Licorice, and Aconite Combination)

Peony	3.0	Licorice	3.0	Aconite	0.5–1.0

Recorded in the *Shang han lun* (傷寒論). Composed of *Shao-yao-kan-tsao-tang* and Aconite. Acute muscular cramping is the main symptom for this formula, but it also treats people with cold limbs with an abnormal fear of becoming chilled. It also is used for a yang conformation that has not been cured after treatment with the perspiration method; instead the patient has developed a fear of chills and/or convulsions, a condition brought on by treating a person with sores with the perspiration method.

Herbs and Actions

Peony and Licorice are both used to nourish yin and replenish fluid. When supplemented by Aconite they strengthen blood circulation and restore normal body temperature by eliminating chills and convulsions.

Indications

Spasms in the back, knee and waist; spasms of the gastrocnemius muscle (leg muscle); sciatica; low back pain; stiff shoulders; muscular rheumatism; intestinal hernia; biliary colic; renal colic; hemorrhoidal colic; pain on urination; rigid tongue.

Discrimination

See *Shao-yao-kan-tsao-tang* (Peony and Licorice Combination).

Szu-Ni-Chia-Jen-Sheng-Tang 四逆加人參湯

(G. L. and Aconite Combination with Ginseng)

Aconite	0.5–1.0	Ginger	2.0	Licorice	3.0
Ginseng	2.0				

Szu-ni-chia-jen-sheng-tang, a combination of *Szu-ni-tang* (Aconite and G.L. Combination) with Ginseng, is recorded in *Shang han lun* (傷寒論) of the Han dynasty. This formula is used for treating severe fatigue, severe anemia, chills in the hands and feet ephidrosis, rapid respiration, and weak and sunken pulse.

Herbs and Actions

Aconite dispels chills. Ginger warms the body and dispels chills. Licorice nourishes the *ch'i*. Ginseng nourishes the body and *ch'i*.

Indications

Febrile diseases, acute vomiting and diarrhea, and dysentery.

Discrimination

Please refer to the section on *Szu-ni-tang*.

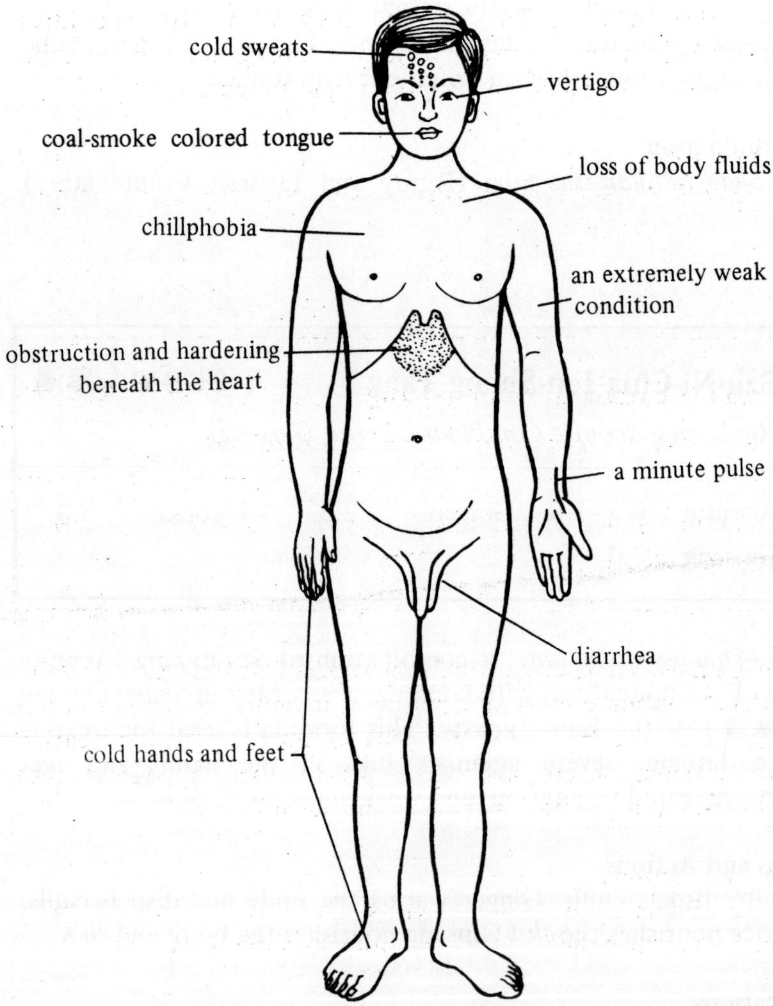

Szu-Ni-Tang 四逆湯

(Aconite and G. L. Combination)

Licorice	3.0	Ginger	2.0	Aconite	0.5–1.0

Recorded in *Shang han lun* (傷寒論) and *Chin kuei yao lueh* (金匱要略) of the Han dynasty. Used for treating cold hands and feet, severe chills throughout the body, pallor, diarrhea, vomiting, abdominal pain, weak pulse, facial redness, and superficial fever.

Herbs and Actions
Aconite is a stimulant that can increase vitality. Ginger dispels chills. Licorice is an analgesic, expectorant, and antidysenteric.

Indications
Influenza, intestinal fever, cholera, diarrhea, neurotic vomiting, indigestion, edema, jaundice, weak heart brought on by excessive bleeding, and cold hands and feet.

Discrimination
Jen-sheng-tang (Ginseng and Ginger Combination): diarrhea, chilling, obstruction and hardness beneath the heart, splashing sound beneath the heart, and excessive urine.
Kan-tsao-kan-chiang-tang (Licorice and Ginger Combination): cold hands and feet, no vomiting, submerged and weak pulse.
Wu-chu-yu-tang (Evodia Combination): cold hands and feet. (Vomiting is the chief symptom and diarrhea the subordinate one.)
Tao-hua-tang (Kaolin and Oryza Combination): diarrhea and stools containing pus and blood.
Tang-kuei-szu-ni-chia-wu-chu-yu-sheng-chiang-tang (*Tang-kuei,* Evodia, and Ginger Combination): coldness of the extremities in the absence of diarrhea.
Chen-wu-tang (Vitality Combination): diarrhea, splashing sound beneath the heart, decreased urine, vertigo, and shivering.
Kuei-chih-jen-sheng-tang (Ginseng and Cinnamon Combination): diarrhea with a floating, weak and quick pulse.

Surface-fever and interior-chill conformation

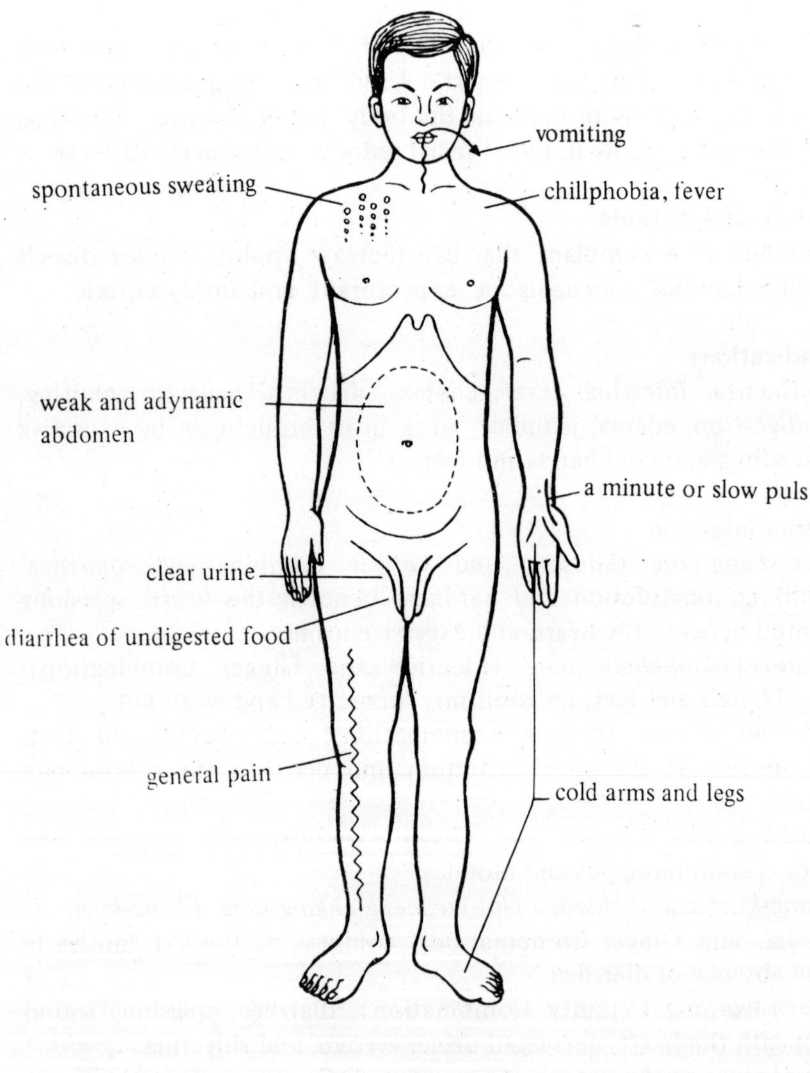

Ta-Chien-Chung-Tang 大建中湯

(Major Zanthoxylum Combination)

Zanthoxylum	2.0	Ginseng	3.0	Ginger	5.0
Maltose	20.0				

Recorded in *Chin kuei yao lueh* (金匱要略) of the Han dynasty. Used for treating internal chills, abdominal pain, weak abdomen, stagnant water, stagnant *ch'i*, vomiting, weak pulse, and chills in the hands and feet.

Herbs and Actions

Zanthoxylum and Ginger increase vitality. Ginseng nourishes the stomach and intestines, and increases digestive absorption. Maltose is a tonic.

Indications

Intestinal constriction, intestinal flaccidity, peritonitis, abdominal pain due to round worms, intestinal colic, acute appendicits, and bladder and kidney stones.

Discrimination

Fu-tzu-keng-mi-tang (Aconite and Oryza Combination): abdominal pain and "chilling" hernia, gas with cutting pain involving the chest and ribs, and vomiting.

Szu-ni-tang (Aconite and G. L. Combination): abdominal fullness and pain, cold hands and feet, diarrhea, chills.

Kuei-chih-chia-shao-yao-tang (Cinnamon and Peony Combination): abdominal fullness and pain; no peristalsis, anxiety and uneasiness; a mild condition.

Ta-huang-mu-tan-pi-tang (Rhubarb and Moutan Combination): abdominal aching and fullness; firm conformation; no peristalsis, uneasiness; tense pulse.

Hsiao-chien-chung-tang (Minor Cinnamon and Peony Combination): abdominal pain, spasms of the abdominal skin, without peristalsis and uneasiness, a mild condition.

Internal weakness conformation

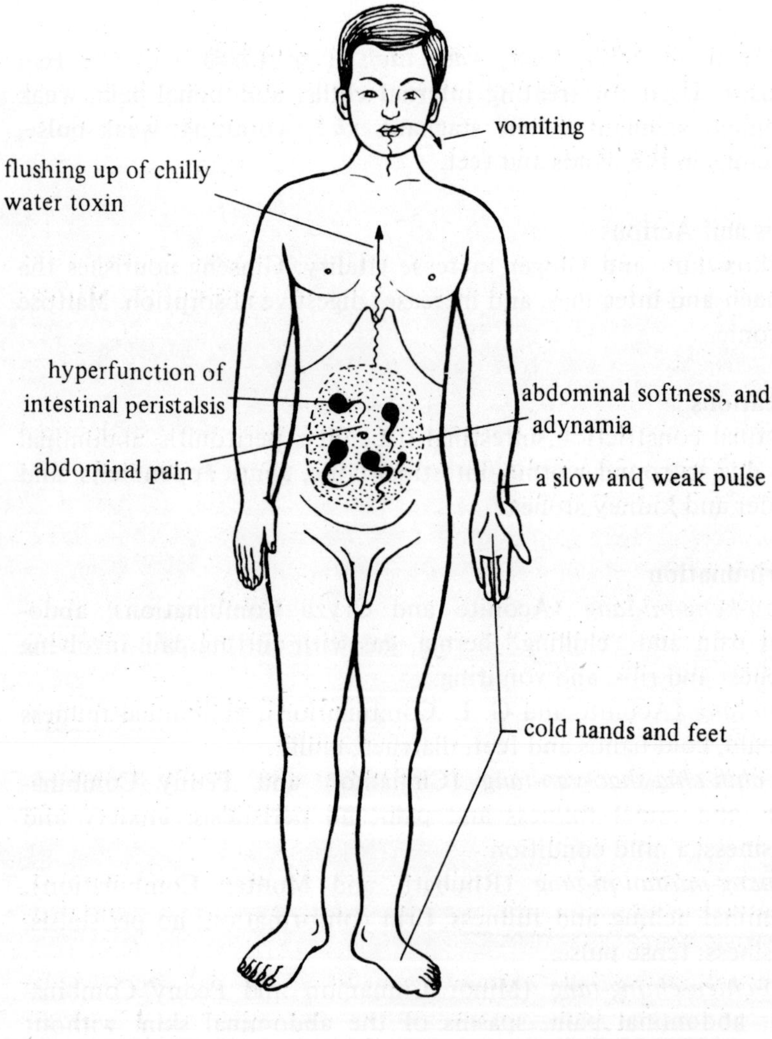

Tang-Kuei-Chien-Chung-Tang 當歸建中湯

(Tang-kuei, Cinnamon, and Peony Combination)

Peony	5.0	*Tang-kuei*	4.0	Cinnamon	4.0
Ginger	4.0	Jujube	4.0	Licorice	2.0

Tang-kuei-chien-chung-tang is recorded in *Chin kuei yao lueh* (金匱要略) of the Han dynasty. This is a combination of *Kuei-chih-tang* (Cinnamon Combination) and *Tang-kuei*. This formula is used for treating those of delicate constitution with severe anemia, continuous abdominal pain, bleeding, abdominal weakness, and abdominal spasms.

Herbs and Actions

Cinnamon and Ginger are stimulants, improve blood circulation, warm the body, and reinforce the functioning of the internal organs. Peony is a sedative which in combination with Licorice can relieve tension and eliminate pain. Jujube and Licorice are tonics. *Tang-kuei* is a blood tonic, nutritive and sedative.

Indications

Abdominal pain in women, postpartum abdominal pain, peritonitis, uterine bleeding, sciatica, lumbago, hernia, gangrene, renal calculi, tubercular kidney, hemorrhoids, and prolapse of the rectum.

Discrimination

Tang-kuei-shao-yao-san (*Tang-kuei* and Peony Formula): abdominal pain, no convulsions in the rectus abdominis muscle, splashing sound beneath the heart. This formula is often given for abdominal pain during pregnancy.

Tang-kuei-szu-ni-tang (*Tang-kuei* and Jujube Combination): abdominal pain, cold hands and feet, thin pulse that tends to die out.

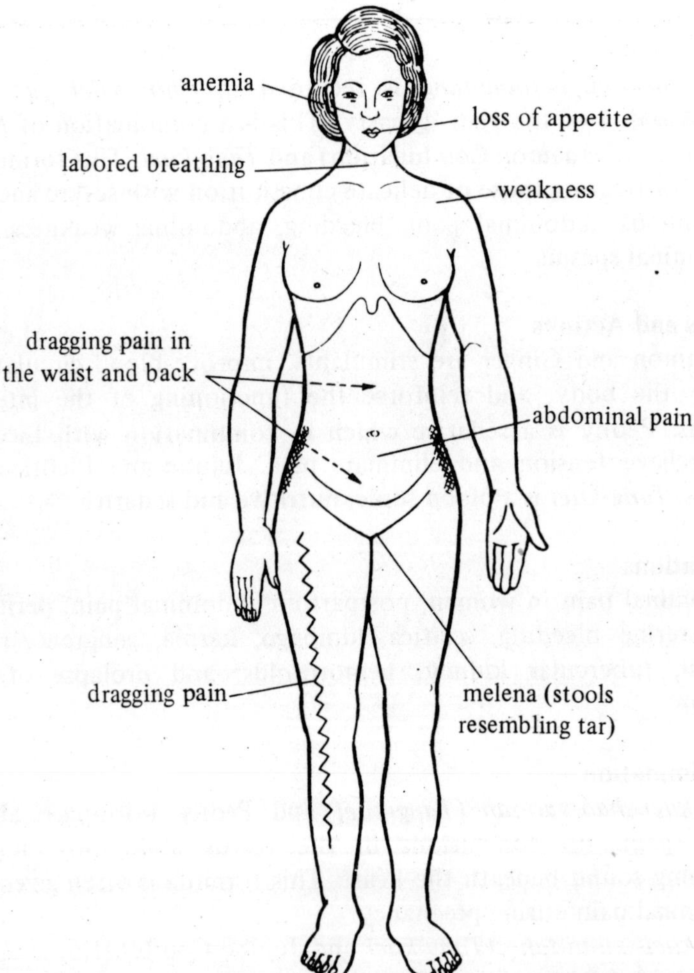
anemia
loss of appetite
labored breathing
weakness
dragging pain in
the waist and back
abdominal pain
dragging pain
melena (stools
resembling tar)

Tang-Kuei-Szu-Ni-Chia-Wu-Chu-Yu-Sheng-Chiang-Tang 當歸四逆加吳茱萸生薑湯

(Tang-kuei, Evodia, and Ginger Combination)

Tang-kuei	3.0	Cinnamon	3.0	Peony	3.0
Asarum	2.0	Licorice	2.0	Akebia	3.0
Jujube	5.0	Evodia	2.0	Ginger	4.0

Recorded in *Shang han lun* (傷寒論) by Chang Chung-ching of the Han dynasty. Used for treating patients having "internal water poisoning" with chest distention, vomiting, acute pain around the waist and in the abdomen, diarrhea, chills in the hands and feet, and a weak pulse.

Herbs and Actions

Tang-kuei and Peony nourish the blood and increase blood circulation. Cinnamon and Asarum remove internal chills. Akebia increases blood circulation. Jujube and Licorice nourish *ch'i*. Evodia remedies flushing-up, increases blood circulation, halts vomiting and headaches. Ginger, an acrid stomachic, relieves vomiting, too.

Indications

Weak pulse, chills in the hands and feet due to a febrile disease, and excessive sweating; chilblains; callouses and corns; sciatica; gangrene; hernia; skin diseases; petechia; uterine pain; chills; and diarrhea.

Discrimination

Pai-hu-tang (Gypsum Combination): cold hands and feet; sweating, extreme thirst; yang-firmness conformation; slippery, massive, and big pulse.
Szu-ni-san (Bupleurum and *Chih-shih* Formula): cold arms and legs, rectus abdominis muscle tension, thoraco-costal distress.
Szu-ni-tang (Aconite and G.L. Combination): cold arms and legs, diarrhea of undigested food, submerged and slow pulse.
Tang-kuei-shao-yao-san (*Tang-kuei* and Peony Formula): chills,

abdominal pain, anemia, stagnant water in the stomach, water and blood symptoms, abdominal muscle convulsion.
Hsiao-chien-chung-tang (Minor Cinnamon and Peony Combination): abdominal pain, abdominal laxity, gas, peristaltic instability.

Stagnant chills in the interior

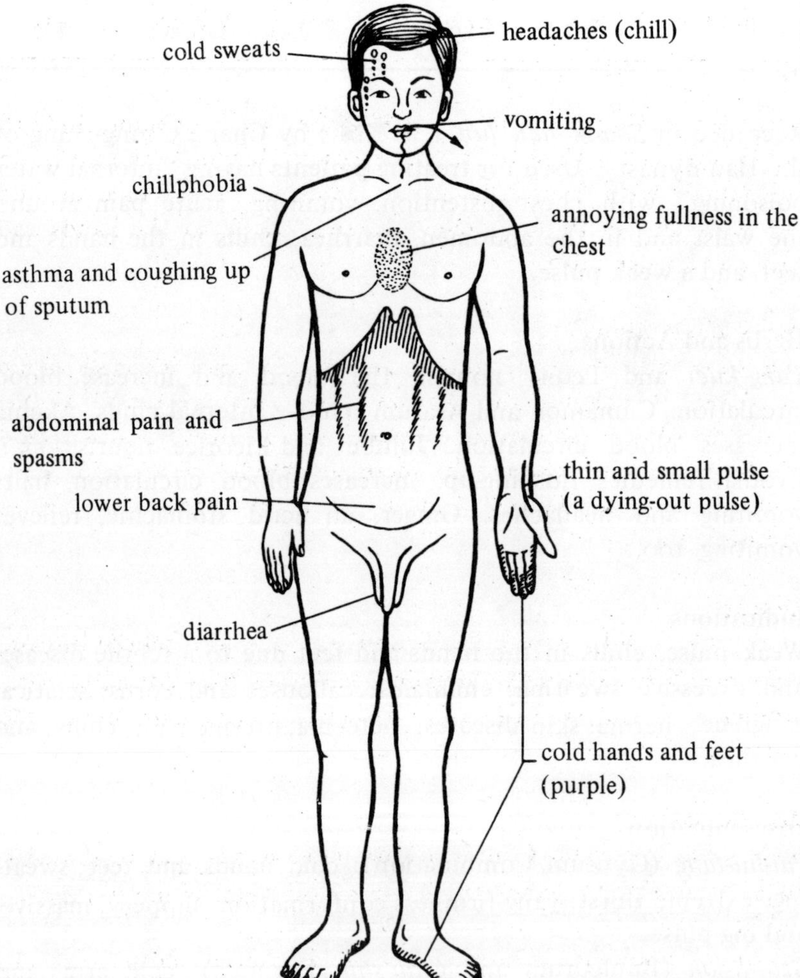

Tang-Kuei-Szu-Ni-Tang 當歸四逆湯

(Tang-kuei and Jujube Combination)

Tang-kuei	3.0	Cinnamon	3.0	Peony	3.0
Akebia	3.0	Jujube	5.0	Asarum	2.0
Licorice	2.0				

Tang-kuei-szu-ni-tang was recorded in the *Shang han lun* (傷寒論) during the Han dynasty. This formula is used for treating cold hands and feet, a weak pulse, ephidrosis during febrile disease, abdominal distention, weak abdomen, and abdominal cramps.

Herbs and Actions

Tang-kuei improves blood circulation and acts as a hematinic. Cinnmon regulates the *ch'i* and when combined with *Tang-kuei*, improves blood circulation. Asarum warms the body and dispels chills. Akebia dispels "stagnant *ch'i*" and "stagnant blood" and works with Asarum to relieve ascites and increase the flow of urine. Jujube improves blood circulation.

Indications

Frostbite, calluses and corns, sciatica, hernia, midline pain, gangrene, stagnant blood in the skin, intestinal colic, uterine pain, abdominal cramps in women, chills, and diarrhea.

Discrimination

Pai-hu-tang (Gypsum Combination): cold hands and feet; sweating; extreme thirst; anxiety; yang-firmness conformation; slippery, massive, and big pulse.

Szu-ni-san (Bupleurum and *Chih-shih* Formula): coldness in arms and legs, tension in the rectus abdominis muscle, thoraco-costal distress.

Szu-ni-tang (Aconite and G. L. Combination): cold arms and legs, diarrhea of undigested food, submerged and slow pulse.

Tang-kuei-shao-yao-san (*Tang-kuei* and Peony Formula): chills, abdominal pain, anemia, stagnant water in the stomach, watery blood conformation, abdominal spasms.

Ta-chien-chung-tang (Major Zanthoxylum Combination): abdominal pain, abdominal laxity, gas, peristaltic instability.

Weak conformation

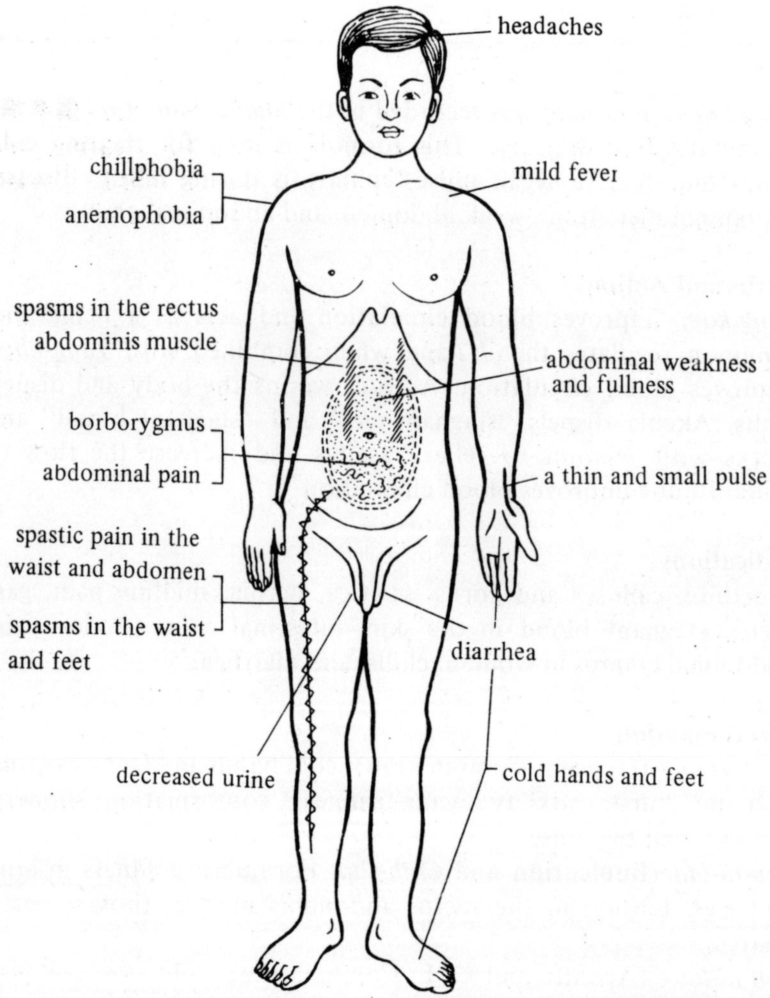

Tung-Mo-Szu-Ni-Tang 通脈四逆湯

(Licorice, Aconite, and Ginger Pulse Combination)

Licorice	3.0	Ginger	4.0	Aconite	0.5–1.0

Formed by doubling the amount of dry ginger in *Szu-ni-tang* (Aconite, Ginger, and Licorice Combination). Used to treat the *Szu-ni-tang* conformation in which vomiting, diarrhea, and cold limbs are exceedingly severe and the pulse is failing rapidly. This formula takes advantage of the warming property of dry ginger by warming yang, reinforcing the insides, and restoring yang, thus normalizing pulsation.

Herbs and Actions

Aconite is extremely acrid and hot. Its warmth revitalizes yang and disperses chills. Dry ginger acts with Aconite to warm the insides and to disperse chills; thus it helps Aconite restore yang vitality. Licorice enriches the insides and warms and nourishes yang.

Indications

Influenza, typhoid fever, diarrhea, autointoxication, appendicitis, gastrointestinal inflammation, dyspepsia, jaundice, hyperhydrosis, and a buoyant pulse in a weak conformation.

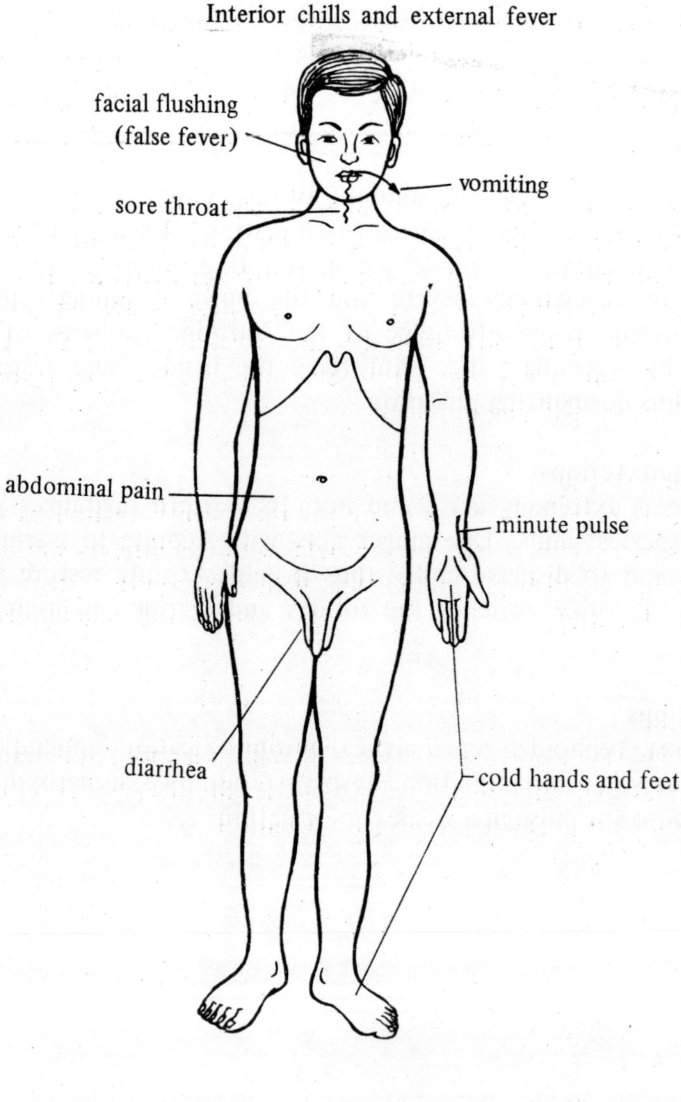
Interior chills and external fever
facial flushing
(false fever)
vomiting
sore throat
abdominal pain
minute pulse
diarrhea
cold hands and feet

Wu-Chu-Yu-Tang *(Evodia Combination)*					吳茱萸湯
Evodia	4.0	Ginseng	3.0	Jujube	3.0
Ginger	6.0				

Wu-chu-yu-tang was recorded in the *Shang han hun* (傷寒論) during the Han dynasty. This formula is used for treating chills in the liver and stomach, vomiting, restlessness, headache, subcardiac distention, cold hands and feet, and a sinking pulse.

Herbs and Actions

Evodia is a tonic that dispels stagnant water. Ginger dispels "internal chills" and eliminates flushing up. Ginseng and Jujube are both tonics effective for eliminating subcardiac distention and increasing vitality.

Indication

Vomiting, eclampsia, acute vomiting and diarrhea, headache, migraine, food poisioning, dyspepsia, gastroptosis, and beriberi.

Discrimination

Pan-hsia-hsieh-hsin-tang (Pinellia Combination): vomiting, obstruction and hardness beneath the heart, gas, belching, yang firm conformation.

Wu-ling-san (Hoelen Five Herb Formula): vomiting and decreased urine; yang conformation with adverse water congestion.

Hsiao-chai-hu-tang (Minor Bupleurum Combination): vomiting, thoraco-costal distress, alternating chills and fever, yang firm conformation.

Szu-ni-tang (Aconite and G. L. Combination): vomiting without headache, severe adversity in the arms and legs.

Pan-hsia-pai-chu-tien-ma-tang (Pinellia and Gastrodia Combination): vomiting, headache, mild and chronic symptoms, and vertigo.

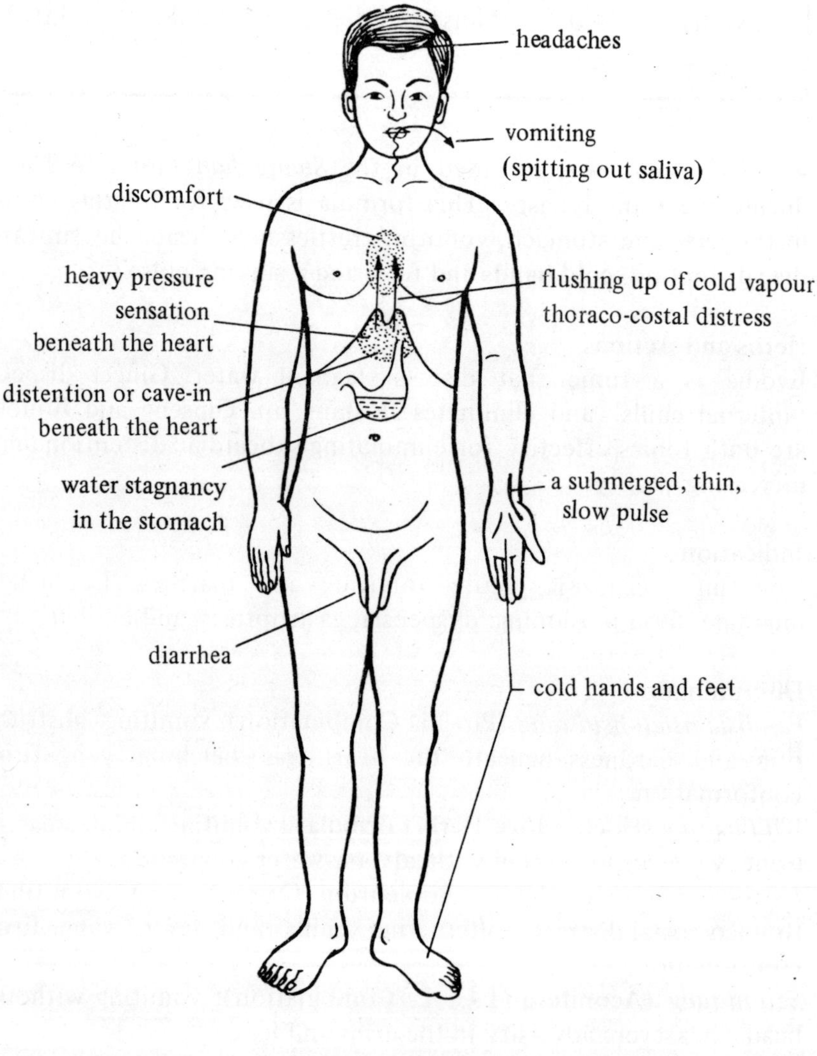
headaches
vomiting
(spitting out saliva)
discomfort
heavy pressure
sensation
beneath the heart
flushing up of cold vapour
thoraco-costal distress
distention or cave-in
beneath the heart
water stagnancy
in the stomach
a submerged, thin,
slow pulse
diarrhea
cold hands and feet

Wu-Tou-Kuei-Chih-Tang 烏頭桂枝湯

(Wu-tou and Cinnamon Combination)

Wu-tou	0.5–1.0	Cinnamon	4.0	Ginger	4.0
Jujube	4.0	Peony	4.0	Licorice	2.0

Essentially for those whose main complaints are abdominal pain, cold arms and legs, paralysis of the arms and legs, or general aching. Abdominal pain is a primary symptom of a hernia. Cold limbs indicate the exhaustion of yang, causing poor circulation. Limb paralysis is caused by extreme coldness. General aching is due to a cold body surface which causes discord between the *ying* and the *wei* (constructive and defensive energies or systems). Thus, chills of both the inside and the outside of the body need to be treated simultaneously. *Wu-tou-kuei-chih-tang* serves this purpose.

Herbs and Actions

Wu-tou removes chills and kills pain. Cinnamon harmonizes the *ying* and the *wei* energies and disperses outside chills.

Indications

Acute or chronic appendicitis, chronic intestinal stenosis, gastric ulcers, gallstones, pancreatitis, and ascariasis that causes chills and aching. Neuralgia, arthritis, myelitis, periostitis, tumors of the spine, gangrene with somatic and limb chills or weakness accompanied by severe pain.

Discrimination

Kuei-chih-chia-fu-tzu-tang (Cinnamon and Aconite Combination) is for abdominal pain, cold symptoms, limb paralysis, spontaneous perspiration, and anemophobia.

Tang-kuei-szu-ni-chia-wu-chu-yu-sheng-chiang-tang (*Tang-kuei*, Evodia and Ginger Combination) is for abdominal pain, chills in the limbs, thoracic irritation and distention, cold sweats, and vomiting.

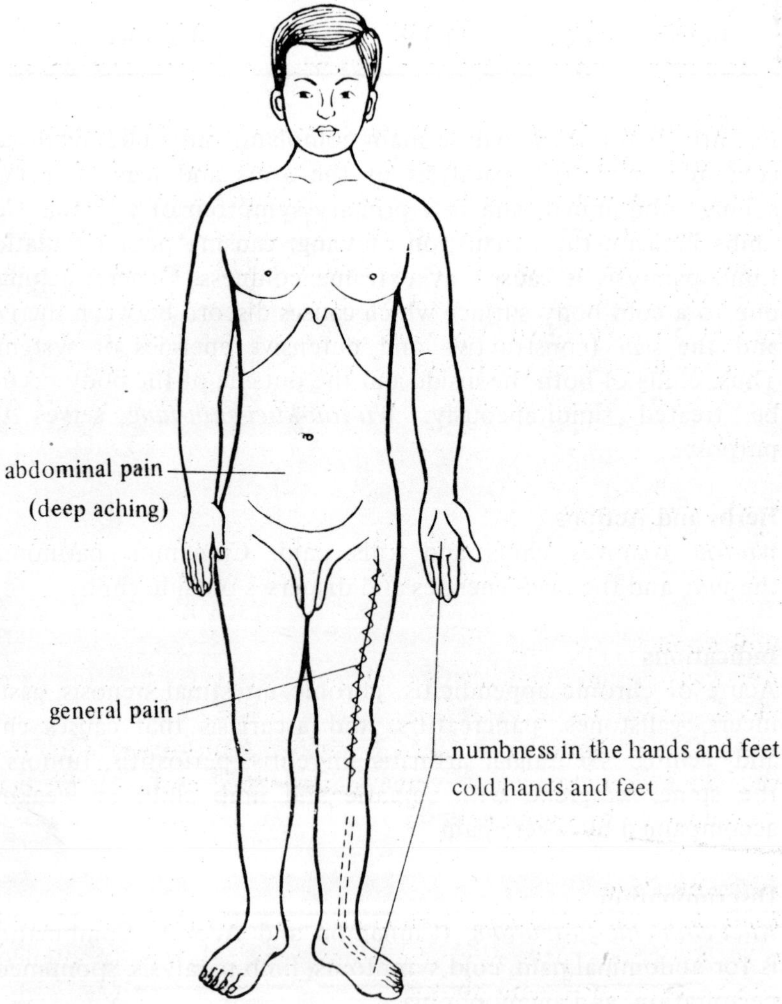
abdominal pain
(deep aching)
general pain
numbness in the hands and feet
cold hands and feet

11.
Kai Chiao Tung Kuan Chi
(開竅通關劑, Smelling Salts, Inhalants)

Formulas composed chiefly of aromatic and "penetrative" herbs treat unconsciousness or a coma and are called *kai chiao tung kuan chi* or *fang hsiang kai kung chi.*

Unconsciousness and comas are differentiated into heat and chill closure. Accordingly, in clinical practice, the formulas are also divided into cool and warm. Cool-opening formulas are composed of aromatic herbs together with fever reducing and detoxicant herbs or with blood cooling and antispasmodic herbs. The formulas cleanse the heart, relieve faintness, lower fevers, and detoxify. The herbal formulas used in the warm-opening method are composed of aromatic herbs together with acrid, warm, *ch'i*-moving, and obstruction-dissolving herbs. They awaken the patient and dissolve turbidity by means of the smell of the herbs.

Before using smelling salts, the doctor must determine whether the conformation is chilly or hot; whereupon the decision to use a cool or warm formula can be made. Moreover, no matter which awakening method, this type of formula is only suitable for an "obstruction conformation" in which harmful toxin is thriving and the patient's *ch'i* is full. Unconscious patients with toneless hands, incontinence, feeble and minute respiration, and spontaneous perspiration – a "prostration" conformation – cannot be treated with these formulas even in the presence of delirium and coma.

An-Kung-Niu-Huang-Wan 安宮牛黃丸

(Bos and Curcuma Formula)

Bos	4.0	Curcuma	4.0	Scute	4.0
Coptis	4.0	Gardenia	4.0	Realgar	4.0
Cinnabar	4.0	Borneol	1.0	Musk	1.0
Pearl	2.0	Rhinoceros horn	4.0		

Pulverized into powder and mixed with honey to form pills weighing 4g each. Dose: one pill each time.

Recorded in *Wen ping tiao pien* (溫病條辨) compiled by Wu Chu-tung who formulated this remedy on the basis of Wan's *Niu-huang-ching-hsin-wan-chia-wei*. Indicated for warm ailments such as summer heatstroke, epidemic heteropathies, internally obstructed sputum, lockjaw, dizziness, delirium, and spasmatic or comatose convulsions resulting from fever.

Herbs and Actions

Bos and Rhinoceros horn clean the heart, open the cavities, and detoxify poisons. Musk and Borneol open the cavities. These components are the chief elements of this formula. Curcuma clears extravasation and opens cavities. Scute, Coptis, Gardenia, and Realgar purge fire and poisons and work as ancillary components. The remaining components, Cinnabar and Pearl, act as a tranquilizer and a sedative, respectively.

Indications

Epidemic encephalitis, septicemia, chronic diarrhea, infectious hepatitis, and hepatic coma – all of which belong to the fever-toxin type coma. In addition to these diseases, uremic coma and coma resulting from cerebral injury are treated with this formula.

Chih-Pao-Tan 至寶丹

(Rhinoceros and Succinum Formula)

Cinnabar	3.2	Realgar	3.2	Succinum	3.2
Musk	0.4	Borneol	0.4	Gold foil	5.0
Silver foil	5.0	Bos	1.6	Benzoin	4.8
Eretmochelys	3.2	Rhinoceros horn	3.2		

Recorded in *Ho chi chu fang* (和劑局方). Chief targets of treatment are apoplexy, apnea (suspension of respiration) as a result of an attack by a noxious toxin, heatstroke, sputum fever of a feverish disease that is shut inside, dizziness, delirium, somatic fever, discomfort, irritability, copious sputum, forceful breathing, red tongue with yellow fur, infantile convulsion, tetanus, heart fever, conditions caused by heteropathy, insomnia, wind toxin salivation, and epilepsy.

Herbs and Actions

It should be noted that the three formulas *An-kung-niu-huang-wan, Chih-pao-tan* and *Tzu-hsueh-tan* have about the same effect. The only difference is that *An-kung-niu-huang-wan* (Bos and Curcuma Formula) is the coolest in nature and is a better expectorant. *Tzu-hsueh-tan* is less cool but is the strongest spasmolytic. As for *Chih-pao-tan,* it is only moderately cool and is less spasmolytic than the other two but is superior to the others in opening up the body cavities.

Rhinoceros horn, Bos, and eretmochelys purge fever, eliminate sputum, and calm someone who has been frightened. They are also antidotes. Realgar cleans and detoxifies. Borneol, Musk, and Benzoin are aromatic cavity opening agents. Cinnabar, Succinum, and Gold and Silver foil tranquilize the mind and calm the spirit.

Indications

Epidemic encephalitis, intoxication, diarrhea, hepatic coma, and the coma caused by cerebral injury. All of these illnesses are classified as sputum-fever conformations.

Niu-Huang-Ching-Hsin-Wan 牛黃清心丸

(Bos and Musk Formula)

Dioscorea	26.3	Licorice	18.8	Ginseng	9.4
Bulrush	9.4	Rhinoceros	7.5	*Shen-chu*	9.4
Cinnamon	6.6	Gelatin	6.6	Ophiopogon	5.6
Scute	5.6	*Tang-kuei*	5.6	Siler	5.6
Cinnabar	5.6	Bupleurum	4.7	Platycodon	4.7
Apricot seed	4.7	Musk	3.8	Borneol	3.8
Antelope horn	3.8	Realgar	3.0	Ampelopsis	2.8
Atractylodes	5.6	Bos	4.5	Cnidium	4.7
Hoelen (white)	4.7	Ginger	2.8		
Bean Sprouts (black variety)			6.6		
Gold foil torn in pieces			120		
Jujube torn in pieces			20		

Since ancient times many formuls have born the name *Niu-huang-ching-hsin-wan*. Though they vary in composition, they have the similar actions of cleaning the heart and dispelling fever. This formula, which is recorded in *Ho chi chu fang* (和劑局方), contains a great number of components and is employed for a variety of ailments. It can clean the heart and purge fever as well as expel wind toxin and calm down a person who is suffering from fright. This formula is prescribed for apoplexy, spasmodic limbs, difficulty in speech, distorted mouth and eyes, panic, amnesia, and absent-mindedness, sputum and saliva blockage, mental uneasiness, horror and sorrow, irritability and sleeplessness, perversities (irregular and abnormal pleasure), anger or hysteria, madness, and mental disorders. It may also be given to children who are irritable, have rigidity in the neck and back and have curvature of the spine.

Herbs and Actions

Bovis bezoar (a concretion found in the stomach or intestines of ruminant animals) cleans the heart and opens cavities. Ginseng aids respiration and nourishes the heart, acting in the same way as the cavity-opening herbs in restoring normal breathing and diminishing hypersensitivity. Antelope horn cleans the liver and expels wind toxin. Rhinoceros horn cleans the heart and detoxifies toxins. Realgar is an expectorant and antidoting agent. Gold foil and Cinnabar calm the mind and tranquilize the spirit. Bupleurum together with *Tang-kuei,* Peony and Atractylodes dispel poisons from the liver, dissolve obstructions, and treat dizziness, eye blurring, and aches in the ribs. Dioscorea and Gelatin are tonics. Siler expels wind and arrests spasms. Cnidium expels wind and kills pain. Hoelen calms the mind and soothes the spirit. Cinnamon and Ginger warm the interior. Apricot seed and Platycodon stop coughing and expel sputum. Bean sprouts are diaphoretic (increase perspiration) and diuretic. Ampelopsis and Scute dissipate fever. Licorice harmonizes all the herbs.

Indications

Hypertension, apoplexy, monoplegia, arteriosclerosis, paralysis of the heart, cardiac asthma, acute or chronic convulsions, vertigo, cerebral anemia, unconsciousness, spiritual miasma, schizophrenia, neurasthenia, distorted mouth and eyes, speech problems, and numbness of the limbs.

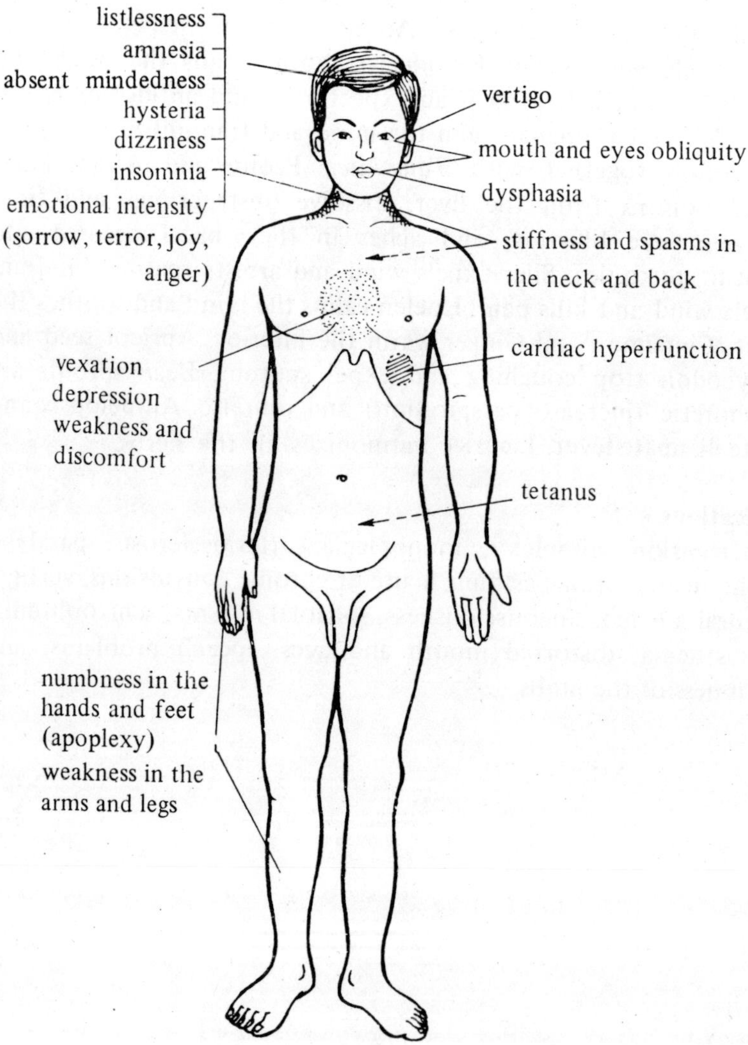
listlessness
amnesia
absent mindedness
hysteria
dizziness
insomnia
emotional intensity (sorrow, terror, joy, anger)
vertigo
mouth and eyes obliquity
dysphasia
stiffness and spasms in the neck and back
vexation
depression
weakness and discomfort
cardiac hyperfunction
tetanus
numbness in the hands and feet (apoplexy)
weakness in the arms and legs

Su-Ho-Hsiang-Wan 蘇合香丸

(Styrax Formula)

Aristolochia	4.0	Rhinoceros	4.0	Cyperus	4.0
Terminalia	4.0	Cinnabar	4.0	Santalum	4.0
Benzoin	4.0	Aquilaria	4.0	Musk	3.1
Clove	4.0	Piper	4.0	Borneol	2.0
Styrax	2.0	Mastic	2.0		

Recorded in *Ho chi chu fang* (和劑局方). The disease apoplexy is classified as either obstructed (firm) or exhausted (weak). The obstructed type is further divided into "cold obstruction" and "heat obstruction". Styrax is warm in nature, and hence it can only be used for the "cold obstruction" type of apoplexy. It treats coma, sputum blockage or abdominal pain, vomiting, diarrhea caused by chill heteropathy, or sputum turbidity that obstructs the air passages.

Apoplectic coma, the main indication for this formula, results from chill heteropathy confined internally or from the pericardium being enveloped by turbid sputum. Thus the method of treatment is to open the cavities, disperse chills, and clear turbidity. The formula gives off aromas that stimulate the respiratory tract. It also expels dirt, breaks up "cold obstructions" and dries excessive fluid. It also can cure thoraco-abdominal distention accompanied by chills that is caused by the breathing in of dirt and noxious air; epidemic cholera; vomiting; and diarrhea caused by the internally obstructed chills and moisture.

Herbs and Actions

Contains ten aromatic components, namely, Aristolochia, Cyperus, Santalum, Benzoin, Aquilaria, Musk, Clove, Styrax, Borneol, and Mastic. The aroma of these constituents opens the obstructed cavities, aids respiration, dissolves occlusion, and lifts melancholia. Piper combined with these aromas disperses chills and removes obstructions. Rhinoceros has detoxicating effects and restores normal heart function. Cinnabar has calming effects because of its heaviness. Terminalia has an astringent effect which prevents excessive penetration of the aromas and the consequential exhaustion of the respiratory system. Thus properly mixed the various components may, by their warmth, channel and open cavities, disperse chills, and dissolve occlusion and turbidity.

Indications
Apoplexy, abrupt coma, lockjaw; breathing dirty and noxious air which causes abdominal and thoracic distention; pain and chills and obstruction of sputum and breathing; epidemic cholera with nausea but inability to vomit; angina pectoris due to respiratory obstructions, hemostasis, and "chill coagulation."

Tung-Kuan-San 通關散

(Gleditsia and Asarum Formula)

Gleditsia	3.0	Asarum	3.0

Included in *Addendum to Tan chi's Mental Ways* (丹溪心法附餘)
Classified as an analeptic for first aid, it stimulates the central nervous system and hence is a restorative. Used for obstructed conformations such as apoplexy, a sudden cessation of breathing and lockjaw due to sputum adversity, and unconsciousness. Taken by placing the fine powder into the nostril to cause sneezing. The lungs control the air supply for the entire body. If the pulmonary air is obstructed then all cavities of the body become clogged and the person loses consciousness. Sneezing allows the pulmonary air to pass and move about freely, enabling the patient to regain consciousness. Therefore, the ancient saying is: "If the patient can be made to sneeze, he can be cured. If he cannot sneeze, he will not recover because the pulmonary air is gone." After coming to, treatment is according to the symptomatic condition.

Herbs and Actions
Gleditsia, acrid and warm in nature, renders expectoration and opens clogged cavities. Asarum, also acrid and warm natured, has a

dispersing effect and opens the nine cavities. When used jointly, the two herbs open the cavities and passageways.

Indications
Apoplexy, lockjaw due to sputum adversity, unconsciousness.

Tzu-Hsueh-Tan *(Rhinoceros and Antelope Horn Formula)*		紫雪丹
Gypsum	Calcite	Talc
Loadstone	Scrophularia	Cimicifuga
Licorice	Mirabilitum	Nitre
Clove	Cinnabar	Aristolochia
Aquilaria	Musk	Rhinoceros
Antelope horn		

(Note: This formula is sold as on OTC drug. Each time take 1.5–3.0g)

An important febrifuge, antidote, and spasmolytic and cavity-opening agent recorded in *Ho chi chu fang* (和劑局方). First appeared in *Chien chin i fang* under the name *Tzu-hsueh,* a formula which contained all the same components except talc. Used essentially to treat fever that has penetrated the depths of the body: high fever, distress, irritability, irrationality, delirium, thirst, dry lips, red urine, constipation, red tongue, and even the severe conditions of convulsion, chilled limbs, and hysteria. It is also used for infantile epileptic convulsions brought on by high fever.

Herbs and Actions
Rhinoceros and Antelope horn, the chief ingredients, open cavities, purge fevers, detoxify, and suppress spasms. Gypsum, Calcite, and Talc are sweet and cold in nature and purge fevers. Scrophu-

laria, Cimicifuga, and Licorice purge fever and detoxify. Cinnabar and Loadstone are heavy and thus settle and calm the mind. Mirabilitum and Nitre lower fevers and disperse obstructions. The actions are further enhanced by Clove, Aquilaria, Aristolochia, and Musk.

Indications

Meningitis, encephalitis, and other acute feverish diseases with the above mentioned symptoms; infantile high fever and convulsions; infantile measles in which the fever toxin is flourishing internally and the color of the macules is purplish red; or in which there are high fever, gasping, a coma, and reddish purple lines in the fingers as a consequence of the incomplete eruption of the measles.

12.

Chen Ching Chi

(鎮靜劑, Sedative Formulas)

Formulas with sedative and tranquilizing effects are called *chen ching chi*. A *chen ching chi* formula reduces pain, arrests spasms, and quiets hysteria. According to origin, pathological mechanism, and herbal action, *chen ching chi* are divided into strong, sedating tranquilizers and heart-nourishing, mind sedatives. The former contains mostly heavy minerals and stones or shells that calm hysteria and tranquilize the mind by means of their heaviness; the latter is composed mainly of herbs that nourish the heart and pacify the mind while enriching the liver.

Because minerals, stones, and shells are detrimental to the spleen and stomach, strong tranquilizers should be used only temporarily.

Chai-Hu-Chia-Lung-Ku-Mu-Li-Tang
柴胡加龍骨牡蠣湯

(Bupleurum and Dragon Bone Combination)

Bupleurum	5.0	Hoelen	3.0	Pinellia	4.0
Rhubarb	1.0	Cinnamon	3.0	Scute	2.5
Jujube	2.5	Ginseng	2.5	Ginger	2.5
Oyster shell	2.5				

In his *Shang han lun* written in A.D. 205. Chang Chung-ching (a famous doctor of the Han dynasty) commented on a sedative, *Chai-hu-chia-lung-ku-mu-li-tang*, which was used in harmonizing the "inside" and "outside" and sedating the mind.

This formula is used to relieve chest and subcardiac distention, palpitation at the abdomen (especially near the umbilicus), insomnia, irritability, melancholia, fearfulness, agitation, unsteadiness, tendency towards mania and convulsions. It is also effective for a tendency toward fatigue and clumsiness of the limbs accompanied by oliguria and constipation.

Herbs and Actions

The principal herbs of this formula are Bupleurum, Dragon bone, and Hoelen.

Bupleurum purges inner heat at the chest. Dragon bone soothes and sedates inner agitation. Hoelen is diuretic and can calm the nerves. Bupleurum and Scute relieve heat and stagnancy in the chest. Dragon bone and Oyster shell decrease chest and abdominal palpitations and relieve cardiac hyperfunction, insomnia, and fearfulness. Cinnamon cures flushing up. A combination of Hoelen, Pinellia, and Ginger dispels fluid accumulation in the stomach. Rhubarb purges the intestines, draws out infection, and produces sedation. Jujube and Ginger assist and reinforce the actions of the other herbs.

Indications

Neurosis, hysteria, epilepsy, neurotic insomnia, climacteric disorders, neurotic palpitation, neurotic impotence, arteriosclerosis, hypertension, apoplexy, valvular disease, angina pectoris, chronic nephritis, nephroatrophy, uremia, beriberi, chronic arthralgia, menoplegia, heat stroke, shoulder stiffness, cirrhosis, and alopecia.

Discrimination

Ta-chai-hu-tang (Major Bupleurum Combination): liver congestion, chills and fever, acute pain beneath the heart, melancholy and irritability, mild emotional distress.

Ling-kuei-chu-kan-tang (Atractylodes and Hoelen Combination): epilepsy, palpitations beneath the heart, stagnant water in the stomach, and submerged pulse.

Ling-kuei-kan-tsao-tang (Hoelen, Licorice, and Jujube Combination): epilepsy, palpitations beneath the umbilicus, submerged and quick pulse.

I-kan-san-chia-chen-pi-pan-hsia (Bupleurum, Pinellia, and Citrus Formula): epilepsy, abdominal movement, mental distress, strong palpitations beside the left umbilicus, weak conformation.

Chai-hu-chiang-kuei-tang (Bupleurum, Ginger, and Cinnamon Combination): liver congestion, abdominal movement, weak conformation.

Kan-mai-ta-tsao-tang (Licorice and Jujube Combination): mania, acute symptoms, severe neurotic behavior, acute pain in the abdominal muscles.

Kuei-chih-chia-lung-ku-mu-li-tang (Cinnamon and Dragon Bone Combination): the same mental distress as *Chai-hu-chia-lung-ku-mu-li-tang,* weak constitution, overwork, no thoraco-costal distress.

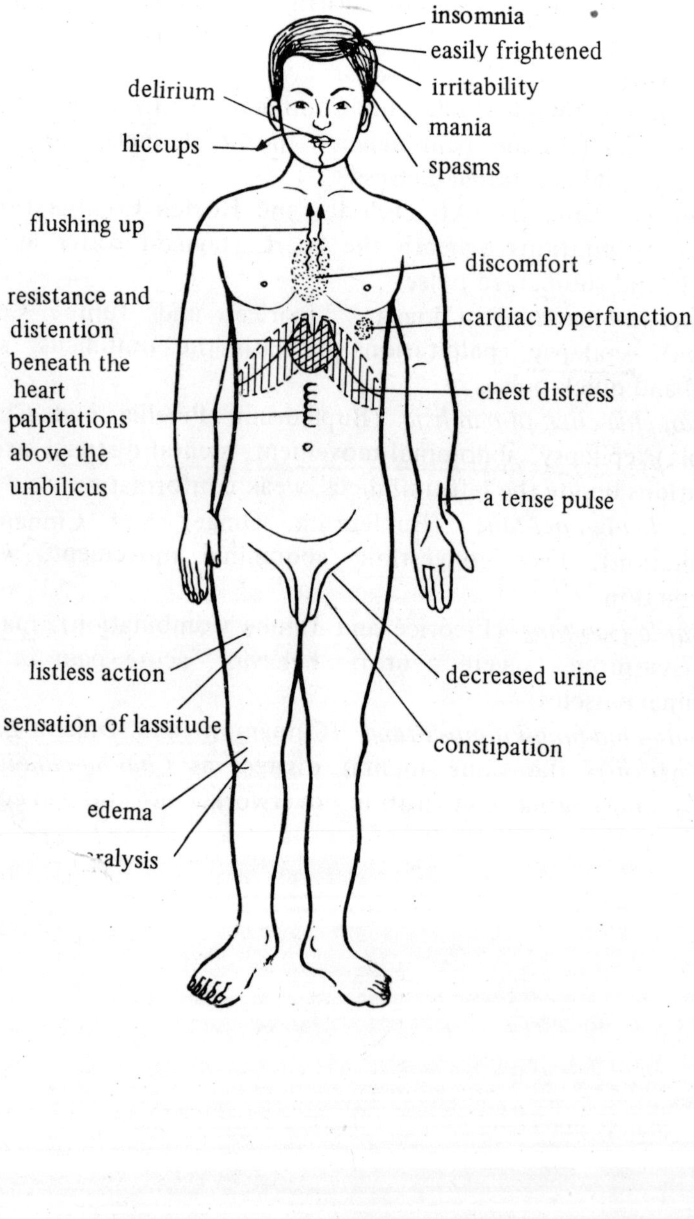
insomnia
easily frightened
irritability
mania
spasms
delirium
hiccups
flushing up
discomfort
resistance and
distention
beneath the
heart
cardiac hyperfunction
chest distress
palpitations
above the
umbilicus
a tense pulse
listless action
sensation of lassitude
decreased urine
constipation
edema
ralysis

Chu-Sha-An-Shen-Wan 硃砂安神丸

(Cinnabar Formula)

Coptis	4.5	Cinnabar	3.0	*Tang-kuei*	3.0
Rehmannia	3.0	Licorice	1.5		

Chu-sha-an-shen-wan was recorded in the *Lan shih mi tsang* (蘭室秘藏) by Li kao during the Yuan dynasty. This formula is used for treating emotional instability, insomnia, "internal heat", nightmares, fever in the chest due to stress, neurasthenia, amnesia, and palpitations.

Herbs and Actions
Cinnabar, a major component of this formula, is a sedative. Coptis is bitter and cooling in nature and acts as an antipyretic. In combination with Cinnabar, it relieves emotional instability. *Tang-kuei* and Rehmannia nourish the heart and blood. Licorice coordinates the actions of the other herbs.

Indications
Insomnia, amnesia, palpitation, and neurasthenia.

I-Kan-San 抑肝散

(Bupleurum Formula)

Tang-kuei	3.0	Gambir	3.0	Cnidium	3.0
Hoelen	4.0	Bupleurum	2.0	Licorice	1.5
Atractylodes	4.0				

Recorded in *Jen chai chih chih fang* (仁齋直指方) by Yang Shih-ying of the Sung dynasty. Used for treating excitability due to liver disturbance, nervousness, irritability, insomnia due to the excitability, and epilepsy. Also suitable for children having internal heat in the liver with fever, rapid heart palpitations due to fear, and convulsions.

Herbs and Actions
Gambir is antispasmodic and sedative. Gambir, Bupleurum, and Licorice relieve nervous excitability. *Tang-kuei* and Cnidium nourish the liver and increase blood circulation. Hoelen and Atractylodes dispel internal heat in the liver and remove any fluid toxins remaining in the stomach.

Indications
Neurosis, epilepsy, hysteria, insomnia, night crying of children, febrile disease, climacteric disorders, rickets, and spasms.

Discrimination
Chai-hu-chia-lung-ku-mu-li-tang (Bupleurum and Dragon Bone Combination): emotional and mental distress, palpitations in the chest and abdomen, thoraco-costal distress, relatively firm conformation.
Pan-hsia-hou-pu-tang (Pinellia and Magnolia Combination): emotional distress, the sensation of broiled meat adhering to the throat, gastrointestinal weakness.
Chia-wei-hsiao-yao-san (Bupleurum and Peony Formula): emotional distress, irritability, weakness and swelling of the abdomen.
Ling-kuei-kan-tsao-tang (Hoelen, Licorice, and Jujube Combination): emotional distress, terror and mania, spasms of the abdominal skin.

Weak conformation

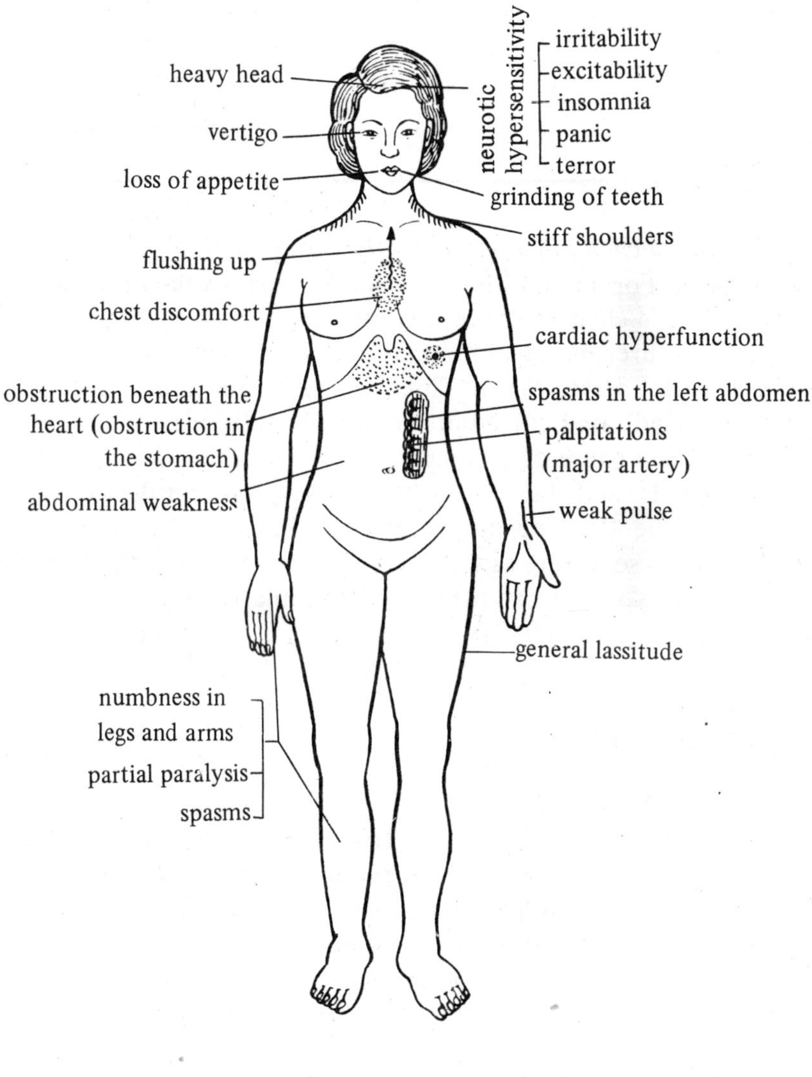

I-Kan-San-Chia-Chen-Pi-Pan-Hsia

抑肝散加陳皮半夏

(Bupleurum and Citrus, Pinellia Formula)

Tang-kuei	3.0	Gambir	3.0	Cnidium	3.0
Hoelen	4.0	Bupleurum	2.0	Licorice	1.5
Atractylodes	4.0	Pinellia	5.0	Citrus	3.0

I-kan-san-chia-chen-pi-pan-hsia is the combination of *I-kan-san* (Bupleurum Formula) with Citrus and Pinellia. *I-kan-san* has a sedative action in children of weak conformation resulting from weak fever of the liver meridian that has caused an excitation syndrome of the brain nerve. When Pinellia and Citrus are added, this formula is indicated for adults (especially those past middle age, either premenopause or postmenopause) with obvious neuropathy and weak pulse and abdomen but strong palpitation (like a gushing spa) from the left side of the naval to beneath the heart. This palpitation is so strong as to be easily detected when the hand is placed on this area. In addition, this formula is also greatly effective in neurotic syndromes with excessive palpitation, phobia, headache, flushing up, dizziness, stiff shoulders, insomnia, and generalized fatigue. The latter use was prescribed by the Japanese physician Asai Nanmei.

Herbs and Actions

Gambir is an antispasmodic effective in relieving spasms of the limbs. *Tang-kuei* nourishes the hepatic blood. Cnidium improves blood circulation. Bupleurum with Licorice and Gambir can enhance sedative function and alleviate excessive liver *ch'i.* Hoelen and Atractylodes are diuretics which can release stagnant water from the stomach. Citrus and Pinellia are expectorants.

Indications

Neurasthenia, hysteria, menopausal neurosis, gout, noctiphobia, insomnia, atrophied limbs, toxemia of pregnancy, and pediatric epilepsy.

Kan-Mai-Ta-Tsao-Tang *(Licorice and Jujube Combination)*					**甘麥大棗湯**
Licorice	5.0	Wheat	20.0	Jujube	6.0

Kan-mai-ta-tsao-tang is mentioned early in a Chinese medical work *Chin kuei yao lueh* by Chang Chung-ching (142-220 A.D.) of the Han dynasty. This formula is good to treat overexcitement, spasms, hysteria, nervousness, insomnia, emotional instability, and frequent yawning.

Herbs and Actions
Licorice and Jujube cure muscular spasm, nervous excitability, and various pains. Wheat relieves excitability.

Indications
Hysteria, nervous exhaustion, neurosis, insomnia, epilepsy, chorea, sleep-walking, gastrointestinal spasms, uterine cramping, spasmodic cough, and night crying.

Discrimination
Pan-hsia-hou-pu-tang (Pinellia and Magnolia Combination): emotional instability, depressed *ch'i,* the sensation of baked meat clinging to the throat.
Chai-hu-chia-lung-ku-mu-li-tang (Bupleurum and Dragon Bone Combination): emotional instability, obstruction and hardness beneath the heart, palpitations above the umbilicus.
Kan-tsao-hsieh-hsin-tang (Pinellia and Licorice Combination): emotional instability, obstruction and hardness beneath the heart, diarrhea and gas.
Ling-kuei-kan-tsao-tang (Hoelen, Licorice, and Jujube Combination): emotional instability and cardiac hyperfunction.

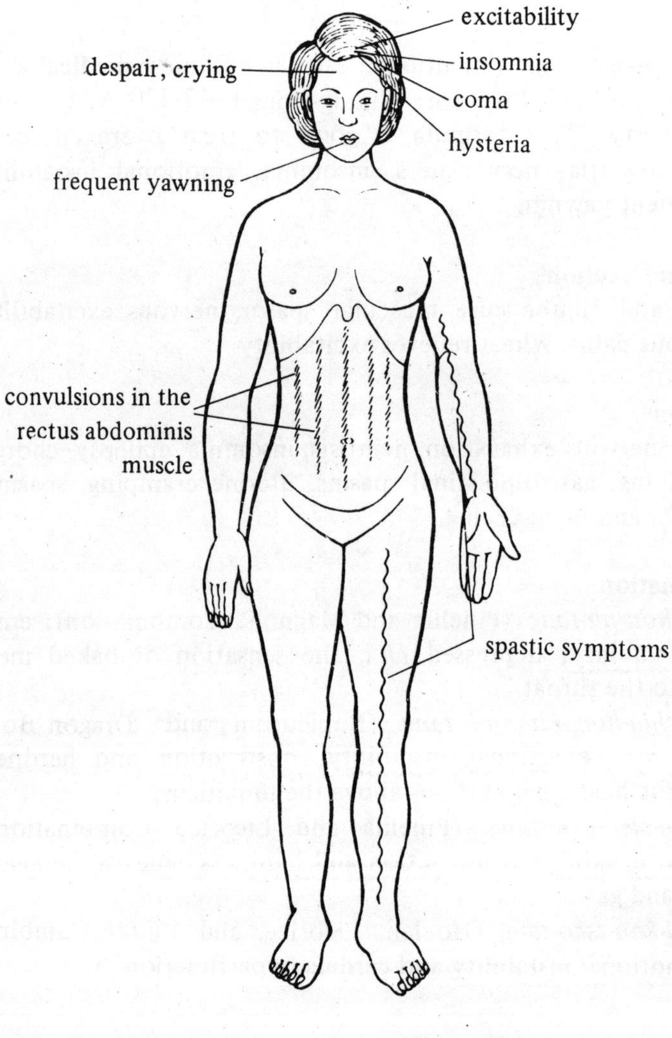
excitability
despair, crying
insomnia
coma
hysteria
frequent yawning
convulsions in the
rectus abdominis
muscle
spastic symptoms

Kan-Tsao-Tang *(Licorice Combination)*	甘草湯
Licorice 8.0	

Kan-tsao-tang is recorded in *Shang han lun* (傷寒論) of the Han dynasty. This formulas is used for treating severe pain in the throat, abdominal pain, and coughing.

Herbs and Actions
Licorice nourishes the spleen and stomach, acts as a detoxifier, eliminates pain, and relieves acute spasms.

Indications
Acute laryngitis, gastric spasm, spasmodic coughing, hoarseness, recurrent abdominal pain, toothache, anuria, dysuria, pain of carbuncles, and food poisoning.

Discrimination
Shao-yao-kan-tsao-tang (Peony and Licorice Combination): pain in the arms and legs. This formula can be used for spasms of deep, smooth muscles.
Hsiao-chien-chung-tang (Minor Cinnamon and Peony Combination): abdominal pain, weak conformation with no acute conditions.

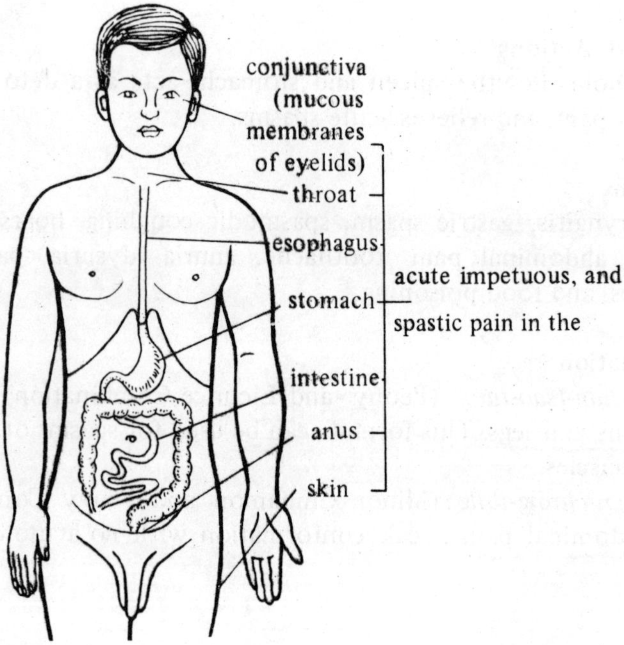
conjunctiva
(mucous
membranes
of eyelids)
throat
esophagus
stomach
intestine
anus
skin
acute impetuous, and
spastic pain in the

Kuei-Chih-Chia-Lung-Ku-Mu-Li-Tang
桂枝加龍骨牡蠣湯
(Cinnamon and Dragon Bone Combination)

Cinnamon	4.0	Peony	4.0	Jujube	4.0
Ginger	4.0	Oyster shell	3.0	Licorice	2.0
Dragon bone	3.0				

Kuei-chih-chia-lung-ku-mu-li-tang is recorded in *Chin kuei yao lueh* (金匱要略) of the Han dynasty. This formula is a combination of *Kuei-chih-tang* (Cinnamon Combination) with Dragon bone and Oyster shell. This formula is used for treating those of delicate constitution with recurrent fever, headache, vertigo, sweating, night sweats, palpitation, spasms in the lower abdomen, chills, and nocturnal emission.

Herbs and Actions
Kuei-chih-tang can remove muscular tension and nourish yin and yang. Cinnamon is a nutrient. Peony nourishes yin. Ginger relieves chills. Licorice and Jujube nourish the spleen and "*ch'i*". Dragon bone constricts yang. Oyster shell constricts yin.

Indications
Nervous exhaustion due to sexual excess, nervousness, palpitation, insomnia, enuresis, and nocturnal emission.

Discrimination
Chai-hu-chia-lung-ku-mu-li-tang (Bupleurum and Dragon Bone Combination): palpitation, insomnia, thoraco-costal distress, and severe mental illness.
Hsiao-chien-chung-tang (Minor Cinnamon and Peony Combination): involuntary emissions, night sweats, cardiac hyperfunction, abdominal pain, fever in the hands and feet, dry throat and mouth.
Kuei-chih-chu-shao-yao-chia-shu-chi-lung-ku-mu-li-tang (Cinnamon, Dichroa, and Dragon Bone Combination): palpitations, mental distress, fire toxin, and severe mental illness.

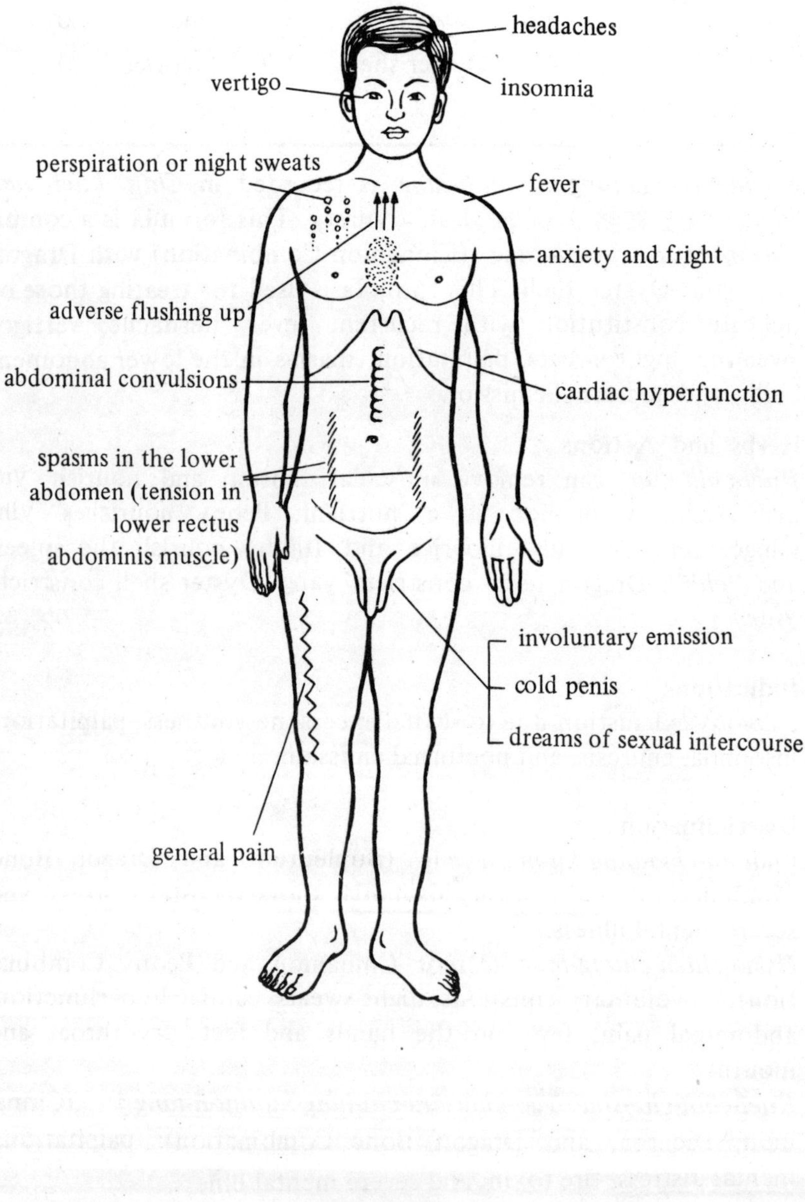
headaches
vertigo
insomnia
perspiration or night sweats
fever
anxiety and fright
adverse flushing up
abdominal convulsions
cardiac hyperfunction
spasms in the lower abdomen (tension in lower rectus abdominis muscle)
involuntary emission
cold penis
dreams of sexual intercourse
general pain

Kuei-Chih-Chu-Shao-Yao-Chia-Shu-Chi-Lung-Ku-Mu-Li-Tang
桂枝去芍藥加蜀漆龍骨牡蠣湯

(Cinnamon and D. D. O. Combination)

Cinnamon	4.0	Ginger	4.0	Dichroa	4.0
Oyster shell	6.0	Licorice	2.0	Jujube	4.0
Dragon bone	5.0				

Generally this formula is employed when neurotic symptoms such as instability, anxiety, terror, hysteria, absent-mindedness, coma, and delirium appear as a result of a fever. Most patients with this conformation have superficial breathing, oliguria, and occasionally hematuria. Such a conformation is termed a fire toxin conformation or fire adversitv. It occurred in ancient times as a result of erroneous treatment with the cauterizing needle or other heating method used to promote sweating. Although such means of treatment are no longer used, the same conformation is encountered in patients suffering from burns, scaldings, or irradiation.

Herbs and Actions

Combines Dichroa, Oyster shell, and Dragon bone with *Kuei-chih-chu-shao-yao-tang* (Cinnamon Minus Peony Combination). The reason that Peony is excluded from *Kuei-chih-tang* (Cinnamon Combination) is to allow the Cinnamon to exert its action specifically so that it rapidly surfaces to harmonize *ying* (constructive energy) and *wei* (defensive energy). Dragon bone and Oyster shell calm the mind and spirit. Dichroa is cold and bitter and eliminates the heteropathic obstruction within the chest.

Indications

Burns, scalds, sunburns, neurotic disorders, and fevers from moxibustion.

Discrimination

Kuei-chih-chia-lung-ku-mu-li-tang (Cinnamon and Dragon Bone Combination) is used for cardiac hyper-function or palpitation, mental instability, impotence, genital chills, and spermatorrhea. *Chai-hu-chia-lung-ku-mu-li-tang* (Bupleurum and Dragon Bone Combination) is used for various neurotic symptoms as well as thoraco-costal distress and lethargy.

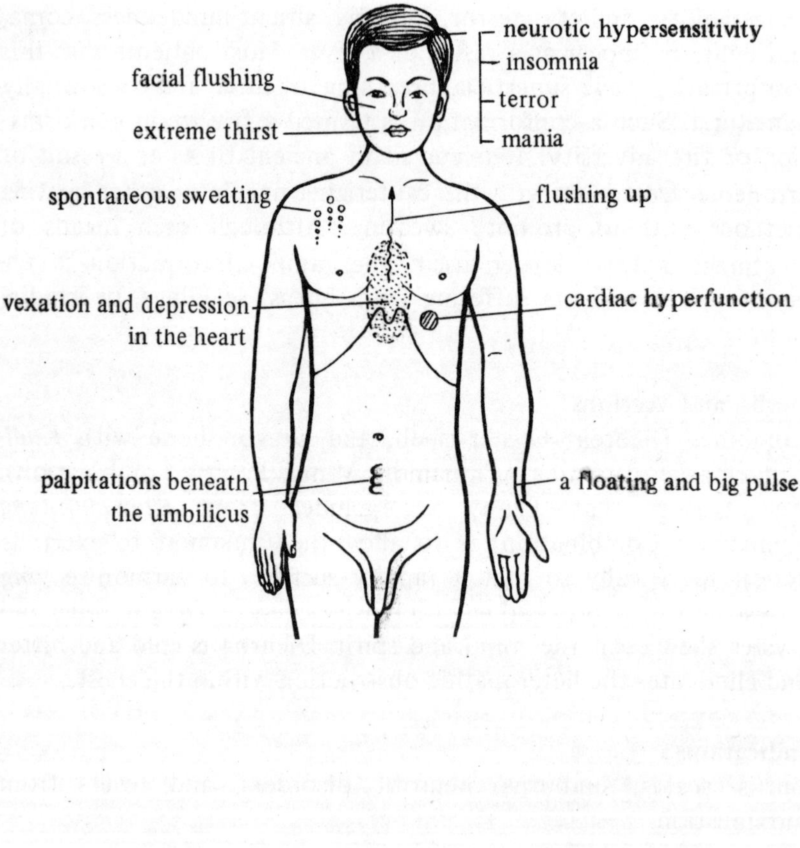

Lung-Ku-Mu-Li-Tang 龍骨牡蠣湯

(Dragon Bone and Oyster Shell Combination)

Dragon bone	5.0	Oyster shell	5.0

Lung-ku-mu-li-tang is an experimental formula which has astringent and sedative actions. It is used for treating palpitation, night swests, chest discomfort, and dyspepsia.

Herbs and Actions
Dragon bone is an astringent, sedative, and aphrodisiac. Oyster shell is an antipyretic, diuretic, aphrodisiac, and sedative.

Indications
Gastroxia, chronic gastritis, neuralgia, and dysuria.

Suan-Tsao-Jen-Tang 酸棗仁湯

(Zizyphus Combination)

Zizyphus	10.0	Hoelen	5.0	Cnidium	3.0
Licorice	1.0	Anemarrhena	3.0		

Recorded in *Chin kuei yao lueh* (金匱要略) of the Han dynasty. Used for treating the delicate constitution with a lack of energy, a weak abdomen, weakness and fatigue, and insomnia due to stress.

Herbs and Actions
Zizyphus nourishes nerves. Anemarrhena is an antipyretic, a sedative, and a general tonic. Cnidium dispels stagnant *ch'i* and relieves headaches. Hoelen is a diuretic, sedative, and tonic. Licorice coordinates the actions of the other herbs.

Indications

Insomnia, sleepiness, nervous exhaustion, night sweats, amnesia, nightmares, and rapid heart palpitations.

Discrimination

Chih-tzu-shih-tang (Gardenia and Soja Combination): insomnia-over stimulation of the brain and heart from inflammatory congestion that leads to insomnia and anxiety.

Hsieh-hsin-tang (Coptis and Rhubarb Combination): insomnia, severe inflammatory congestion, firm conformation.

Chia-hu-chia-lung-ku-mu-li-tang (Bupleurum and Dragon Bone Combination): insomnia, inflammatory congestion, cardiac hyperfunction, thoraco-costal distress, firm conformation.

Chu-ling-tang (Polyporus Combination): insomnia, insomnia due to blood fever, extreme thirst and frequent urination.

Wu-ling-san (Hoelen Five Herb Formula): insomnia, extreme thirst, and excessive urination.

Kan-tsao-hsieh-hsin-tang (Licorice and Pinellia Combination): insomnia, obstruction and hardness beneath the heart, firm fever.

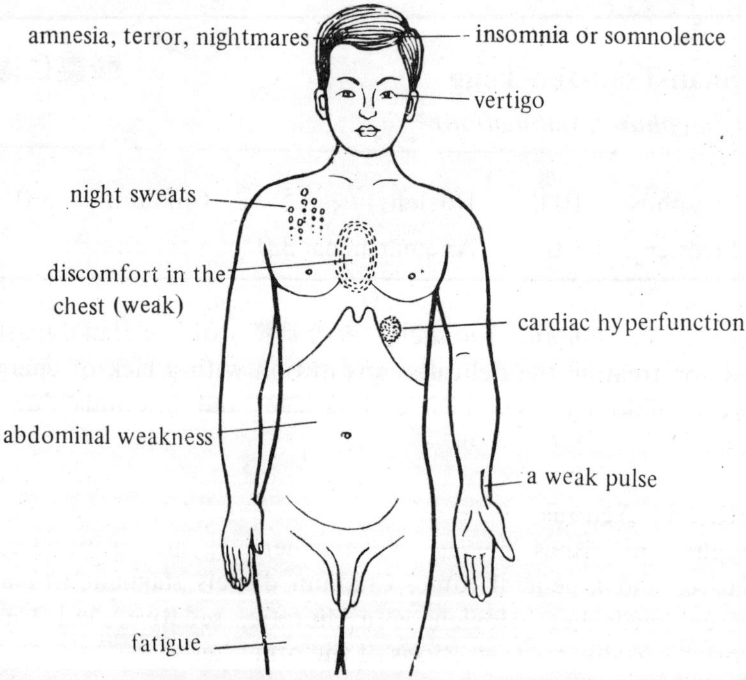

13.

Sho She Chi

(收濇劑, Astringent Formulas)

Formulas composed mainly of astringent and restraining herbs that treat loss, debilitation, wasting, and exhaustion of *ch'i*, blood, or sperm are called *sho she chi.*

An astringent formula is principally used for spontaneous sweating, night sweats, a prolonged cough, mild asthma, chronic diarrhea, spermatorrhea, urinary incontinence, uterine hemorrhage, uterine discharge, and hemorrhoidal bleeding. The classics say: "If there is looseness, we astringe it, and astringency restrains prolapses."

These formulas arrest sweating, coughing, excessive menstrual flow and leukorrhea; tone the skin and muscle and thus restrain prolapses; astringe the lungs and intestines; and stimulate sperm production. They are contraindicated in the presence of fever with hyperhidrosis, sputum stagnancy with asthmatic cough, initial feverish diarrhea, diarrhea due to tainted food, and "fire agitation" that causes spermatorrhea.

Chih-Cho-Ku-Pen-Wan 治濁固本丸

(Hoelen and Polyporus Formula)

Lotus stamen	2.0	Coptis	2.0	Cardamon	1.0
Black cardamon	1.0	Hoelen	1.0	Polyporus	2.0
Phellodendron	1.0	Pinellia	1.0	Licorice	3.0

Chih-cho-ku-pen-wan is recorded in *I fang chi chieh* (醫方集解) of the Ching dynasty. This formula is used for treating the sensation of fever in the stomach which is accompanied by sweating, polyuria, spermatorrhea, chronic prostatitis, chronic cystitis, chronic and simple urethritis. It often acts as an antiphlogistic, diuretic, and antigonorrhoral agent.

Herbs and Actions

Coptis and Phellodendron are antiphlogistics and bactericides. Hoelen with Polyporus acts as a diuretic. Cardamon and Pinellia are stomachics and can dispel moist *ch'i*. Lotus stamen with Black cardamon is a demulcent and tonic. Licorice nourishes the spleen and stomach.

Indications

Gonorrhea, cystitis, urethritis, and chronic prostatitis.

Chih-Shih-Chih-Yu-Yu-Liang-Tang 赤石脂禹餘糧湯

(Kaolin and Limonite Combination)

Kaolin	16.0	Limonite	16.0

Recorded in *Shang han lun* (傷寒論). Extremely effective

for diarrhea caused by pathological changes in the lower torso. Indications are a lax abdomen and pulse, incessant diarrhea with mucous, thick and pus-filled stools, and no fever. However, if the patient has anorexia, nausea, and vomiting–symptoms of the middle torso–and a worsening in his condition, intensive care is needed.

Herbs and Actions
This formula is composed of two components, Kaolin and Limonite. They are heavy, harsh, and sweet substances. The heaviness stops the diarrhea; the harshness prevents prolapse; and the sweetness aids digestion.

Indications
Colitis, rectal ulcer, rectal cancer, dysentery, periproctitis, anal ulcer, intra-anal furunculosis (localized infection) and gangrene.

Discrimination
Szu-ni-tang (Aconite and G. L. Combination) is used for weak conformational diarrhea, somatic pain, chills, and the fear of being chilled.
Pai-tou-weng-tang (Anemone Combination) is indicated for suppurative, bloody stools; feverish diarrhea; tenesmus; and a burning sensation in the anal area.

Chin-Sou-Ku-Ching-Wan 金鎖固精丸

(Lotus Stamen Formula)

Dragon bone	3.0	Tribulus	6.0	Lotus seed	3.0
Oyster shell	3.0	Euryale	6.0		
Lotus stamen	6.0				

Chin-sou-ku-ching-wan is recorded in the Chinese medical text, *I fang chi chieh* (醫方集解). This is a commonly used formula for treating impotence, nocturnal emission, night sweats, anxiety due to stress, pain in the midline, tinnitus, and weakness in the arms and legs.

Herbs and Actions
Tribulus, the main herb in this formula, is used as an aphrodisiac. Lotus seed and Euryale nourish the kidneys and spleen. Lotus stamen, Dragon bone, and Oyster shell are astringents and eliminate the problem of nocturnal emission.

Indications
Impotence, spermatorrhea, nocturnal emission, and enuresis.

Discrimination
Kuei-chih-chia-lung-ku-mu-li-tang (Cinnamon and Dragon Bone Combination): involuntary emissions; weak, void and slow pulse; acute cramping in the lower abdomen.
Ching-hsin-lien-tzu-yin (Lotus Seed Combination): involuntary emissions, thriving upper body and weak lower body, hyperfunctioning of heart life.
Ling-chiang-chu-kan-tang (Ginger and Hoelen Combination): involuntary emissions; incontinence; bed wetting; chills from the lower back radiating downward; a submerged, thin, and minute pulse.

Fu-Tu-Tan 茯菟丹

(Hoelen and Cuscuta Formula)

Cuscuta	10.0	Schizandra	8.0	Hoelen	3.0
Lotus fruit	3.0	Dioscorea	6.0		

Fu-tu-tan is reocrded in *Tai ping huei min ho chi chu fang* (太平惠民和劑局方) of the Ming dynasty. This formula is used for treating nocturnal emission, turbid urine, thirst, and diabetes.

Herbs and Actions
Lotus fruit and Dioscorea are nutritient tonics, Schizandra is an astringent, Cuscuta is a sexual tonic. Hoelen is a diuretic.

Indications
Sexual nervous exhaustion, nocturnal emission, and diabetes.

Sang-Piao-Hsiao-San 桑螵蛸散

(Mantis Formula)

Mantis	3.0	Polygala	3.0	Acorus	3.0
Dragon bone	3.0	Ginseng	3.0	*Fu-shen*	3.0
Tang-kuei	3.0	Tortoise shell	3.0		

Sang-piao-hsiao-san is recorded in *Pen ts'ao yen i* (本草衍義) by Kou Tzung-shih of the Sung dynasty. This formula is used for nourishing the spleen, heart, and kidneys; to tone the *ch'i* and blood; for treating mental instability, amnesia, nocturnal emission, frequent urination, enuresis, polyuria, and diabetes insipidus.

Herbs and Actions
Mantis nourishes the kidneys and treats nocturnal emission and enuresis. Dragon bone is an astringent. Ginseng, Hoelen, Acours, and Polygala are sedatives. *Tang-kuei* nourishes the blood. Tortoise shell nourishes *yin. Tang-kuei* with Ginseng nourish the *ch'i* and blood. Dragon bone with Tortoise shell can regulate the heart and kidneys.

Indications
Frequent urination, chronic nephritis, turbid urine due to cystitis, and amnesia due to nervous exhaustion.

Tao-Hua-Tang 桃花湯

(Kaolin and Oryza Combination)

Kaolin	6.0	Oryza	8.0	Ginger	1.5

Tao-hua-tang was recorded in both the *Shang han lun* (傷寒論) and the *Chin kuei yao lueh* (金匱要略) during the Han dynasty. This formula is used for treating those with a delicate constitution who are afebrile but have cold hands and feet, distention and pain in the abdomen, persistent diarrhea, bloody and purulent stools, and a sinking pulse.

Herbs and Actions

Kaolin is an astringent and hemostatic. Ginger warms the body and dispels "internal chills". Oryza is warm in nature and nourishes the spleen and stomach.

Indications

Dysentery, colitis, rectal ulcer, rectal cancer, hemorrhoids, and periproctitis.

Discrimination

Pai-tou-weng-tang (Anemone Combination): stools with pus and blood; fever conformation with a hot feeling at the anus during bowel movement.

Szu-ni-tang (Aconite and G. L. Combination): diarrhea, yin conformation with cold hands and feet, submerged and weak pulse, no stools with pus and blood.

Chih-shih-chih-yu-yu-liang-tang (Kaolin and Limonite Combination): diarrhea, mucous stools, and lower-warmer originated diarrhea.

Yin conformation

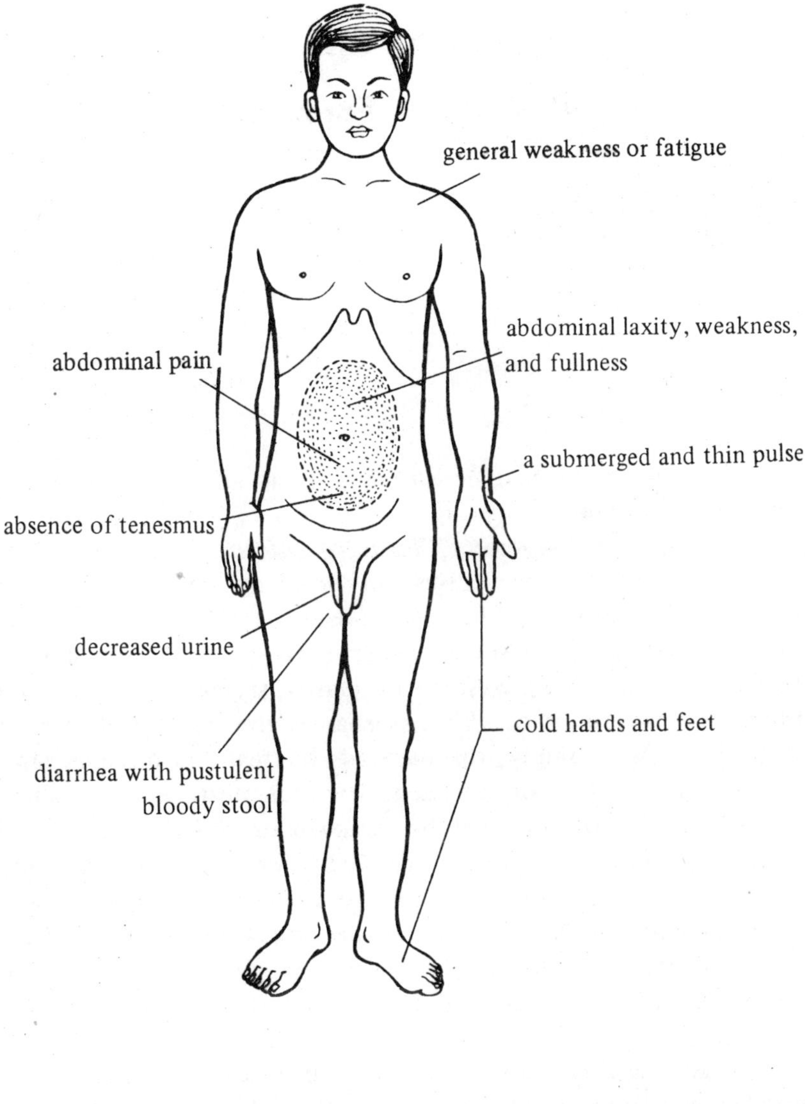

14.
Li Ch'i Chi
(理氣劑, Chi Formulas)

Formulas that balance *ch'i* and treat all *ch'i* diseases are termed *ch'i* formulas.

The Yellow Emperor's Classic of Internal Medicine (黃帝內經) says: "Anger causes an up-rising of *ch'i*, pleasure mollifies *ch'i*, sorrow makes *ch'i* subside, horror makes *ch'i* descend, chills make *ch'i* shrink, fever exhausts *ch'i*, astonishment disturbs *ch'i*, weariness wastes *ch'i*, and worrying obstructs *ch'i*." These nine variations of *ch'i* disturbance give rise to all manner of diseases. Accordingly, the methods to treat *ch'i* diseases vary. For example, a loss or subsidence of *ch'i* must be replenished; an obstruction to *ch'i* must be removed or *ch'i* circulated, and an adversity in *ch'i* must be descended. Clinically there are many ways to treat *ch'i* disorders. These include nourishment and replenishment, discharge and guidance, purgation, expectoration, astringement, and stimulation of blood circulation. Most illnesses cannot be effectively treated without the inclusion of *ch'i* herbs.

When using *ch'i* formulas, the physician has to determine whether the conformation is weak or firm. If the condition calls for supplementation and *ch'i* moving herbs are used instead, *ch'i* will become weaker and empty. If the condition requires circulating *ch'i* but *ch'i* tonics are used instead, the *ch'i* will become further stagnated. If it is a complex condition, so that there is a trace of weakness within firmness, then *ch'i* supplementing and *ch'i*-moving formulas are used concomitantly. Because most *ch'i* formulas contain herbs that are aromatic, arid, bitter, and warm, *ch'i* obstruction accompanied with fluid deficiency and injury is treated deliberately.

An-Chung-San 安中散

(Cardamon and Fennel Formula)

Cardamon	1.0	Fennel	1.5	Cinnamon	4.0
Corydalis	3.0	Oyster shell	3.0	Licorice	1.0
Galanga	0.5				

An-chung-san is listed as a nutritive in the Chinese governmental medical dictionary of the Sung dynasty, *Tai ping huei min ho chi chu fang* (太平惠民和劑局方 A.D. 1107-1110). This formula is used to treat patients of delicate constitution and slender physique with weak pulse and flaccid muslces and skin, abdominal weakness, ascites, palpitation at the umbilicus, subcardiac pain, nausea, vomiting, and pain in the lower abdomen and midline.

Herbs and Actions

Cinnamon nourishes the blood, dispels stagnant blood, and checks abdominal pain. Corydalis is an emmenagogue that also cures pain in the chest and abdomen and relieves neuralgia. Oyster shell relieves chest pain and neutralizes gastric acid. Cardamon cures stagnant *ch'i* and relieves pain. Fennel nourishes the stomach and relieves pain due to chilling of the stomach. Galanga is a stomachic that alleviates "stagnant air" and neuralgia. Licorice coordinates and reinforces the actions of the other herbs.

Indications

Nervous stomach, gastric ulcer, duodenal ulcer, gastroxia, gastroptosis, chronic gastritis, gastric tumor, pyloric obstruction, dysmenorrhea, and pernicious vomiting.

Discrimination

Szu-ni-san (Bupleurum and *Chih-shih* Formula): pain and spasms beneath the heart.

Ta-chai-hu-tang (Major Bupleurum Combination): pain beneath the heart, thoraco-costal distress, firm conformation.

Chai-hu-kuei-chih-tang (Bupleurum and Cinnamon Combination): pain beneath the heart, tension in the abdominal wall.
Shao-yao-kan-tsao-tang (Peony and Licorice Combination): abdominal pain and abdominal muscle spasms.
Chien-chung-tang (Hoelen and Jujube Combination): pain beneath the heart, abdominal muscle tension, vomiting.
Liang-chih-tang (Galanga and *Chih-shih* Combination): pain beneath the heart, slight hardness beneath the heart, spasmodic pain.
Ling-kuei-kan-tsao-tang (Hoelen, Licorice, and Jujube Combination): pain beneath the heart; agitated *ch'i* beside the umbilicus is the chief symptom.
Ting-hsiang-fu-ling-tang (Cloves and Hoelen Combination): pain beneath the heart, weak conformation.
Szu-chun-tzu-tang (Four Major Herb Combination), *Liu-chun-tzu-tang* (Six Major Herb Combination): loss of appetitie, lax abdomen, loss of weight, loss of vitality, suction sound in the lower heart, absence of abdominal pain.
Sheng-chiang-hsieh-hsin-tang (Pinellia and Ginger Combination): obstruction and hardness beneath the heart, vomiting of acid water, no splashing sound beneath the heart.
Jen-sheng-tang (Ginseng and Ginger Combination): thinness, poor complexion, abdominal laxity and weakness, cold hands and feet, noticeable splashing sound beneath the heart.

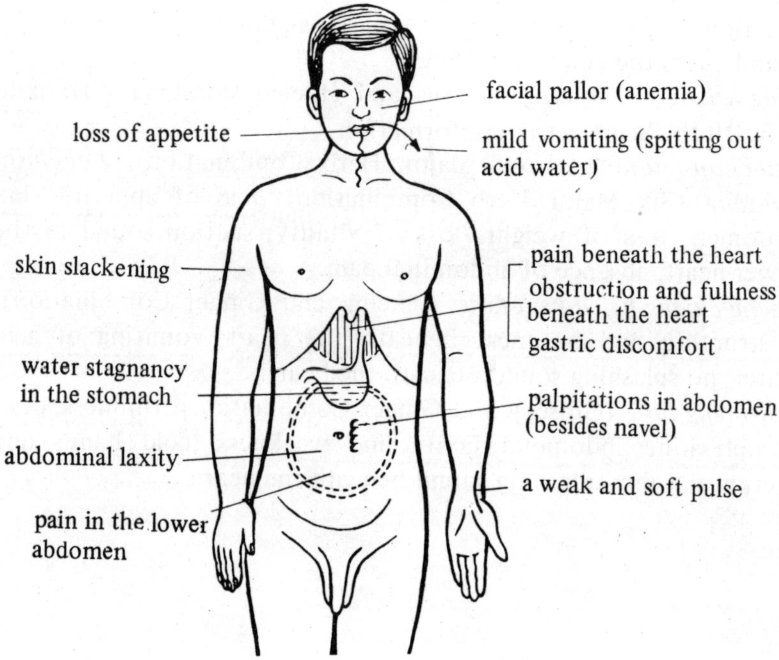
facial pallor (anemia)
loss of appetite
mild vomiting (spitting out acid water)
skin slackening
pain beneath the heart
obstruction and fullness beneath the heart
gastric discomfort
water stagnancy in the stomach
palpitations in abdomen (besides navel)
abdominal laxity
a weak and soft pulse
pain in the lower abdomen

Chen-Chi-Tien-Hsiang-San 正氣天香散

(Lindera and Cyperus Formula)

Cyperus	4.0	Citrus	3.0	Lindera	3.0
Perilla	1.5	Ginger	1.5	Licorice	1.0

Recorded in *I hsueh ju men* (醫學入門) as a general formula for the treatment of *ch'i* occlusion (depression) in women with menopausal neurosis, frustration, blood stagnation, obstruction and stagnation of sputum, extravasated and coagulated blood, laborious and abrupt up-rush of occluded and depressed *ch'i* causing aches beneath the heart or in the lower abdomen, vertigo, vomiting, alternate chills and fever, and submerged pulse with slight cold symptoms. Hence this formula is indicated for various *ch'i* problems in women, vertigo, headache, massess within the stomach, menoxenia, sullenness and various diseases caused by depression, amenorrhea in virgins, and diseases of widows, monks and nuns.

Incompatible with *Chai hu* (Bupleurum) preparations or *Chien-chung-tang* preparation.

Herbs and Actions

Lindera, Cyperus, and Perilla are acrid, warm in nature, and fragrant. Together they disperse stagnated and depressed *ch'i*. Ginger is acrid and hot and makes *ch'i* fluent. Citrus can stabilize ascending and descending *ch'i* in the upper and lower parts of the body. Licorice is sweet and mollifies the dispersing action of the other herbs and helps restore vitality.

Indications

Climacteric neurosis in females, diseases caused by occlusion and stagnation of *ch'i*, hysteria, neurasthenia, prepartum and postpartum neuroses, amenorrhea, melena, neuroses of widows, nuns and monks.

Discrimination

Ta-chai-hu-tang (Major Bupleurum Combination): pain beneath the heart, thoraco-costal distress, constipation, firm conformation.

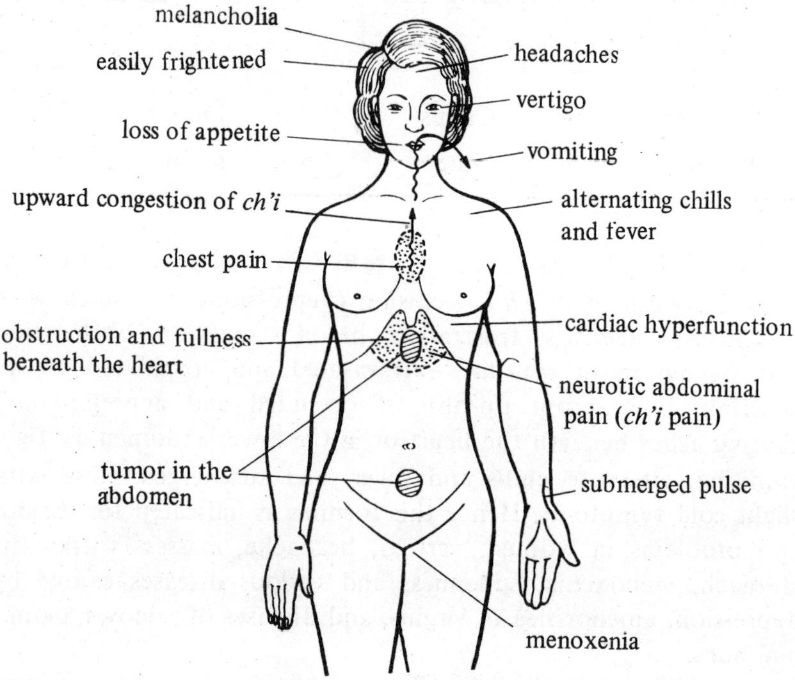

Chen-Hsiang-Tien-Ma-Tang *(Aquilaria and Gastrodia Combination)*					**沈香天麻湯**
Siler	3.0	Black cardamon	2.0	*Tang-kuei*	2.0
Pinellia	3.0	Aquilaria	2.0	*Tu-huo*	3.0
Wu-tou	0.5-1.0	Gastrodia	2.0	Licorice	1.0
Aconite	0.5-1.0	Silk worm	1.5	*Chianghuo*	3.0

Recorded in *Wei sheng pao chien* (衛生寶鑑). Indicated for epilepsy or for convulsions, sputum and noisy, frothing salivation; tongue biting; rolled-up eyes; and rigidity in the neck and back of infants who are scared.

Originally this formula was indicated for weak-conformational epilepsy in children. However, it is also suitable for adults who have hyperfunctioning livers, experience abdominal cramping in the upper torso and weakness in the lower torso, live at a fast pace, and have a quick temper that causes a distortion in the mouth and eyes. It is also good for women giving birth to a second or third child who have repeated bleeding, liver hyperfunction, rapid palpitations, and are easily frightened.

Herbs and Actions

Tu-huo relaxes the neck and relieves paralysis and rheumatism in the feet. *Chianghuo* alleviates rheumatism, relaxes muscles, and activates the circulation of blood. Gastrodia treats epilepsy, convulsions, and head dizziness. Black cardamon tranquilizes the spirit and settles rapid respiration, warms the stomach, and expels hypersensitivity. *Tang-kuei* activates, enlivens, and nourishes the blood. Siler eliminates wind hypersensitivity, relieves convulsions, expels moisture, and kills pain. Pinellia dries moistness and eliminates sputum. Aconite and *Wu-tou* restore yang, drive away cold, expel wind, and dry moisture. Licorice harmonizes the various herbs.

Indications

Weak-conformational epilepsy, acute infantile convulsions, neurasthenia, hysteria, paralysis of facial nerves, uncoordination of autonomic nerves, and the somatic pains of patients with weak physiques.

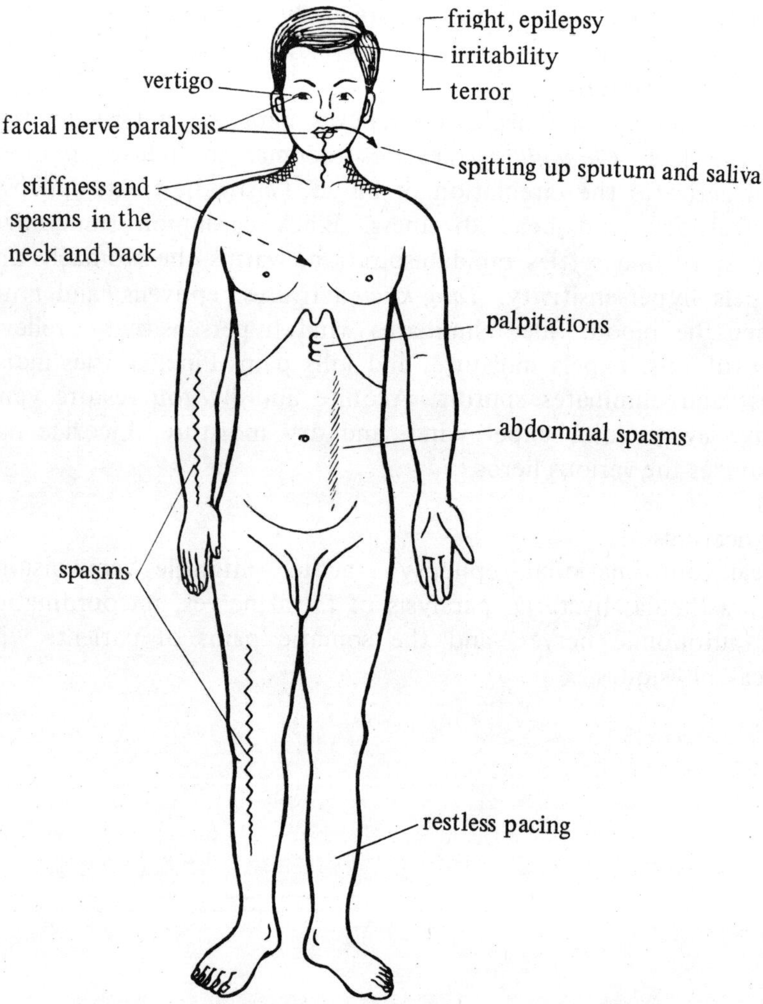
fright, epilepsy
irritability
terror
vertigo
facial nerve paralysis
spitting up sputum and saliva
stiffness and spasms in the neck and back
palpitations
abdominal spasms
spasms
restless pacing

Chih-Shih- Hsieh-Pai-Kuei-Chih-Tang 枳實薤白桂枝湯

(*Chih-shih, Bakeri, and Cinnamon Combination*)

Chih-shih	3.0	Magnolia bark	3.0	Bakeri	4.0
Cinnamon	1.0	Trichosanthes fruit	4.0		

Recorded in *Chin kuei yao lueh* (金匱要略). Used for weak-conformational thoracic paralysis, the symptoms of which are asthma, coughing, drooling, dragging pain in the chest and back, and obstruction and distention beneath the heart; the affliction affects the area of the chest and shoulders down to the epigastrium (upper middle portion of the abdomen) and ribs with air and gas abnormally flushing up from the hypochondrium (area below and lowest rib). This formula may be administered to drain the distention, to settle the flushing gas and air, and to open a passage for yang by breaking the obstruction if yang is not yet weakened in the patient.

Herbs and Actions

Bakeri warms the interior, disperses obstructions and smooths blocked air and gas; hence it treats heart and chest pain, asthma, sputum, and drooling. Trichosanthes fruit expels sputum and disperses obstructions. The addition of *Chih-shih*, Magnolia bark, and Cinnamon enhances the actions of channeling the yang, calming the up-rushing air, and eliminating obstructions and distention.

Indications

Intercostal neuralgia, angina pectoris, and cardiac colic.

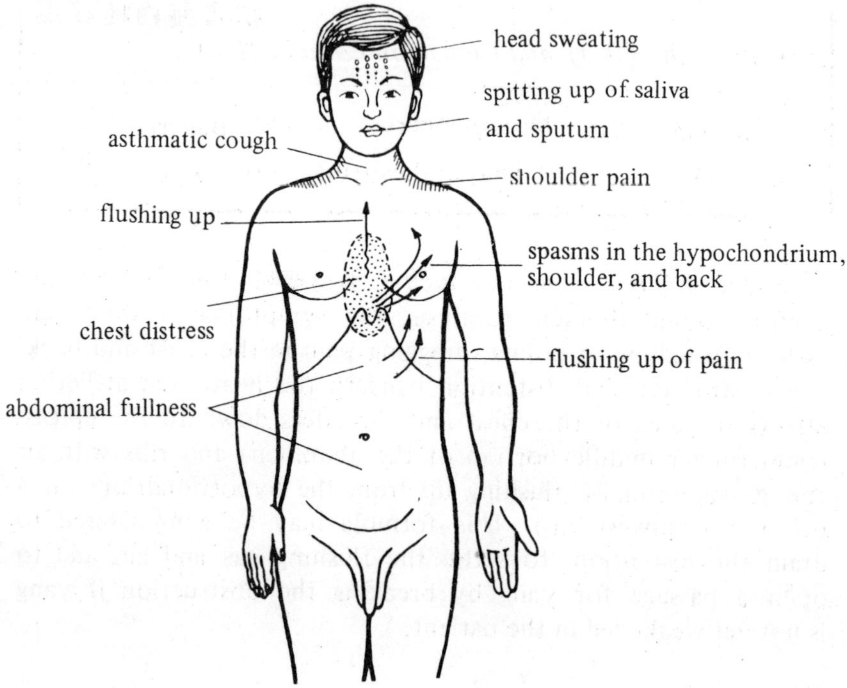

Chu-Pi-Chu-Ju-Tang *(Aurantium and Bamboo Combination)*					**橘皮竹茹湯**
Aurantium	4.0	Ginger	6.0	Bamboo	2.0
Jujube	6.0	Licorice	3.0	Ginseng	1.5

Chu-pi-chu-ju-tang was recorded in the *Chin kuei yao lueh* (金匱要略) during the Han dynasty. This formula is effective for patients of delicate constitution (due to prolonged illness) who have "internal heat" in the stomach, flushing up, eructation, and vomiting. According to Western medicine, eructation is caused by spasms in the diaphragm, but in Chinese medicine it is said to be caused by "weak chills" and "weak heat" in the stomach.

Herbs and Actions
Ginseng, Jujube, and Licorice are tonics which increase stomach *ch'i*. Aurantium and Ginger are antiemetics that also alleviate flushing up. Bamboo dispels "internal heat" in the stomach.

Indications
Eructation, morning sickness, persistent eructation after abdominal surgery, and chronic gastric disease.

Discrimination
Shih-ti-tang (Kaki Combination): hiccups, weakness and chills in the stomach.

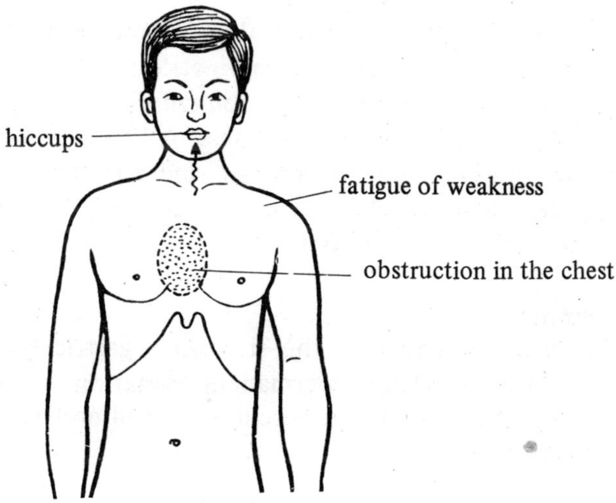

Chuan-Szu-Chun-Tzu-Tang 喘四君子湯

(Atractylodes and Cardamon Combination)

Ginseng	2.0	Atractylodes	4.0	*Tang-kuei*	4.0
Hoelen	4.0	Citrus	2.0	Cardamon	1.0
Perilla fruit	2.0	Magnolia bark	2.0	Aquilaria	1.0
Morus	1.5	Saussurea	1.0	Licorice	1.0

A remedy for weak-conformational asthma. Commonly used for aged or debilitated individuals who have drastic stridor and labored breathing due to upward attacking weak fire and excessive sputum.

Herbs and Actions
As the name implies, this formula is a modification of *Szu-chun-tzu-tang* (Four Major Herb Combination). Ginseng, Atracylodes, Hoelen, and Licorice constitute *Szu-chun-tzu-tang*, which is used to treat splenic and gastric weakness. All the other herbs together have the functions of moving air and gas, treating the insides and settling adversity: the whole formula is thus a good remedy for weak-conformational asthma.

Indications
Gastroptosis (prolapse of the stomach), gastric laxity, bronchial asthma, bronchiectasis (permanent dilatation of one or more bronchi), pulmonary tuberculosis, pulmonary emphysema, pulmonary edema.

Discrimination
Hsiao-ching-lung-tang (Minor Blue Dragon Combination) is for asthma; stagnated water beneath the heart; copious, thin sputum; and epigastric rigidity.

Fen-Hsin-Chi-Yin 分心氣飲

(Citrus and Perilla Combination)

Citrus	2.0	Cinnamon	1.5	Peony	1.5
Akebia	1.5	Pinellia	1.5	Areca	2.0
Hoelen	2.0	*Chianghuo*	2.0	Morus	2.0
Juncus	1.5	Perilla	2.0	Jujube	1.5
Blue citrus peel	2.0	Licorice	1.5	Ginger	1.5

Fen-hsin-chi-yin is recorded in *Tai ping huei min ho chi chu fang* (太平惠民和劑局方) of the Ming dynasty. This formula is used for treating vomiting, distention, vertigo, fatigue, dry tongue, loss of appetite, emaciation, and anxiety due to stress.

Herbs and Actions

Citrus, Blue citrus peel, and Areca can regulate the *ch'i* and remove distention. Pinellia and Morus are expectorants. Cinnamon and Peony dispel stagnant blood. Licorice coordinates the actions of the other herbs. Hoelen dispels "stagnant water" beneath the heart. Perilla is an expectorant and antitussive, and it increases the *ch'i. Chianghuo* is helpful for rheumatism and is an anodyne. Akebia and Juncus dispel internal heat of the lungs. Ginger and Jujube coordinate the actions of the other herbs.

Indications

Nervous exhaustion, edema, peritonitis, mastitis, cough during pregnancy, and anorexia.

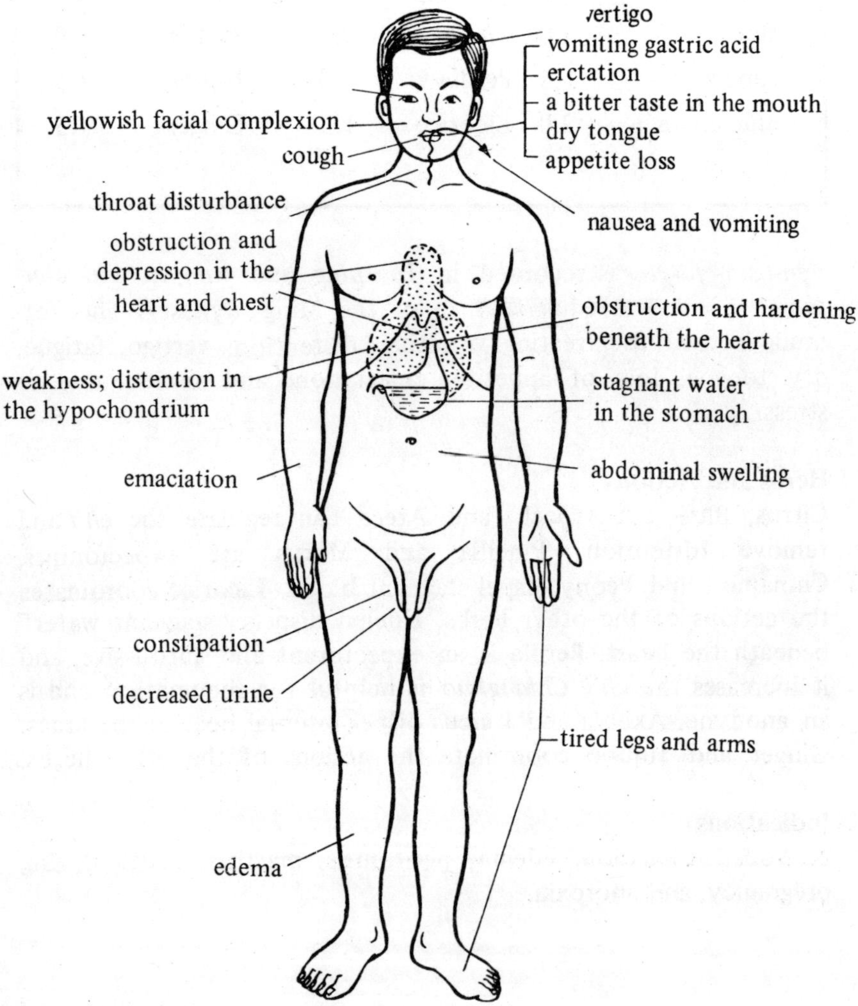
vertigo
vomiting gastric acid
erctation
a bitter taste in the mouth
dry tongue
appetite loss
yellowish facial complexion
cough
throat disturbance
nausea and vomiting
obstruction and depression in the heart and chest
obstruction and hardening beneath the heart
weakness; distention in the hypochondrium
stagnant water in the stomach
emaciation
abdominal swelling
constipation
decreased urine
tired legs and arms
edema

Hou-Pu-San-Wu-Tang *(Magnolia Three Combination)*					**厚朴三物湯**
Magnolia bark 8.0	Rhubarb	4.0	*Chih-shih*	3.5	

Recorded in *Chin kuei yao lueh* (金匱要略). Basically the same composition as *Hsiao-cheng-chi-tang* (Minor Rhubarb Combination). Both are used for firm fevers, internal accumulations, impeded respiration, abdominal distention, and obstructed stools. However, this formula treats abdominal distention that is more severe than that treated with *Hsiao-cheng-chi-tang*, which is primarily intended to cleanse the accumulation. The major action of *Hsiao-cheng-chi-tang* comes from Rhubarb, the dominant ingredient, which is then said to play the Emperor's role. *Hou-pu-san-wu-tang*, on the other hand, aims mainly at restoring respiration and Magnolia bark assumes the emperor's role by being the dominant herb of the formula. Therefore, this formula is suitable for an internally firm conformation where respiration is obstructed.

Herbs and Actions

Magnolia bark eliminates distention and aids normal respiration. *Chih-shih* dissolves turgidity and breaks up the impediments. Rhubarb cleanses a firm fever in the middle warmer (part of the abdomen).

Indications

Habitual constipation, hypertension, air (pneumata) of the feet rushing toward the heart, food intoxication, pediatric convulsion, schizophrenia, obstructed urine, and asthma.

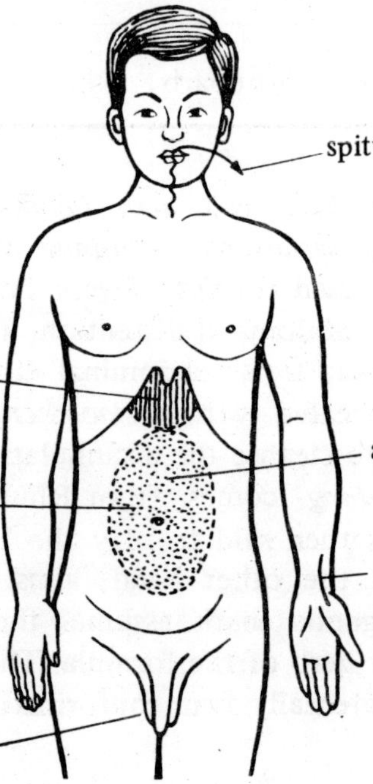

Hou-Pu-Sheng-Chiang-Pan-hsia-Kan-Tsao-Jen-Sheng-Tang 厚朴生薑半夏甘草人參湯

(Magnolia Five Combination)

Magnolia bark	3.0	Pinellia	4.0	Ginseng	1.5
Licorice	2.5	Ginger	1.0		

Recorded in *Shang han lun* (傷寒論). Prescribed for patients who have been treated with diaphoretics or cathartics, the treatment resulting in internal weakness, disharmony of the gastric air, gas and water obstruction, and accumulations within the abdomen leading to a weakness distention and turgidity. In other words, this formula has as its therapeutic targets the symptoms of thoracic and abdominal distention, subcardiac obstruction and distention, vomiting, and a reduced appetite.

Herbs and Actions

Magnolia bark disperses the trapped air (pneumata) which relieves the weak or firm distention of the abdomen or releases the gas obstruction. Ginseng and Licorice nourish internal weakness. Pinellia calms rising air in the system (belching) and in collaboration with Ginger suppresses vomiting.

Indications

Gastroptosis, gastrectasis, or abdominal engorgement and peritonitis caused by gas stagnation; vomiting with subcardiac obstruction and distention or with eructation; excessive stomach acidity; abdominal distention and nausea that remains after vomiting; and diarrhea from food poisoning.

Discrimination

Kuei-chih-chia-shao-yao-tang (Cinnamon and Peony Combination) is indicated for abdominal distention accompanied by abdominal pain.

Pan-hsia-hou-pu-tang (Pinellia and Magnolia Combination) is a carminative that treats gas problems and the feeling that something is clinging to the throat.

Sheng-chiang-hsieh-hsin-tang (Pinellia and Ginger Combination) is indicated for vomiting, eructation, gastric hyperacidity, subcardiac turgidity, and a firm conformation.

Wu-chu-yu-tang (Evoida Combination) is indicated for vomiting, regurgitation, headache, discomfort, irritability, and cold limbs.

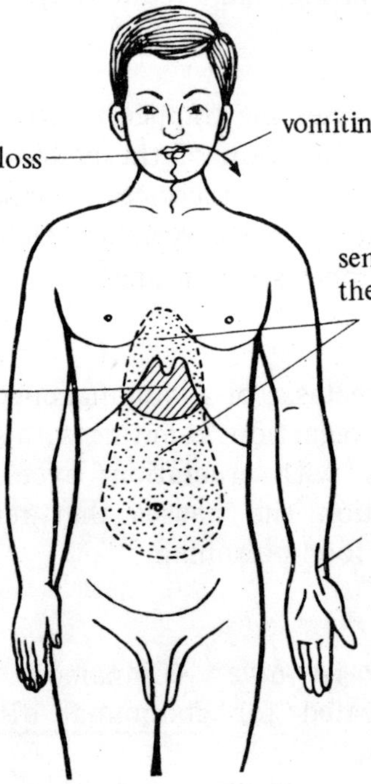

Hsing-Chi-Hsiang-Su-San *(Cyperus, Perilla, and Citrus Formula)*					**行氣香蘇散**
Perilla	2.0	Citrus	2.5	Cyperus	2.5
Lindera	2.5	*Chianghuo*	2.5	Cnidium	2.5
Ma-huang	2.0	*Chih-ko*	2.0	Ginger	1.0
Licorice	1.0				

Hsing-chi-hsiang-su-san is recorded in *Wan ping hui chun* (萬病回春) of the Ming dynasty. This formula is used for treating internal injury caused by raw and cold substances with a strong odor; diseases initiated by external factors such as wind, chill, and moisture; severe chills with fever; and abdominal distention and fullness. It is also effective for stagnant *ch'i* in any part of the body, illness due to foods, and abdominal distress and pain that were not initiated by external factors. This formula is suitable for those whose illness is due to excessive food and drink, external factors such as wind and chills, chillphobia, high fever, headache, hernia, and abdominal pain.

Herbs and Actions
Perilla, *Chianghuo,* and *Ma-huang* block the effects of the external factors. Cyperus, Citrus, Lindera, Cnidium, and *Chih-ko* regulate the stagnant *ch'i.* Licorice supplements the spleen *ch'i.*

Indications
Common cold, gastritis, hernia, intestinal hernia, dysmenorrhea, and muscular rheumatoid arthritis.

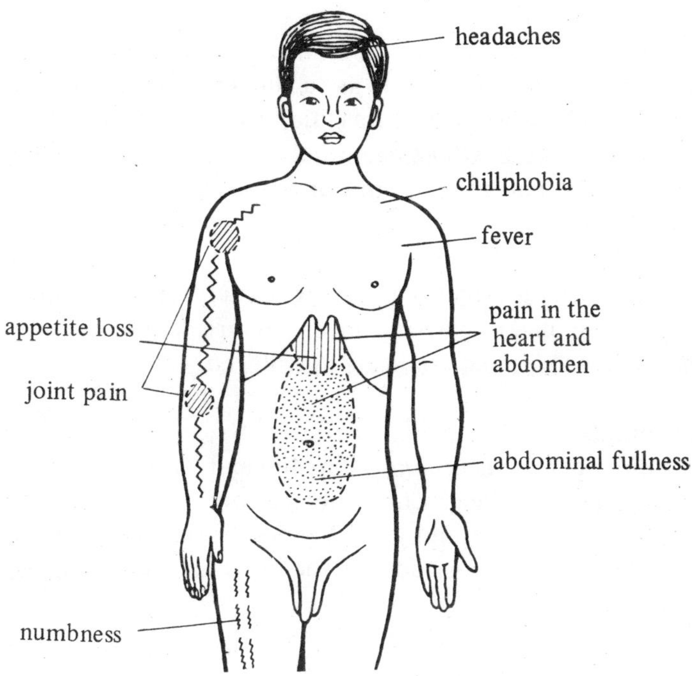

Hsuan-Fu-Hua-Tai-Che-Shih-Tang 旋覆花代赭石湯

(Inula and Hematite Combination)

Inula	3.0	Hematite	3.0	Jujube	3.0
Licorice	2.0	Ginseng	2.0	Pinellia	5.0
Ginger	4.0				

Hsuan-fu-hua-tai-che-shih-tang is recorded in *Shang han lun* (傷寒論) of the Han dynasty. This formula is good for treating gastrointestinal weakness, "stagnant water" beneath the heart, distention beneath the heart, flushing up, sour stomach, vomiting, frequent eructation, delicate constitution, and weak pulse.

Herbs and Actions

Inula is a stomachic; in combination with Hematite, it can relieve eructation and act as a hemotonic, hemostatic, and astringent. Ginseng is a stomachic, tonic, and nutrient. Pinellia and Ginger arrest vomiting. Jujube is a tonic and emollient. Licorice coordinates the actions of the other herbs.

Indications

Sour stomach, gastrectasia, gastric distention, gastroptosis, gastritis, gastric ulcer, gastric cancer, pyloric constriction, toxemia during pregnancy, and vomiting in children.

Discrimination

Sheng-chiang-hsieh-hsin-tang (Pinellia and Ginger Combination): vomiting, gas, diarrhea, firm conformation.

An-chung-san (Cardamon and Fennel Formula): vomiting, pain beneath the heart, lassitude of the arms and legs, and weak conformation.

Weak conformation

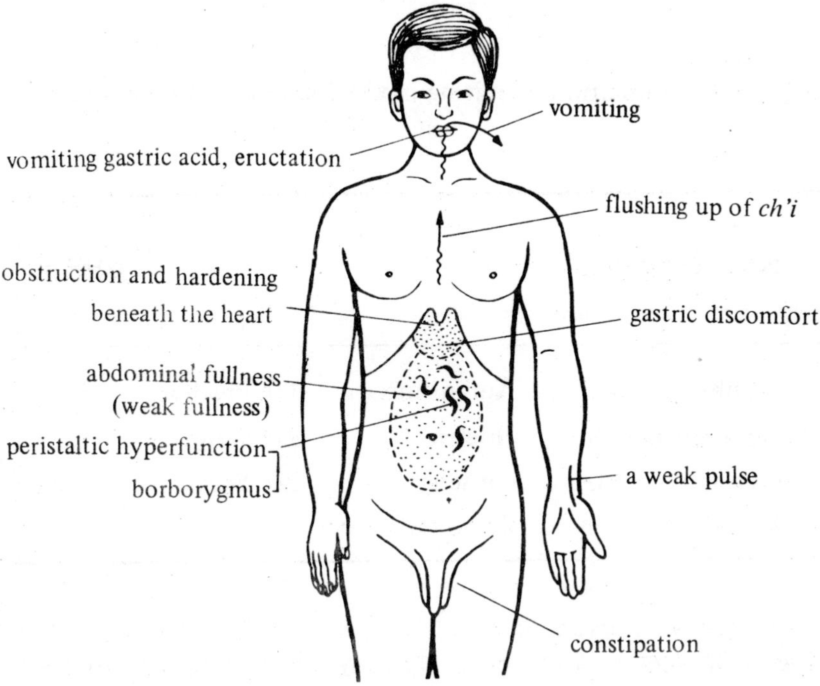

Kan-Chiang-Jen-Sheng-Pan-Hsia-Wan

乾薑人參半夏丸

(G. P. and Ginseng Formula)

Ginger	3.0	Ginseng	3.0	Pinellia	6.0

Recorded in *Chin kuei yao lueh.* Regulates *ch'i,* warms the insides, harmonizes the stomach, and stops vomiting. Mainly indicated for the constant, severe nausea and vomiting of some pregnancies. Suitable also for the vomiting in patients with a deteriorated stamina.

Herbs and Actions

Pinellia is an anti-emetic, treating mainly the symptoms of nausea and vomiting and also hiccups. Ginseng is effective as a hematinic to increase hemoglobin and as a strengthening agent. Dry ginger acts as an antiemetic and a stomachic.

Indications
Hyperemia gravidarum, vomiting in the debilitated, gastroenteritis.

Kou-Teng-San 鈎藤散

(Gambir Formula)

Gambir	3.0	Aurantium	3.0	Pinellia	3.0
Ophiopogon	3.0	Hoelen	3.0	Ginger	1.0
Gypsum	5.0	Ginseng	2.0	Siler	2.0
Licorice	1.0	Chrysanthemum	2.0		

Kou-teng-san is listed in the Chinese medical work, *Pen shih fang* (本事方) of the Sung dynasty. This formula is used for treating obese patients who are exceptionally nervous and are experiencing irritability, flushing up, subcardiac distention, muscle spasms in the shoulders and back, orbital and conjunctival congestion, headache, vertigo, tinnitus, palpitation, and insomnia.

Herbs and Actions
Gambir removes stagnant *ch'i* from the liver and "internal heat" from the heart, and it calms high nervous excitement. Ginseng and Hoelen improve vitality and eliminate emotional instability. Chrysanthemum, Aurantium, Pinellia, and Ophiopogon relieve flushing up. Siler and Chrysanthemum remove stagnant *ch'i* from the upper body and dispel "internal heat". Gypsum is a sedative that dispels "stagnant heat" in the body.

Indications
Neuroses, headache, vertigo, aching shoulders, climacteric dis-

turbances, arteriosclerosis, hypertension, chronic nephritis, and cerebrovascular diseases.

Discrimination

Wu-chu-yu-tang (Evodia Combination): headaches, flushing up of *ch'i*, stagnant water in the stomach, vomiting, anxiety. *Chia-wei-hsiao-yao-san* (Bupleurum and Peony Formula); vertigo, mental instability, drifting feverish feeling, facial flushing, chillpnobia in the back.

Weak conformation

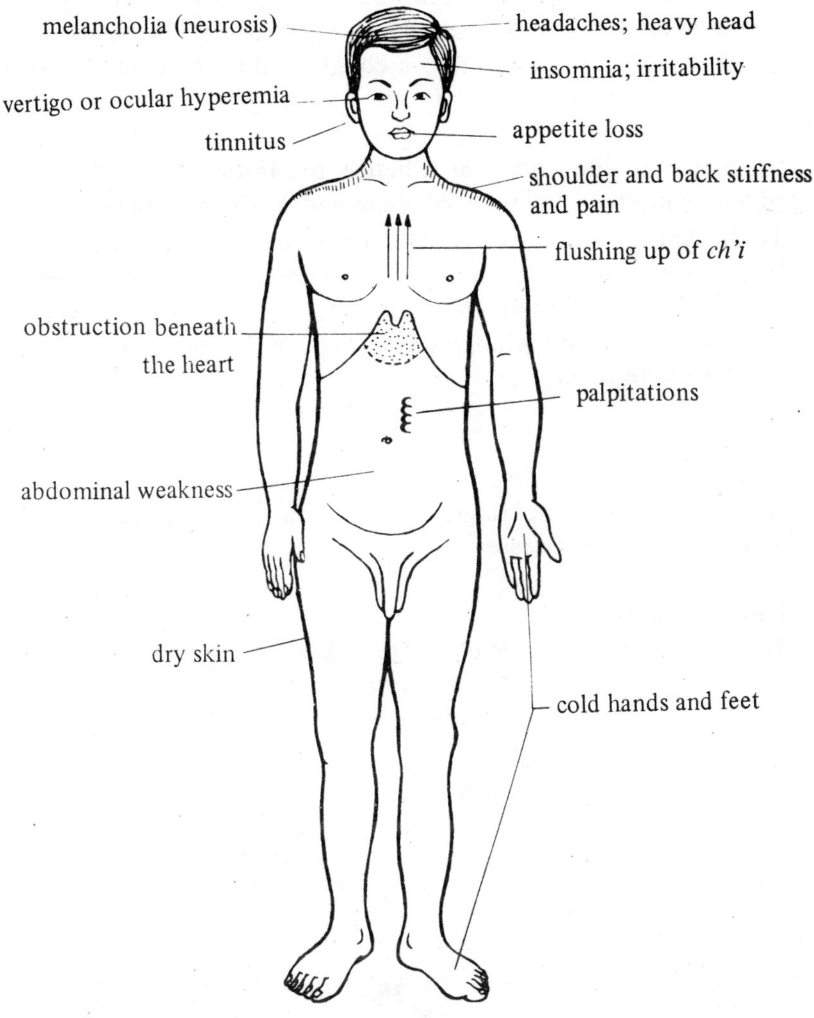

Kua-Lou-Hsieh-Pai-Pai-Chiu-Tang 栝樓薤白白酒湯

(Trichosanthes, Bakeri, and Vinegar Combination)

Bakeri 4.5 Trichosanthes fruit 2.0

Vinegar(Boil 400ml. of vinegar until 150ml. remains)

Treats thoracic paralysis which exhibits the chief symptoms of a sensation of blockage in the chest accompanied by paroxysmal, colicky aching which radiates out from the heart to the upper shoulders, neck, back, and epigastrium. In addition, the patient suffers from asthma, a cough, and mucous in the throat.

Herbs and Actions

Blockage of the chest, and hence respiration, by an irritation of yin, will stop the flow of yang and lead to thoracic paralysis. Trichosanthes fruit cleans the lungs and breaks the blockage. Bakeri stimulates the heart and aids general functioning of the organs. Vinegar speeds the circulation of blood and oxygen in the body Once breathing is free and unobstructed, the thoracic paralysis is relieved.

Indications

Cardiac asthma, cardiac neurosis, cardiac infarction, angina pectoris, intercostal neuralgia, cardiac valvular disease, pleuritis, and other cardiac diseases.

Discrimination

Ta-hsien-hsiung-tang (Rhubarb and *Kan-sui* Combination) is used for aching in the heart and chest, subcardiac hardness, and stiffness and cramping in the back and shoulders.

Ta-chai-hu-tang (Major Bupleurum Combination) is used for cardiac and thoracic blockage, surface conformations, thoracocostal distress, and constipation.

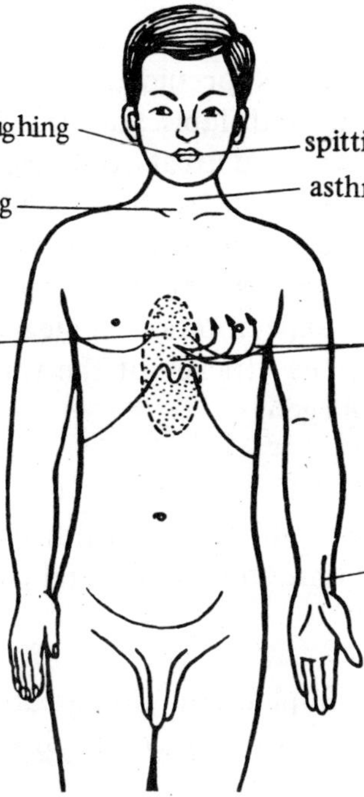

Kua-Lou-Hsieh-Pai-Pan-Hsia-Tang 栝樓薤白半夏湯

(Trichosanthes, Bakeri, and Pinellia Combiantion)

Trichosanthes fruit	3.0	Bakeri	4.5	Pinellia	6.0

Recorded in *Chin kuei yao lueh* under thoracic paralysis as "a condition in which the patient is unable to lie down and pains in the heart are so strong that they penetrate to the back." Thoracic paralysis is equivalent to today's angina pectoris. Symptoms indicative of this formula include pains occurring in the heart and pericordio-epigastric region and radiating pain in the back accompanied by asthma, coughing, spitting, labored breathing, intra-thoracic distress, and vomiting. In most cases, the abdominal symptoms mainfest subcardiac turgidity and rigidity.

Herbs and Actions

Trichosanthes fruit eliminates occulded fever within the chest and diaphragm, moistens and lubricates the heart and lungs, removes sputum stagnancy, and treats thoracic paralysis. Bakeri warms the insides, disperses obstructions, and eases breathing; thus it treats cardio-thoracic pain, asthma, and overproduction of sputum. Pinellia suppresses vomiting, opens diaphragmatic obstruction, and renders expectoration. Vinegar promotes blood circulation and augments the efficacy of the various herbs; hence it is used as the decoction agent.

Indications

Angina pectoris, cardiac insufficiency, cardiac neurosis, cardiac valvular disease, cardiac infarction, inter-costal neuralgia.

Discrimination

Ta-chai-hu-tang (Major Bupleurum Combination) is used for a firm conformation with thoraco-costal distress and cardiac-thoracic obstruction.

Ta-hsien-hsiung-tang (Rhubarb and *Kan-sui* Combination) is used for cardiac-thoracic pain and severe symptoms, thoracic distention, stone-like hardness beneath the heart, and cramping and stiffness in the back and shoulders.

Chih-tzu-shih-tang (Gardenia and Soja Combination) is used for an abnormal heart beat, a weak conformation, and insomnia.

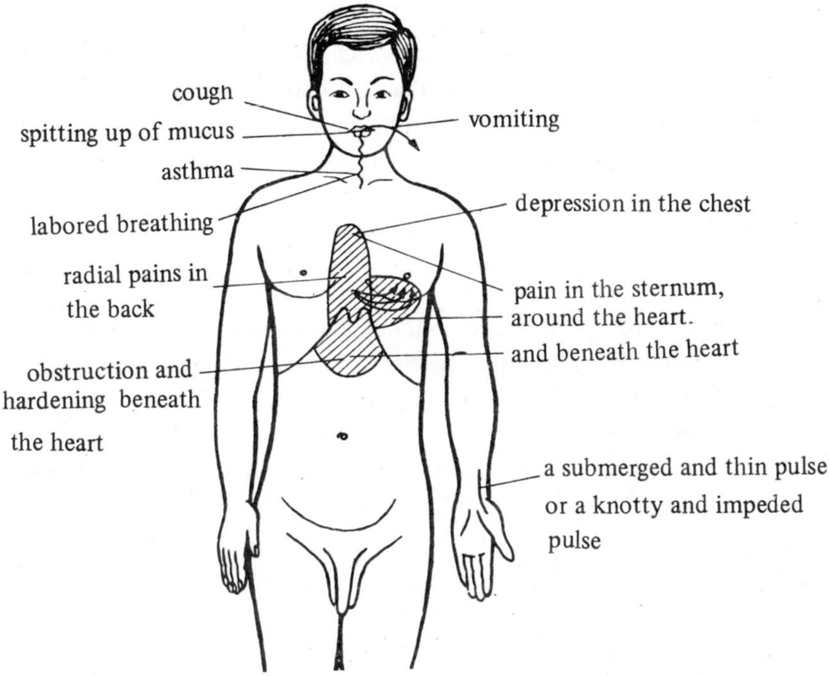

Liang-Chih-Tang 良枳湯

(Galanga and Chih-shih Combination)

Hoelen	6.0	Pinellia	6.0	Cinnamon	4.0
Jujube	4.0	Licorice	2.0	Galanga	1.0
Chih-shih	2.0				

Originated in *Liao chih ta kai* (療治大概) and included in most Japanese medical books. Used mostly for subcardiac or abdominal convulsive pain accompanied by vomiting. Sufferers of these symptoms mostly have a weak constitution with chronic, weak conformations; a weak and soft pulse; a weak and thin abdominal wall, and a hard mass situated beneath the heart or at the umbilicus where the pain begins and then moves upward.

Herbs and Actions

Composed of *Ling-kuei-kan-tsao-tang* (Hoelen, Licorice, and Jujube Combination) plus Pinellia, *Chih-shih* and galanga. *Ling-kuei-kan-tsao-tang* treats the moving pain that starts from around the navel; Pinellia settles gas in stomach pneumata; *Chih-shih* channels obstructed air and gas and breaks up firm obstructions. Galanga disperses chills and warms the stomach.

Indications

Gastrectasis, gastric ulcer, duodenal ulcer, gastric cancer, gastroptosis, cholelithiasis, pancreatitis.

Discrimination

Ling-kuei-kan-tsao-tang (Hoelen, Licorice, and Jujube Combination); pain beneath the heart, flushing up or vomiting, weak conformation.

Chien-chung-tang (Hoelen and Jujube Combination): pain beneath the heart, weak conformation, thin and tense abdominal wall.

Ta-chai-hu-tang (Major Bupleurum Combination): pain beneath the heart, thoraco-costal distress, firm conformation.

Weak conformation

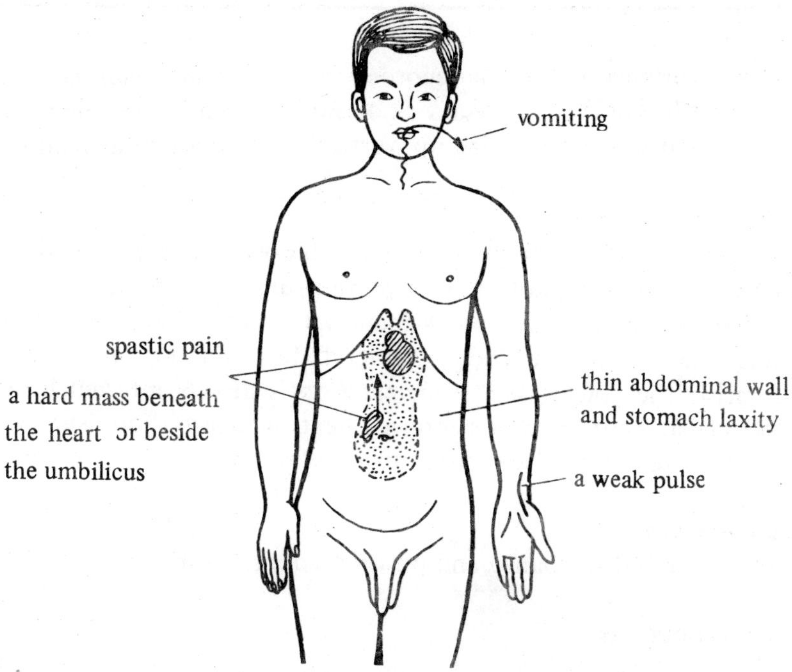

Nu-Shen-San 女神散

(Tang-kuei and Cyperus Formula)

Tang-kuei	3.0	Cnidium	3.0	Cinnamon	2.0
Atractylodes	3.0	Saussurea	1.5	Scute	2.0
Coptis	1.5	Ginseng	2.0	Licorice	1.5
Cyperus	3.0	Areca seed	2.0	Clove	1.0
Rhubarb	0.5-1.0				

An experimental formula recorded in *Wu wu fang han ko chueh* (勿誤方函口訣) by Asata S. of Japan. Used for treating neurosis, blood disease, flushing up, vertigo, and menopausal symptoms.

Herbs and Actions

Tang-kuei and Cnidium nourish the blood and stimulate circulation. Cinnamon quiets flush up. Saussurea dispels stagnant *ch'i*. Clove improves *ch'i*. Cyperus increases vitality. Areca seed dispels stagnant *ch'i* in the chest. Atractylodes, Ginseng, and Licorice nourish the spleen and stomach. Coptis dispels internal heat in the chest. Scute removes internal heat. Rhubarb diminishes fever but may be omitted if there is no constipation.

Indications

Menopausal disturbance and postnatal depression.

Discrimination

Chia-wei-hsiao-yao-san (Bupleurum and Peony Formula); women's diseases, headache, vertigo, weak conformation with mild symptoms.

Kuei-chih-fu-ling-wan (Cinnamon and Hoelen Formula): flushing up, vertigo, firm conformation with blood occlusion in the lower abdomen.

Kou-teng-san (Gambir Formula): mental distress, headaches, vertigo, shoulder pain, hypertension.

Half-weak, half-firm conformation

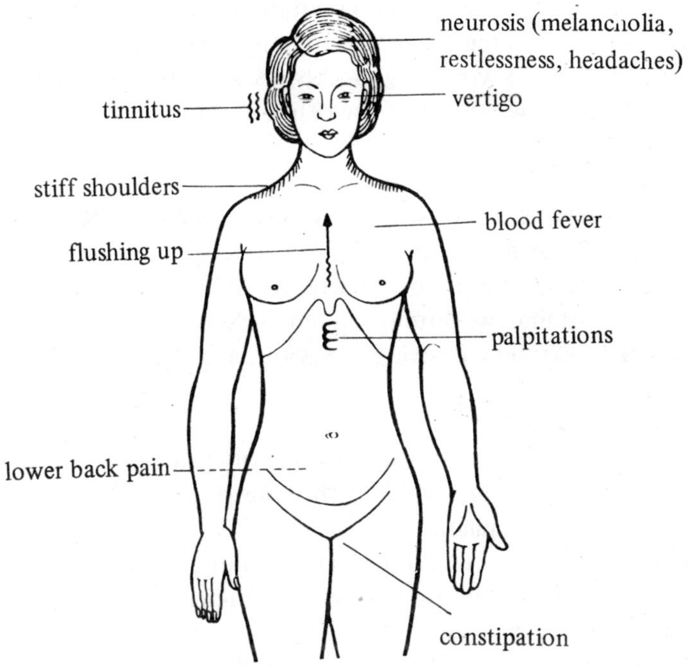

Pan-Hsia-Hou-Pu-Tang *(Pinellia and Magnolia Combination)*					**半夏厚朴湯**
Pinellia	6.0	Magnolia bark	3.0	Hoelen	5.0
Ginger	4.0	Perilla	2.0		

Pan-hsia-hou-pu-tang is mentioned early in the Chinese medical work *Chin kuei yao lueh* of the 1800-year Han dynasty. This formula is used to treat stress reactions, gastrointestinal weakness, muscular and skin flaccidity, abdominal fullness, ascites, floating or sunken pulse, emotional instability, delicate constitution,and a tendency towards fatigue.

Herbs and Actions

Pinellia and Hoelen relieve abdominal ascites, cure nausea and vomiting, and increase blood circulation. Magnolia bark cures abdominal fullness and increases vitality. Perilla has a tranquilizing effect and increases gastrointestinal function. Ginger acts as a diuretic, cures vomiting, increases gastrointestinal function, and coordinates the action of the other herbs.

Indications

Neurosis, nervous exhaustion, hysteria, nervousness, insomnia, fearfulness, neurotic esophageal constriction, recurrent palpitations, esophageal spasm, bronchitis, hoarseness due to the common cold, asthma, whooping cough, toxemia during pregnancy, blood vessel disorders, gastric relaxation, and edema.

Discrimination

Fu-ling-yin (Hoelen Combination): obstruction beneath the heart, splashing sound, agitated thriving of *ch'i*, noticeable water stagnancy in the stomach.

Kan-mai-ta-tsao-tang (Licorice and Jujube Combination): depressed *ch'i*, acute conditions; water stagnancy in the stomach, no throat discomfort.

Tang-kuei-shao-yao-san (*Tang-kuei* and Peony Formula): fatigability, mental instability, blood disease, no throat discomfort.

Ling-kuei-chu-kan-tang (Atractylodes and Hoelen Combination): vertigo, water stagnancy in the stomach, submerged and tense pulse, unstable *ch'i*.

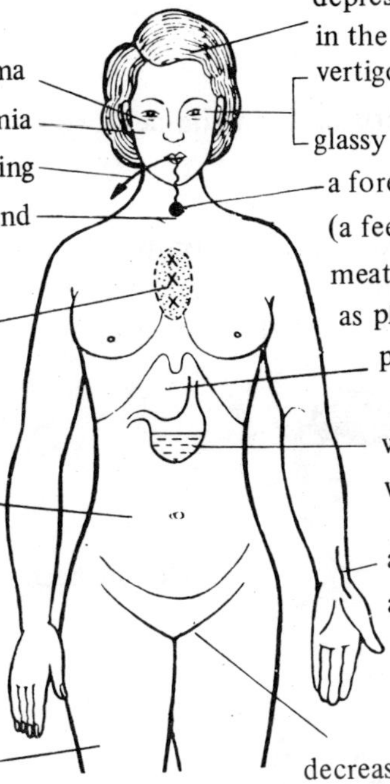

Pien-Chih-Hsin-Chi-Yin 變製心氣飲

(Areca and Evodia Combination)

Hoelen	5.0	Pinellia	5.0	Akebia	3.0
Cinnamon	2.5	Areca seed	2.5	Perilla fruit	2.0
Chih-shih	2.0	Morus	1.0	Licorice	1.0
Evodia	1.0	Tortoise shell	2.0		

Pien-chih-hsin-chi-yin is an experimental formula used for treating cardiac asthma, palpitatoin in the chest cavity, a sensation of hardness beneath the heart, stiffness in the shoulders and back, dyspnea, and hepatomegaly.

Herbs and Actions

Hoelen, Pinellia, and Akebia are diuretics. Morus, Perilla fruit, Tortoise shell, *Chih-shih*, and Areca seed are expectorants and antitussives. Cinnamon and Evodia dispel chills and pain in the chest and abdomen.

Indications

Cardiac asthma, chronic bronchitis, and angina pectoris.

Discrimination

Mu-fang-chi-tang (Stephania and Ginseng Combination): labored breathing, cardiac palpitations, obstruction and hardness beneath the heart, absence of palpitations beneath the heart.

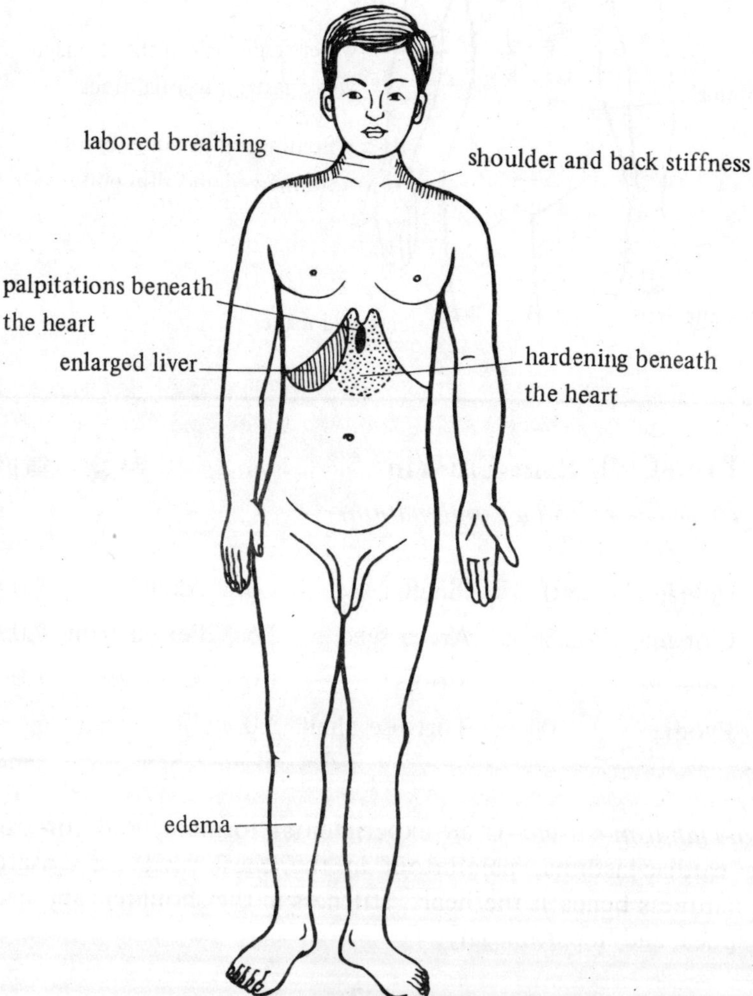

San-Ho-San 三和散

(Aquilaria and Perilla Formula)

Aquilaria	2.0	Perilla	2.0	Areca	2.0
Atractylodes	3.0	Cnidium	3.0	Saussurea	1.5
Citrus	1.5	Areca seed	1.5	Ginger	1.5
Chaenomeles	1.5	Licorice	1.0		

San-ho-san is used for treating stagnant blood and stagnant *ch'i,* distention beneath the heart, tension spasms, abdominal distention, pain in the waist and back, dysuria, constipation, facial edema, edema in the hands and feet, beriberi. Those having a weak pulse, abdominal weakness, and gastrointestinal weakness should not take this formula.

Herbs and Actions
Aquilaria, Saussurea, Citrus, Perilla, Areca, and Areca seed can smooth the *ch'i.* Cnidium eliminates pain. Atractylodes nourishes the spleen, relieves spasms, and acts as a diuretic. Chaenomeles corrects beriberi. Licorice relieves spasms and coordinates the actions of the other herbs.

Indications
Intestinal colic, abdominal pain, peritonitis, rheumatism, beriberi, constipation, anuria, edema, tendon spasms, and spasmodic pain in the scrotal area.

Discrimination
Su-Tzu-chiang-chi-tang (Perilla Fruit Combination): obstruction and fullness beneath the heart, edema, constipation, copious sputum causing flushing up, gasping, cold feet. These symptoms are commmon in senile and debilitated people.

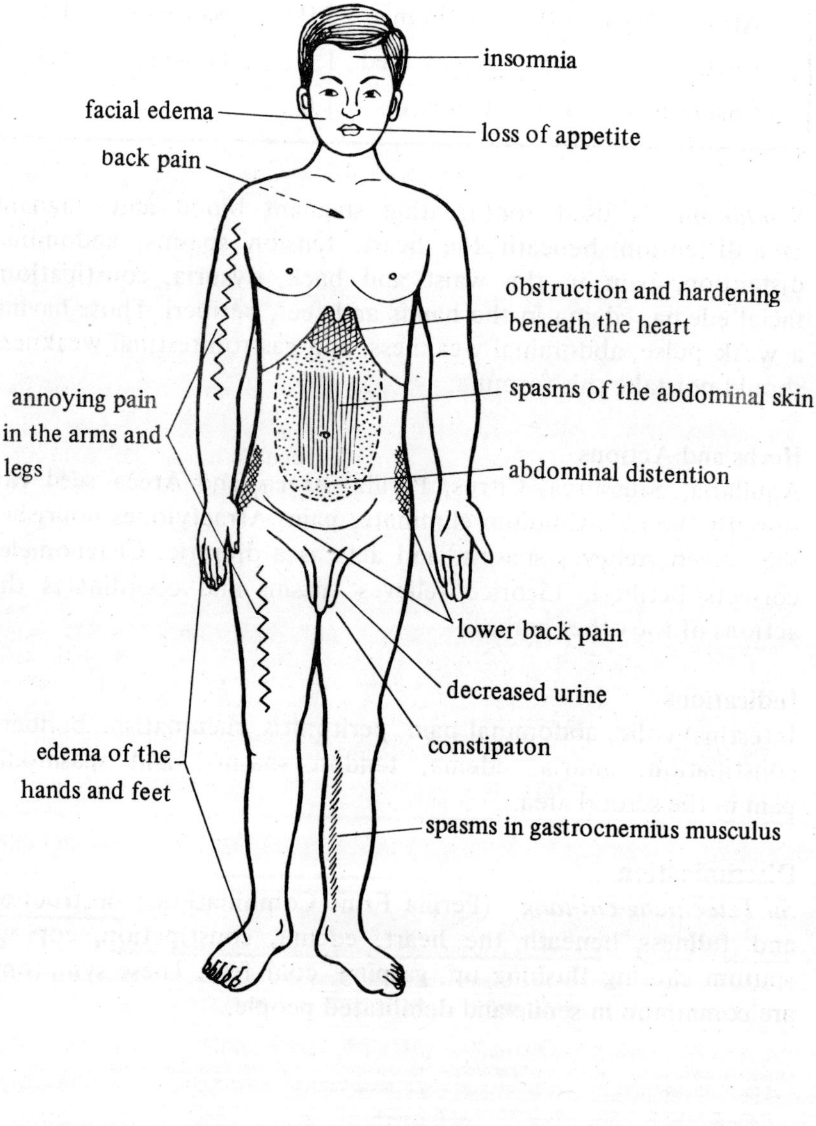
insomnia
facial edema
loss of appetite
back pain
obstruction and hardening beneath the heart
spasms of the abdominal skin
annoying pain in the arms and legs
abdominal distention
lower back pain
decreased urine
constipaton
edema of the hands and feet
spasms in gastrocnemius musculus

Shen-Mi-Tang 神秘湯

(Ma-huang and Magnolia Combination)

Ma-huang	5.0	Perilla	1.5	Citrus	2.5
Apricot seed	4.0	Magnolia bark	3.0	Licorice	2.0
Bupleurum	2.0				

Shen-mi-tang was first recorded in the *Wai tai mi yao* (外臺秘要) by Wang Tao during the Tang dynasty. This formula is used for treating a persistent cough, abodminal weakness, slight chest distention, little sputum, dyspnea, and neuroses.

Herbs and Actions
Ma-huang is a diaphoretic which relieves asthmatic coughing. Apricot seed dispels water toxins in the chest. Citrus is an antitussive and expectorant. Magnolia bark is an expectorant which also relieves flushing up and gasping. Perilla is a carminative. Bupleurum dispels "internal heat" and chest distention. Licorice coordinates the actions of the other herbs.

Indications
Bronchial asthma, asthma in children, and pulmonary emphysema.

Discrimination
Ma-hsing-kan-shih-tang (*Ma-huang* and Apricot Seed Combination): asthma, perspiring during a seizure, extreme thirst, and abnormally increased appetite before the seizure.
Hsiao-ching-lung-tang (Minor Blue Dragon Combination): asthma, water vapour beneath the heart, expectoration of thin sputum.
Hsiao-chai-hu-ho-pan-hsia-hou-pu-tang (Minor Bupleurum Combination with Pinellia and Magnolia Combination): asthma. This formula is suitable for the neurotic asthamtic with thoracocostal distress.
Wu-hu-erh-chen-tang (Gypsum, Citrus, and Pinellia Combination): asthma, and appetite loss; the conformation resembles *Ma-hsing-kan-shih-tang*. This formula is suitable for prolonged administration.

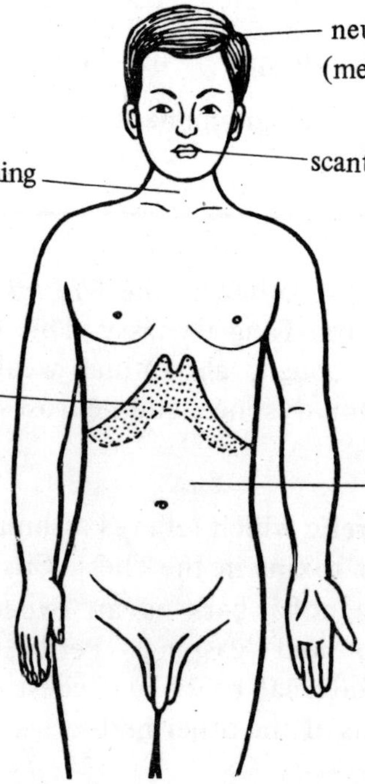

Shih-Liu-Wei-Liu-Chi-Yin 十六味流氣飲

(Tang-kuei Sixteen Herb Combination)

Tang-kuei	3.0	Cnidium	3.0	Peony	3.0
Cinnamon	3.0	Ginseng	3.0	Angelica	2.0
Platycodon	3.0	Astragalus	2.0	Saussurea	2.0
Lindera	2.0	Magnolia bark	2.0	*Chih-ko*	2.0
Areca seed	2.0	Perilla	2.0	Siler	2.0
Licorice	2.0				

Shih-liu-wei-liu-chi-ying is derived from the "carbuncle" category in *Wan ping hui chun* (萬病回春) of the Ming dynasty. This formula is used for treating a severe abscess of unknown etiology, carbuncles, and breast cancer. It is especially effective for undiagnosible intestinal diseases.

This formula is suitable for disintegrating unknown toxic tumors; swelling of shoulders, neck or limbs; and emphysema. It is effective for fibrocystic disease, intraductal papillomas, and breast cancer.

Herbs and Actions

Ginseng, Astragalus and Licorice supplement the *ch'i. Tang-kuei,* Peony and Cnidium nourish the blood. Saussurea, Areca seed, *Chih-ko,* Magnolia bark, and Perilla can regulate the *ch'i.* Lindera and Siler destroy stagnant *ch'i.* Cinnamon and Angelica disperse stagnant blood. Platycodon disperses pus and heightens the effectiveness of the other herbs.

Indications

Fibrocystic disease, breast cancer, intraductal papillomas, goiter, and cervical lymphadenoma.

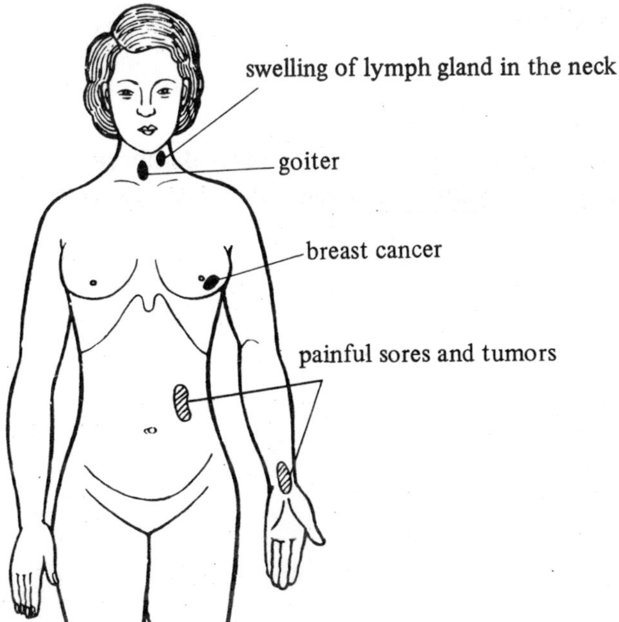

Shih-Ti-Tang *(Kaki Combination)*					柿蒂湯
Clove	1.5	Kaki pedicle	5.0	Ginger	4.0

Recorded in *Chi sheng fang* (濟生方). Warms the stomach, disperses chills, settles harmful gas and air, and stops hiccups. The principal indication for this formula is hiccups caused by abnormal respiration due to a cold stomach. It also treats cold limbs and a submerged and thin pulse.

Herbs and Actions

The chief component, Kaki pedicle, calms moving gas and air. The formula is the sacred remedy for hiccups. When subordinated to Ginger, Kaki breaks up obstructions and disperses chills. Cloves warm the stomach and drive away the wind (dispel gas); hence they are suitable for hiccups. If hiccups are hot, then it is proper to administer *Chu-pi-chu-ju-tang* instead.

Indications

Hiccups.

Discrimination

Chu-pi-chu-ju-tang (Aurantium and Bamboo Combination) is for hiccups, stomach emptiness, and hiccups caused by weakness fever.

Su-Tzu-Chiang-Chi-Tang 蘇子降氣湯

(Perilla Fruit Combination)

Perilla fruit	3.0	Pinellia	4.0	Citrus	2.5
Magnolia	2.5	Peucedanum	2.5	Cinnamon	2.5
Tang-kuei	2.5	Jujube	1.5	Licorice	1.0
Ginger	1.5				

Su-tzu-chiang-chi-tang is recorded in the Chinese medical text, *Tai ping huei min ho chi chu fang* (太平惠民和劑局方) of the Sung Dynasty. This formula is used as treatment for chilling of the legs, dyspnea, weakness below the umbilicus, dysuria, copious sputum, hyperpnea, flushing up, tense pulse, and subcardiac distention.

Herbs and Actions

Perilla fruit, Peucedanum, Magnolia bark, Citrus, Pinellia, and Cinnamon alleviate flushing up and relieve congestion. *Tang-kuei* is a hematinic. Licorice coordinates the actions of the other herbs.

Indications

Chronic bronchitis, bronchial asthma, pulmonary emphysema, tinnitus, hemoptysis, epistaxis, pyorrhea, mastitis, edema, and beriberi.

Discrimination

Hsiao-ching-lung-tang (Minor Blue Dragon Combination): cough and asthma, thin sputum which can be easily expectorated, stagnant water in the stomach, floating and quick pulse.

Ling-kan-chiang-wei-hsin-hsia-jen-tang (Hoelen and Schizandra Combination): cough and asthma; chilling; no internal conformation; weak condition; decreased urine; submerged pulse.

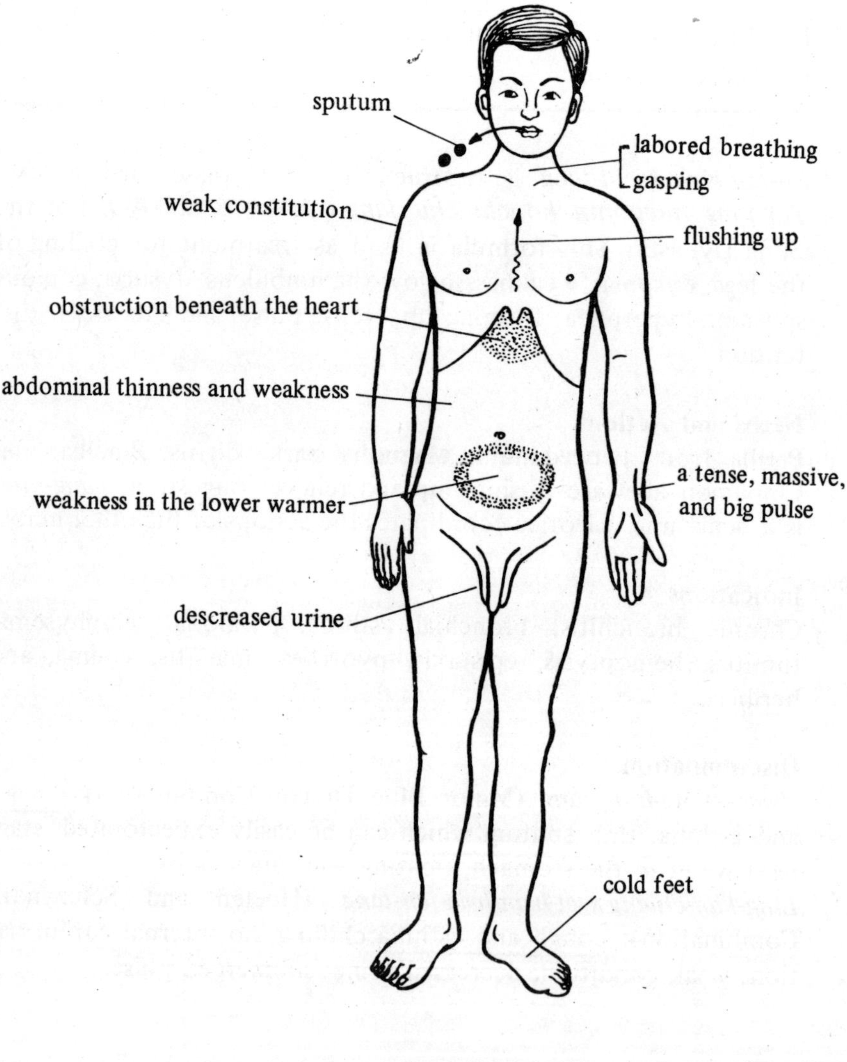
sputum
labored breathing
gasping
weak constitution
flushing up
obstruction beneath the heart
abdominal thinness and weakness
a tense, massive, and big pulse
weakness in the lower warmer
descreased urine
cold feet

Ting-Hsiang-Shih-Ti-Tang 丁香柿蒂湯

(Clove and Kaki Combination)

Clove	2.5	Kaki	6.0	*Tang-sheng*	3.0
Ginger	6.0				

Ting-hsiang-shih-ti-tang is recorded in *Cheng yin mai chih* (證因脈治). This formula is used for treating those whose delicate constitution is due to prolonged illness. It can relieve the problems of eructation due to gastric weakness, loss of appetite, chest distention, white coating on the tongue, and sunken pulse.

Herbs and Actions

Clove and *Kaki* treat eructation and vomiting, and they warm the stomach. *Tang-sheng* nourishes the *ch'i.* Ginger dispels chills and eliminates eructation.

Indications

Eructation.

Ting-Chuan-Tang 定喘湯

(Ma-huang and Ginkgo Combination)

Ma-huang	3.0	Pinellia	3.0	Morus	1.8
Apricot seed	1.8	Perilla fruit	1.8	Ginkgo	4.8
Scute	0.6	Tussilago	3.0	Licorice	0.6

Ting-chuan-tang is recorded in a Chinese medical work. *I fang chi chieh* (醫方集解) of the Ching dynasty as being effective for asthma, for removing internal heat in the lungs, and for dispeling sputum. This formula cures cough with sputum, rapid respirations, and wheezing due to the common cold with internal heat.

Herbs and Actions

Ma-huang and Morus relieve internal heat in the lungs and stop dyspnea. Apricot seed, Perilla fruit, and Ginkgo improve the function of the lungs and cure asthma. Pinellia with Tussilago dispels sputum. Scute with Morus relieves internal heat. Licorice synthesizes the action of all the other herbs.

Indications

Acute and chronic bronchitis, common cold, cough, asthma, and bronchial asthma and cough.

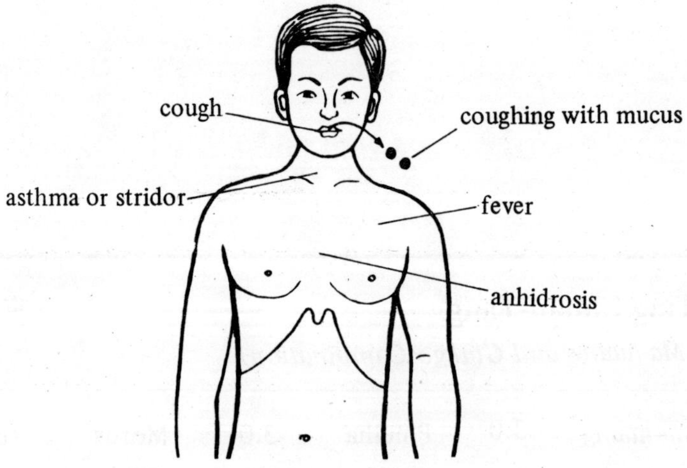

Wu-Yao-Shun-Chi-San 烏藥順氣散
(Lindera Formula)

Lindera	2.5	*Ma-huang*	2.5	Citrus	2.5
Silkworm	2.5	Ginger	2.5	Cnidium	2.5
Chih-ko	2.0	Platycodon	2.5	Angelica	1.5
Licorice	1.5				

Wu-yao-shun-chi-san is listed in the *Tai ping huei min ho chi chu fang* (太平惠民和劑局方, A.D. 1107-1110). This formula is used for stroke followed by arthralgia, aphasia, Bell's palsy, congestion, asthma, and flushing up.

Herbs and Actions
Ma-huang and Platycodon are diaphoretics that also dispel chills. Cnidium and Angelica are carminatives and hematinics. *Chih-ko* and Citrus improve vitality and dispel sputum. Silkworm aids in expectoration of tenacious sputum. Ginger is an emmenagogue. Licorice regulates the action of other herbs. Lindera dispels stagnant *ch'i*.

Indications
Apoplexy, cerebromalacia, monoplegia, 40 years' wrist, 50 years' shoulder, palsy of the hands and feet, trigeminal neuralgia, beriberi, and senility.

Discrimination
Hsu-ming-tang (*Ma-huang* and Ginseng Combination): apoplexy, difficulty in speaking, weak blood, internal fever, and extreme thirst.

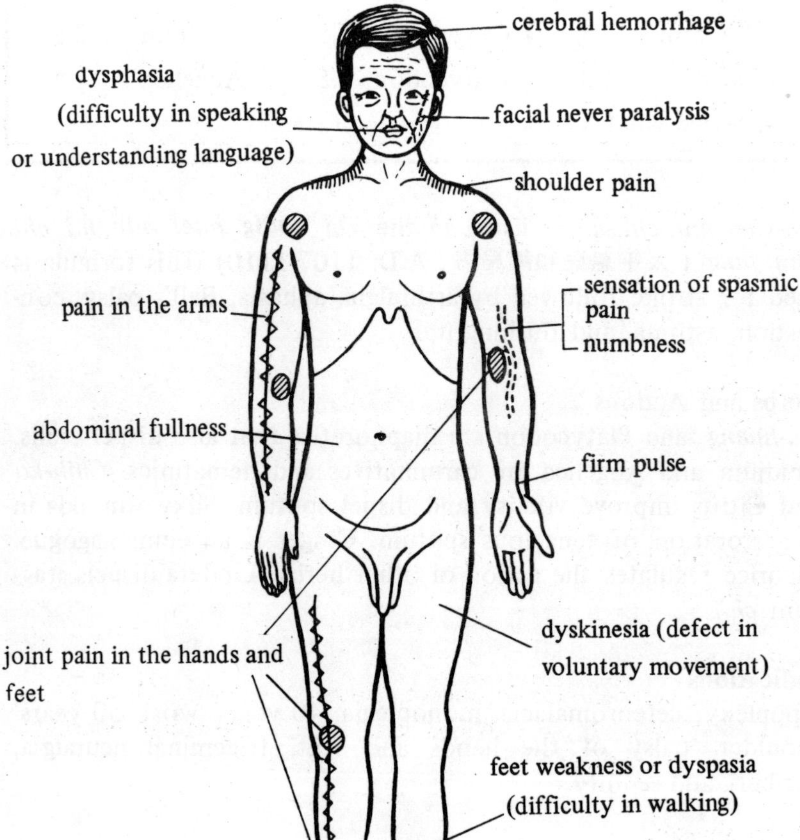
cerebral hemorrhage
dysphasia
(difficulty in speaking
or understanding language)
facial never paralysis
shoulder pain
sensation of spasmic
pain
numbness
pain in the arms
abdominal fullness
firm pulse
dyskinesia (defect in
voluntary movement)
joint pain in the hands and
feet
feet weakness or dyspasia
(difficulty in walking)

Yen-Nien-Pan-Hsia-Tang 延年半夏湯

(Evodia and Pinellia Combination)

Ginseng	2.0	Pinellia	5.0	Platycodon	3.0
Chih-shih	1.0	Ginger	2.0	Areca seed	3.0
Evodia	1.0	Tortoise shell	3.0	Peucedanum	3.0

Yen-nien-pan-hsia-tang is recorded in *Wai tai mi yao* (外臺秘要). This formula is used for treating chronic gastrointestinal disorder, pain in the chest, shoulder stiffness, chilled feet, gastroptosis, gastric distention, gastric ulcer, abdominal weakness, and lack of vigor.

Herbs and Actions

Chih-shih, Peucedanum, Areca seed, and Tortoise shell are expectorants which also smooth the *ch'i* and treat distention. Pinellia removes "stagnant sputum" in the stomach. Platycodon removes phlegm from the chest. Evodia dispels chills and treats hernia. Ginseng nourishes the *ch'i* and stomach. Ginger dispels chill and warms the body.

Indications

Gastric ulcer, duodenal ulcer, chronic gastritis, intercostal neuralgia, sour stomach, chronic pancreatitis, shoulder stiffness, neurosis, chest pain, and loss of appetite.

Discrimination

Ta-chai-hu-tang (Major Bupleurum Combination): chest pain, obstruction and hardness beneath the heart, thoraco-costal distress, firm chest.

Chih-so-erh-chen-tang (*Chih-shih* and Cardamon Combination): pain in the chest and back, radiating to the lower back, congestion in the heart.

Chai-hu-kuei-chih-tang (Bupleurum and Cinnamon Combination): tension of abdominal muscles and thoraco-costal distress.

Chai-hu-pieh-chia-tang (Bupleurum and Tortoise Shell Combination): pain in the chest and back; acute cramping in the chest, back, and abdomen.

Liang-chih-tang (Galanga and *Chih-shih* Combination): chest pain, pain beneath the heart, and belching.

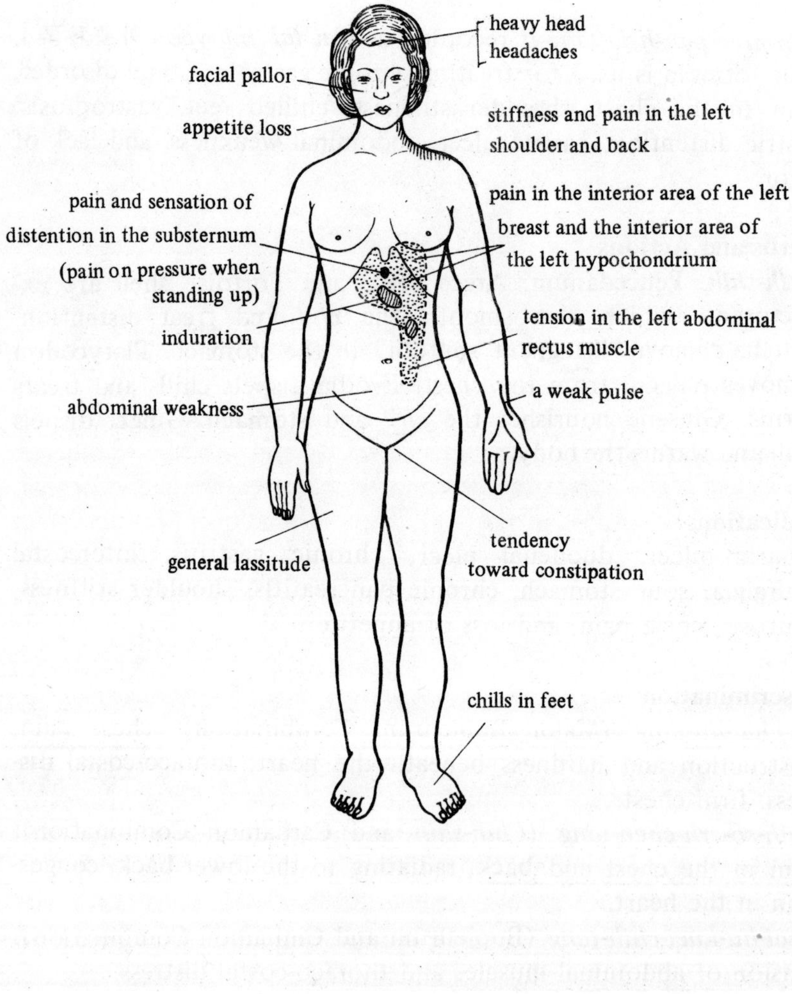

15.

Li Hsieh Chi

(理血劑, Blood Formulas)

Formulas that circulate the blood and treat blood diseases are termed *li hsieh chi.*

The blood carries the nutrients to all parts of the body. An ancient adage says: "When the blood is weak, the body deteriorates, but with healthy blood the eyes can see, the ears can hear, the palms can grip, and the feet can walk." Blood formulas treat poor circulation, occlusion or stagnancy, extravasation and the consequent hemoptysis (hemorrhage of the larynx, trachea, bronchi or lungs), hematemesis (vomiting blood), hematuria (bloody urine), and bloody feces. The contents of a blood formula varies according to its action. Blood formulas can be divided into hematinic (increasing hemoglobin), hemostatic (stopping bleeding), cooling, and warming types. The hematinic and cooling types are discussed in the sections on *pu yang chi* (補養劑) and *ching je chi* (清熱劑). Here the hemostatic and deobstruent formulas are introduced.

This type of formula belongs to the "attacking" type and should not be used excessively, otherwise *ch'i* will be injured. "Blood flowing within the vessels" is the normal condition. Pathological changes sometimes cause the blood to overflow or pool, resulting in hemorrhage, nosebleeds, bloody urine, or bloody feces. Each condition must be treated with the proper formula with respect to whether the condition is chills, fever, weakness, or firmness: for example, an acute condition uses the palliative hemostasis method; a firm fever calls for a hemostatic as well as a fever-reducing formula; and a weak chill conformation needs a hemostatic formula together with a yang-warming formula. Both the principal and subordinate symptoms have to be noted before a correct treatment can be prescribed.

Chi-Li-San 七厘散

(Musk and Catechu Formula)

Carthamus	0.6	Cinnabar	0.5	Calamus gum	5.0
Musk	0.05	Borneol	0.05	Mastic	0.6
Myrrh	0.6	Catechu	1.0		

Chi-li-san is a well-known formula for external and internal injuries. This formula was recorded in the *Liang fang chi yueh yeh ho pi* (良方集月夜合璧) by Hsieh Yueh-ching during the Ching dynasty. It is used for treating external injuries, contusions, fractures, stagnant blood with pain, hemorrhage, stab wounds, swelling due to unknown causes, and burns. Pregnant woman should not take this formula.

Herbs and Actions

Calamus gum and Carthamus dispel stagnant blood and act as hematinics. Mastic and Myrrh increase vitality, dispel stagnant *ch'i*, relieve swelling, and ease pain. Catechu is an antipyretic and hemostatic. Cinnabar is a sedative. Musk and Borneol increase vitality, improve blood circulation, and ease pain.

Indications

External and internal injuries, stagnant blood, and general pain.

Chi-Wu-Chiang-Hsia-Tang 七物降下湯

(Tang-kuei and Gambir Combination)

Tang-kuei	3.0	Peony	3.0	Cnidium	3.0
Rehmannia	3.0	Astragalus	3.0	Gambir	4.0
Phellodendron	2.0				

Chi-wu-chiang-hsia-tang was recorded in the Japanese medical text, *Han fang chu fang chieh so* (漢方處方解說). The original prescription for this formula was devised by Otsuka Keisetsu of Japan. It is a combination of *Szu-wu-tang* (*Tang-kuei* Four Combination) with Phellodendron, Gambir, and Astragalus. It is used for treating hypertension in patients of weak conformation who have kidney disorders and experience flushing up, aching shoulders, tinnitus, and heaviness in the head.

Herbs and Actions

Tang-kuei, Peony, Cnidium, and Rehmannia are hematinics that also improve the heart and liver functions. Phellodendron dispels moisture and removes "internal heat". Astragalus nourishes the *ch'i.* Gambir dispels "internal heat" in the heart and acts as a sedative.

Indications

Essential hypertension, chronic nephritis, and arteriosclerosis.

Chia-Wei-Kuei-Pi-Tang 加味歸脾湯

(Ginseng, Longan, and Bupleurum Combination)

Ginseng	3.0	Atractylodes	3.0	Hoelen	3.0
Jujube	1.0	Longan	3.0	*Tang-kuei*	2.0
Astragalus	2.0	Polygala	1.0	Licorice	1.0
Saussurea	1.0	Jujube	1.0	Ginger	1.0
Bupleurum	3.0	Gardenia	2.0		

Chia-wei-kuei-pi-tang is recorded in *Chi sheng fang* (濟生方). This is a combination of *Kuei-pi-tang* (Ginseng and Longan Combination) with Bupleurum and Gardenia. This formula is used for treating those of delicate constitution who have a mild fever, gastrointestinal weakness, fatigue, tendency to bleed, anemia, amnesia, and neurotic symptoms.

Herbs and Actions
Ginseng, Astragalus, Atractylodes, Hoelen, Jujube, and Licorice can nourish the spleen and stomach. Longan, Polygala, and Jujube nourish the heart and nerves and act as sedatives. Saussurea increases the vigor. *Tang-kuei* treats anemia, and in combination with Ginseng is a blood tonic. Bupleurum treats chest distention, recurrent fever and chills, and abdominal pain, and it acts as an antipyretic and stomachic. Gardenia treats stress symptoms, generalized fever, insomnia, and mental instability; it also acts as an antiphlogistic, sedative, and hemostatic.

Indications
Severe anemia, amnesia, neurotic palpitation, loss of appetite, menstrual irregularities, hysteria, nervous exhaustion, nocturnal emission, and chronic gonorrhea.

Chiao-Ai-Szu-Wu-Tang 膠艾四物湯

(Gelatin and Artemisia Four Combination)

Tang-kuei	2.0	Cnidium	2.0	Peony	2.0
Rehmannia	2.0	Gelatin beads	2.0	Scute	2.0
Atractylodes	2.0	Artemisia	2.0	Cyperus	2.0
Cardamon	2.0	A handful of Oryza			

Recorded in *Wan ping hui chun* (萬病回春). Composed of *Szu-wu-tang* (*Tang-kuei* Four Combination) along with a hemostatic and fetal-stabilizing agent. Hence it has the actions of replenishing blood, smoothing respiration, stabilizing the fetus, and arresting bleeding. It is commonly used for menoxenia; menorrhagia; uterine bleeding or fetal agitation and instability that is causing abdominal pain and bleeding during pregnancy; and anemia. This formula also may be used for other kinds of bleeding.

Herbs and Actions

Tang-kuei, Cnidium, Peony, and Rehmannia constitute *Szu-wu-tang* which is capable of nourishing the respiratory system and blood. Gelatin enriches blood. Cyperus, Artemisia, Atractylodes, Cardamon, and Scute are helpful in stabilizing the fetus.

Indications

Bleeding during pregnancy, a sign of imminent abortion, accompanied by abdominal pain; postpartum bleeding, intestinal bleeding, hemorrhoidal bleeding, hematuria, internal bleeding caused by an external injury and the resulting anemia; purpura.

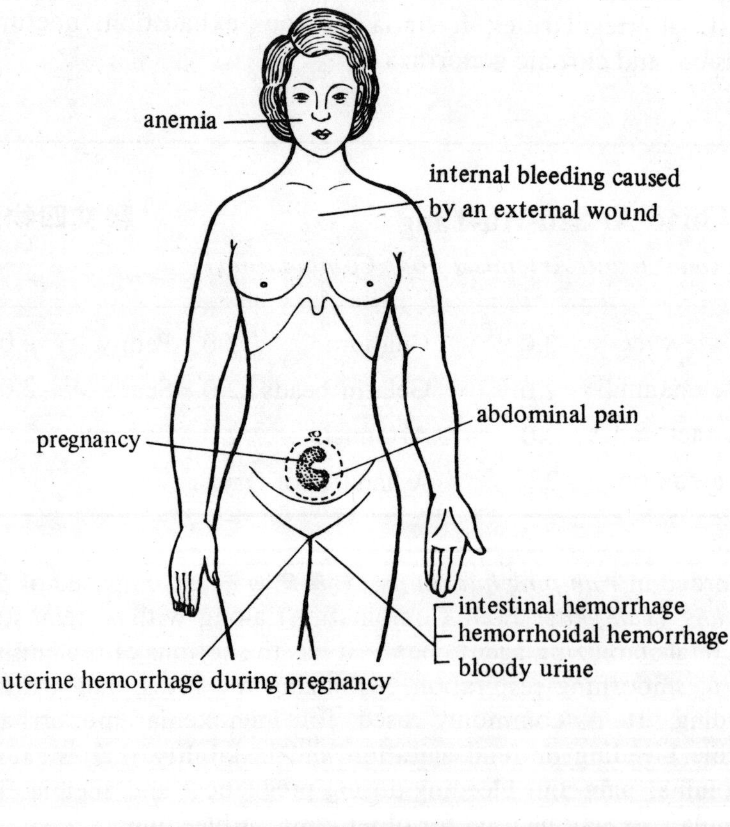

Fu-Yuan-Huo-Hsieh-Tang 復元活血湯

(Tang-kuei and Persica Combination)

Bupleurum	12.0	*Tang-kuei*	9.0	Carthamus	6.0
Licorice	6.0	Persica	12.0	Rhubarb	9.0
Trichosanthes root	9.0			Anteater scales	9.0

Fu-yuan-huo-hsieh-tang is recorded *I hsueh fa ming* (醫學發明). This formula is used for treating chest pain and stagnant blood and pain due to swelling of external injuries.

Herbs and Action

Bupleurum nourishes the liver and *ch'i. Tang-kuei* nourishes the blood. Anteater Scales dispels stagnant blood. Rhubarb, Persica, and Carthamus nourish the blood and dispel stagnant blood. Trichosanthes root is an antipyretic and antiphlogistic. Licorice is a sedative which also coordinates the action of the other herbs.

Indications

Pain due to external injuries; stagnant blood in the abdomen; and severe pain.

Huang-Tu-Tang 黃土湯

(Fu-lung-kan Combination)

Fu-lung-kan	7.0	Rehmannia	3.0	Gelatin	3.0
Scute	3.0	Licorice	2.0	Aconite	0.5–1.0
Atractylodes	3.0				

Huang-tu-tang was recorded in the *Chin kuei yao lueh*(金匱要略) during the Han dynasty. This formula is used for treating hemorrhage, hemoptysis, and epistaxis in patients of delicate constitution with coarse skin, a weak abdomen, flushing up, restlessness, a sensation of heat in the palms, body fever, severe chills, dysuria, abdominal pain, and diarrhea.

Herbs and Actions

Huang-tu-tang is a hemostatic and antiemetic which is especially useful for pernicious vomiting. Gelatin and Rehmannia function as hematinics, hemostatics, and nutritives. Licorice and Aconite improve metabolism. Scute and Atractylodes improve gastric function.

Indications

Intestinal bleeding, rectal ulcer, rectal cancer, hemorrhoids, endometritis, uterine bleeding, epistaxis, and hemoptysis.

Note: *Huang-tu* (yellow soil) is a kind of burned clay, found after use of a special type of stove in China.

Discrimination

Chiung-kuei-chiao-ai-tang (Gelatin and *Tang-kuei* Combination): uterine bleeding, weak and chilling blood occlusion, abdominal tension.

Huang-lien-ah-chiao-tang (Coptis and Gelatin Combination): various hemorrhaging, yang weakness conformation.

San-huang-hsieh-hsin-tang (Coptis and Rhubarb Combination): all hemorrhages, tension beneath the heart, flushing up, firm conformation.

Kuei-chih-fu-ling-wan (Cinnamon and Hoelen Formula): abdominal mass, blood occlusion, firm conformation.

Kuei-pi-tang (Ginseng and Longan Combination): various hemorrhages and blood weakness in the heart and spleen.

Pa-wei-wan (Rehmannia Eight Formula): annoying fever, no hemorrhaging.

Chih-kan-tsao-tang (Baked Licorice Combination): annoying fever, yang-weakness conformation, abdominal tension.

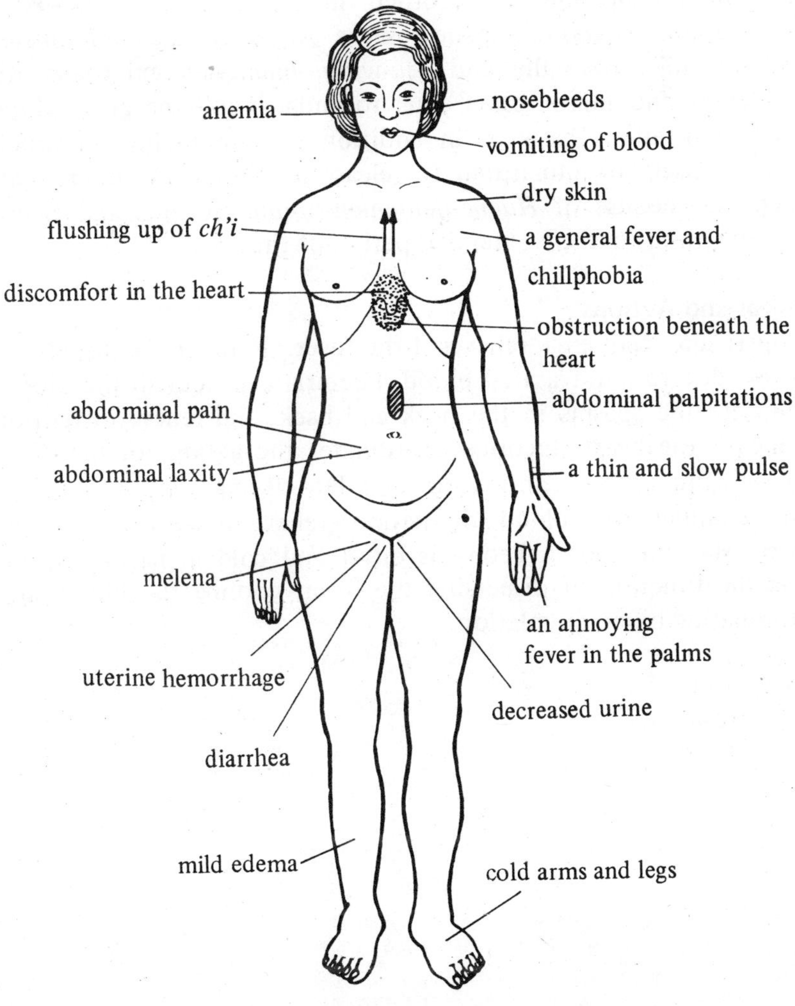

Ko-Ken-Hung-Hua-Tang 葛根紅花湯

(Pueraria and Carthamus Combination)

Pueraria	3.0	Peony	3.0	Rehmannia	3.0
Coptis	1.5	Gardenia	1.5	Carthamus	1.5
Rhubarb	1.0	Licorice	1.0		

Ko-ken-hung-hua-tang is recorded in *Fang yu ni* (方輿輗). This formula is good for acne rosacea. In severe cases, administer this formula internally and *Szu-wu-liu-huang-san* externally. In moderate and minor cases, this formula should be given alone on a continuous basis or in addition to acupuncture in which blood vessels are punctured to release bad blood. Another treatment is the use of *Huang-lien-chieh-tu-tang* (Coptis and Scute Combination) over an extended period of time.

Herbs and Actions

Coptis and Gardenia relieves firm fever. Rehmannia dispels all fevers due to extravasated blood. Pueraria can nourish the blood, alleviate the spasms in the neck and back, and relieve distention beneath the heart. Licorice coordinates the actions of the other herbs. Rhubarb is an antipyretic and detoxifying agent. Carthamus can stimulate the blood circulation, relieve hypermia, and disperse stagnant blood. Peony is bitter and cold in nature, and it has the function of dispersing the fever, cooling the blood, and stimulating blood circulation.

Indication

Acne rosacea.

Kuei-Chih-Fu-Ling-Wan 桂枝茯苓丸

(Cinnamon and Hoelen Formula)

Cinnamon	4.0	Hoelen	4.0	Persica	4.0
Peony	4.0	Moutan	4.0		

Kuei-chih-fu-ling-wan is recorded in the Chinese medical work *Chin kuei yao lueh* (A.D. 205) as a treatment for gynecological disorders with stagnant blood and also as a drug for men. This formula is good to treat those of strong constitution with a flushed face, protruding abdomen, resistant pressing pain at the umbilicus, tense and sunken pulse, headache, shoulder stiffness, vertigo, and chills in the feet.

Herbs and Actions

Cinnamon checks blood flushing up and coordinates the effects of the other herbs on blood circulation. Hoelen with Cinnamon cures abdominal palpitation and is diuretic. Persica removes stagnant blood and increases blood circulation. Moutan also removes stagnant blood and increases vitality. Peony causes stagnant blood to be expelled.

Indications

1. Gynecological diseases: endometritis, ovaritis, inflammation of the oviduct, uterine myoma, climacteric disorders, menstrual irregularity, leukorrhea, lumbago, shoulder stiffness and headache.
2. Dermatopathy: eczema, urticaria, dermatitis, black spots, pimples, and frigorism.
3. Neuropathy: nervousness, neurosis, and hysteria.
4. Ophthalmology: hordeolum, hemophthalomos, blepharitis, and keratitis.
5. Other ailments: prostatomegaly, hypertension, arthritis, neuralgia and rheumatism.

Discrimination

Tao-ho-cheng-chi-tang (Persica and Rhubarb Combination): blood occlusion, noticeable upward congestion, and cold feet.

Ta-huang-mu-tan-pi-tang (Rhubarb and Moutan Combination): blood occlusion, acute localized symptoms in the right lower abdomen, a tendency toward suppuration.

Ti-tang-tang (Rhubarb and Leech Combination): blood occlusion, mental excitation, and amnesia.

Hsia-yu-hsieh-tang (Persica and Eupolyphaga Combination): prolonged blood occlusion and coarse skin.

Tang-kuei-shao-yao-san (*Tang-kuei* and Peony Formula): blood occlusion, weak conformation.

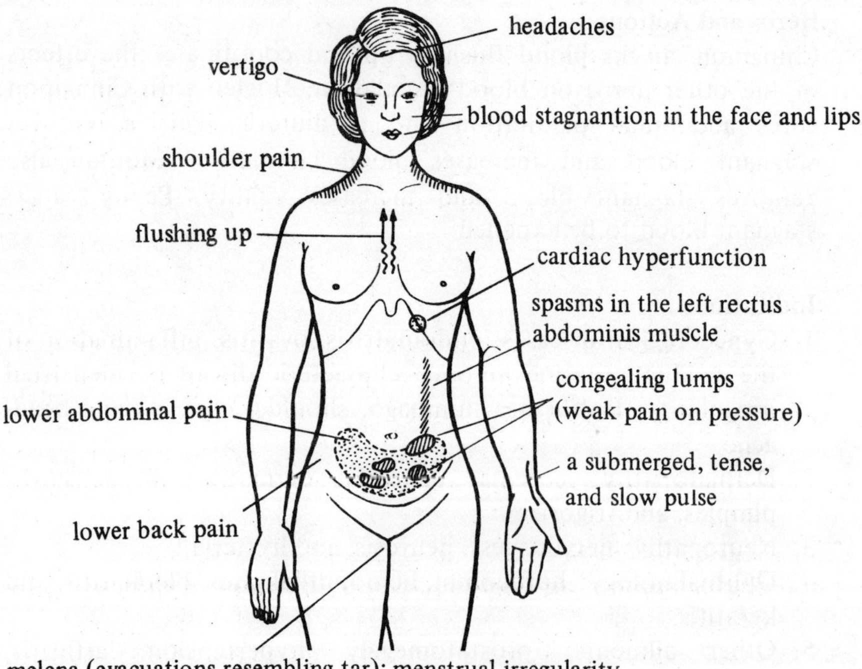

Kuei-Pi-Tang 歸脾湯

(Ginseng and Longan Combination)

Astragalus	2.0	Ginseng	3.0	Hoelen	3.0
Atractylodes	3.0	Zizyphus	3.0	Longan	3.0
Tang-kuei	2.0	Ginger	1.0	Jujube	1.0
Polygala	1.0	Licorice	1.0	Saussurea	1.0

Kuei-pi-tang is recorded in *Chi sheng fang* by Yen Yung-ho of the Sung dynasty. This formula is used to treat bleeding due to gastrointestinal weakness in those of delicate constitution, convalescent debility and fatigue, anemia, amnesia, palpitations, insomnia, excessive perspiration, night sweats, recurrent fevers, pallor, weak pulse and abdomen, lack of vigor, fatigue, and mild neurosis – all without inflammation or congestion. This formula is also good for those having gastric distention after taking *Pu-chung-i-chi-tang* (Ginseng and Astragalus Combination) or *Shih-chuan-ta-pu-tang* (Ginseng and *Tang-kuei* Ten Combination).

Herbs and Actions

Ginseng, Astragalus, Atractylodes, Hoelen, Jujube, and Licorice nourish the spleen and stomach. Longan, polygala, and Zizyphus seed are hematinics and sedatives. Saussurea cures mental instability. Ginger is stomachic. *Tang-kuei* nourishes the blood.

Indications

Anemia, bleeding, amnesia, insomnia, nervous exhaustion, neurotic palpitation, gastric ulcer, leukemia, irregular menstruation, uterine carcinoma, endometritis, itching in the genital area, nocturnal emission, impotence and chronic gonorrhea.

Discrimination

Shih-chuan-ta-pu-tang (Ginseng and *Tang-kuei* Ten Combination): anemia, weakness of *ch'i* and blood. This formula is indicated when there is only occasional mental distress.

Liu-chun-tzu-tang (Six Major Herb Combination): weakness of the spleen and stomach, stagnant water in the stomach.
Pu-chung-i-chi-tang (Ginseng and Astragalus Combination): weakness of *ch'i* and insufficiency of stomachic or splenic *ch'i*.
Huang-tu-tang (*Fu-lung-kan* Combination): hemorrhaging, chillphobia, abdominal palpitations, numbness beneath the umbilicus, yin-weakness conformation.

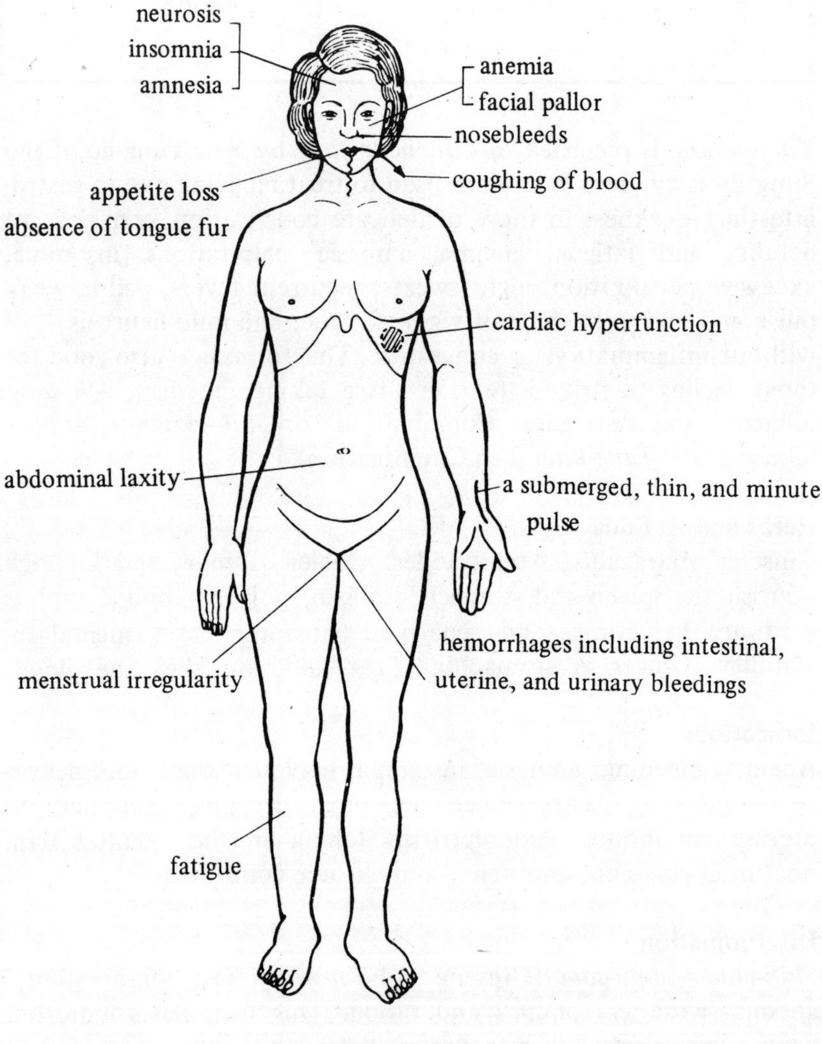

Lien-Chu-Yin 連珠飲

(Tang-kuei and Atractylodes Combination)

Hoelen	5.0	Cinnamon	4.0	*Tang-kuei*	3.0
Cnidium	3.0	Peony	3.0	Rehmannia	3.0
Atractylodes	3.0	Licorice	2.0		

Lien-chu-yin is a combination of *Szu-wu-tang* (*Tang-kuei* Four Combination) and *Ling-kuei-chu-kan-tang* (Atractylodes and Hoelen Combination). This formula is used for treating anemia with palpitation, vertigo, tinnitus, and facial edema. Patients with gastrointestinal weakness; a tendency toward diarrhea; and paleness of the lips, conjunctiva, and fingernails should not take this formula. If the patient experiences anorexia or diarrhea after using this formula, the treatment should be discontinued.

Herbs and Actions

Tang-kuei, Peony, Cnidium, and Rehmannia of *Szu-wu-tang* nourishes the liver, spleen, heart, and kidneys. *Ling-kuei-chu-kan-tang* is effective for flushing up and vertigo (sensation of swinging).

Indications

Anemia, palpitations and tinnitus due to anemia, valvular disease, and chlorosis.

Discrimination

Chih-kan-tsao-tang (Baked Licorice Combination): palpitations, knotty and alternating pulse, and annoying fever in the hands and feet.

Chiung-kuei-chiao-ai-tang (Gelatin and *Tang-kuei* Combination): anemia, diarrhea, and uterine bleeding.

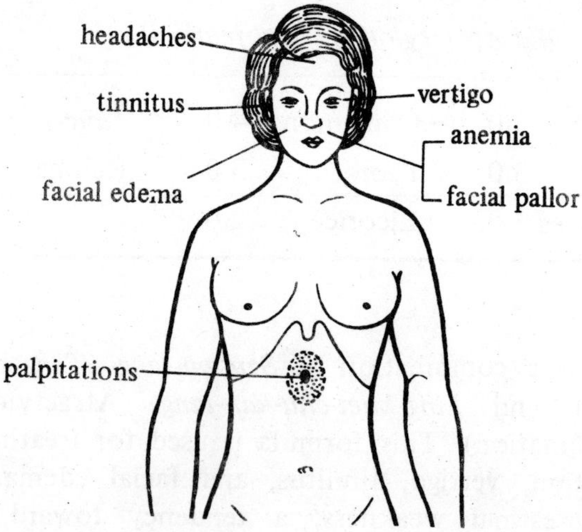

Shao-Yao-Tang 芍藥湯

(Peony Combination)

Peony	4.0	Scute	2.0	Rhubarb	1.0
Cinnamon	1.0	Licorice	1.0	Areca seed	1.0
Saussurea	1.0	*Tang-kuei*	2.0	Coptis	2.0

Shao-yao-tang is recorded in *Cheng chih chuen sheng* (證治準繩) of the Ming dynasty. This formula is a combination of *Hsiang-lien-wan* (Saussurea and Coptis Formula) with *San-huang-hsieh-hsin-tang* (Coptis and Rhubarb Combination) and *Shao-yao-kan-tsao-tang* (Peony and Licorice Combination). This formula is used in the initial stage of diarrhea in those of firm conformation without outside conformations. It is effective for disentery with bloody pus, abdominal pain, and tenesmus. Experience has shown that it is more effective when Citrus is substituted for Cinnamon. If the patient has thirst, the Cinnamon should be removed.

Herbs and Actions

Peony, a main herb of this formula, can relieve discomfort and pain in the abdomen. Cinnamon can regulate the *ch'i* and act as an analgesic. *Tang-kuei* nourishes the blood; in combination with Peony it relieves diarrhea and abdominal pain. Rhubarb, Scute, and Coptis relieve stagnation in the body and act as dessicants and antipyretics. Areca seed has a direct effect on the lower *ch'i*. Saussurea relieves abdominal pain and acts as an aromatic, stomachic, bactericide, and antiseptic. Licorice is an analgesic and neutralizing agent.

Indications

Acute colitis, bacterial enteritis, diarrhea, and tenesmus.

Shu-Ching-Huo-Hsieh-Tang 疏經活血湯

(Clematis and Stephania Combination)

Tang-kuei	2.0	Rehmannia	2.0	Atractylodes	2.0
Cnidium	2.0	Persica	2.0	Hoelen	2.0
Peony	2.5	Achyranthes	1.5	Clematis	1.5
Siler	1.5	Gentiana	1.5	Ginger	1.5
Citrus	1.5	Angelica	1.0	Licorice	1.0
Stephania	1.5	*Chianghuo*	1.5		

Shu-ching-huo-hsieh-tang is a formula used for increasing blood circulation, dispeling stagnant blood, and treating rheumatism. It was recorded in *Wan ping hui chun* by Kung Ting-hsien of the Ming Dynasty. This formula is suitable for stagnant blood and water toxemia and for severe pain in the muscles, joints, and nerves, especially with pain below the waist. All these symtoms are due to excessive alcohol intake, sexual indulgence, or internal or external injuries.

Herbs and Actions

Tang-kuei, Peony, Cnidium, and Rehmannia are *Szu-wu-tang*;

the addition of Persica dispels stagnant blood in the lower abdomen. Hoelen, Atractylodes, Citrus, *Chianghuo*, Angelica, Clematis Stephania, and Gentiana cure rheumatism in the waist and legs. Achyranthes dispels moisture and relieves pain in the waist and legs.

Indications

Gout, mucoid arthritis, lumbago, sciatica, numbness in the legs, beriberi, edema, purpura, monoplegia, hypertension, postpartum pain.

Discrimination

Shu-ching-li-an-san (Clematis and Carthamus Formula): multiple arthralgia.

Kan-tsao-fu-tzu-tang (Licorice and Aconite Combination): arthritic rheumatism with violent, acute, multiple pains accompanied by anemophobia; spontaneous sweating; decreased urine with a floating, weak and quick pulse or a big and weak pulse.

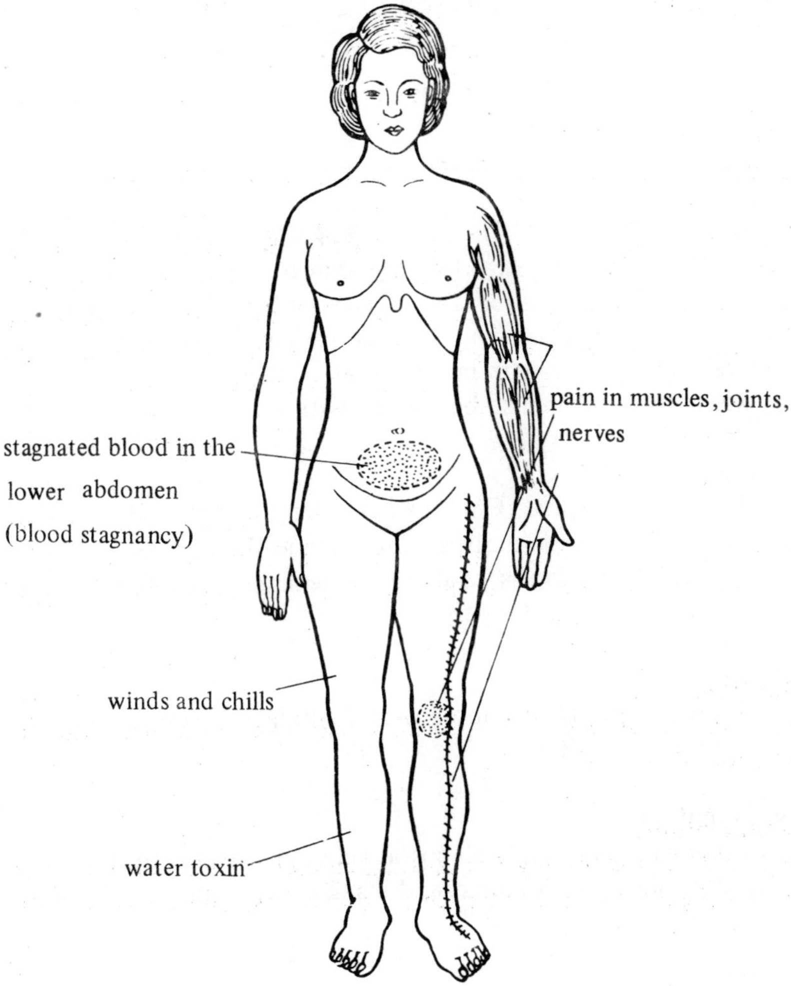

pain in muscles, joints, nerves
stagnated blood in the lower abdomen (blood stagnancy)
winds and chills
water toxin

Shu-Kan-Tang 疏肝湯

(Bupleurum and Evodia Combination)

Bupleurum	5.0	*Tang-kuei*	5.0	Persica	3.0
Peony	3.0	Cnidium	3.0	*Chih-ko*	2.0
Coptis	1.0	Carthamus	1.0	Evodia	0.5
Blue citrus peel	3.0				

Recorded in *Wan ping hui chun* (萬病回春). A remedy chiefly used for pain in the lower left ribs due to hepatic hemostasis or for anger that has injured the *ch'i* (vitality) or for a contusion that has caused internal wounds that are giving rise to the aching. A left abdominal straight muscle that is tensive with a resistant pain when pressed can also be treated with this formula.

Herbs and Actions

Tang-kuei, Peony, and Cnidium are hemopoeitics; Persica and Carthamus are exsanguinatives; *Chih-ko* and Blue citrus peel break up stagnated *ch'i;* Coptis cools and quenches heart fever; Peony disperses chills and arrests pain.

Indications

Pain in the lower left ribs, intercostal neuralgia, costal pains due to contusion, pancreatitis.

Discrimination

Use *Chai-hu-shu-kan-tang* for costal ache, an adverse flush-up that causes a headache, shoulder and back aches, and extravasation pain.

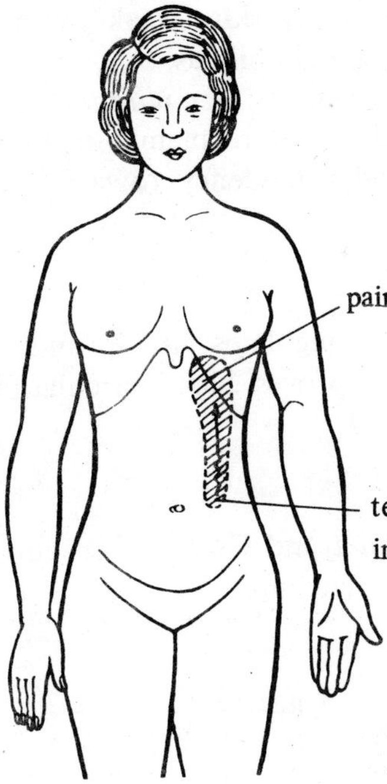

Szu-Wu-Tang 四物湯

(Tang-kuei Four Combination)

Tang-kuei	4.0	Peony	4.0	Cnidium	4.0
Rehmannia	4.0				

Szu-wu-tang, the all-purpose herb tea for gynecological diseases, has been mainly used by women, but is sometimes given to men as well. First recorded in the medical dictionary of the Sung dynasty *Tai ping huei min ho chi chu fang* (A.D. 1107-1110), it can cure weaknesses in various parts of the body or fevers due to loss of blood, menstrual irregularity, paroxysmal pain at the umbilicus and abdomen, uterine bleeding, abdominal pain during pregnancy, intestinal or anal bleeding, and postpartum blood clots or bleeding. It may cure the diseases of blood insufficiency, and its general indications are anemia with dry skin, weak pulse, abdominal weakness, and palpitation at the umbilicus.

Although it is a formula for anemia, *Szu-wu-tang* with its nourishing action may not be used for severe anemia in which pale lips, gastrointestinal weakness, and a tendency towards diarrhea are present.

Herbs and Actions

Rehmannia is hematinic; *Tang-kuei* regulates vitality and supplements the blood; and Cnidium improves blood circulation and vitality. Peony harmonizes the blood.

Discrimination

Chiung-kuei-chiao-ai-tang (*Tang-kuei* and Gelatin Combination): blood disease. This formula arrests bleeding.

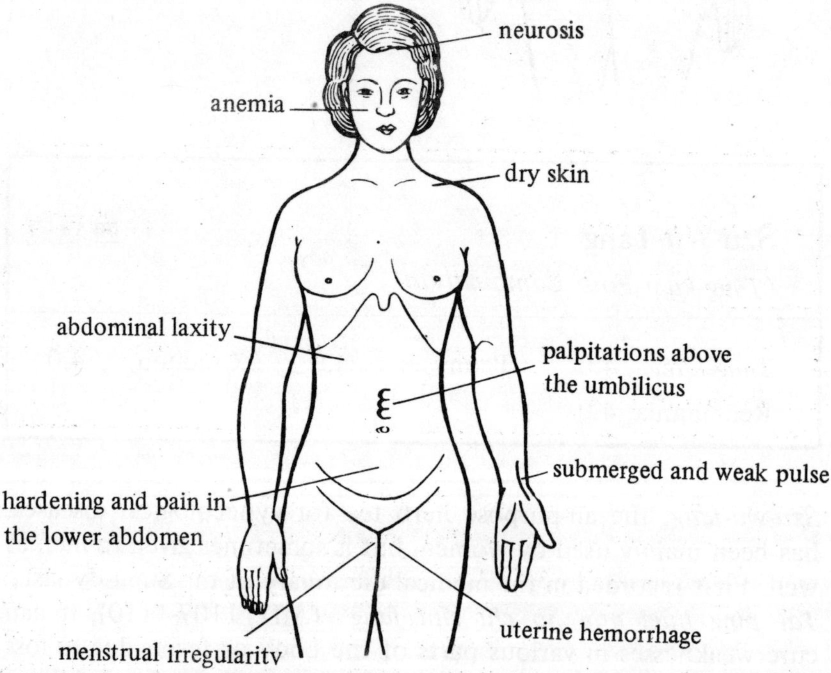

Tao-Ho-Cheng-Chi-Tang 桃核承氣湯

(Persica and Rhubarb Combination)

Persica	5.0	Rhubarb	3.0	Cinnamon	4.0
Mirabilitum	2.0	Licorice	1.5		

Tao-ho-cheng-chi-tang was first recorded in *Shang han lun* (傷寒論, A.D. 205) by Chang Chung-ching of the Han dynasty This formula is used for treating stagnant blood with marked flushing up, headache, vertigo, tinnitus, insomnia, palpitation, constipation, polyuria, emotional instability, general febrile sensation, chills in the waist and feet, and palsy.

Herbs and Actions

Persica and Cinnamon dispel stagnant blood in the lower abdomen and improve blood circulation. Cinnamon in combination with Licorice relieves flushing up. Rhubarb and Mirabilitum dispel "internal heat".

Indications

1. Menstrual irregularity, dysmenorrhea, climacteric disorders, endometritis, ovaritis, habitual abortion, hemorrhaging due to retained placenta, and stillbirth.
2. Cystitis, gallstones, renal calculus, urethritis, prostatitis, prostatomegaly.
3. Dermatitis, eczema, urticaria, acne, athelete's foot, ringworm, frostbite, and warts.
4. Blepharitis, conjunctivitis, retinitis, keratitis, trachoma, hemopthalmia, and glaucoma.
5. Hemoptysis, hematuria, and bleeding of the conjunctiva, tongue, intestine, anus, and uterus.
6. Habitual constipation, hypertension, arteriosclerosis, and pyorrhea.

Discrimination

Kuei-chih-fu-ling-wan (Cinnamon and Hoelen Formula): mild

blood occlusion, blood stagnancy without acute cramping.

Ta-huang-mu-tan-pi-tang (Rhubarb and Moutan Combination): blood occlusion, resistance and tumor and pain in the right lower abdomen.

Ti-tang-tang (Rhubarb and Leech Combination): stale, obstinate blood occlusion that causes amnesia; no acute cramping in the lower abdomen.

Tang-kuei-shao-yao-san (*Tang-kuei* and Peony Formula): fatigability; blood occlusion, emaciation, and mild anemia in a weak constitution; the abdominal conformation of blood occlusion is occasionally not apparent.

Occluded blood, firm conformation

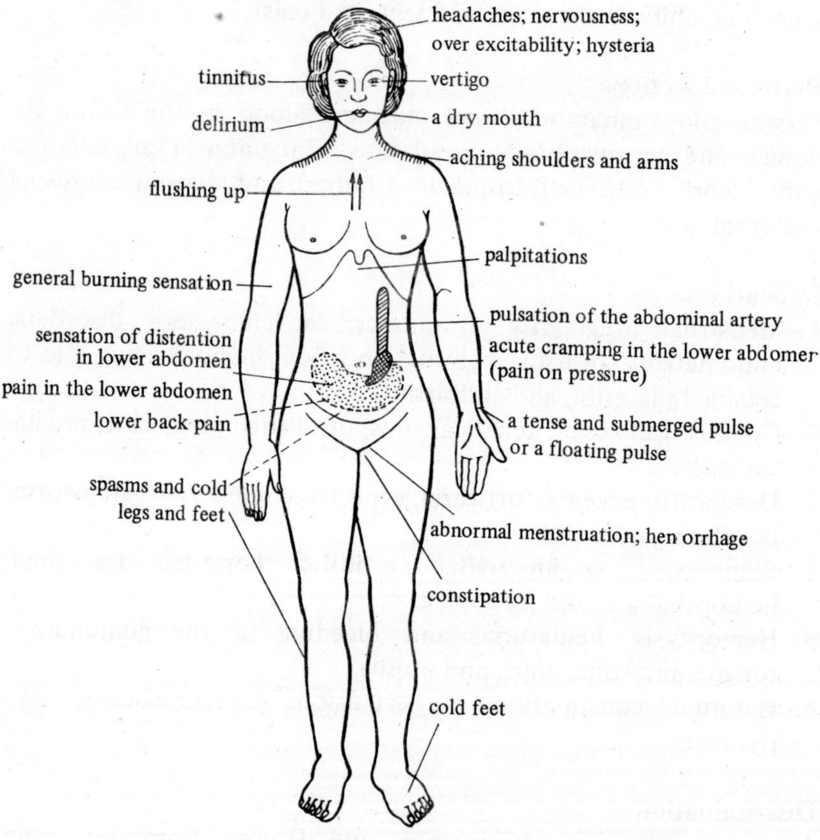

Ti-Tang-Tang *(Rhubarb and Leech Combination)*					**抵當湯**
Leech	1.0	Gadfly	1.0	Persica	1.0
Rhubarb	3.0				

Recorded in *Shang han lun* (傷寒論) and *Chin kuei yao lueh* (金匱要略) of the Han dynasty. Used for treating stagnant blood, distention in the lower abdomen, resistance and pain when pressed in the abdomen, polyuria, dark stools, amnesia, and anxiety.

Herbs and Actions
Leech removes stagnant blood and Gadfly also dispels it. Persica is anti-inflammative and dispels stagnant blood in the abdomen.

Indications
Amenorrhea, menstrual irregularity, uterine myoma, gangrene, amnesia, anxiety, and external injuries.

Discrimination
Tao-ho-cheng-chi-tang (Persica and Rhubarb Combination): blood occlusion, firm fever, acute cramping in the lower abdomen, severe flushing up.
Kuei-chih-fu-ling-wan (Cinnamon and Hoelen Formula): mild blood occlusion in a medium constitution that is neither weak nor firm.
Tang-kuei-shao-yao-san (*Tang-kuei* and Peony Formula): blood occlusion, weak conformation, anemia.

Tung-Tao-San 通導散

(Tang-kuei and Carthamus Formula)

Tang-kuei	3.0	Rhubarb	3.0	*Chih-shih*	3.0
Mirabilitum	4.0	Magnolia bark	2.0	Citrus	2.0
Akebia	2.0	Carthamus	2.0	Licorice	2.0
Sappan wood	2.0				

Tung-tao-san is recorded in *Wan ping hui chun* (萬病回春) of the Ming dynasty as useful "to treat severe contusions, dysuria and dyschezia, stagnant blood, abdominal distention, and a feeling of tension and strong up-rushing beneath the heart. The patient with these symptoms may die as a result of a blocked and disordered abdomen". In summary, the above-mentioned formula is used mainly for treating severe cases of internal bleeding resulting from contusion. The condition is manifested by extravasated blood in the lower abdomen as well as a feeling of tension and strong up-rushing beneath the heart. It is the only anti-extravasated blood agent of later experimental formulas, and it can compare with the ancient formula of *Tao-ho-cheng-chi-tang* (Persica and Rhubarb Combination).

Herbs and Actions

Tang-kuei can nourish and stimulate the blood circulation. Carthamus is used to clear the extravasated blood. Magnolia bark and *Chih-shih* treat abdominal distention. Akebia is a diuretic and antiphlogistic. Rhubarb and Mirabilitum are antiphlogistics and laxatives. Sappan wood can clear the extravasated blood and act as an analgesic. Citrus can smooth the *ch'i*. Licorice coordinates the actions of the other herbs.

Indications

Menoxenia, dysmenorrhea, climacteric disorder, contusion, and the complications of hypertension (headache, vertigo, and shoulder stiffness).

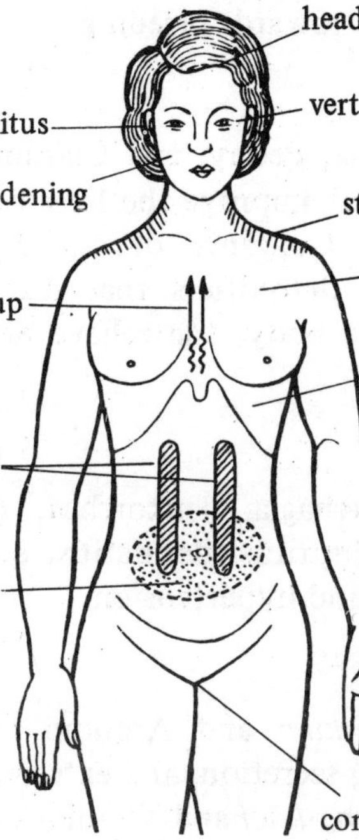

Wen-Ching-Yin *(Tang-kuei and Gardenia Combination)*					溫清飲
Tang-kuei	4.0	Rehmannia	4.0	Peony	3.0
Cnidium	3.0	Coptis	1.5	Scute	3.0
Phellodendron	1.5	Gardenia	2.0		

Wen-ching-yin is recorded in the *Wan ping hui chun*(萬病回春) and is a combination of the *Szu-wu-tang* (*Tang-kuei* Four Combination) and *Huang-lien-chieh-tu-tang* (Coptis and Scute Combination). This formula is used for treating dark-brown coarse skin, severe pruritus, ulcers of the mucous membrane, flushing up, nervous excitement, resistance in the abdomen, liver disorders, severe uterine bleeding, menorrhagia, persistent leukorrhea, underweight due to bleeding occurring in various parts of the body, and a tendency towards bleeding.

Herbs and Actions

Tang-kuei, Rehmannia, Peony, and Cnidium of the *Szu-wu-tang* nourish the blood and improve the liver function. Coptis, Scute, Phellodendron, and Gardenia of the *Huang-lien-chieh-tu-tang* are refrigerants and detoxifiers that dispel "internal heat" in the blood and whole body, tne relieve neurotic symptoms and emotional instability.

Indications

Metrorrhagia, menorrhagia, leukorrhea, peptic and duodenal ulcers, hemorrhage, pruritus, dermatitis, eczema, urticaria, tinea, emotional disorders, and hypertension.

Discrimination

Hsiao-feng-san (*Tang-kuei* and Arctium Formula): pruritus, internal fever, scabbing, secretion, and extreme thirst.
Tang-kuei-yin-tzu (*Tang-kuei* and Tribulus Combination): pruritus, blood weakness, wind fever, and "dry blood".
Pai-hu-chia-jen-sheng-tang (Ginseng and Gypsum Combination): pruritus, dryness, extreme thirst.
Huang-lien-chieh-tu-tang (Scute and Coptis Combination): pruritus, congestion, firm fever, inflammation.
Shih-wei-pai-tu-tang (Bupleurum and Schizonepeta Combination): pruritus, thoraco-costal distress, purulence.

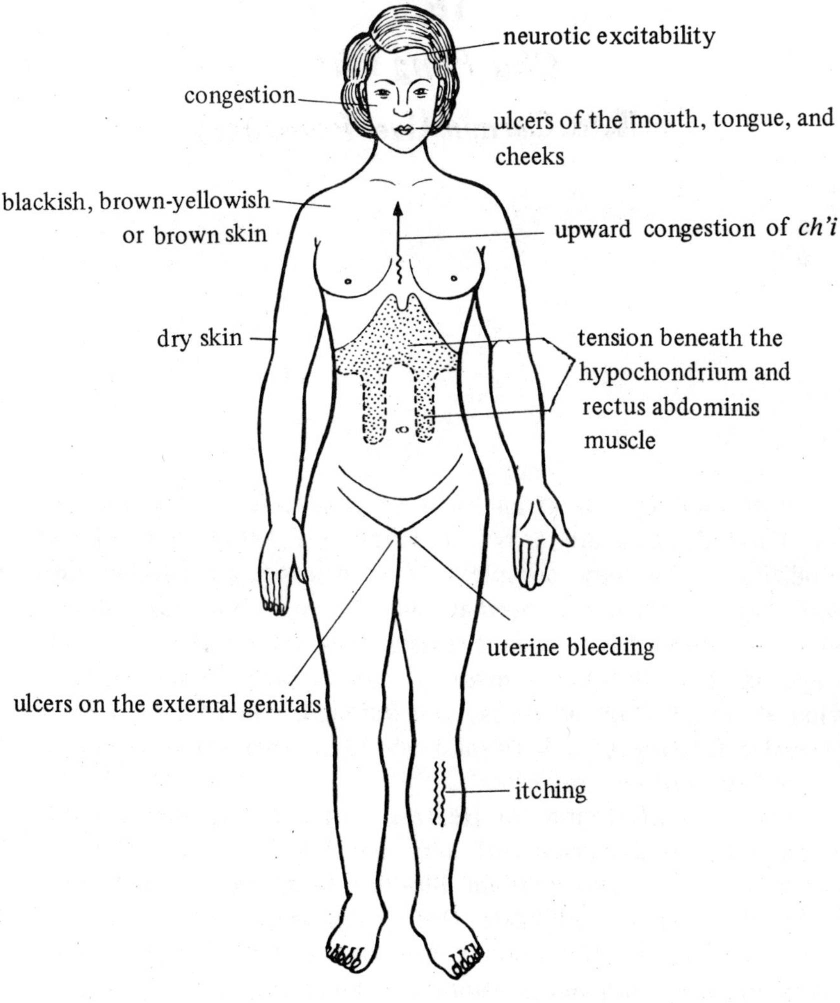
neurotic excitability
congestion
ulcers of the mouth, tongue, and cheeks
blackish, brown-yellowish or brown skin
upward congestion of *ch'i*
dry skin
tension beneath the hypochondrium and rectus abdominis muscle
uterine bleeding
ulcers on the external genitals
itching

16.
Chu Feng Chi
(祛風劑, Carminative Formulas)

Formulas that treat all kinds of wind diseases are *chu feng chi*. Wind diseases are broad in scope, the variation in disease condition being very complex. Wind diseases are divided into two major categories: internal and external. Whereas external wind is caused by the six excesses that invade the body and lodge in the meridians, muscles, sinews, and bones, internal wind develops from weakness and deficiency in blood, or from excessive thriving of a harmful fever toxin that causes disorders in circulation of *ch'i* and blood.

The rule of thumb for treatment of external wind diseases is that they are dispersed with acrid and arid herbs. The formulas prescribed must also contain blood nourishing and activating herbs in order to subjugate the strong aridity of such herbs. Internal wind diseases should not be treated with dispersing herbs but with cool and moistening or lubricating herbs. However, if moistening herbs are used in excess, they may hinder the stomach's function. Therefore, every aspect of a patient's condition must be considered before prescribing a formula.

Ching-Shang-Chuan-Tung-Tang 清上蠲痛湯

(Ophiopogon and Asarum Combination)

Tang-kuei	2.5	Cnidium	2.5	Angelica	2.5
Chianghuo	2.5	*Tuhuo*	2.5	Siler	2.5
Atractylodes	2.5	Ophiopogon	2.5	Scute	3.0
Vitex	1.5	Chrysanthemum	1.5	Asarum	1.0
Licorice	1.0	Ginger	1.0		

Ching-shang-chuan-tung-tang is recorded in *Sou shih pao yuan* (壽世保元) of the Ming dynasty. This formula is used mainly for all types of headache. It is also suitable for facial pain.

Herbs and Actions

Ophiopogon, Asarum, and Siler treat flushing up. Cnidium, Angelica, Chrysanthemum, and Vitex can regulate the *ch'i* and blood circulation in the head. *Tuhuo*, Siler, and Atractylodes act as diaphoretics and dessicants. *Tang-kuei*, Asarum, and Ginger dispel internal chills and warm the body. Scute can remove internal heat.

Indications

All types of headaches, including chronic headache, trigeminal neuralgia, and pain due to maxillary cancer.

Chuan-Pi-Tang 蠲痺湯

(Chianghuo and Turmeric Combination)

Chianghuo	4.5	Turmeric	4.5	*Tang-kuei*	4.5
Peony	4.5	Astragalus	4.5	Siler	4.5
Licorice	1.5	Ginger	1.0	Jujube	1.0

Chuan-pi-tang is recorded in *I fang chi chieh* (醫方集解) of the Ching dynasty. This formula is used for increasing vitality, promoting blood circulation, and acting as a carminative and dessicant. It is suitable for limited joint mobility due to "wind evil," pain in the limbs, neck spasms, difficulty in movement, and muscular spasms in the limbs.

This combination and *Tu-huo-chi-sheng-tang* are used to treat limited joint mobility. But the former is more suitable for the weakness of "*yin ch'i*" and "*wei ch'i*" and for numbness in the upper limbs, while the latter is effective for liver and kidney weakness and numbness in the lower limbs.

Herbs and Actions

Tang-kuei and Peony nourish blood. Astragalus and Licorice improve vitality. *Chianghuo* is an antirheumatic which increases joint mobility. Siler can dispel wind evil and cure gout. Turmeric is good for treating rheumatic pain in the arms and body; it also acts as a carminative. Ginger and Jujube are stomachics and tonics.

Indications

Muscular pain, 50 years' shoulders, 40 years' wrists, and lumbago.

Hsiao-Feng-San 消風散

(Tang-kuei and Arctium Formula)

Tang-kuei	3.0	Rehmannia	3.0	Gypsum	3.0
Anemarrhena	1.5	Sesame	1.5	Arctium	2.0
Atractylodes	2.0	Siler	2.0	Akebia	2.0
Licorice	1.0	Cicada	1.0	Sophora	1.0
Schizonepeta	1.0				

Hsiao-feng-san is listed in the Chinese medical work, *Wai k'o cheng tzung* (外科正宗 , A.D. 1617) of the Ming dynasty. This formula is used to treat skin diseases with "internal heat", copious discharge, and pruritis. It is particularly suitable for recalcitrant eczema with desquamation, continuous pruritis, dermatitis, and thirst.

Herbs and Actions

Tang-kuei, Rehmannia, and Sesame nourish the blood. Sophora eliminates the "internal heat" in the blood and relieves itching due to scabies. Anemarrhena and Gypsum also dispel "internal heat" in the blood, and relieve thirst. Arctium and Cicada cure "internal heat" and sloughing ulcer. Schizonepeta and Siler eliminate "internal heat" and cure scabies. Akebia and Atractylodes dispel stagnant blood. Licorice synthesizes the actions of the other herbs.

Indications

Recalcitrant eczema, chronic urticaria, pruritus, prickly heat, scabies, and skin diseases which become aggravated by hot weather.

Discrimination

Tang-kuei-yin-tzu (*Tang-kuei* and Tribulus Combination): itching blood weakness, wind fever, and blood dryness.
Pai-hu-chia-jen-sheng-tang (Ginseng and Gypsum Combination):

itching with reddening of skin, dryness, and extreme thirst.
Tao-ho-cheng-chi-tang (Persica and Rhubarb Combination): itching, blood occlusion, blood stagnancy, constipation, and firm conformation.
Huang-lien-chieh-tu-tang (Scute and Coptis Combination): itching, firm fever, inflammation and congestion.

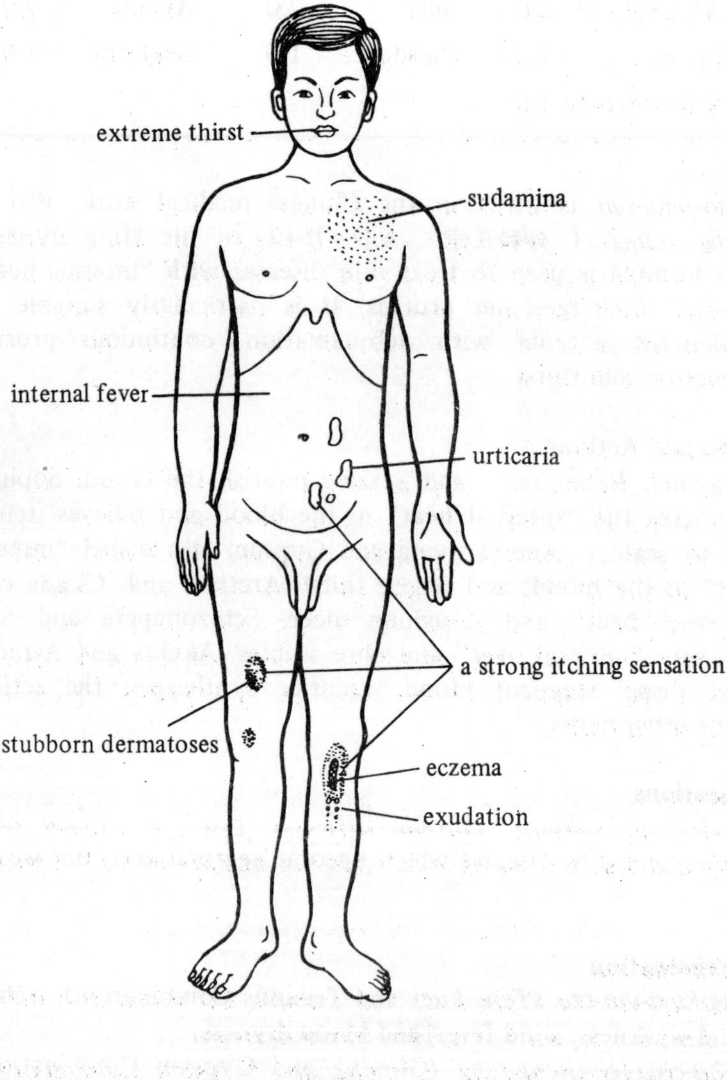

Hsiao-Hsu-Ming-Tang 小續命湯

(Ma-huang and Peony Combination)

Siler	4.5	*Ma-huang*	3.0	Stephania	3.0
Ginseng	3.0	Scute	3.0	Cinnamon	3.0
Licorice	3.0	Peony	3.0	Cnidium	3.0
Apricot seed	3.0	Aconite	1.5	Ginger	9.0

Hsiao-hsu-ming-tang is recorded in *Chien chin yao fang* (千金要方) by Sun Szu-miao of the Tang dynasty. This formula is used for treating apoplexy, sensory confusion, monoplegia, spasms, convulsions, speech disturbances, rheumatism, low back pain, and febrile sputum. It is to be taken for weaker conformations than those requiring *Hsu-ming-tang* (*Ma-huang* and Ginseng Combination).

Herbs and Actions

Ma-huang and Apricot seed treat *"shang han"* of the greater yang diseases. Cinnamon and Peony treat "superficial evil" of greater yang diseases. Ginseng and Licorice nourish the *ch'i.* Cnidium and Peony are hemotonics. Siler treats the "internal penetration of wind". Stephania treats the "internal penetration of moisture". Aconite treats the "internal penetration of chills". Scute treats the "internal penetration of heat".

Indications

Apoplexy, cerebromalacia, hypertension, neuralgia, monoplegia, facial palsy, arthritis, migraine, asthma, and edema.

Hsu-Ming-Tang 續命湯

(Ma-huang and Ginseng Combination)

Apricot seed	4.0	*Ma-huang*	3.0	Cinnamon	3.0
Ginseng	3.0	*Tang-kuei*	3.0	Cnidium	2.0
Ginger	2.0	Licorice	2.0	Gypsum	6.0

Hsu-ming-tang is recorded in *Chin kuei yao lueh* (金匱要略) of the Han dynasty. This formula is used for treating apoplexy, paralysis, speech disturbances, generalized pains, convulsions, cough, flushing up, edema, sensory disorders, and fever.

Herbs and Actions

Ma-huang, Cnidium, and Cinnamon ease muscular tension and relieve rheumatism. *Tang-kuei* and Ginseng nourish the blood. Gypsum and Apricot seed cure ailments caused by cold. Licorice and Ginger increase vitality.

Indications

Apoplexy, cerebromalacia, hypertension, neuralgia, monoplegia, facial palsy, arthritis, edema and bronchitis.

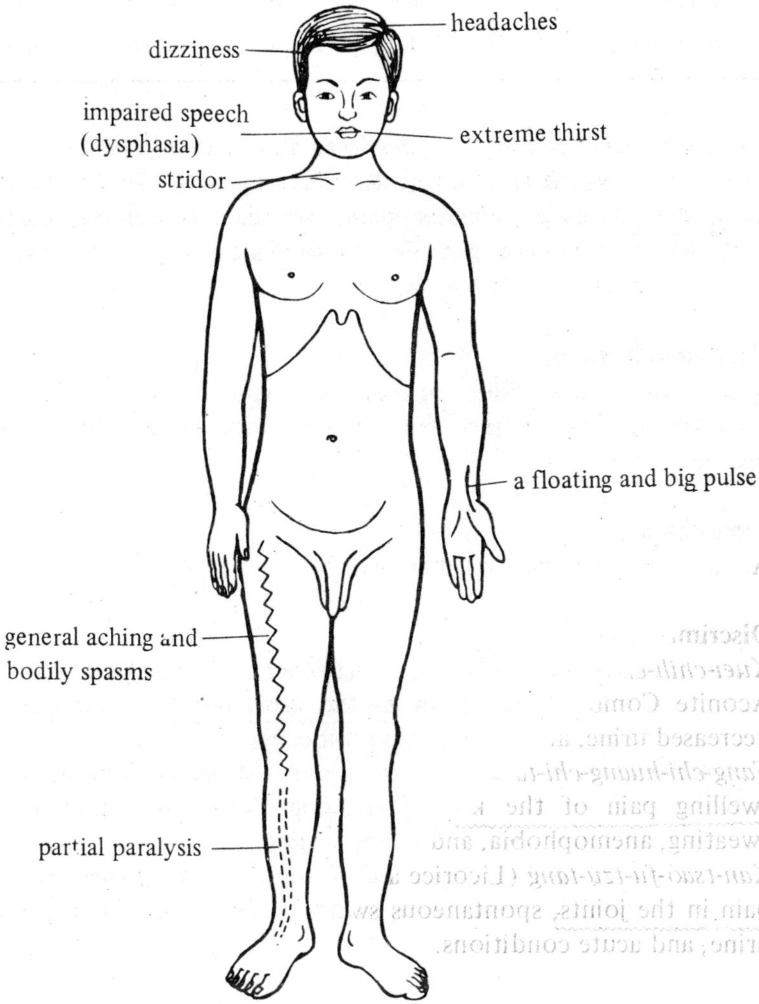
headaches
dizziness
impaired speech (dysphasia)
extreme thirst
stridor
a floating and big pulse
general aching and bodily spasms
partial paralysis

Kuei-Chih-Shao-Yao-Chih-Mu-Tang 桂枝芍藥知母湯

(Cinnamon and Anemarrhena Combination)

Cinnamon	3.0	Anemarrhena	3.0	Siler	3.0
Ginger	3.0	Peony	3.0	*Ma-huang*	3.0
Aconite	0.5-1.0	Atractylodes	4.0	Licorice	1.5

Kuei-chih-shao-yao-chih-mu-tang was recorded in the *Chin kuei yao lueh* (金匱要略) during the Han dynasty. This formula is used for treating general pain, vertigo, hyperpnea, nausea, arthralgia, rheumatism, pain due to swelling of the joints, paresthesia, and muscle atrophy in the legs.

Herbs and Actions

Atractylodes and Siler nourish the spleen. Peony, Aconite, and Anemarrhena adjust the yin and yang. Ginger counteracts nausea.

Indications

Arthritis and rheumatoid arthritis.

Discrimination

Kuei-chih-chia-ling-chu-fu-tang (Hoelen, Atractylodes, and Aconite Combination): pain in the arms and legs, chillphobia, decreased urine, and cardiac hyperfunction.

Fang-chi-huang-chi-tang (Stephania and Astragalus Combination): swelling pain of the knee joint, decreased urine, spontaneous sweating, anemophobia, and heavy feeling.

Kan-tsao-fu-tzu-tang (Licorice and Aconite Combination): swelling pain in the joints, spontaneous sweating, anemophobia, decreased urine, and acute conditions.

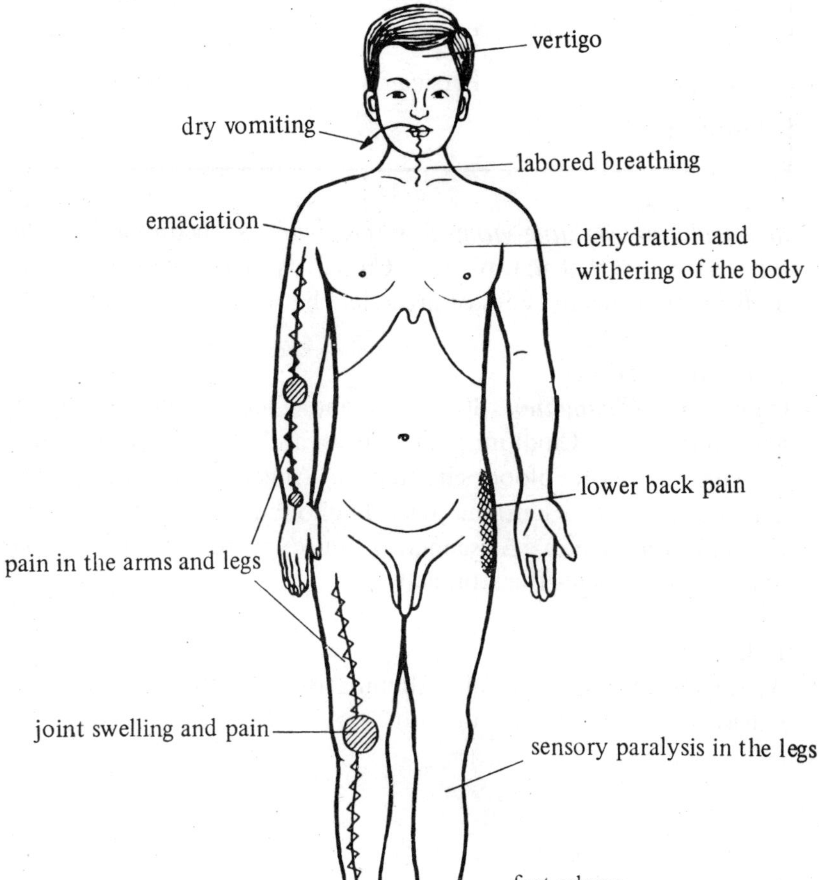
vertigo
dry vomiting
labored breathing
emaciation
dehydration and
withering of the body
lower back pain
pain in the arms and legs
joint swelling and pain
sensory paralysis in the legs
feet edema

Shang-Chung-Hsia-Tung-Yung-Tung-Feng-Wan 上中下通用痛風丸

(Cinnamon and Angelica Formula)

Phellodendron	20	Atractylodes	20	*Chianghuo*	3.0
Shen-chu	10	Cnidium	10	Clematis	3.0
Gentiana	10	Stephania	10	Cinnamon	3.0
Arisaema	20	Persica	10	Carthamus	2.0
Angelica	10				

Shang-chung-hsia-tung-yung-tung-feng-wan is recorded in *I fang chi chieh* (醫方集解) of the Ching dynasty. This formula is used for treating all types of articular rheumatism.

Herbs and Actions

Cinnamon, *Chianghuo*, Stephania and Clematis are antipyretics and analgesics. Cnidium, Carthamus, and Persica can regulate *ch'i* and promote blood circulation. Angelica and Atractylodes act as analgesics. Gentiana with Phellodendron is an antiphlogistic and antipyretic. Arisaema is an expectorant and sedative. *Shen-chu* nourishes the stomach.

Indications

Acute and chronic articular rheumatism, all other types of rheumatism with arthralgia, and gout.

Shih-Wei-Tsuo-San 十味挫散

(Astragalus and Aconite Formula)

Tang-kuei	3.0	Peony	3.0	Cnidium	3.0
Rehmannia	3.0	Hoelen	3.0	Astragalus	3.0
Atractylodes	3.0	Cinnamon	3.0	Siler	3.0
Aconite	0.5-1.0				

Shih-wei-tsuo-san is recorded in *I chien fang* (易簡方) by Wang Shuo of the Sung dynasty. This formula is a combination of *Shih-chuan-ta-pu-tang* (Ginseng and *Tang-kuei* Ten Combination) with Aconite and Siler instead of Ginseng and Licorice. It is suitable for pain in the arms, weak feet, painful joints, body aches, and difficulty in walking. It is especially good for 50 years' shoulders and for anemia in the elderly.

Herbs and Actions
Tang-kuei, Rehmannia, Peony, and Cinnamon [all of *Szu-wu-tang* (*Tang-kuei* Four Combination)] promote blood circulation. Atractylodes and Hoelen nourish the spleen. Astragalus and Cinnamon nourish the muscles and improve blood circulation. Siler is an antirheumatic agent which effectively treats paralysis. Aconite improves circulation, thereby increasing resistance to chilling.

Indications
Beriberi, 40 years' wrists, 50 years' shoulders, gout, rheumatism, arthralgia, and hemiplegia.

Discrimination
Shih-chuan-ta-pu-tang (Ginseng and *Tang-kuei* Ten Combination): blood weakness, spasmodic pain, weakness in the blood and *ch'i*, heart weakness, general lassitude, a desire to press the abdomen with the hands.

Shu-Chin-Li-An-San 舒筋立安散

(Clematis and Carthamus Formula)

Siler	1.2	*Chianghuo*	1.2	*Tuhuo*	1.2
Cnidium	1.2	Hoelen	1.2	Angelica	1.2
Rehmannia	1.2	Atractylodes	1.2	Carthamus	1.2
Persica	1.2	Arisaema	1.2	Citrus	1.2
Pinellia	1.2	Achyranthes	1.2	Clematis	1.2
Stephania	1.2	Chaenomeles	1.2	Forsythia	1.2
Aconite	0.5-1.0	Akebia	1.2	Licorice	1.2
Bamboo	1.2	Gentiana	1.2	Scute	1.2
White atractylodes		1.2			

Shu-chin-li-an-san was recorded in the *Wan ping hui chun* (萬病回春) by Kung Ting-hsien during the Ming dynasty. This formula is used for treating arthritic pain in the arms and legs.

Herbs and Actions

Siler and *Chianghuo* relieve rheumatic spasms in the joints. Clematis, Arisaema, Atractylodes, and *Tuhuo* are carminatives that relieve rheumatic pain. Hoelen and Peony are tonics. Stephania, Scute, Gentiana, Forsythia, Akebia, and Bamboo are antiphlogistics, antipyretics, and purgatives. Atractylodes, Pinellia, and Citrus are expectorants and dispel stagnant *ch'i.* Carthamus, Persica, and Rehmannia are blood tonics that dispel stagnant blood. Aconite, Cnidium, and Angelica are hematinics and carminatives. Chaenomeles is an analgesic effective for rheumatism and beriberi. Licorice is also a carminative.

Indications

Acute and chronic rheumatoid arthritis, palsy, monoplegia, and chronic beriberi.

Shu-Feng-Huo-Hsieh-Tang 疏風活血湯

(Stephania and Carthamus Combination)

Tang-kuei	2.5	Cnidium	2.5	Clematis	2.5
Angelica	2.5	Stephania	2.5	Arisaema	2.5
Phellodendron	2.5	*Chianghuo*	2.5	Cinnamon	2.5
Atractylodes	2.5	Carthamus	1.0	Ginger	1.0

Shu-feng-huo-hsieh-tang is recorded in *Shen shih chuen sheng shu* (沈氏尊生書) of the Ching dynasty. This formula is used to treat aching limbs; movable and stinging pain in the joints due to air, moisture, sputum, or blood occlusion; and swelling or reddening of the joint. It is effective in the primary stage of rheumatic purpura, rheumatism, and platelet purpura not due to platelet insufficiency.

Herbs and Actions

Clematis, Arisaema, Atractylodes, and *Chianghuo* can relieve rheumatism and pain in the joints. *Tang-kuei*, Cnidium, and Angelica can promote blood circulation by stimulating the blood and increasing the yang. Stephania and Phellodendron are antiphlogistics, antipyretics, and antirheumatics. Carthamus can expel extravasated blood and form new blood. Cinnamon coordinates the actions of the other herbs, warms the uterus and increases circulation throughout the body, and releases the pulse.

Indications

Neuralgia of the limbs, rheumatism, gout, rheumatic purpura, and platelet purpura not due to platelet insufficiency.

Discrimination

Shu-ching-huo-hsieh-tang (Clematis and Stephania Combination): pain in the arms and legs, blood occlusion, and pain below the waist.

Firm conformation

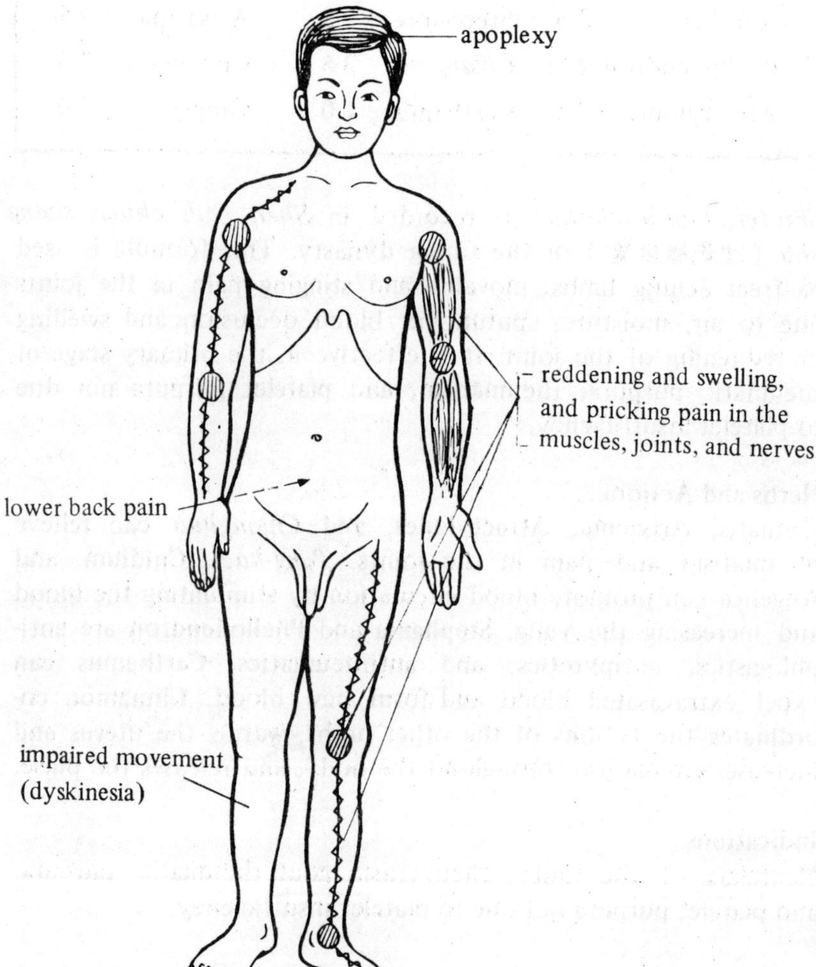

Ta-Fang-Feng-Tang 大防風湯

(Major Siler Combination)

Tang-kuei	3.0	Peony	3.0	Rehmannia	3.0
Siler	3.0	Astragalus	3.0	Eucommia	3.0
Atractylodes	3.0	Cnidium	3.0	Ginseng	1.5
Chianghuo	1.5	Achyranthes	1.5	Licorice	1.5
Jujube	1.5	Aconite	1.5-1.0	Ginger	1.5

Ta-fang-feng-tang is recorded in *Tai ping huei min ho chi chu fang* (太平惠民和劑局方) of the Ming dynasty. This formula is used for nourishing blood and *ch'i*; for treating paralysis, stiffness, swelling, pain in the knees and feet; and for paralysis in the lower limbs because of postpartum weakness, paralysis of the lower limbs due to apoplexy, and paralysis due to beriberi. This formula is suitable for those of weak conformation only.

Herbs and Actions

Tang-kuei, Peony, Cnidium, and Rehmannia of *Szu-wu-tang* (*Tang-kuei* Four Combination) can nourish the blood and improve blood circulation. Atractylodes, Ginseng, and Licorice nourish the spleen and muscles. Siler and *Chianghuo* relieve muscule pain. Achyranthes and Eucommia relieve pain in the waist and feet and act as tonics. Astragalus nourishes the muscles, Aconite eliminates pain and dispels moisture.

Indications

Arthritis, rheumatoid arthritis, myelophthisis, myelitis, monoplegia, beriberi, paralysis of the lower limbs, and neuralgia.

Discrimination

Kuei-chih-shao-yao-chih-mu-tang (Cinnamon and Anemarrhena Combination): swelling pain in the knees. This formula is used for a mild conformation when the weakness of *ch'i* and blood is not serious.

Yin weakness conformation

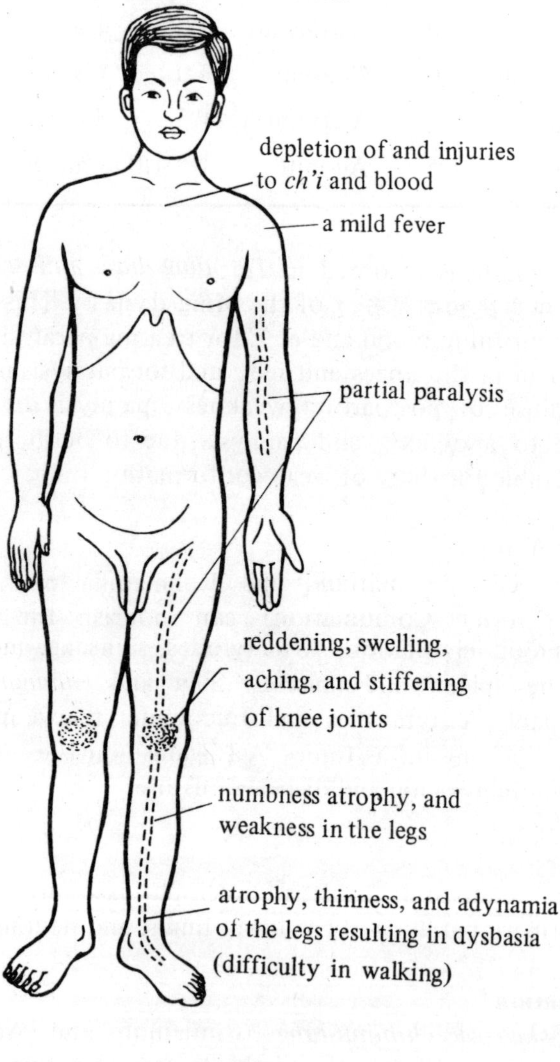

Tu-Huo-Chi-Sheng-Tang 獨活寄生湯

(Tuhuo and Vaeicum Combination)

Tuhuo	4.5	Loranthus	4.5	*Chin-chiu*	4.5
Siler	4.5	Asarum	4.5	*Tang-kuei*	3.0
Peony	3.0	Cnidium	4.5	Rehmannia	3.0
Eucommia	4.5	Achyranthes	4.5	Ginseng	4.5
Hoelen	4.5	Licorice	3.0	Cinnamon	4.5

Tu-huo-chi-sheng-tang is recorded in the Chinese medical classic *Chien chin fang* (千金方) of the Tang dynasty. This formula is used for nourishing the liver, kidneys, and blood; for increasing vitality; for relieving rheumatism, and for checking spasmodic pain in the midline and knees.

Herbs and Actions

Tuhuo alleviates rheumatism, arthritis, and palsy in the legs. Loranthus nourishes the liver and kidneys, and relieves arthritis and rheumatism. Eucommia, Rehmannia, Achyranthes, and Loranthus nourish the waist, the kidneys, and the bones. *Tang-kuei,* Peony, and Cnidium are hematinics. When combined with *Tuhuo*, Asarum nourishes the kidneys and checks pain. Cinnamon nourishes the blood and kidneys, and eliminates chills and pain. Gentiana and Siler relieve rheumatism and arthritis.

Indications

Chronic arthritis, chronic pain near the waist and in the legs, sciatica due to degenerative joint disease, and pain in the midline and the back during pregnancy.

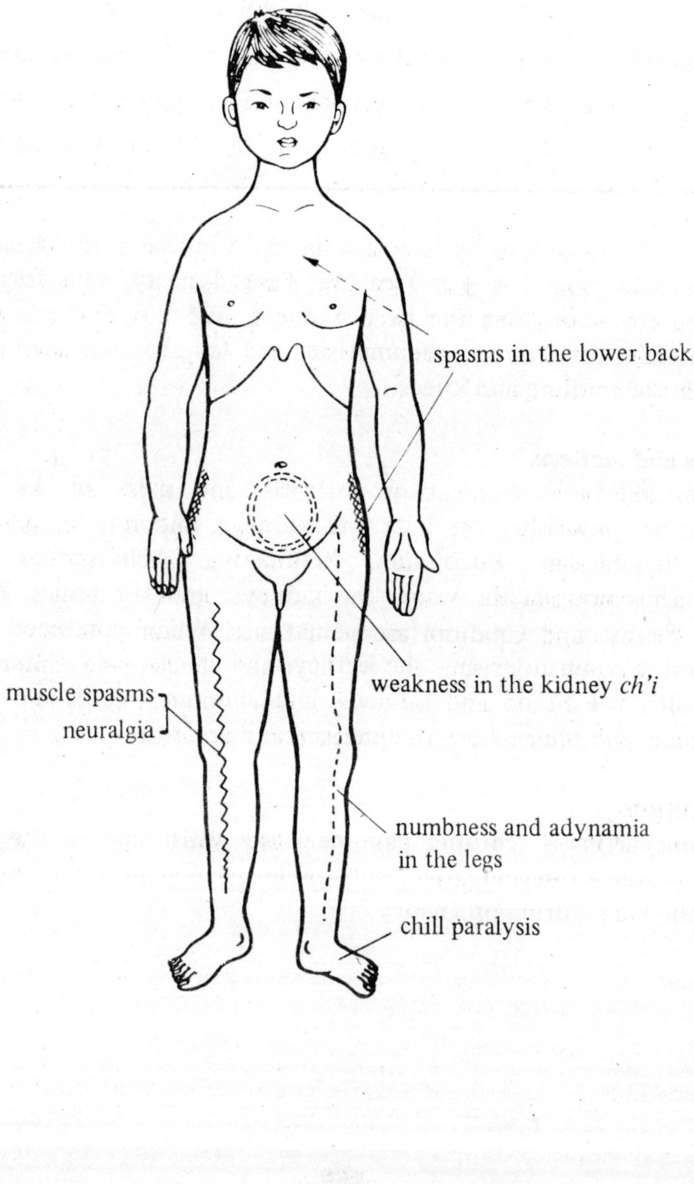
spasms in the lower back
weakness in the kidney ch'i
muscle spasms
neuralgia
numbness and adynamia in the legs
chill paralysis

Wei-Feng-Tang 胃風湯

(Atractylodes and Setaria Combination)

Tang-kuei	3.0	Peony	3.0	Cnidium	3.0
Ginseng	3.0	Atractylodes	3.0	Hoelen	4.0
Cinnamon	2.0	Setaria	2.0		

Wei-feng-tang was recorded in the *Tai ping huei min ho chi chu fang* (太平惠民和劑局方) during the Sung dynasty. This formula is used to treat chronic enteritis and persistent diarrhea in patients of weak conformation. It is suitable for those having gastrointestinal weakness with a tendency toward diarrhea during cold weather, soft stools, watery stools, and a weak abdomen.

Herbs and Actions
Hoelen, Atractylodes, and Ginseng dispel water poisoning in the stomach and intestines. *Tang-kuei,* Peony, and Cnidium are hemostatics and hematinics that also improve the stomach and spleen. Cinnamon regulates the actions of the other herbs. Setaria strengthens flaccid intestinal ducts.

Indications
Chronic enteritis, chronic proctitis, ulcerative colitis, tendency toward rectal prolapse in the winter, tendency toward bleeding in winter, and chronic diarrhea.

Discrimination
Pan-hsia-hsieh-hsin-tang (Pinellia Combination): diarrhea, obstruction and hardness beneath the heart, vomiting.
Tuan-li-tang (Pinellia and Jujube Combination): diarrhea, water stagnancy beneath the heart in the yin region.
Chen-wu-tang (Vitality Combination): diarrhea, watery stools, palpitations beneath the heart, abdominal pain, decreased urine.
Tao-hua-tang (Kaolin and Oryza Combination): diarrhea with pus and blood; the patient is weakened.
Kuei-chih-jen-sheng-tang (Cinnamon and Ginseng Combination):

diarrhea with external fever and obstruction beneath the heart.
Jen-sheng-tang or *Li-chung-tang* (Ginseng and Ginger Combination): diarrhea, obstruction beneath the heart, severe gastric illness.
Sheng-ling-pai-chu-san (Ginseng and Atractylodes Formula): diarrhea, gastrointestinal weakness, loss of appetite, and fermentation.

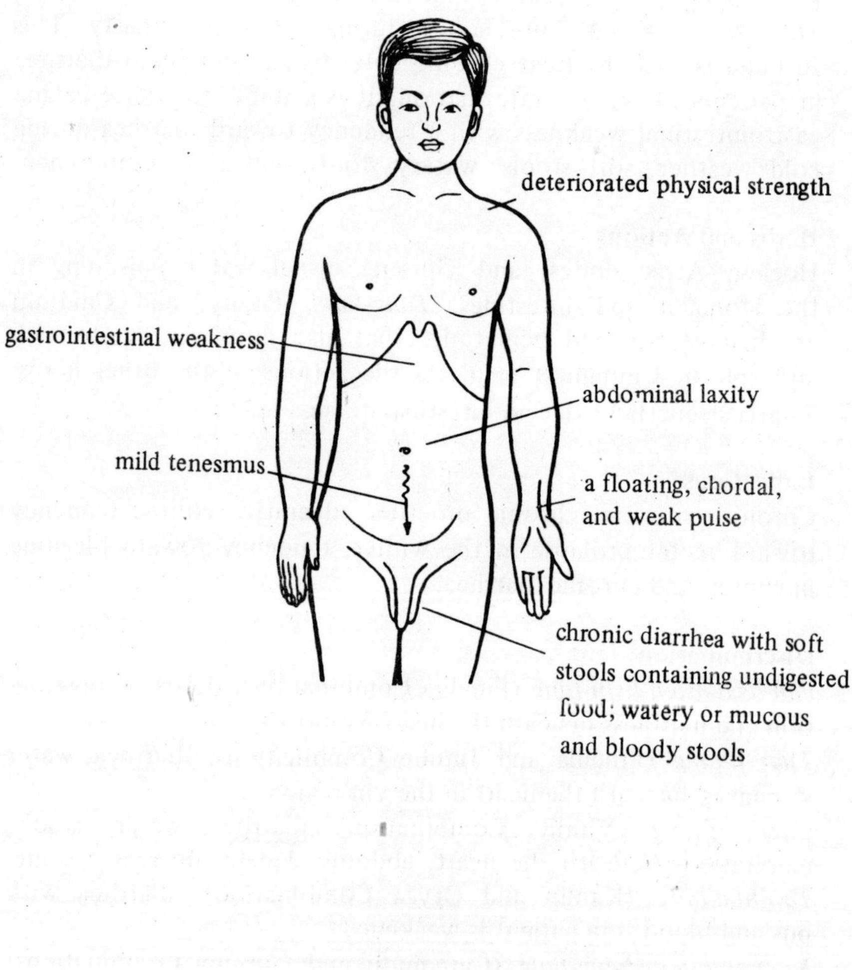

17.
Chu Shih Chi
(祛濕劑, Diuretics)

Formulas that treat body fluids are called *chu shih chi.*

Fluids are either yin chilly, heavily turbid, or sticky and poisonous. They are divided into internal and external fluids, or water. Internal fluids are further differentiated into upper, middle, and the lower. The fluid may also be affected by the fever toxin generated by wind, chills, heat, and fever. Therapeutically the location of the toxin is determined and treated accordingly. Diuretics increase water flow and discharge, relieve urinary stuttering, and bring about the excretion. Depending on whether the condition is humid and warm, formulas are prescribed according to the presence of diarrhea, dysentery, edema, or jaundice.

In treating a water conformation, attention must be given to a yin-weakness or saliva drying-up conformation for which a diuretic formula is contraindicated. Because a diuretic will dry salivation, it is necessary to incorporate other herbs. This is especially true for bitter and arid herbs which should be used with extreme care. For example, post-illness edema due to splenic weakness or foot edema in pregnant women are conditions calling for diuresis, but the prescription must incorporate spleen-strengthening tonics in order to protect *ch'i.*

Chai-Ling-Tang 柴苓湯

(Bupleurum and Hoelen Combination)

Bupleurum	5.0	Pinellia	4.0	Scute	2.5
Ginseng	2.5	Jujube	2.5	Ginger	4.0
Licorice	2.0	Cinnamon	2.5	Polyporus	2.5
Atractylodes	2.5	Hoelen	2.5	Alisma	4.0

Chai-ling-tang was recorded in the *Shih i te hsiao fang* (世醫得效方) by Wei I-lin during the Yuan dynasty. This formula is a combination of *Hsiao-chai-hu-tang* (Minor Bupleurum Combination) and *Wu-ling-san* (Hoelen Five Herb Formula) and is suitable for treating those symptoms alleviated by *Hsiao-chai-hu-tang* and *Wu-ling-san* as well as thirst, dysuria, edema, diarrhea, and infectious diseases which appear during the summer.

Herbs and Actions
Bupleurum relieves chest distention. Bupleurum and Scute are antiphlogistics that dispel chest distention. Pinellia and Ginger serve as antiemetics and appetizers. Ginseng, Licorice, and Jujube improve gastric function and relieve chest distention. Alisma, Polyporus, Hoelen, and Atractylodes dispel "stagnant water" in the stomach and intestines, increase the flow of urine, and eliminate edema. Cinnamon dispels superficial fever, alleviates flushing up, and coordinates the diuretic actions of the other herbs.

Indications
Common cold, heatstroke, acute gastroenteritis, pyelitis, nephritis, edema, and liver and gallbladder disorders.

Chi-Ming-San 雞鳴散

(Areca Seed and Chaenomeles Formula)

Areca seed	4.0	Chaenomeles	3.0	Ginger	3.0
Aurantium	2.5	Platycodon	2.5	Perilla	1.0
Evodia	1.0				

Chi-ming-san is recorded in *Shih fang ko kua* (時方歌括) by Chen Hsiu-yuan of the Ching dynasty. This formula is used for treating moist beriberi with bitter taste and distention in the chest, difficulty in breathing, palpitations, flushing up, and edema.

Herbs and Actions

Evodia relieves chills. Areca seed increases *ch'i* and dispels moisture. Chaenomeles dispels moisture in the lower body. Ginger and Perilla warm the body, relieve chills, and remove moisture. Aurantium removes moisture. Platycodon improves "internal *ch'i*" in the lungs.

Indications

The initial stage of beriberi, edematous beriberi, nephritis, and edema.

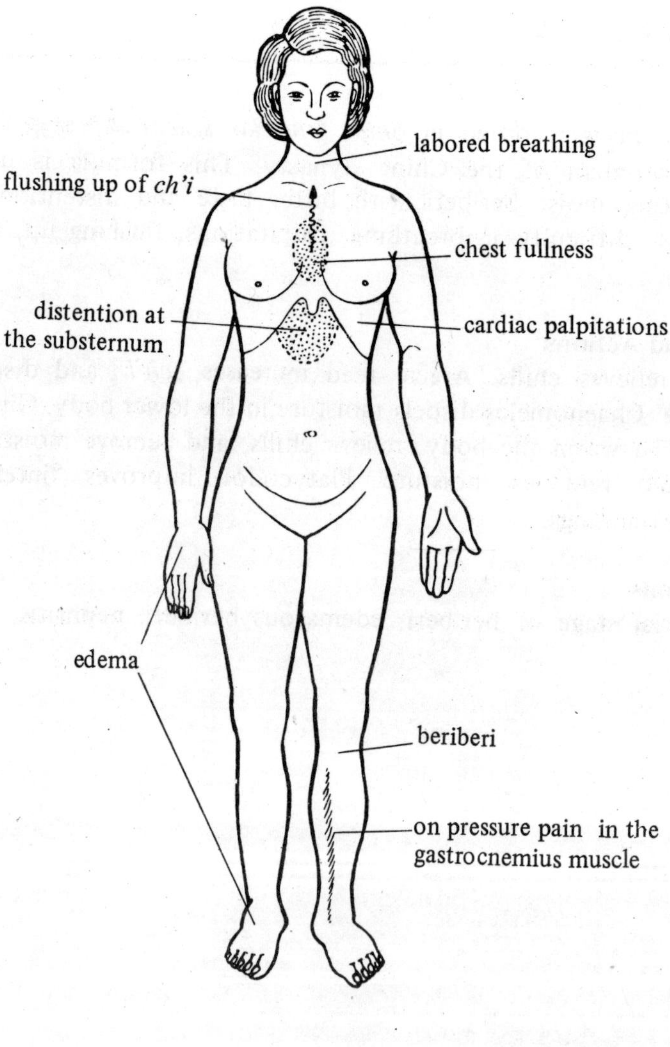
labored breathing
flushing up of *ch'i*
chest fullness
distention at the substernum
cardiac palpitations
edema
beriberi
on pressure pain in the gastrocnemius muscle

Chien-Chung-Tang 堅中湯

(Hoelen and Jujube Combination)

Pinellia	5.0	Hoelen	5.0	Cinnamon	4.0
Jujube	3.0	Peony	3.0	Ginger	3.0
Licorice	1.0				

Chien-chung-tang is a modification of *Hsiao-chien-chung-tang* (Minor Cinnamon and Peony Combination) and is recorded in *Chien chin yao fang* (千金要方) of the Tang dynasty. This formula is used for treating peptic ulcer, chronic gastritis, thinned abdominal wall, abdominal atony, stagnant water in the stomach, colic, hiccups, and vomiting after meals. It is suitable for those of weak conformation.

Herbs and Actions

Peony coordinates with Licorice to supplement the blood and *ch'i* and regulate the stagnant blood. Jujube functions to nourish and strengthen. Cinnamon combined with Licorice calms excessive palpitations. Pinellia is an antiemetic and sedative. Hoelen is a cardiotonic, diuretic, and sedative; it also expels stagnant water from the stomach and relieves excessive palpitation. Ginger is an antiemetic and stomachic which can increase tissue tone, promote blood circulation, and renew vigor and strength.

Indications

Peptic ulcer, chronic gastritis, gastrectasia, and abdominal pain.

Discrimination

Szu-ni-san (Bupleurum and *Chih-shih* Formula): pain beneath the heart, discomfort beneath the heart, and thoraco-costal distress.

Ta-chai-hu-tang (Major Bupleurum Combination): pain beneath the heart and thoraco-costal distress, firm conformation.

Chai-hu-kuei-chih-tang (Bupleurum and Cinnamon Combination):

pain beneath the heart, abdominal tension, and distention beneath the heart.

Liang-chih-tang (Galanga and *Chih-shih* Combination): pain beneath the heart, hardness beneath the heart, spasmodic pain.

An-chung-san (Cardamon and Fennel Formula): pain beneath the heart, weak chills, lingering pain traveling from the lower abdomen to the lower back during the night.

Weak conformation

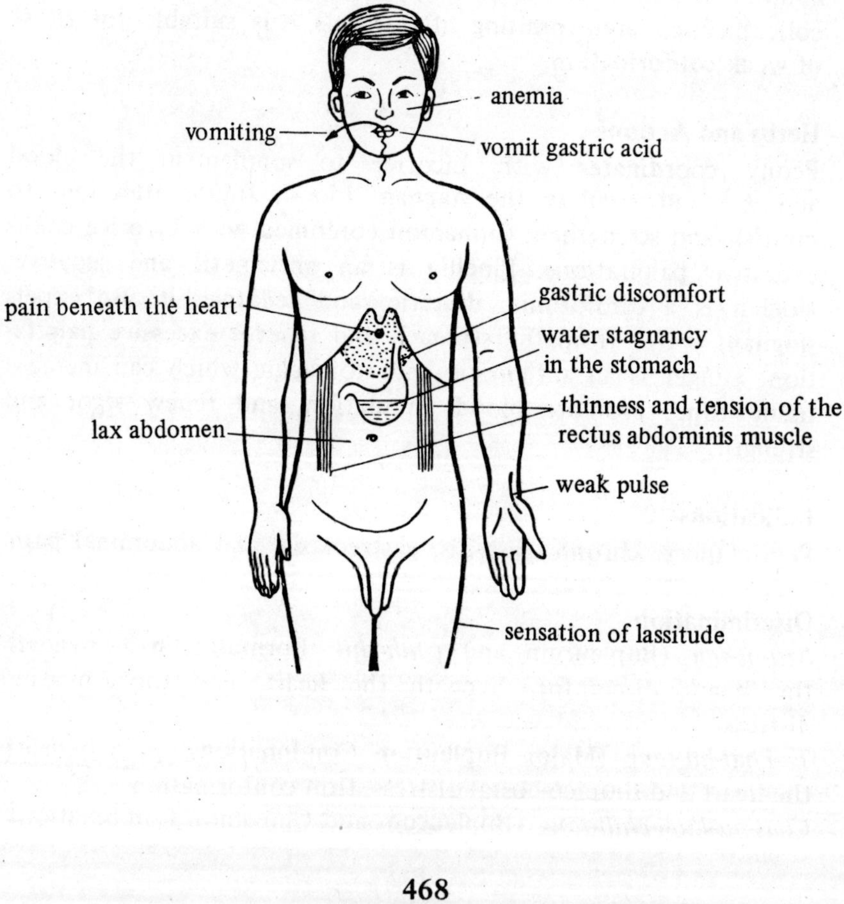

Chih-Tzu-Po-Pi-Tang *(Gardenia and Phellodendron Combination)*					**梔子蘗皮湯**
Gardenia	3.0	Phellodendron	1.0	Licorice	1.0

Chih-tzu-po-pi-tang was recorded in the *Shang han lun* (傷寒論) during the Han dynasty. This formula is used for treating "internal moisture", febrile disease, and jaundice. It is contraindicated for patients with gastrointestinal weakness and diarrhea as well as for patients who do not suffer from constipation and abdominal distention.

Herbs and Actions
Phellodendron is a bitter refrigerant that dispels "moist heat". Gardenia is also a bitter refrigerant and dispels stagnant "moist heat". Licorice coordinates the actions of the other herbs.

Indications
Jaundice and pruritus.

Discrimination
Yin-chen-hao-tang (Capillaris Combination): yellowish body color and fever, abdominal fullness, constipation, internal firm condition.
Mu-huang-lien-chiao-chih-hsiao-tou-tang (*Ma-huang*, Forsythia, and Phaseolus Combination): yellowish body color, fever, no sweating, external conformation.

Chiu-Ping-Wu-Fu-Tang 九檳吳茯湯

(Areca Seed Combination)

Areca seed	4.0	Magnolia bark	3.0	Cinnamon	3.0
Aurantium	3.0	Perilla	1.5	Licorice	1.0
Ginger	1.0	Saussurea	1.0	Rhubarb	1.0
Evodia	1.0	Hoelen	3.0		

Chiu-ping-wu-fu-tang was recorded in the *Chien tien fang han* (淺田方函) by Asata S. of Japan. This formula is used for treating beriberi, nervous diseases, fatigue in the legs, numbness, palpitation, edema in the legs, subcardiac distention, and a tendency toward constipation.

Herbs and Actions

Areca seed dispels "stagnant *ch'i*" and acts as a diuretic and expectorant. Aurantium regulates the *ch'i* and dispels "internal moisture". Magnolia bark is used to treat distention and dispel "internal moisture". Saussurea is effective for flushing up. Perilla relieves flushing up and distention. Evodia dispels "internal moisture". Cinnamon improves blood circulation. Hoelen is a diuretic. Rhubarb promotes evacuation.

Indications

Emotional disorders due to beriberi; chest pain; multiple neuritis; hypertension; Basedow's disease.

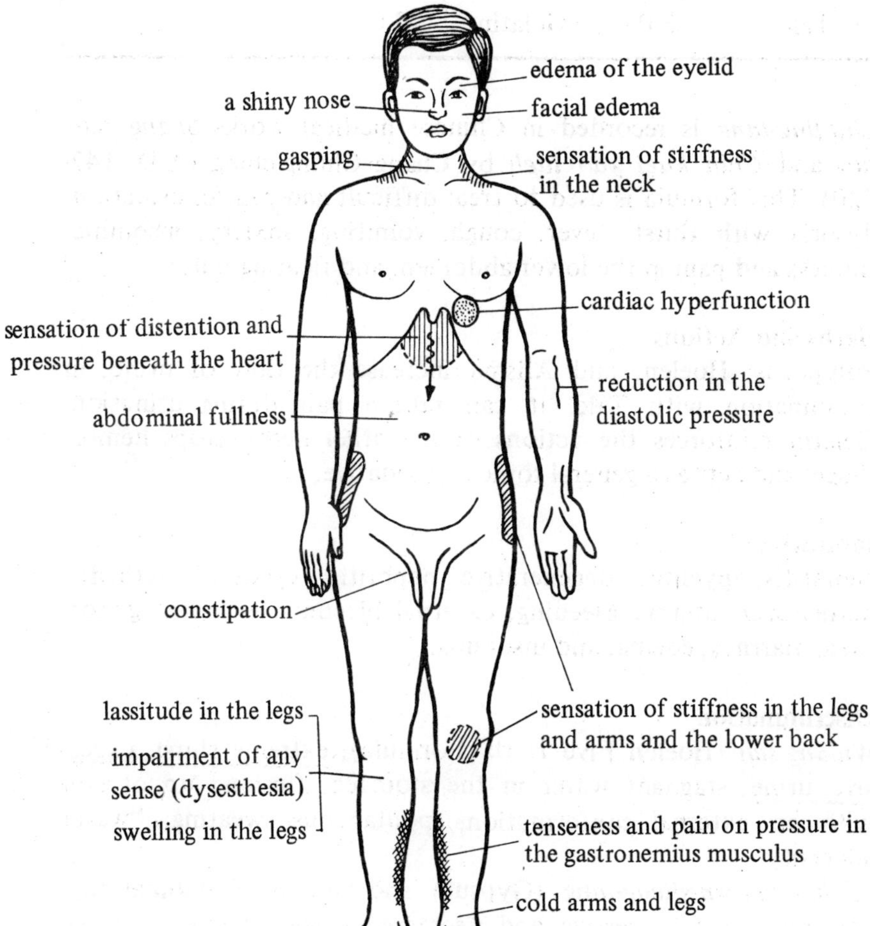
edema of the eyelid
a shiny nose
facial edema
gasping
sensation of stiffness in the neck
cardiac hyperfunction
sensation of distention and pressure beneath the heart
reduction in the diastolic pressure
abdominal fullness
constipation
lassitude in the legs
impairment of any sense (dysesthesia)
swelling in the legs
sensation of stiffness in the legs and arms and the lower back
tenseness and pain on pressure in the gastronemius musculus
cold arms and legs

Chu-Ling-Tang 豬苓湯

(Polyporus Combination)

Polyporus	3.0	Hoelen	3.0	Alisma	3.0
Talc	3.0	Gelatin	3.0		

Chu-ling-tang is recorded in Chinese medical works *Shang han lun* and *Chin kuei yao lueh* by Chang Chung-ching (A.D. 142-220). This formula is used to treat difficult and painful urination, dysuria with thirst, fever, cough, vomiting, anxiety, insomnia, fullness and pain in the lower abdomen, and floating pulse.

Herbs and Actions

Polyporus, Hoelen, and Alisma increase the flow of urine; in combination with Talc, it can relieve pain during urination. Gelatin reinforces the actions of the other herbs, stops hemorrhage, and acts as a general tonic and sedative.

Indications

Nephritis, pyelitis, degenerative nephritis, cystitis, urethritis, hermaturia, uterine bleeding, external bleeding, enteritis, gonorrhea, diarrhea, edema, and insomnia.

Discrimination

Wu-ling-san (Hoelen Five Herb Formula); extreme thirst, excessive urine, stagnant water in the stomach, flushing up of *ch'i* with an external conformation, spontaneous sweating, "water adversity".

Pai-hu-chia-jen-sheng-tang (Gypsum and Ginseng Combination): extreme thirst, excessive and decreased urine, massive and big pulse.

Pa-wei-wan (Rehmannia Eight Herb Formula): extreme thirst, excessive urine, numbness in the lower abdomen, lower back pain, and tense or weak pulse.

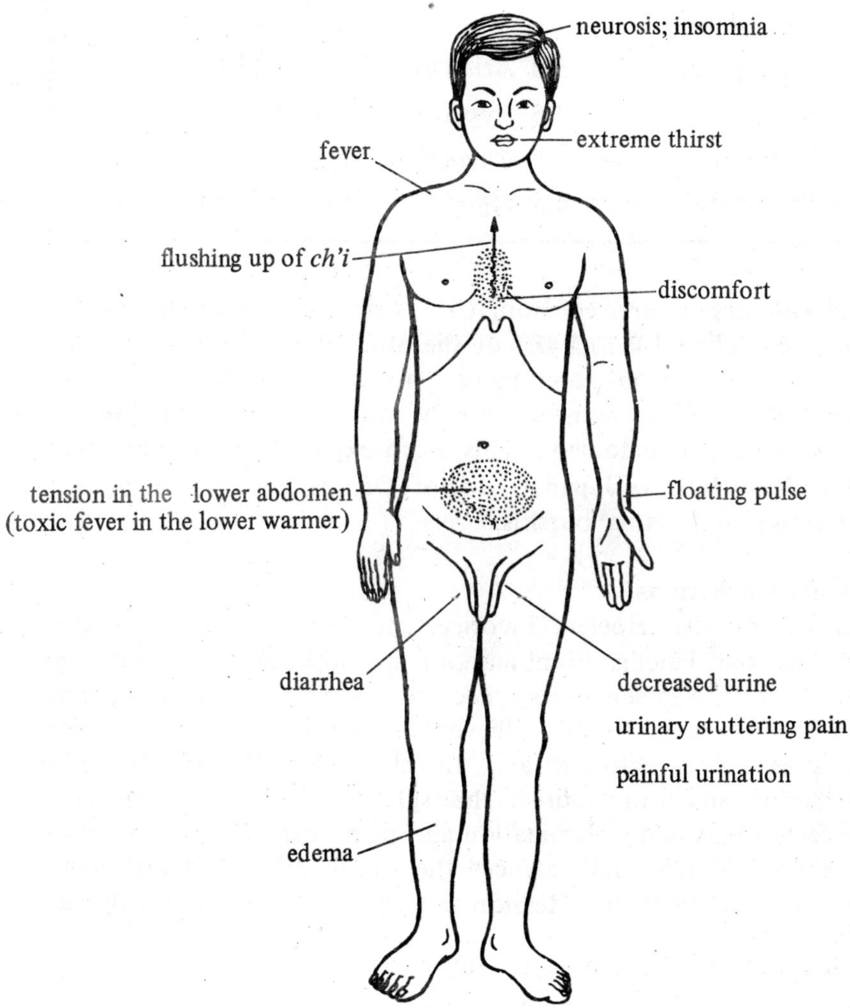
neurosis; insomnia
extreme thirst
fever
flushing up of ch'i
discomfort
tension in the lower abdomen
(toxic fever in the lower warmer)
floating pulse
diarrhea
decreased urine
urinary stuttering pain
painful urination
edema

Erh-Chu-Tang 二朮湯

(Atractylodes and Arisaema Combination)

Atractylodes	3.0	Arisaema	2.5	Citrus	2.5
Hoelen	2.5	Cyperus	2.5	Scute	2.5
Clematis	2.5	*Chianghuo*	2.5	Licorice	1.0
White atractylodes	2.5	Ginger	1.0	Pinellia	4.0

Erh-chu-tang is derived from the "Armache" Category in *Wan ping hui chun* (萬病回春) of the Ming dynasty. It is used for treating congestion accompanied by aching in the arms, and discomfort in the arms due to the wet sputum of the *shang-chiao* (upper abdomen). This is an experimental combination developed by the Japanese doctor Otsuka keisetsu. It is very effective in treating bursitis.

Herbs and Actions

Citrus, Pinellia, Hoelen, Licorice, and Ginger of *Erh-chen-tang* (Citrus and Pinellia Combination) are dessicants, effective regulators of the spleen and stomach functions, and expectorants of moist sputum. *Chianghuo* relieves rheumatic joint pain. Arisaema acts as an expectorant and antirheumatic. Atractylodes is a dessicant and can nourish the spleen and stomach. Clematis relieves rheumatic inflammation and pain, increases circulation in the upper torso, and balances the *ch'i* in the meridians. Scute is an antipyretic and dessicant. Cyperus acts as an analgesic.

Indications

Shoulder bursitis, forearm neuralgia.

Fang-Chi-Fu-Ling-Tang *(Stephania and Hoelen Combination)*					防己茯苓湯
Stephania	3.0	Astragalus	3.0	Cinnamon	3.0
Hoelen	5.0	Licorice	1.5		

Fang-chi-fu-ling-tang was recorded in the *Chin kuei yao lueh* (金匱要略) during the Han dynasty. This formula is used for treating muscle spasms, convulsions, edema of the arms and legs, dysuria, floating pulse, and numbness due to "water poisoning".

Herbs and Actions

Stephania is a diuretic, and in combination with Hoelen it serves to dispel edema. Astragalus is a tonic. Cinnamon dispels "superficial evil" and acts as a tonic.

Indications

Nephritis, eclampsia, edema of the hands and feet, convulsions, numbness, beriberi, uremia, and epilepsy.

Discrimination

Fang-chi-huang-chi-tang (Stephania and Astragalus Combination): edema, sweating, external and internal water (abnormal retention of water). This formula aims at external water, i.e., puffiness, muscular aches and pains.

Ling-kuei-chu-kan-tang (Hoelen, Licorice, and Atractylodes Combination): water toxin, vertigo, cardiac hyperfunction, submerged pulse.

Chen-wu-tang (Vitality Combination): trembling, decreased urine, yin weak conformation, submerged and minute pulse.

Yin conformation

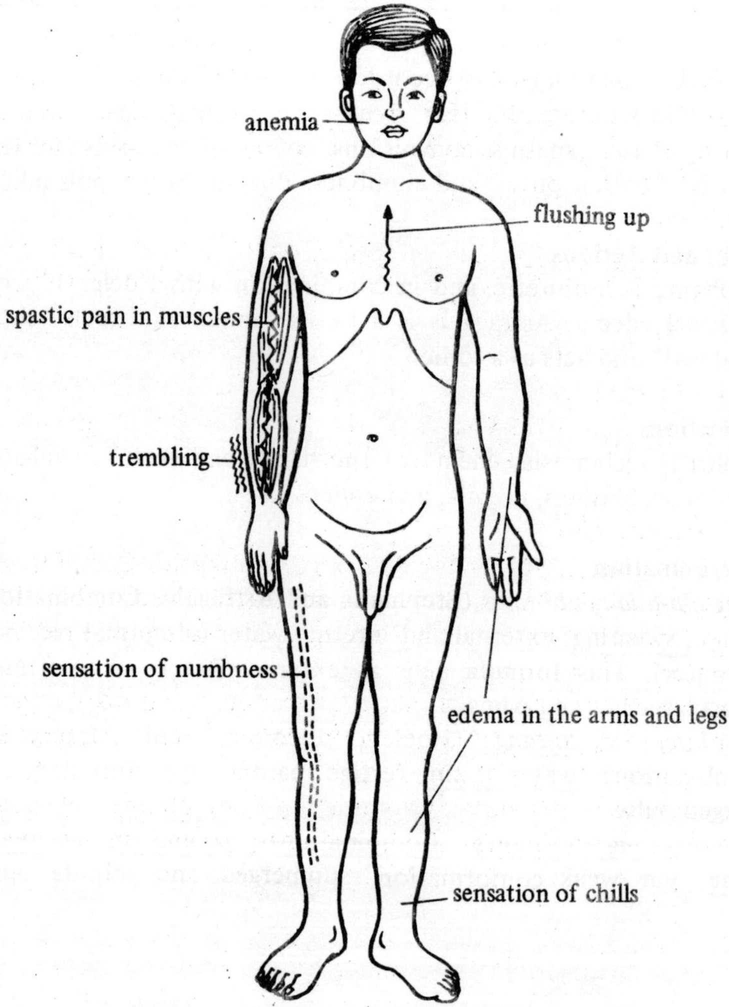

Fang-Chi-Huang-Chi-Tang 防己黃耆湯

(Stephania and Astragalus Combination)

Stephania	5.0	Astragalus	5.0	Licorice	1.5
Atractylodes	3.0	Jujube	3.0	Ginger	3.0

Fang-chi-huang-chi-tang is recorded in *Chin kuei yao lueh* (Summaries on Household Drugs) by Chang Chung-ching (A.D. 142-220) of the Han dynasty. It is effective for stimulating spleen function, improving general vitality, increasing the flow of urine, and reducing swelling. It cures ephidrosis and weakness, and it improves blood circulation in the legs. This formula is to be taken by those of obese constitution with a tendency towards fatigue, ephidrosis, difficulty in urination, edema in the lower limbs, and arthralgia in the knees.

Herbs and Actions

Stephania and Atractylodes cure edema, stop excessive sweating, increase the flow of urine, and relieve pain. Astragalus and Licorice nourish the skin. Jujube and Licorice improve the taste and coordinate the actions of other herbs. Ginger acts as a stomachic.

Indications

Rheumatism, arthritis, ephidrosis, obesity, nephritis, hydrocele of the testis, edema in the legs, and menstrual irregularity.

Discrimination

Kuei-chih-tang (Cinnamon Combination): floating pulse, perspiration, anemophobia, fever, flushing up, dry vomiting.
Yueh-pei-chia-chu-tang (Atractylodes Combination): edema, perspiration, weak feet, submerged pulse.
Ma-hsing-i-kan-tang (*Ma-huang* and Coix Combination): external water, rheumatism, floating pulse, lack of sweat, general pain.
Fang-chi-fu-ling-tang (Stephania and Hoelen Combination): edema, spasms, trembling, numbness.

Ling-chiang-chu-kan-tang (Ginger and Hoelen Combination): cold lower back, excessive urination, submerged and thin pulse.

Rheumatism, surface weakness, lower warmer weakness

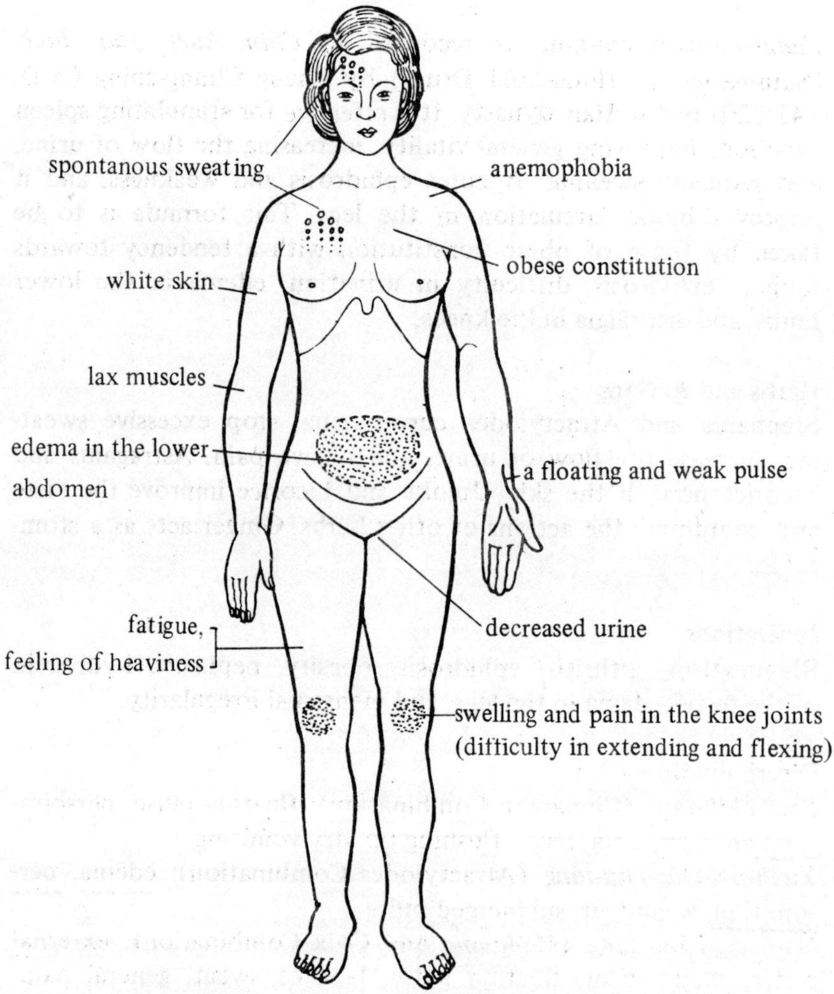

Fu-Ling-Kan-Tsao-Tang 茯苓甘草湯

(Licorice and Hoelen Combination)

Hoelen	6.0	Cinnamon	4.0	Ginger	3.0
Licorice	1.0				

Recorded in *Shang han lun* (傷寒論): "*Shang han* conditions which have the symptoms of sweating and thirst are treated with *Wu-ling-san*. If there is no thirst, *Fu-ling-kan-tsao-tang* is used." In other words, this formula is for fever diseases which show no surface fever, and no thirst, but do show a buoyant pulse, spontaneous sweating, and oliguria. It is also used when the patient has a fever but his arms and legs are cold and he has rapid palpitations of the heart. It may also be used for common miscellaneous diseases that present cardiac palpitation and a splashing sound beneath the heart due to "water toxin."

Herbs and Actions

Hoelen drains fluids and encourages diuresis. Cinnamon harmonizes the outside of the body. Ginger warms the insides and disperses stagnated fluids. Licorice nourishes and harmonizes the insides.

Indications

Valvular diseases of the heart, irritability, palpitation, cardiac hyperfunction, circulation disturbances.

Discrimination

Wu-ling-san (Hoelen Five Herb Formula) is indicated for a buoyant pulse, sweating, dysuria, thirst, fluid disturbances, and vomiting.

Ling-kuei-chu-kan-tang (Atractylodes and Hoelen Combination) is used for gastric fluid stagnancy, dysuria, flushing-up of gas, and static dizziness.

Chih-kan-tsao-tang (Baked Licorice Combination) is for cardiac palpitation and hyperfunction, feverish limbs, and a knotty and alternating pulse.

Weak conformation

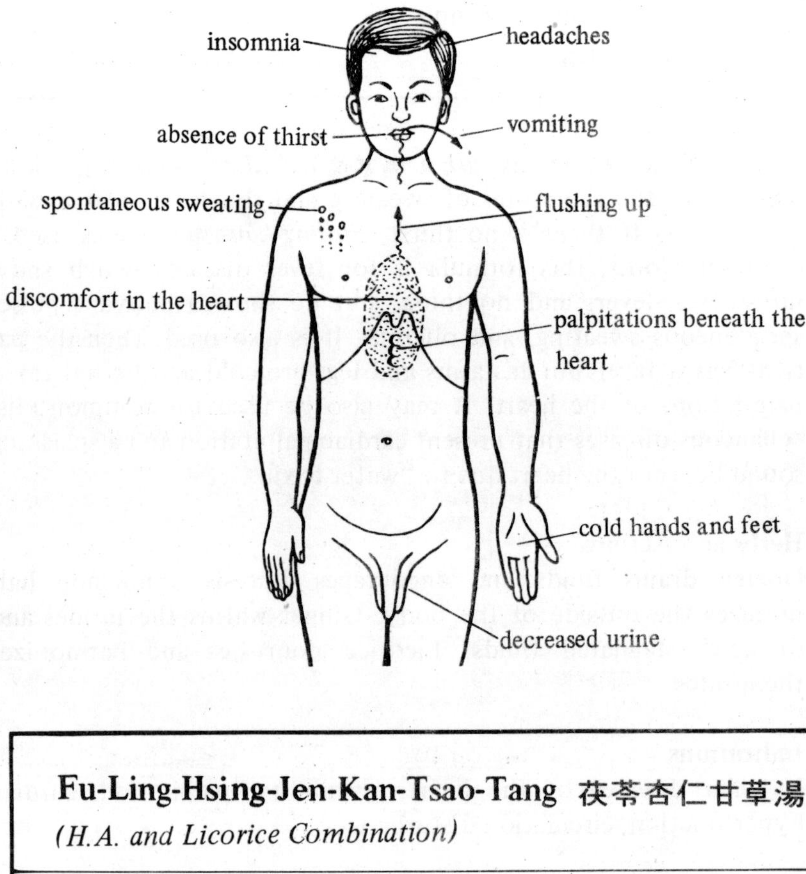

Fu-Ling-Hsing-Jen-Kan-Tsao-Tang 茯苓杏仁甘草湯 *(H.A. and Licorice Combination)*					
Hoelen	6.0	Apricot seed	4.0	Licorice	1.0

Fu-ling-hsing-jen-kan-tsao-tang is recorded in *Chin kuei yao lueh* (金匱要略) of the Han dynasty. This formula is used for treating chest distention, rapid respiration, palpitation, asthma, chest pain, pain in the back, and difficulty in breathing.

Herbs and Actions

Hoelen removes stagnant water from the stomach and relieves flushing up. Apricot seed dispels stagnant water in the chest, relieves flushing up, and is effective treatment for asthma. Licorice coordinates the actions of the other herbs.

Indications

Bronchial asthma, cardiac asthma, pulmonary emphysema, pleurisy, intercostal neuralgia, angina pectoris, myocardial infarction, valvular disease, cardiac neurosis, and pharyngeal contraction.

Discrimination

Kua-lu-hsieh-pai-pai-chiu-tang (Trichosanthes, Bakeri, and Vinegar Combination): chest paralysis, asthma, pain in the chest and back.
Chih-kan-tsao-tang (Baked Licorice Combination): cardiac hyperfunction, dry skin, fever in the hands and feet, knotty and alternate pulse.
Chu-yeh-shih-kao-tang (Bamboo Leaf and Gypsum Combination): labored breathing, adverse cough with less *ch'i*, yang disease, adverse vomiting, and dry mouth and tongue.

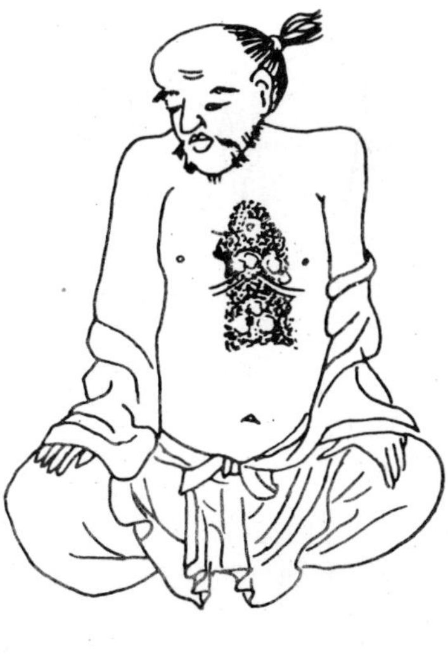

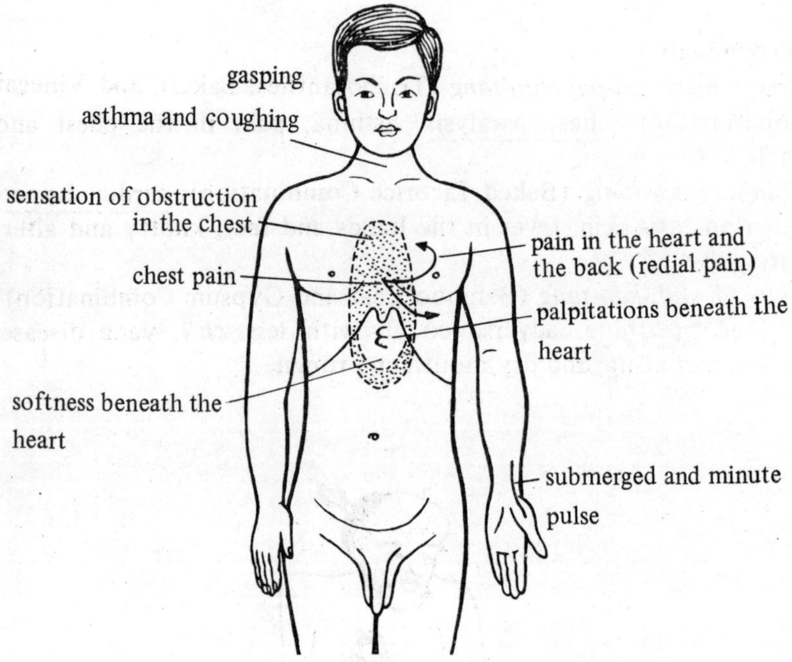
gasping
asthma and coughing
sensation of obstruction
in the chest
chest pain
softness beneath the
heart
pain in the heart and
the back (redial pain)
palpitations beneath the
heart
submerged and minute
pulse

Fu-Ling-Tse-Hsieh-Tang 茯苓澤瀉湯

(Alisma and Hoelen Combination)

Hoelen	4.0	Alisma	4.0	Cinnamon	2.0
Atractylodes	3.0	Ginger	3.0	Licorice	1.5

Fu-ling-tse-hsieh-tang was recorded in the *Chin kuei yao lueh* (金匱要略) during the Han dynasty. This formula is used for treating gastric distress with vomiting and thirst, oliguria, palpitation, flushing up, headache, vertigo, abdominal distention, and abdominal pain.

Herbs and Actions

Hoelen and Alisma relieve stagnant water in the stomach. Atractylodes and Licorice nourish the spleen and act as sialogagues. Ginger stops vomiting. Cinnamon relieves flushing up and increases salivation.

Indications

Abdominal distention, gastroptosis, gastromegaly, gastric ulcer, gastric cancer, eclampsia, regurgitation of milk in young children, and pyloric obstruction.

Discrimination

Wu-ling-san (Hoelen Five Herb Formula): vomiting, extreme thirst, vomiting after drinking water, floating pulse.

Hsiao-pan-hsia-chia-fu-ling-tang (Minor Pinellia and Hoelen Combination): vomiting which occurs after extreme thirst.

Ling-kuei-chu-kan-tang (Hoelen and Atractylodes Combination): stagnant water in the stomach, decreased urine, palpitations beneath the heart, vertigo, submerged pulse.

Fu-ling-yin (Hoelen Combination): vomiting, apparent water stagnancy in the stomach, expectoration of over night water, and congested chest.

Pan-hsia-hsieh-hsin-tang (Pinellia Combination): vomiting, obstruction and hardness beneath the heart, gas, firm conformation.

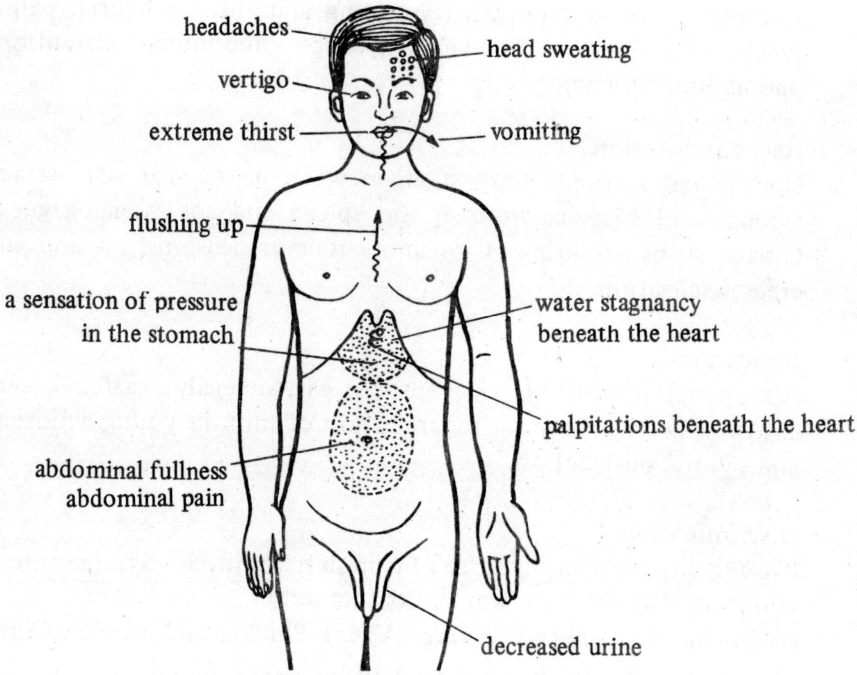

headaches
head sweating
vertigo
extreme thirst
vomiting
flushing up
a sensation of pressure in the stomach
water stagnancy beneath the heart
palpitations beneath the heart
abdominal fullness
abdominal pain
decreased urine

Fu-Ling-Yin 茯苓飲

(Hoelen Combination)

Hoelen	5.0	Ginseng	3.0	*Chih-shih*	1.5
Atractylodes	4.0	Citrus	3.0	Ginger	3.0

Recorded in *Chin kuei yao lueh* (金匱要略) of the Han dynasty. Used for treating stagnant fluids and *ch'i* in the stomach, nausea, and mild resistance beneath the heart.

Herbs and Actions

Hoelen and Atractylodes remove stagnant water in the stomach. Ginseng reinforces gastric function. Citrus and *Chih-shih* are bitter stomachics; they dispel stagnant water and *ch'i*, increase the appetite, and reduce gastric distention. Ginger coordinates the actions of the other herbs.

Indications

Gastritis, gastroptosis, enlargement of the stomach, gastroxia, and gastrointestinal exhaustion.

Discrimination

Jen-sheng-tang (Ginseng and Ginger Combination): a weak conformation with stagnant water in the stomach, severe weakness, chills, and mild gastric distention.

Wu-chu-yu-tang (Evodia Combination): obstruction beneath the heart, severe upward congestion of chills and *ch'i*, vomiting, headache, and anxiety.

Sheng-chiang-hsieh-hsin-tang (Pinellia and Ginger Combination): obstruction beneath the heart, firm conformation.

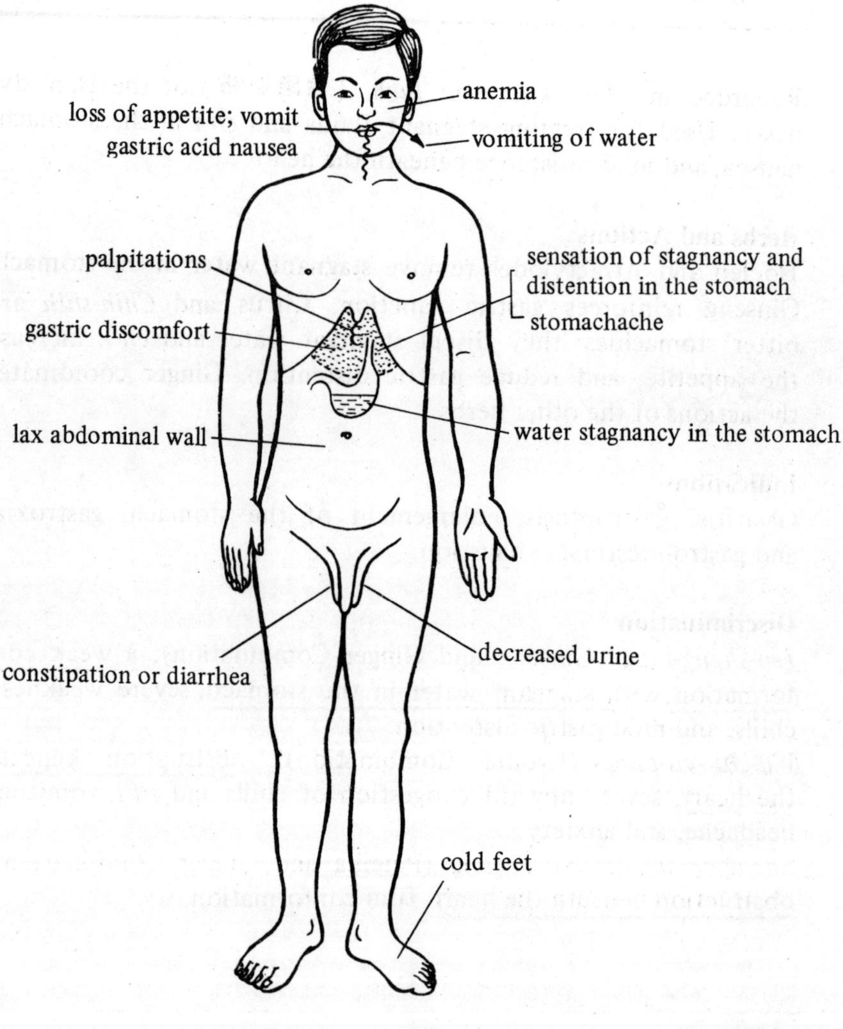
anemia
loss of appetite; vomit
gastric acid nausea
vomiting of water
palpitations
sensation of stagnancy and
distention in the stomach
stomachache
gastric discomfort
lax abdominal wall
water stagnancy in the stomach
decreased urine
constipation or diarrhea
cold feet

Hsiao-Pan-Hsia-Chia-Fu-Ling-Tang 小半夏加茯苓湯

(Minor Pinellia and Hoelen Combination)

Pinellia	8.0	Ginger	5.0	Hoelen	5.0

Hsiao-pan-hsia-chia-fu-ling-tang was recorded in the *Chin kuei yao lueh* (金匱要略) during the Han dynasty. This formula is used for treating vomiting due to stagnant water in the stomach, eclampsia, flushing up, nausea, subcardiac distention, vertigo, and palpitation.

Herbs and Actions
Pinellia is an expectorant and antiemetic. Ginger is a stomachic. Hoelen and Pinellia eliminate stagnant water in the stomach and increase the flow of urine.

Indications
Pernicious vomiting, acute gastroenteritis, gastroptosis, beriberi, and pleurisy.

Discrimination
Hsiao-pan-hsia-tang (Minor Pinellia Combination): vomiting, water stagnancy in the stomach, no thirst.
Hsiao-chai-hu-tang (Minor Bupleurum Combination): vomiting, distressed chest, bitter taste in the mouth.
Wu-chu-yu-tang (Evoida Combination): vomiting, headache, water stagnancy in the stomach, cold hands and feet, distress and irritability, submerged and slow pulse.
Wu-ling-san (Hoelen Five Herb Formula): vomiting, water congestion, severe thirst, decreased urine, headache, irritability, floating pulse.
Fu-ling-tse-hsieh-tang (Alisma, Hoelen, and Ginger Combination): vomiting, flushing up, extreme thirst, vertigo, sensation of stagnancy in the stomach, nausea.

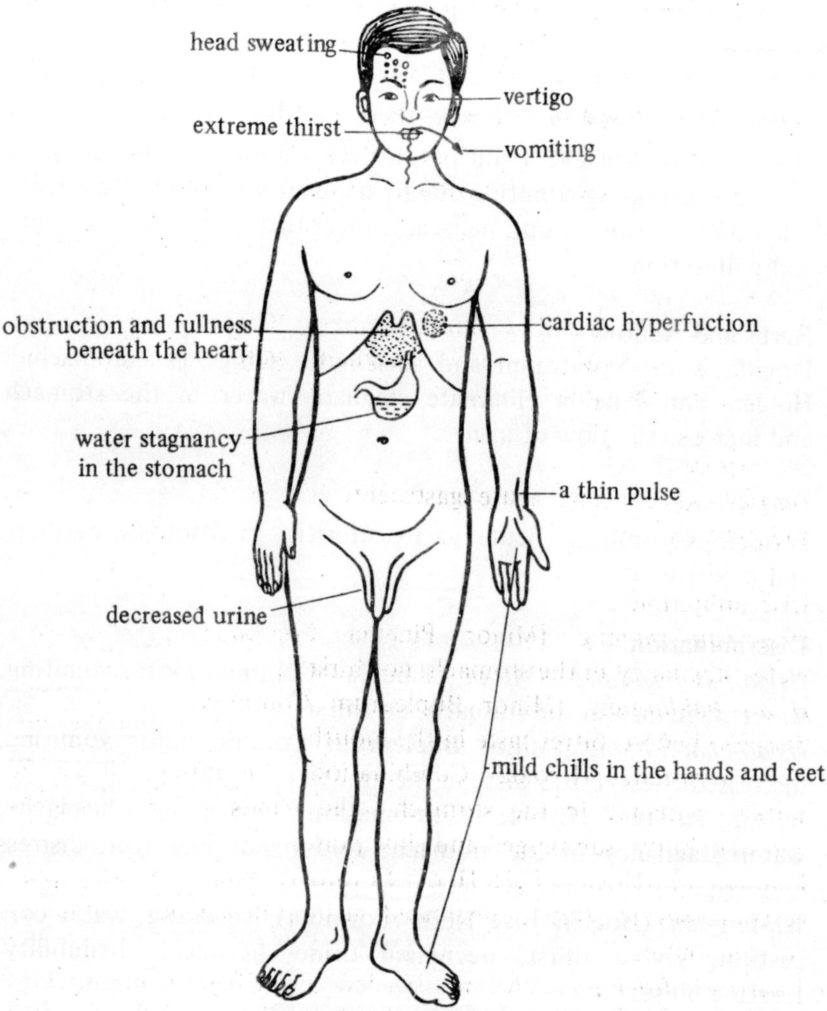
head sweating
vertigo
extreme thirst
vomiting
obstruction and fullness beneath the heart
cardiac hyperfuction
water stagnancy in the stomach
a thin pulse
decreased urine
mild chills in the hands and feet

I-Yi-Jen-Tang *(Coix Combination)*					薏苡仁湯
Ma-huang	4.0	*Tang-kuei*	4.0	Coix	8.0
Atractylodes	4.0	Cinnamon	3.0	Peony	3.0
Licorice	2.0				

Rheumatism and arthritis have been two recalcitrant diseases in modern medicine. Recently, paranephric cortical hormone has been used with excellent short-term results; however, excess use causes severe side effects. The Chinese formula, *I-yi-jen-tang* is a complete treatment and is without side effects. *I-yi-jen-tang* corrects the disturbance in blood circulation, dispels fluid accumulated in the joints and tissues, and relieves muscular tension. The effect of *I-yi-jen-tang* on arthritis and rheumatism has been recorded in many Chinese medical classics. *Chien chin fang* (千金方, Precious Formulas A.D. 652) of the Tang dynasty, states that it "cures muscular spasm"; *Ming i chih chang* (明醫指掌, A.D. 1502) of the Ming dynasty states that it "cures aching, numbness, and slackness of the limbs"; and *Chang shih i tung* (張氏醫通. A.D. 1693) of the Chin dynasty also states that it "cures apoplexy, rheumatism, and arthralgia". It is used for arthralgia, swelling, and chronic fever in the arms and legs.

Herbs and Actions

Tang-kuei and Peony promote good blood circulation, synthesize the actions of all the herbs, and relieve pain. Coix helps rheumatism, increases the secretion and flow of urine, and dispels accumulated fluid.

Indications

Polyrheumatism, mucoid arthritis, tubercular arthritis, muscular rheumatism, beriberi, nephritis, pulmonary edema, and pleurisy.

Discrimination

Ma-huang-chia-chu-tang (*Ma-huang* and Atractylodes Combination): generalized aching, arthralgia in the initial stage when the symptoms are mild.

Ma-hsing-i-kan-tang (*Ma-huang* and Coix Combination): generalized aching, and arthralgia in the initial stage when the symptoms are yet mild.

Kuei-shao-chih-mu-tang (Cinnamon and Anemarrhena Combination): chronic arthralgia symptoms, severe stiffness and emaciation.

Shu-ching-li-an-san (Clematis and Carthamus Formula): chronic arthralgia and blood occlusion.

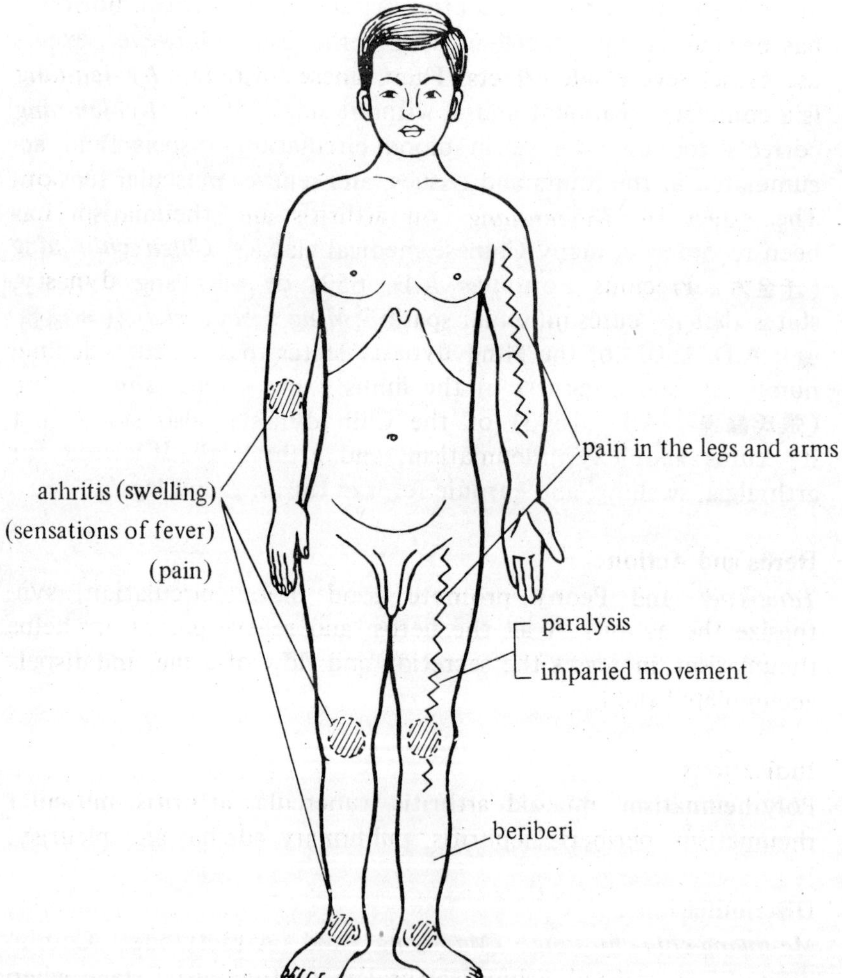

Ling-Chiang-Chu-Kan-Tang 苓薑朮甘湯

(Ginger and Hoelen Combination)

Hoelen	6.0	Ginger	3.0	Licorice	2.0
Atractylodes	3.0				

Ling-chiang-chu-kan-tang is recorded in *Chin kuei yao lueh* (金匱要略) of the Han dynasty. This formula is used for treating the feeling of being chilled below the waist, pain due to chills, fatigue and weakness in the abdominal wall.

Herbs and Actions

Ginger is warm in nature and acts as a diuretic. Hoelen and Atractylodes increase the *ch'i* and dispel "surface water". Licorice and Ginger are tonics and stop polyuria.

Indications

Feeling of being chilled below the waist, lumbago, sciatica, diurnal and nocturnal enuresis, and leukorrhea.

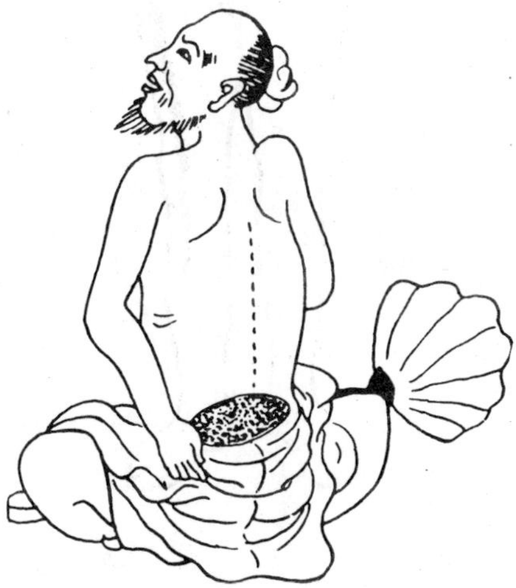

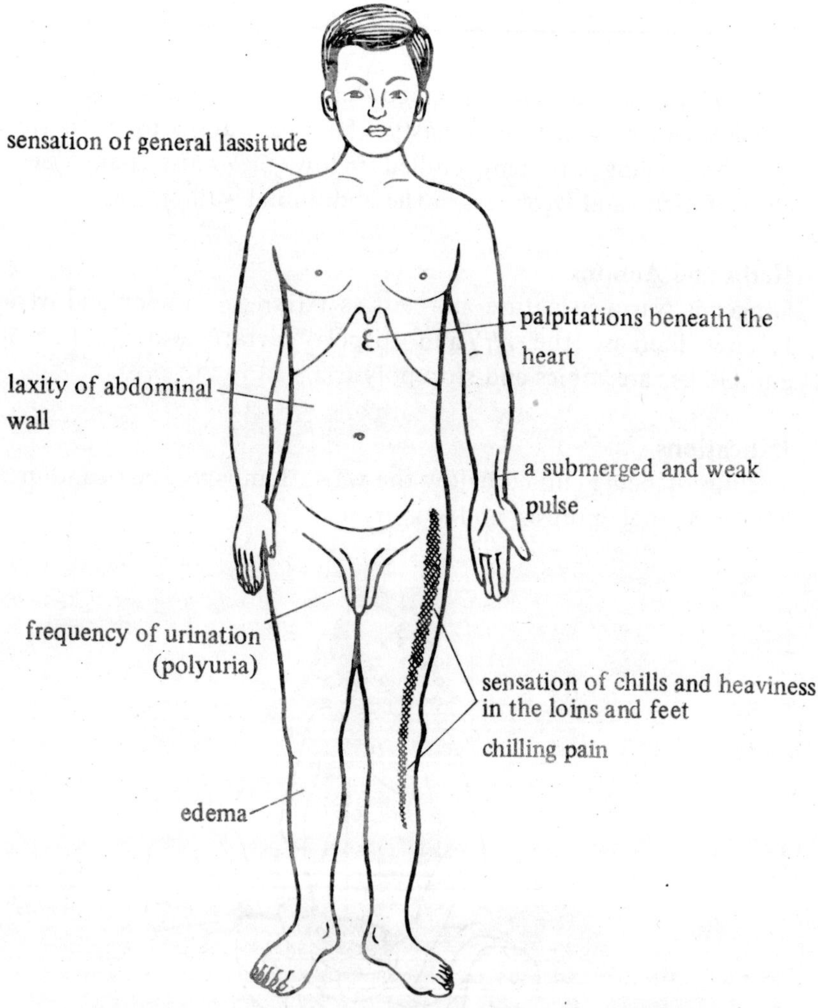
sensation of general lassitude
palpitations beneath the heart
laxity of abdominal wall
a submerged and weak pulse
frequency of urination (polyuria)
sensation of chills and heaviness in the loins and feet
chilling pain
edema

Ling-Kuei-Chu-Kan-Tang *(Atractylodes and Hoelen Combination)*					苓桂朮甘湯
Hoelen	6.0	Cinnamon	4.0	Licorice	2.0
Atractylodes	3.0				

Ling-kuei-chu-kan-tang was recorded during the Han dynasty in both the *Shang han lun* (傷寒論) and the *Chin kuei yao lueh* (金匱要略) by Chang Chung-ching. This formula is used for palpitations, hyperpnea, distention in the chest near the heart, vertigo when standing, dysuria, mild edema, headache, cold feet, a sinking pulse, a weak abdomen, and treating flushing up due to water poisoning.

Herbs and Actions
Hoelen dispels ascites. Atractylodes assists Hoelen to improve metabolic function. Cinnamon relieves flushing up. Licorice is an adjuvant to Cinnamon.

Indications
Nervous disorders: neurasthenia, anxiety, hysteria, cardiac palpitations, instability of the autonomic nervous system, and motion sickness.
Heart disease: valvular disease, cardiac asthma, neurogenic palpitations, and Basedow's disease.
Eye ailments: conjunctivitis, chronic optic nerve disorders, optic atrophy, and nebula.
Kidney diseases: chronic nephritis, anascara, and renal atrophy.
Others: hypertension, sinusitis, anemia, and rhinitis.

Discrimination
Wu-ling-san (Hoelen Five Herb Formula): decreased urine, water toxin, floating pulse, extreme thirst, adverse water congestion, and vomiting.
Chen-wu-tang (Vitality Combination): palpiations, vertigo, cold hands and feet, submerged and weak pulse, and a yin and weak conformation.

Tang-kuei-shao-yao-san (*Tang-kuei* and Peony Formula): palpitations, vertigo, weak pulse, blood disease, anemia.
Ling-chiang-chu-kan-tang (Ginger and Hoelen Combination): palpitations beneath the heart, chills in the lower back and feet, escessive urination, submerged and weak pulse.

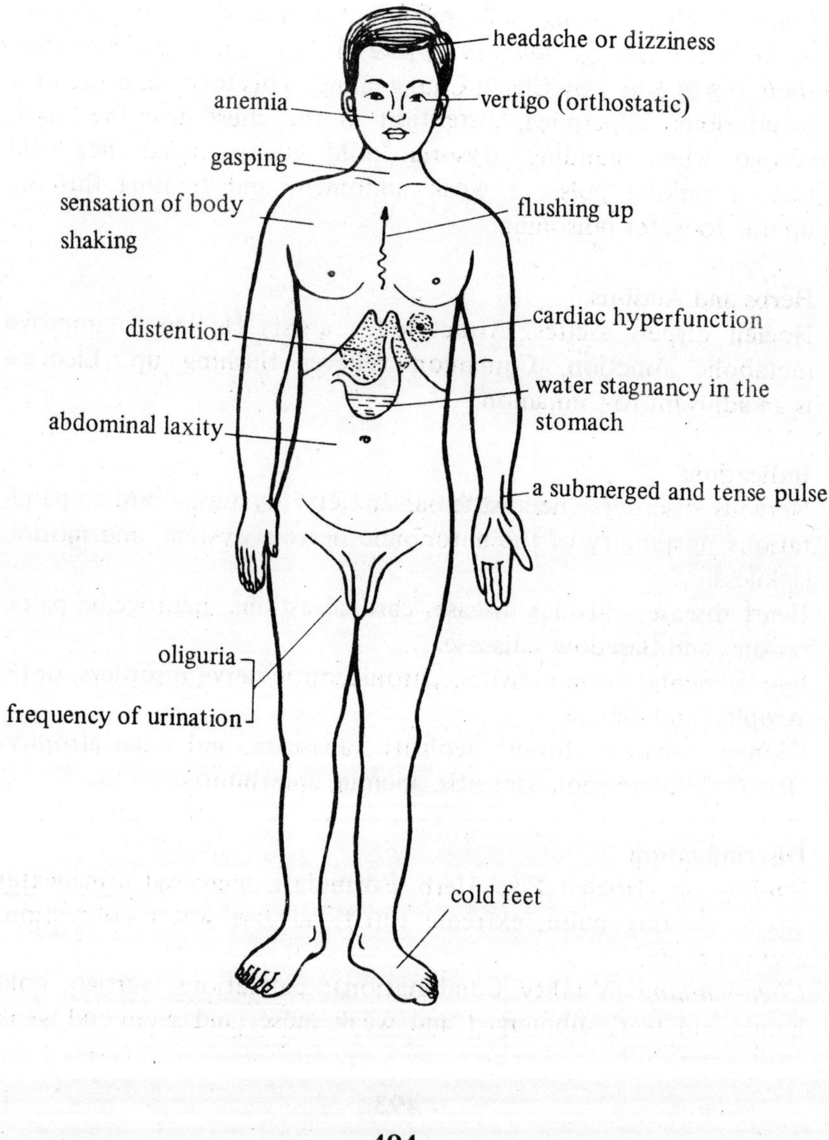

Ling-Kuei-Kan-Tsao-Tang *(Hoelen, Licorice, and Jujube Combination)*					苓桂甘棗湯
Cinnamon	4.0	Licorice	2.0	Hoelen	6.0
Jujube	4.0				

Recorded in the *Shang han lun* (傷寒論) of the Han dynasty. Used for treating hysteric palpitation of the heart, labored breathing, and severe abdominal pain.

Herbs and Actions
Cinnamon with Licorice treats palpitation. Hoelen and Jujube are sedatives and diuretics and coordinate the actions of Cinnamon and Licorice.

Indications
Cardiac neurosis, neurotic palpitation, nervous exhaustion, hysteria, uterine spasms, gastric spasms, and epilepsy.

Discrimination
Kuei-chih-chia-kuei-tang: treats flushing up causing cardiac palpitations, palpitations beneath the heart, headache, head sweating, anxiety, floating, big and weak pulse.
Fu-ling-kan-tsao-tang (Hoelen and Licorice Combination): flushing up, cardiac palpitations, palpitations beneath the heart, vomiting, decreased urine, discomfort, spontaneous sweating, harsh pulse.
Ling-kuei-chu-kan-tang (Atractylodes and Hoelen Combination): flushing up, palpitations, adverse distention beneath the heart, orthostatic vertigo, a submerged and tense pulse.
Kan-mai-ta-tsao-tang (Licorice and Jujube Combination): emotional instability, hysteria, acute conditions, and acute cramping in the rectus abdominis muscle.
Ling-kuei-wei-kan-tang (Schizandra, Licorice, and Hoelen Combination): flushing up, palpitations beneath the heart, congestion in the chest and throat, cough, and the common cold.

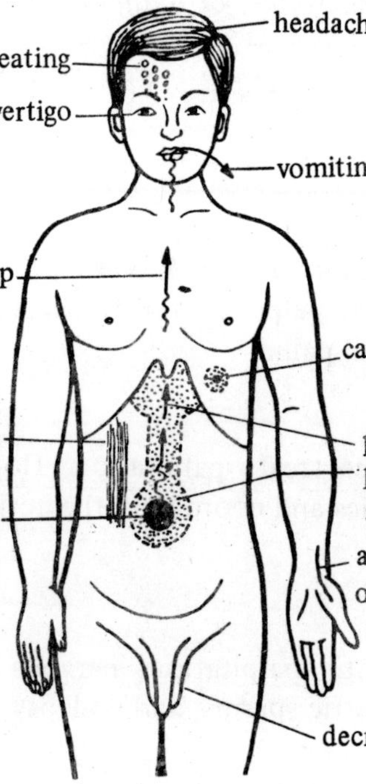

Ling-Kuei-Wei-Kan-Tang 苓桂味甘湯

(Hoelen, Licorice and Schizandra Combination)

Hoelen	6.0	Cinnamon	4.0	Schizandra	3.0
Licorice	2.0				

Recorded in *Chin kuei yao lueh* (金匱要略). Formed by substituting Schizandra for Atractylodes in *Ling-kuei-chu-kan-tang* (Atractylodes and Hoelen Combination). Used for patients having chills in their limbs, and up-rushing air and gas causing a ruddy facial complexion and headache. These symptoms are accompanied by a cough and cardiac hyperfunction, along with a submerged and small pulse. Oliguria (abnormally small amount of urine) is the main symptom treated by this formula and *Ling-kuei-chu-kan-tang*.

Herbs and Actions

Schizandra together with Cinnamon treats headaches caused by the adverse up-rushing of air and gas, and suppresses coughs. Hoelen, together with Cinnamon and Licorice, treats cardiac hyperfunction and restores urination to normal.

Indications

Bronchitis, exudative otitis media, pulmonary emphysema, edema.

Ma-Huang-Lien-Chiao-Chih-Hsiao-Tou-Tang

麻黃連翹赤小豆湯

(Ma-huang, Forsythia, and Phaseolus Combination)

Ma-huang	3.0	Forsythia	3.0	Morus	3.0
Ginger	3.0	Jujube	3.0	Phaseolus	10.0
Apricot seed	4.0	Licorice	1.0		

Ma-huang-lien-chiao-chih-hsiao-tou-tang is recorded in *Shang han lun* (傷寒論) of the Han dynasty. This formula acts as an antipyretic an diuretic, and is used for treating "moist heat", fever, severe chills, anhidrosis, coughing, edema, mild abdominal distention, dysuria, and generalized itching.

Herbs and Actions

Ma-huang removes stagnant blood. Forsythia dispels internal heat. Phaseolus removes internal moisture. Morus dispels "moist heat" of the muscle. Apricot seed nourishes the lungs. Licorice coordinates the actions of the other herbs. Ginger and Jujube are nutrients.

Indications

Jaundice, edema, eczema, urticaria, generalized pruritis, and nephritic dermatitis.

Discrimination

Chih-tzu-po-pi-tang (Gardenia and Phellodendron Combination): fever and yellowish body, no external conformation.
Yin-chen-hao-tang (Capillaris Combination): fever and yellowish body, internal firm conformation.

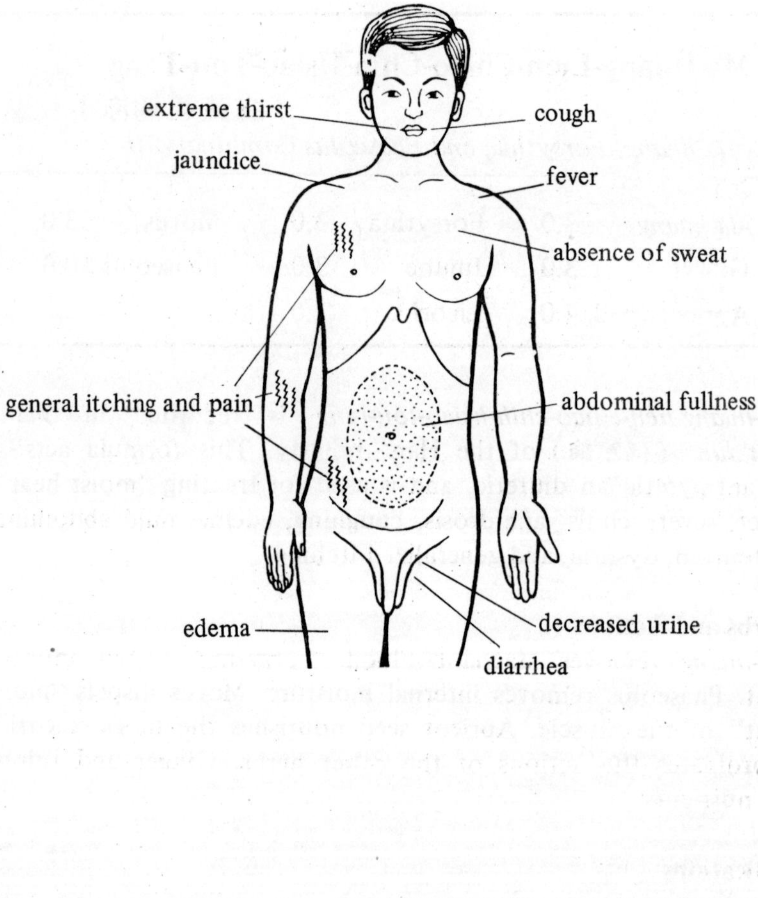

Mi-Niao-Chien 泌尿煎

(Hoelen and Akebia Combination)

Hoelen	1.0-2.0	Akebia	1.0-2.0	Nuphar	1.0-2.0
Atractylodes	1.0-2.0				

Mi-niao-chien is an experimental formula of Nagakura Pharmaceutical Company of Japan. This formula is used for treating albuminuria and urosis. It is suitable for difficult urination, enuresis, dysuria, turbid urine, hematuria alone or with pus, vesical or renal ulcer, and edema.

Herbs and Actions

Hoelen and Atractylodes relieve thirst and act as diuretics and dessicants. Akebia is a refrigerant and diuretic. Nuphar acts as an extravasated blood agent.

Indications

Nephritis, pyelitis, cystitis, urethritis, and edema during pregnancy.

Mu-Fang-Chi-Tang 木防己湯

(Stephania and Ginseng Combination)

Stephania	4.0	Cinnamon	3.0	Ginseng	3.0
Gypsum	10.0				

Recorded in *Chin kuei yao lueh* (金匱要略) of the Han dynasty. Used for treating heart trouble, stagnant water in the chest, rapid breathing, asthma, palpitations, distention beneath the heart, abdominal pain, dysuria (painful urination), edema, and a sunken and tight pulse.

Herbs and Actions
Stephania increases blood circulation and dispels stagnant water in the chest. Gypsum and Ginseng remove stress, thirst, and distention beneath the heart. Gypsum dispels stagnant water in the chest. Cinnamon removes flushing up and increases the flow of urine.

Indications
Valvular disease, heart trouble, cardiac asthma, nephritis, dropsy, beriberi, and bronchial asthma.

Discrimination
Ta-ching-lung-tang (Major Blue Dragon Combination): asthmatic cough, yang diseases, serious discomfort, floating and tense pulse.
Ta-chai-hu-tang (Major Bupleurum Combination): chest fullness, distressed chest, firm fever, submerged and firm pulse.
Ta-hsien-hsiung-tang (Rhubarb and *Kan-sui* Combination): cough, asthma, the stone-like sensation and pain on pressure beneath the heart, submerged and tense pulse.
Chih-kan-tsao-tang (Baked Licorice Combination): palpitations, gasping, knotty and alternate pulse, irritation and fever in the hands and feet, spontaneous sweating.

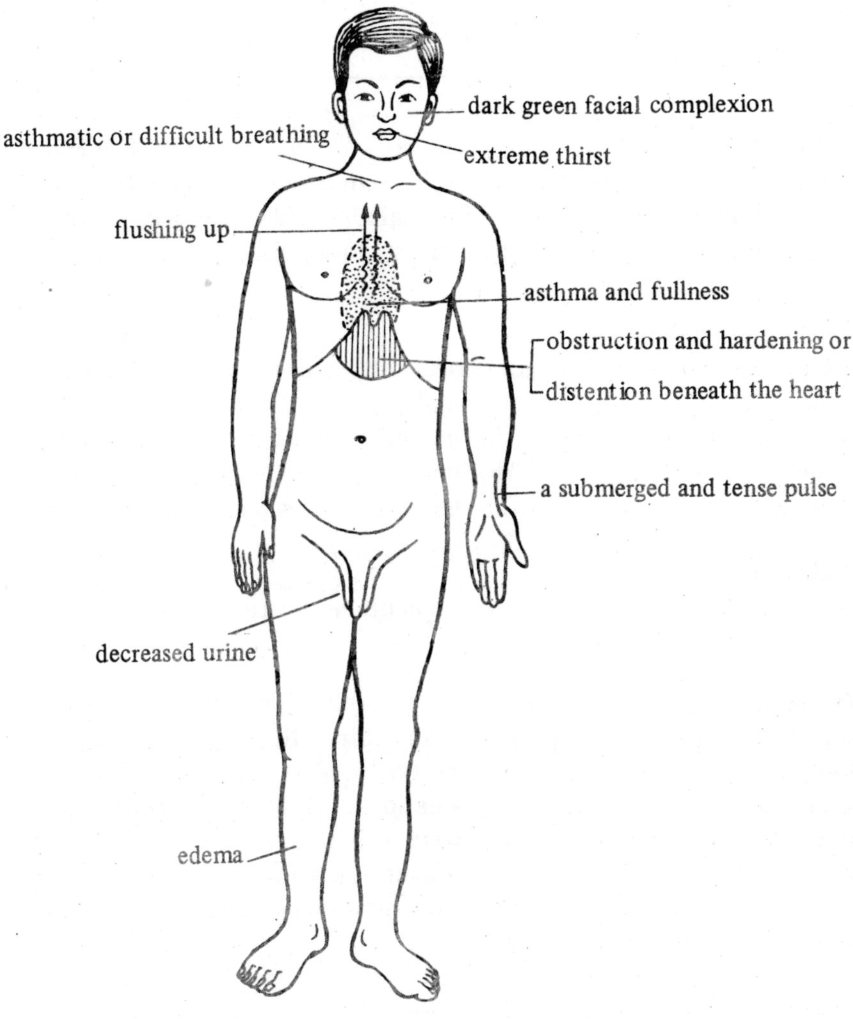
dark green facial complexion
asthmatic or difficult breathing
extreme thirst
flushing up
asthma and fullness
obstruction and hardening or
distention beneath the heart
a submerged and tense pulse
decreased urine
edema

Pa-Cheng-San 八正散
(Dianthus Formula)

Plantago	1.5	Akebia	3.0	Dianthus	3.0
Polygonum	3.0	Licorice	1.5	Gardenia	3.0
Rhubarb	1.0	Juncus	2.0	Talc	5.0

Recorded in *Tai ping huei min ho chi chu fang* (太平惠民和劑局方) of the Sung dynasty. Acts as an antipyretic and diuretic. It is suitable for acute abdominal pain, turbid urine, pain during urination, enuresis, dry mouth, thirst, fast pulse, and gonococcal infections with fever.

Herbs and Actions

Dianthus is a diuretic, gonococcicide, and antipyretic. Akebia is a diuretic and antipyretic. Polygonum, Plantago, Talc, and Juncus dispel internal heat and moisture and increase the flow of urine. Gardenia and Rhubarb remove internal heat. Licorice coordinates the actions of the other herbs and eases pain.

Indications

Goncoccus, urinary infections, and acute nephritis.

Discrimination

Ching-hsin-lien-tzu-yin (Lotus Seed Combination): urinary stuttering, frequency of urination, extreme thirst, thriving in the upper body and weakness in the lower body.

Chu-ling-tang (Polyporus Combination): diminished urine, pain due to urinary stuttering, extreme thirst, anxiety, and edema.

Pa-wei-wan (Rehmannia Eight Formula): diminished urine, extreme thirst, numbness beneath the umbilicus, irritating fever in the palms and feet, fatigability.

Wu-ling-san (Hoelen Five Herb Formula): diminished urine, extreme thirst, vomiting, edema, and headaches.

Lung-tan-hsieh-kan-tang (Gentiana Combination): urinary stuttering, frequent urination, dark skin, tension in the abdominal muscles.

Firm conformation

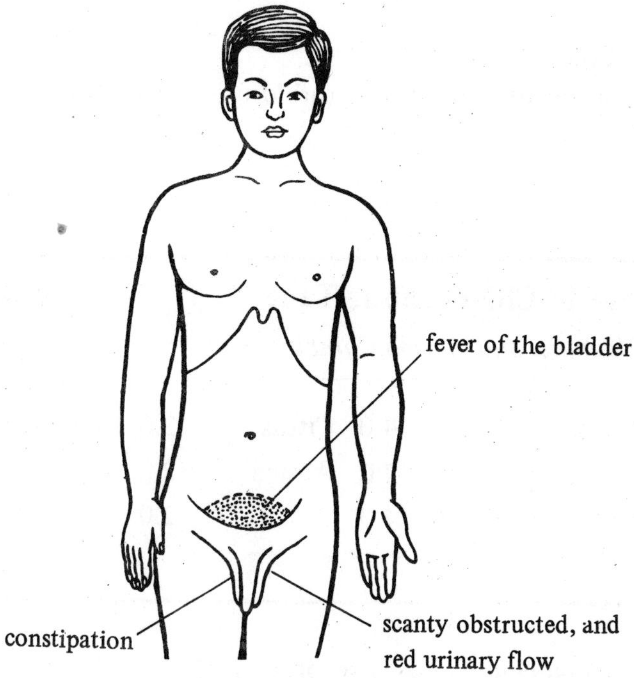

Pi-Hsieh-Fen-Ching-Yin 萆薢分清飲

(Tokoro Combination)

Tokoro	4.0	Lindera	4.0	Acorus	4.0
Black cardamon	4.0				

Pi-hsieh-fen-ching-yin was recorded in the *Tan chi hsin fa* (丹溪心法) edited by Chen Chung during the Ming dynasty. This formula is used for treating cloudy urine, polyuria, and urethritis.

Herbs and Actions

Tokoro is effective for cloudy urine. Black cardamon nourishes the spleen and kidneys. Lindera nourishes the kidney *ch'i*. Acorus is a diuretic.

Indications

Polyuria, cystitis, urethritis, turbid urine, and chronic gonorrhea.

Pu-Chi-Chien-Chung-Tang 補氣健中湯

(Magnolia and Alisma Combination)

Hoelen	4.0	Citrus	3.0	Ginseng	4.0
Magnolia bark	2.0	Alisma	2.0	Ophiopogon	2.0
White atractylodes	4.0	Scute	2.0	Atractylodes	3.0

Pu-chi-chien-chung-tang is recorded in *Chi sheng fang* (濟生方). This formula is used for treating edema and ascites in those of "weak conformation". Patients in whom edema increases after taking *Hsiao-chien-chung-tang* (Minor Cinnamon and Peony Combination) or *Pu-chung-i-chi-tang* (Ginseng and Astragalus Combination) should use this formula.

Herbs and Actions

Ginseng, Atractylodes, and Hoelen of *Szu-chun-tzu-tang* (Major Four Herb Combination) nourish the spleen and stomach, and improve gastric functioning. Atractylodes, Magnolia bark, and Citrus of *Ping-wei-san* (Magnolia and Ginger Formula) remove stagnant water in the stomach. Scute dispels internal heat, Alisma and Ophiopogon are diuretics, and they coordinate the actions of Atractylodes and Hoelen to eliminate edema. Magnolia bark returns the stagnant *ch'i* to normal.

Indications

Edema, ascites, swelling, cirrhosis, chronic peritonitis, chronic nephritis, and edema due to valvular disease.

Weak conformation

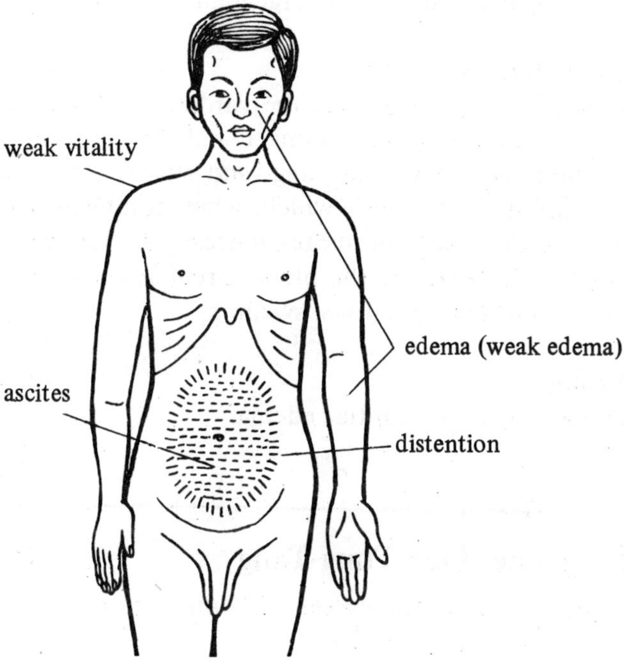

Shih-Pi-Yin					實脾飲
(Magnolia and Atractylodes Combination)					
Magnolia bark	4.0	Atractylodes	4.0	Areca	4.0
Chaenomeles	4.0	Aconite	4.0	Hoelen	4.0
Saussurea	4.0	Ginger	4.0	Licorice	2.0
Cochin Cardamon	4.0				

Shih-pi-yin is recorded in *Chi sheng fang* (濟生方) of the

Sung dynasty. This formula is used to warm the yang, strengthen the spleen, dissipate moisture, and reduce swelling. It is suitable for edema due to yang weakness of the spleen and kidneys. The conformation is manifested by anascara, distention in the chest and abdomen, chills in the limbs, lack of thirst, watery stool, and copious and clear urine. In addition, there is white and wet tongue fur and a submerged and slow pulse.

Herbs and Actions

Atractylodes, Saussurea, Cochin cardamon, Magnolia bark and Licorice are all stomachics. Ginger and Aconite warm the body, dispel chills, stimulate the yang, and suppress the yin. Chaenomeles is an alterative herb which, when combined with Aconite, strengthens the heart, promotes diuresis, stimulates all the body functions, and regulates the blood circulation. Areca and Hoelen are diuretics which can reduce swelling.

Indications

Chronic nephritis and cardiac edema.

Tang-Kuei-Lien-Tung-Tang 當歸拈痛湯

(Tang-kuei and Anemarrhena Combination)

Tang-kuei	2.5	Anemarrhena	2.5	*Chianghuo*	2.5
Capillaris	2.5	Atractylodes	2.0	Scute	2.5
Polyporus	2.5	Alisma	2.5	Siler	2.0
Pueraria	2.0	Ginseng	2.0	Sophora	1.0
White atractylodes	2.5	Licorice	1.0	Cimicifuga	1.0

Tang-kuei-lien-tung-tang is recorded in *Lan shih mi tsang* (蘭室秘藏). This formula is used for treating arthralgia due to "moist heat", dermatitis of the legs with suppuration; generalized pain; shoulder stiffness; chest pain; melasma; gonorrhea; and eczema in the genital areas.

Herbs and Actions
Siler, *Chianghuo*, and Cimicifuga are antiphlogistics. Alisma, Polyporus, and Atractylodes are diuretics. Pueraria, Scute, Sophora, Anemarrhena, Licorice, and Capillaris are antipyretics. *Tang-kuei* is an anti-inflammative and analgesic. Ginseng nourishes the body and *ch'i.* Atractylodes nourishes the spleen and dispels moisture.

Indications
Arthralgia with swelling, generalized swelling and pain, dermatitis in the lower limbs, beriberi, and scabies.

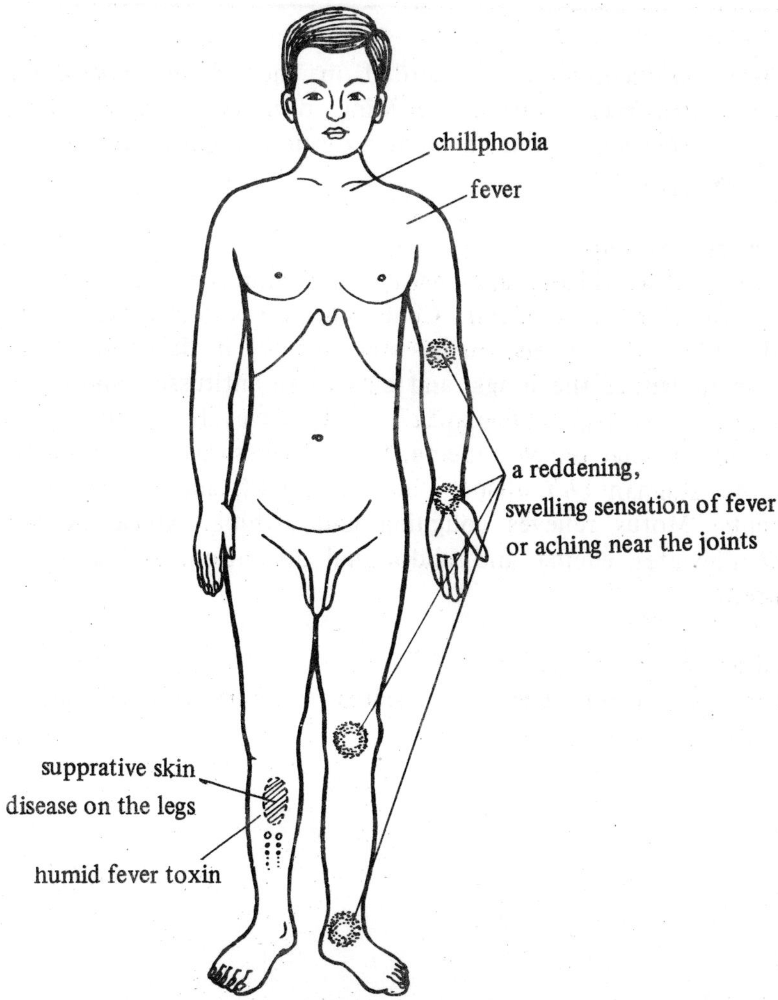

Tao-Shui-Fu-Ling-Tang 導水茯苓湯

(Hoelen, Atractylodes, and Areca Combination)

Hoelen	3.0	Atractylodes	3.0	Alisma	3.0
Morus	1.0	Ophiopogon	5.0	Perilla	1.0
Areca	1.0	Cardamon	3.0	Saussurea	1.0
Juncus	1.0	Chaenomeles	2.0	Areca seed	2.0
Citrus	1.5				

Tao-shui-fu-ling-tang was recorded in the *Cheng chih chuen sheng* (證治準繩) during the Ming dynasty. This formula is used for treating asthma, anascara, dysuria, oliguria, and kidney diseases.

Herbs and Actions

Hoelen, Atractyldoes, and Alisma are diuretics that eliminate excessive thirst and edema. Chaenomeles is effective for edema and beriberi. Areca seed dispels stagnant *ch'i* in the chest. Ophiopogon nourishes the lungs, and acts as an antitussive and expectorant. Perilla dispels stagnant *ch'i* and relieves distention. Juncus is a diuretic that relieves edema. Citrus, Saussurea, and Cardamon remove stagnant *ch'i*, dispel "internal heat", and act as expectorants. Morus relieves coughing and asthma. Areca increases *ch'i*, alleviates edema and abdominal distention, and acts as a diuretic.

Indications

Nephritis, chronic nephritis, ascites, beriberi, and edema due to valvular disease.

Edema of a semi-weak and a semi-firm conformation

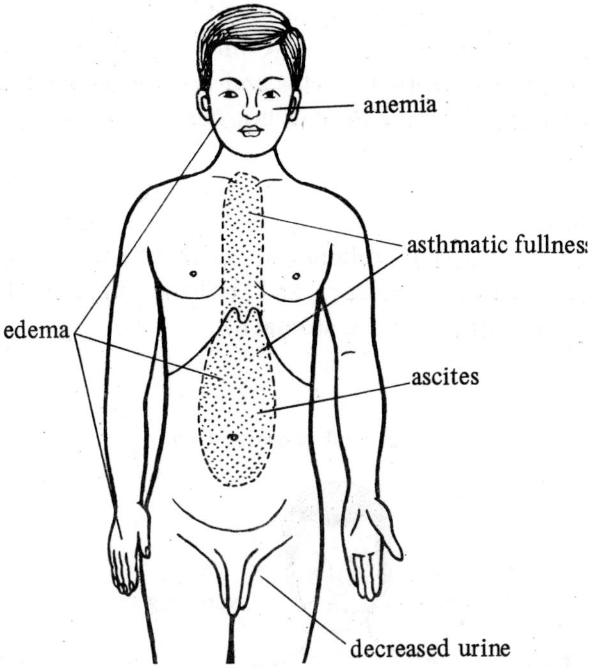

Ting-Hsiang-Fu-Ling-Tang *(Clove and Hoelen Combination)*				丁香茯苓湯	
Hoelen	6.0	Pinellia	6.0	Cinnamon	3.0
Citrus	3.0	Ginger	1.5	Cardamon	1.5
Clove	1.0	Aconite	0.5		

Used to treat gastric water stagnancy and stagnated sour water that causes aching. Commonly used for vomiting of phlegm or sour water and the inability to eat, in patients with gastric ulcers who have a soft and weak pulse, a weak abdomen, extreme debility, and thinness.

Herbs and Actions

Clove treats heart and abdominal pain. Pinellia, Hoelen, and Citrus remove subcardiac water stagnancy. Cardamon harmonizes the stomach, opens obstructed breathing passages, helps digestion, and arrests vomiting. Cinnamon warms and stimulates the pulse rate. Aconite activates and revives reduced and deteriorated metabolism. Dry ginger, a hot herb, also revives the metabolic function.

Indications

Gastric ulcers, gastric dilatation, gastroptosis (prolapse of the stomach), stomach cancer, and pyloric stenosis (obstruction of the pyloric orifice of the stomach).

Weak and chill conformation

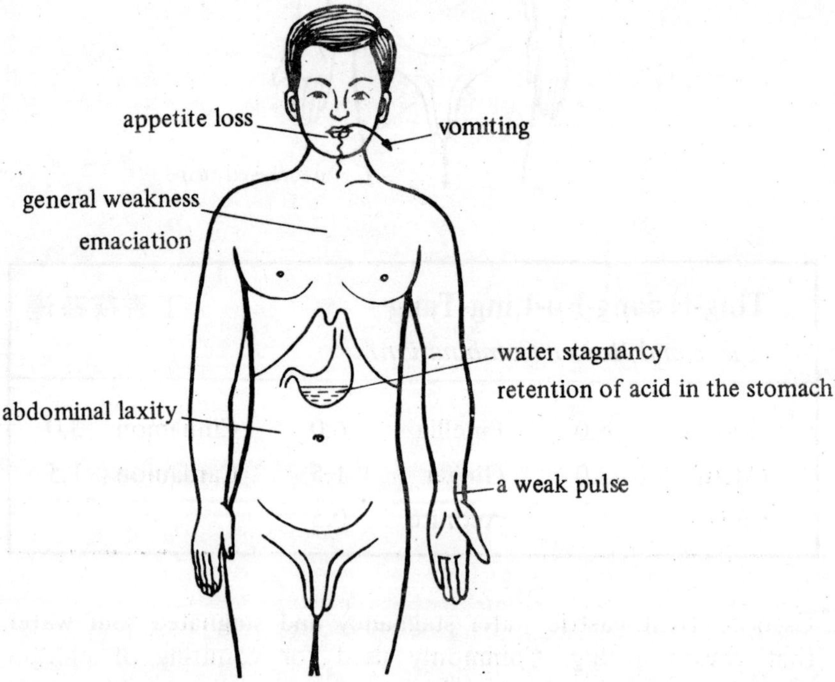

Tse-Hsieh-Tang 澤瀉湯

(Alisma Combination)

Alisma	5.0	Atractylodes	2.0

Tse-hsieh-tang was recorded in the *Chin kuei yao lueh* (金匱要略) during the Han dynasty. This formula is used for treating severe vertigo and a feeling of excess fluid in the epigastric area which is thought to be due to an imbalance in all the body fluids.

Herbs and Actions
Alisma, the major herb in this formula, acts as a diuretic to dispel "water poisoning" and relieve vertigo. Atractylodes nourishes the *ch'i* in the spleen.

Indications
Vertigo, chronic headaches, Meniere's disease, gastroptosis, abdominal distention, and hypertension.

Discrimination
Ling-kuei-chu-kan-tang (Atractylodes and Hoelen Combination): congestion beneath the heart, vertigo, distention and obstruction in the chest, stagnant water in the stomach, a shaky feeling.
Hsiao-pan-hsia-chia-fu-ling-tang (Minor Pinellia and Hoelen Combination): stagnant water beneath the heart, vertigo, palpitations, vomiting.

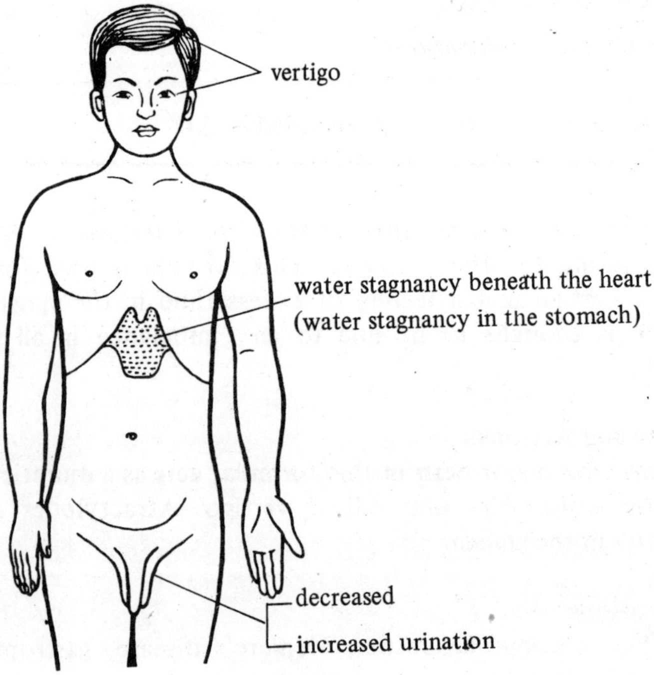

Wei-Ling-Tang *(Magnolia and Hoelen Combination)*					胃苓湯
Atractylodes	2.5	Magnolia	2.5	Citrus	2.5
Jujube	1.5	Ginger	1.5	Licorice	1.0
Hoelen	2.5	Polyporus	2.5	Alisma	2.5
Cinnamon	2.0	White atractylodes	2.5		

Wei-ling-tang is recorded in the three Chinese medical works of the Ming dynasty; *Ku chin i chien* (古今醫鑑), *Wan. ping hui chun* (萬病回春), and *Cheng chih chuen sheng* (證治準繩). This formula is suitable for water toxin with diarrhea due to acute gastritis or heatstroke, abdominal pain, abdominal distention, thirst, edema, and dysuria.

Herbs and Actions

This formula is a combination of the *Ping-wei-san* (Magnolia and Fennel Formula) and *Wu-ling-san* (Hoelen Five Herb Formula). Atractylodes, Magnolia, Citrus, Jujube, Ginger, and Licorice in *Ping-wei-san* regulate *ch'i*, nourish the stomach, improve digestion, and dispel sputum. Atractylodes, Hoelen, Polyporus, Alisma, and Cinnamon in *Wu-ling-san* can dispel moisture and nourish the spleen.

Indications

Acute gastritis, acute enteritis, colitis, acute nephritis, abdominal pain, diarrhea, edema, and attacks of neuralgia during the summer.

Discrimination

Ping-wei-san (Magnolia and Ginger Formula): disharmony between spleen and stomach, abdominal pain, mild diarrhea, no thirst.

Wei-feng-tang (Atractylodes and Setaria Combination): watery stools, stools with blood, and spasms of the hands and feet.

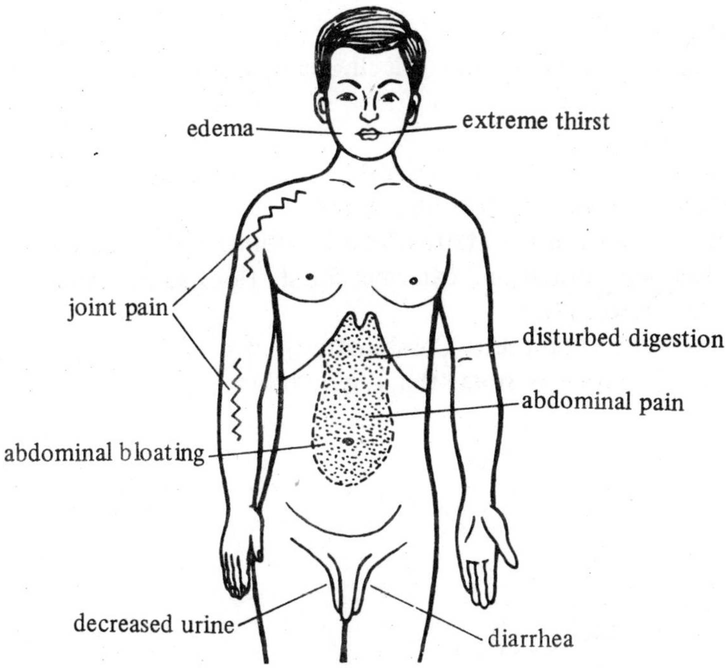

Wu-Lin-San 五淋散

(Gardenia and Hoelen Formula)

Hoelen	6.0	*Tang-kuei*	3.0	Licorice	3.0
Peony	2.0	Gardenia	2.0		

Wu-lin-san was recorded in the *Tai ping huei min ho chi chu fang* (太平惠民和劑局方) during the Sung dynasty. This formula is used for treating "internal heat" in the bladder, dysuria, acute pain in the umbilicus and abdomen, fatigue, urinary gravel, dark colored urine, and hematuria.

Herbs and Actions
Hoelen is an antipyretic, antiphlogistic, and diuretic. *Tang-kuei* and Peony relieve "blood dryness". Gardenia is a diuretic and antiphlogistic that reduces chest distention and improves liver function. Licorice nourishes the *ch'i*.

Indications
Urethritis, cystitis, vesical calculi, renal calculi, and gonorrhea.

Discrimination
Pa-cheng-san (Dianthus Formula): urinary stuttering, bladder fever, constipation, firm conformation.
Ching-hsin-lien-tzu-yin (Lotus Seed Combination): urinary stuttering, frequent urination, extreme thirst, flourishing upper body but weak lower body.
Chu-ling-tang (Polyporus Combination): decreased urine, painful urinary stuttering, extreme thirst, irritability, edema.

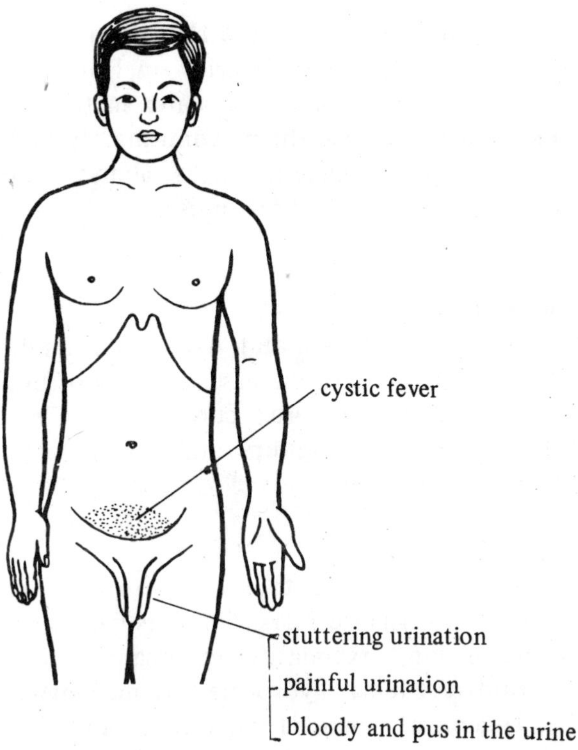
cystic fever
stuttering urination
painful urination
bloody and pus in the urine

Wu-Ling-San 五苓散

(Hoelen Five Herb Formula)

Polyporus	4.5	Hoelen	4.5	Alisma	6.0
Atractylodes	4.5	Cinnamon	3.0		

Both the medical dictionary of the Han dynasty, *Shang han lun* and *Chin kuei yao lueh* (Summaries on Household Drugs, 205 A.D.) list *Wu-ling-san* for stagnant water in the stomach due to watery metabolic disorder, thirst, vomiting, dysuria, flushing up, palpitations, vertigo, anxiety, headache, abdominal pain, diarrhea, edema, fever, and floating and fast pulses.

Herbs and Actions

Alisma, Polyporus, Hoelen, and Atractylodes relieve fluid accumulation in the stomach, increase the flow of urine, and dispel edema. Alisma and Polyporus cure thirst. Cinnamon dispels surface heat, cures flushing up, and acts in conjunction with the other herbs as a diuretic.

Indications

Vomiting and diarrhea due to a common cold, acute gastroenteritis, gastrectosis, gastric relaxation, gastroptosis, diabetes, seasickness, indigestion, toxemia during pregnancy, hypersalivation, nephritis, cardiac edema, hydrocele, uremia, migraine, recurrent headache, trigeminal neuralgia, vital conjunctivitis, dacrocystitis, nyctalopia, blisters, and varicella.

Discrimination

Chu-ling-tang (Polyporus Combination): decreased urine; extreme thirst; dry mouth, tongue, and skin; distress; pain on urination; blood disease; discomfort at night; no water congestion.
Fu-ling-tse-hsieh-tang (Alisma, Hoelen, and Ginger Combination): extreme thirst, water stagnancy in the stomach, vomiting, and alternation of temperament.

Pa-wei-wan (Rehmannia Eight Formula): extreme thirst, decreased urine, numbness beneath the umbilicus.
Pai-hu-chia-jen-sheng-tang (Ginseng and Gypsum Combination): extreme thirst, massive and big pulse, no vomiting.
Ling-kuei-chu-kan-tang (Atractylodes and Hoelen Combination): vertigo, water stagnancy in the stomach, submerged and tense pulse, no thirst or vomiting.
Fu-ling-kan-tsao-tang (Licorice and Hoelen Combination): water stagnancy in the stomach, cold hands and feet, cardiac palpitations, palpitations beneath the heart.
Wu-chu-yu-tang (Evoida Combination): headache, water stagnancy in the stomach, cold hands and feet, severe irritability, severe vomiting, submerged and slow pulse.
Yin-chen-hao-tang (Capillaris Combination): decreased urine, extreme thirst, irritability, mild abdominal distention.
Yueh-pei-chia-chu-tang (Atractylodes Combination): fever, asthmatic cough, no fever, edema, spontaneous perspiration, decreased urine.
Hsiao-ching-lung-tang (Minor Blue Dragon Combination): pallid facial complexion, obesity, cough and asthma due to the common cold, fever due to kidney disease, dry vomiting, edema, decreased urine.

Surface fever and interior water conformation

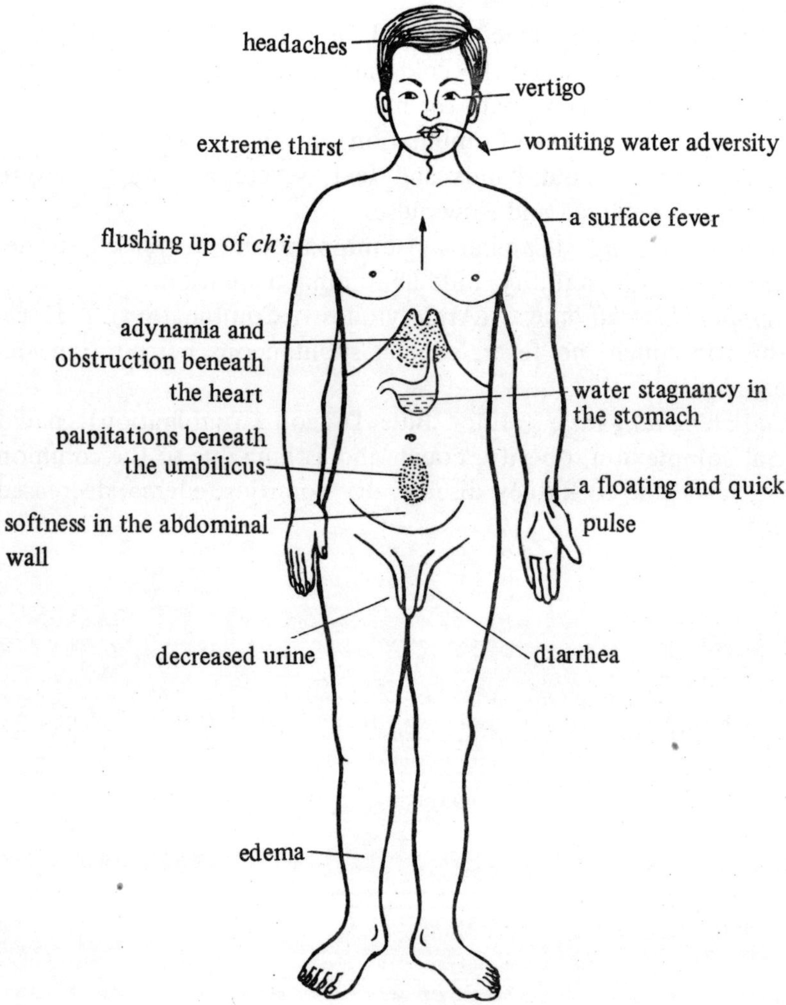

Wu-Pi-Yin 五皮飲

(Hoelen and Areca Combination)

Hoelen	9.0	Citrus	6.0	Morus	6.0
Areca	9.0	Ginger	3.0		

Wu-pi-yin is recorded in *Tang tou ko chueh* (湯頭歌訣). This formula acts as an antiphlogistic and is used for treating dropsy, distention in the chest and abdomen, rapid breathing, dysuria, and generalized edema during pregnancy.

Herbs and Actions

Hoelen is a diuretic. Morus is an antipyretic and diuretic, and it is an effective treatment for asthma. Areca is also a diuretic. Citrus and Ginger are stomachics and diaphoretics.

Indications

Generalized edema, asthma, nephritis, cardiac edema, and edema during pregnancy.

Yin-Chen-Hao-Tang 茵陳蒿湯

(Capillaris Combination)

Capillaris	4.0	Gardenia	3.0	Rhubarb	1.0

Yin-chen-hao-tang was recorded in the Chinese medical works *Shang han lun* (傷寒論) and *Chin kuei yao lueh* (金匱要略) during the Han dynasty. This formula is used for treating jaundice, distention in the upper abdomen, discomfort in the chest cavity, nausea, thirst, dysuria, constipation, and dark-colored urine.

Herbs and Actions

Capillaris is an antiphlogistic and diuretic, effective for stagnant heat and jaundice. Gardenia is also an antiphlogistic and diuretic, effective for stagnant heat, jaundice, and distention in the chest near the heart. Rhubarb is a laxative and antipyretic.

Indications

Jaundice, acute hepatitis, nephritis, edema, beriberi, stomatitis, urticaria, pruritus, gingivitis, ophthalmic disorders, and uterine bleeding.

Discrimination

Yin-chen-wu-ling-san (Capillaris and Hoelen Formula): jaundice, mild weak conformation, extreme thirst and decreased urine. *Hsiao-chai-hu-tang* (Minor Bupleurum Combination), *Ta-chai-hu-tang* (Major Bupleurum Combination): hardness and fullness beneath the heart and hypochondrium; thoraco-costal distress and vomiting.

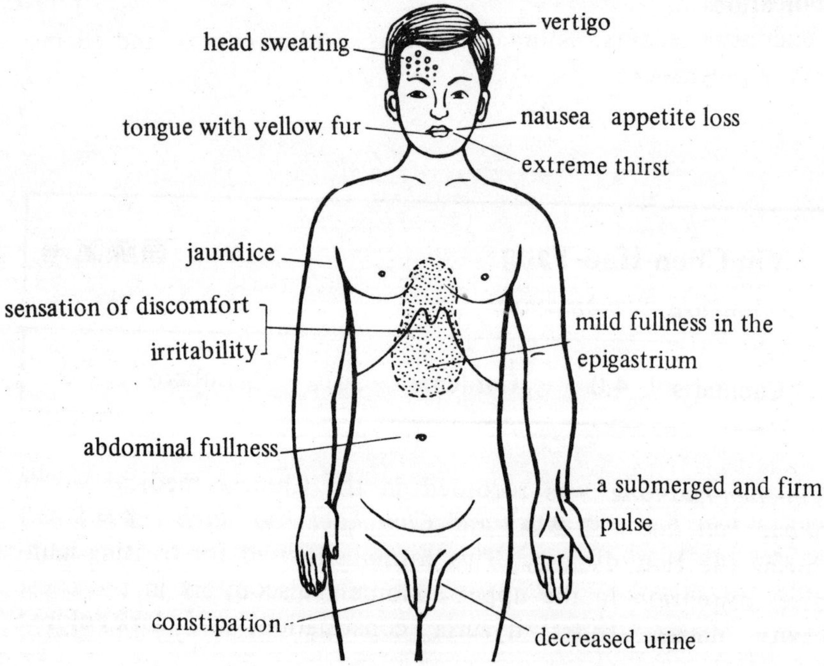

Yin-Chen-Wu-Ling-San 茵陳五苓散

(Capillaris and Hoelen Formula)

Capillaris	6.0	Cinnamon	3.0	Polyporus	4.5
Hoelen	4.5	Atractylodes	4.5	Alisma	4.0

Yin-chen-wu-ling-san is a combination of *Wu-ling-san* (Hoelen Five Herb Formula) with Capillaris and is recorded in both *Chin kuei yao lueh* (金匱要略) and *Cheng chih chuen sheng* (證治準繩). This formula is used to treat liver disturbances, jaundice, thirst, dark-colored urine, abdominal bloating, restlessness, and fever.

Herbs and Actions

Capillaris is an antiphlogistic and diuretic that is effective for jaundice. Alismà, Polyporus, Hoelen, and Atractylodes remove stagnant water from the stomach and intestine. Alisma and Polyporus cure excessive thirst. Cinnamon relieves the sensation of surface fever and synthesizes the actions of the other herbs.

Indications

Jaundice, hepatitis, nephritis, kidney atrophy, and stagnant water in the stomach.

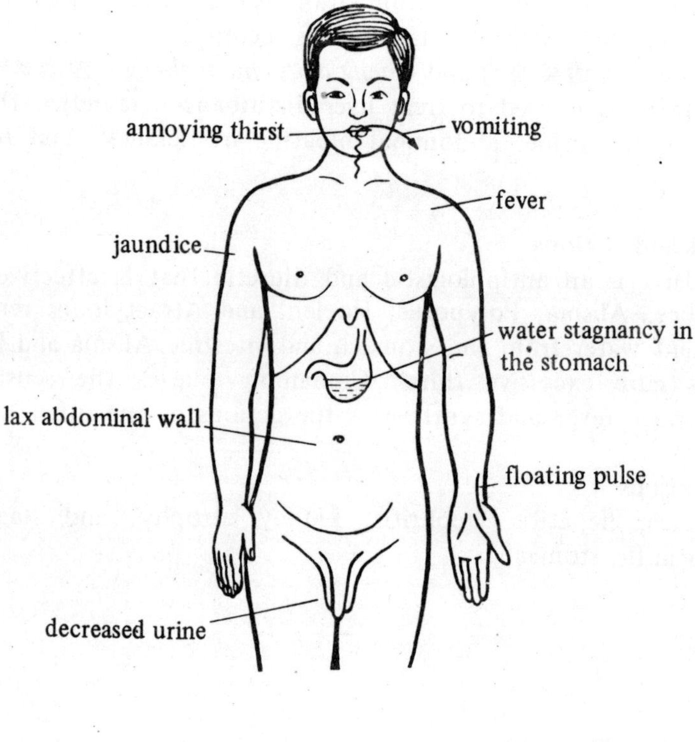
annoying thirst
vomiting
fever
jaundice
water stagnancy in the stomach
lax abdominal wall
floating pulse
decreased urine

Yueh-Pi-Chia-Chu-Tang *(Atractylodes Combination)*					越婢加朮湯
Ma-huang	6.0	Gypsum	8.0	Jujube	3.0
Licorice	2.0	Atractylodes	4.0	Ginger	3.0

Recorded in *Chin kuei yao lueh* (金匱要略) of the Han dynasty. Used for treating dysuria, skin problems, hidrosis, and weakness in the waist and feet.

Herbs and Actions

Ma-huang nourishes the lungs. *Ma-huang* together with Gypsum is an antihidrotic. Gypsum removes internal heat. Gypsum with Ginger relieves muscular swelling. Jujube and Licorice nourish the spleen and stomach.

Indications

Nephritis, dermatic nephritis, beriberi, arthritis, rheumatism, hydrocele, keratitis, nebula, inguinal tinea, polyps, weak and aching feet, and jaundice.

Discrimination

Mu-fang-chi-tang (Stephania and Ginseng Combination): edema, obstruction and hardness beneath the heart.

Ta-ching-lung-tang (Major Blue Dragon Combination): edema, floating pulse, asthmatic cough, anxiety.

Pa-wei-wan (Rehmannia Eight Formula): weakness of the feet, numbness beneath the umbilicus.

Fang-chi-huang-chi-tang (Stephania and Astragalus Combination): edema, flabby skin, weak conformation.

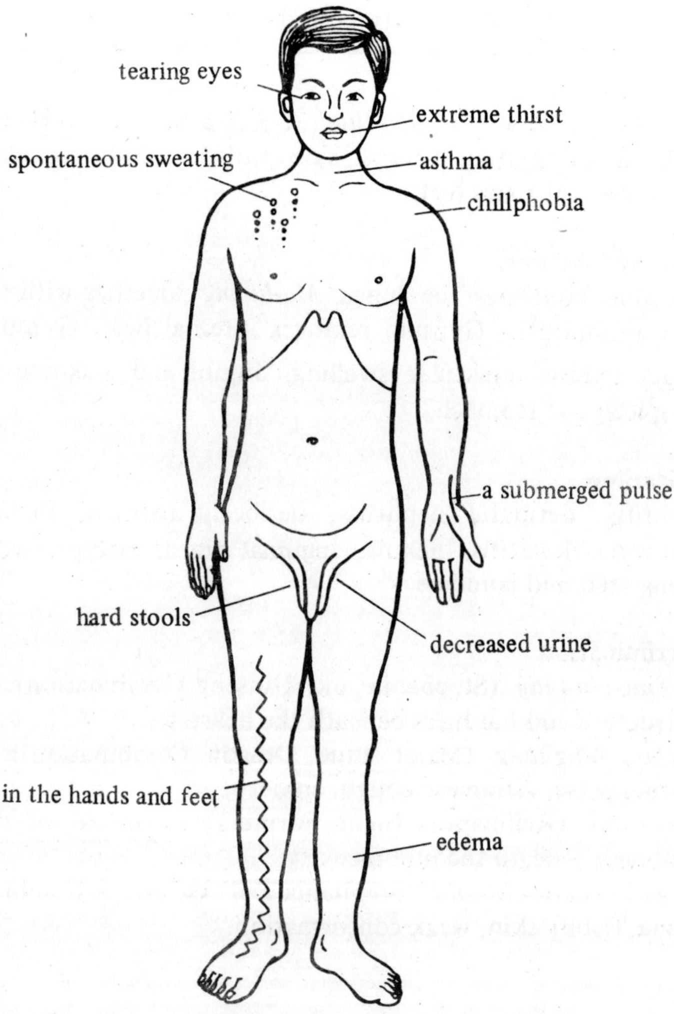
tearing eyes
extreme thirst
spontaneous sweating
asthma
chillphobia
a submerged pulse
hard stools
decreased urine
pain in the hands and feet
edema

Yueh-Pi-Chia-Pan-Hsia-Tang 越婢加半夏湯

(Ma-huang, Gypsum and Pinellia Combination)

Ma-huang	6.0	Gypsum	8.0	Ginger	3.0
Jujube	3.0	Licorice	2.0	Pinellia	5.0

Recorded in *Chin kuei yao lueh* (金匱要略): "The external contraction of wind and heat with the internal action of water stagnancy causes pulmonary distention and an up-rushing of fluids accompanied by a fever. As a consequence the patient will have a cough, up-flushing of gas, asthma, bulging eyes, and a buoyant and big pulse. *Yueh-pi-chia-pan-hsia-tang* disperses the blockage in the lungs, expels the fever, calms the adverse air and gas, and suppresses the asthma."

Herbs and Actions

High doses of *Ma-huang* and Gypsum, which are acrid and cooling, are capable of evaporating water and cleansing internal fever. Ginger and Pinellia disperse water and settle adverse air and gas. Licorice and jujube harmonize all the herbs and stabilize the insides.

Indications

Asthma, chronic bronchitis, pulmonary emphysema, "pregnancy kidney," a severe cough that causes facial edema and ocular swelling and thirst, and oliguria.

Yueh-Pi-Tang 越婢湯

(Ma-huang and Gypsum Combination)

Ma-huang	6.0	Gypsum	8.0	Jujube	3.0
Licorice	2.0	Ginger	3.0		

Yueh-pi-tang is recorded in *Chin kuei yao lueh* (金匱要略) of the Han dynasty. This formula is used for treating the initial stage of dropsy in which there is a floating pulse, diaphoresis, edema, asthma, coughing, dysuria, and thirst.

Herbs and Actions
Ma-huang and Gypsum are anhidrotics. Gypsum relieves internal heat, and a combination with Ginger can decrease muscular swelling. Jujube and Licorice nourish the *ch'i* of the spleen and stomach.

Indications
Dropsy, primary nephritis, dermatic nephritis, arthritis of the lower limbs, carbuncles, beriberi, and edema.

Discrimination
Ta-ching-lung-tang (Major Blue Dragon Combination): asthmatic cough, anxiety, extreme thirst, sweating, floating and tense pulse.
Ma-hsing-kan-shih-tang (*Ma-huang* and Apricot Seed Combination): asthma, extreme thirst in the absence of edema.
Hsiao-ching-lung-tang (Minor Blue Dragon Combination): asthmatic cough and external fever.
Fang-chi-huang-chi-tang (Stephania and Astragalus Combination): edema, spontaneous sweating, obesity, feeling of body heaviness, submerged pulse.

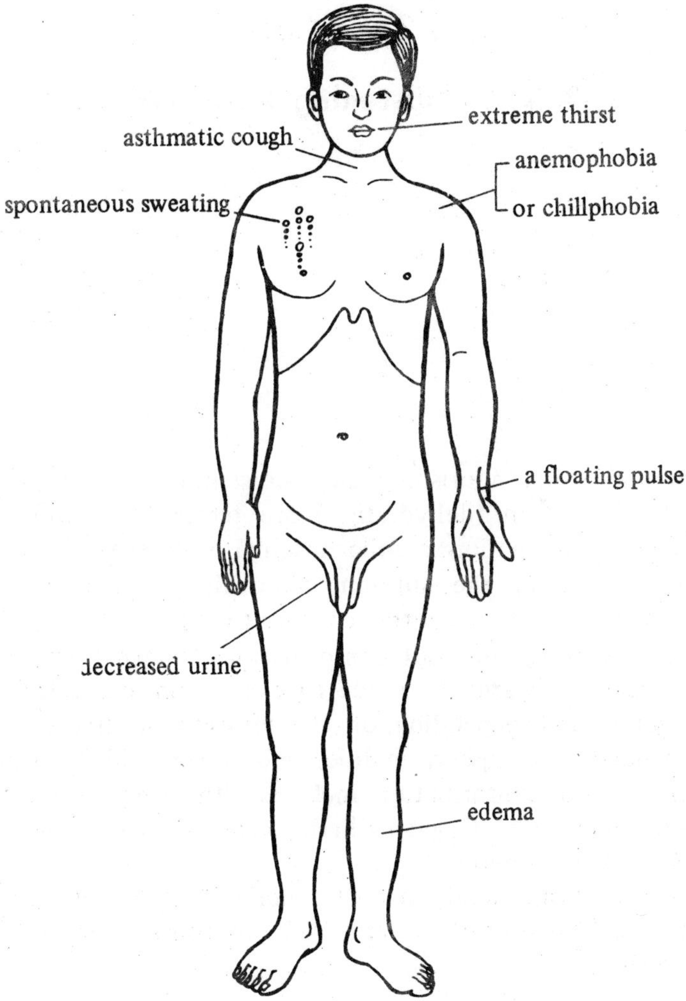
extreme thirst
asthmatic cough
anemophobia
or chillphobia
spontaneous sweating
a floating pulse
decreased urine
edema

18.
Jun Tsao Chi
(潤燥劑, Moistening Formulas)

Formulas using nourishing and moistening herbs to treat an arid conformation (dehydration) are termed *jun tsao chi.*

An arid conformation is either internal or external. External aridity occurs during the autumn. Since the autumn weather may be warm or cool, a contracted harmful toxin will manifest itself in either warm or cool conformations. Internal aridity is also either cool or warm. It is due to exhaustion and a lack of visceral fluids, and depending on the location of illness, it is further divided into upper, middle, and lower aridity. Treatment for an arid conformation includes either moistening the aridity with light herbs dispersing herbs or moistening the aridity with sweet and chilly herbs.

Obviously both acrid, aromatic herbs that exhaust saliva and bitter, chilly herbs that harm *ch'i* are contraindicated for aridity diseases.

Chih-Kan-Tsao-Tang 炙甘草湯

(Baked Licorice Combination)

Baked licorice	3.0	Jujube	3.0	Gelatin	2.0
Ginger	3.0	Ginseng	3.0	Rehmannia	6.0
Linum	3.0	Ophiopogon	6.0	Cinnamon	3.0

Chih-kan-tsao-tang was recorded in the *Shang han lun* (傷寒論) during the Han dynasty. This formula is used for treating palpitations, hyperpnea, stagnant pulse, irregular pulse, coarse skin, fever in the hands and feet due to stress, a tendency toward fatigue, and thirst.

Herbs and Actions

Licorice alleviates acute symptoms in the heart and lungs. Jujube nourishes the heart and relieves hyperpnea. Ophiopogon nourishes the lungs. Linum promotes evacuation. Rehmannia dispels "internal heat" in the heart and the blood. Gelatin alleviates stress and checks bleeding. Ginseng is a sialagogue. Cinnamon nourishes the blood. Ginger nourishes *ch'i.*

Indications

Valvular disease, palpitations, anemia, endocarditis, Basedow's disease, anxiety, hypertension, arteriosclerosis, tuberculosis, and postpartum fever.

Discrimination

Chu-yeh-shih-kao-tang (Bamboo Leaf and Gypsum Combination): gasping and excessive thirst.

Huang-lien-an-chiao-tang (Coptis and Gelatin Combination): discomfort, feverish peeling, anxiety, abdominal pain, and black stools.

Hsiao-chien-chung-tang (Minor Cinnamon and Peony Combination): weakness, fatigability, acute pain in the abdomen and abdominal skin.

Kuei-chih-chia-lung-ku-mu-li-tang (Cinnamon and Dragon Bone

Combination): weakness, fatigability, palpitations in the chest and abdomen and beneath the umbilicus.

Pa-wei-wan (Rehmannia Eight Formula): weakness, fatigability, numbness beneath the umbilicus, decreased urine.

Chai-hu-kuei-chih-kan-chiang-tang (Bupleurum, Cinnamon, and Ginger Combination): palpitations, stagnancy beneath the hypochondrium, head sweating.

San-wu-huang-chin-tang (Scute Three Herb Combination): discomfort in the heart and chest, annoying fever in the arms and legs, and abdominal weakness.

Mai-men-tung-tang (Ophiopogon Combination): gasping and the severe upward congestion of *ch'i*.

Weak yang conformation

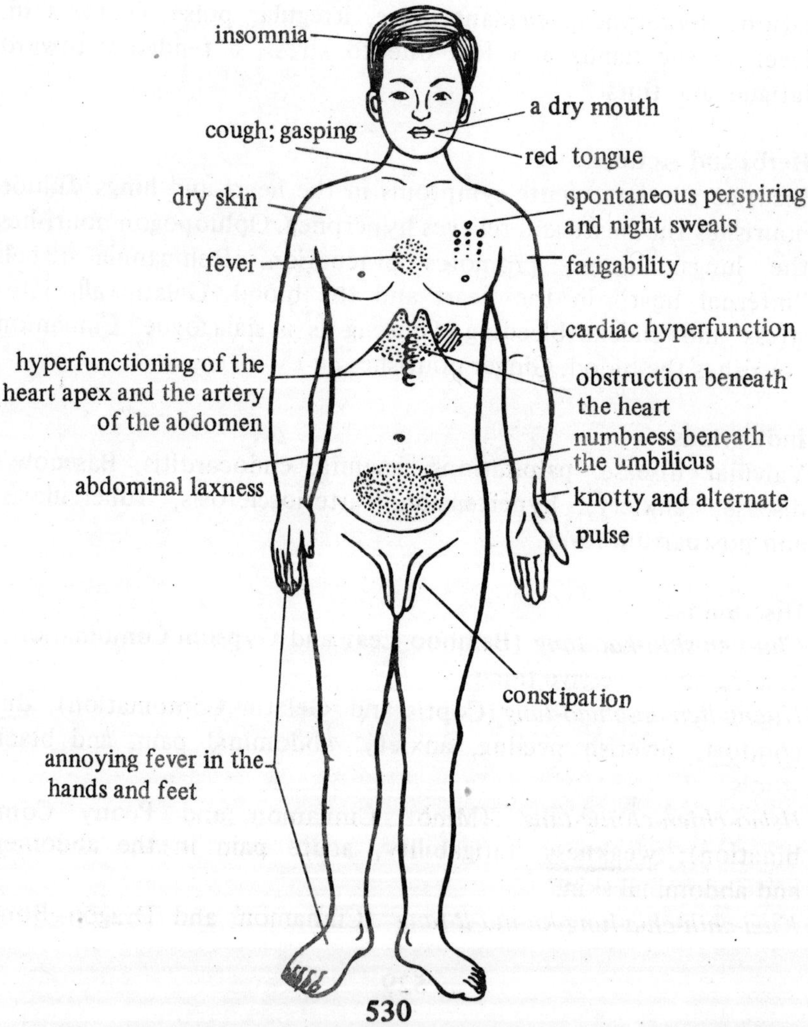

Ching-Je-Pu-Hsieh-Tang 清熱補血湯

(Cnidium and Moutan Combination)

Tang-kuei	3.0	Peony	3.0	Cnidium	3.0
Anemarrhena	1.5	Rehmannia	3.0	Ophiopogon	3.0
Phellodendron	1.5	Figwort	1.5	Moutan	1.5
Schizandra	1.5	Bupleurum	1.5		

Ching-je-pu-hsieh-tang is recorded in *Cheng chih chuen sheng* (證治準繩) of the Ming dynasty. This formula is a hematinic, nourishing the blood and expelling fever from it. It is suitable for treating stomatitis, anemia,lack of stamina, dry skin, and fever in the blood.

Herbs and Actions

Tang-kuei, Peony, Cnidium, and Rehmannia of *Szu-wu-tang* (*Tang-kuei* Four Combination) are hematinics which nourish the blood. Schizandra and Ophiopogon produce an increase of body fluids, thereby relieving dryness. Figwort, Anemarrhena, and Coptis relieve the fever in the stomach. Figwort is especially effective in reducing fever of the mouth and throat while also acting as a nutritive. Bupleurum reduces fever in the liver. Moutan reduces blood fever.

Indications

Ulcerative stomatitis, ulcerated tongue due to aphthous stomatitis or postnatal blood dryness, and pyelitis; ulcerative stomatitis due to Behcet's diseases and Vincent's infection.

Discrimination

Pa-wei-wan (Rehmannia Eight Formula): tongue erosion, postpartum blood fever, annoying fever in the soles, and extreme thirst.

Chia-wei-hsiao-yao-san (Bupleurum and Peony Formula): tongue and mouth abscesses which occur during pregnancy; depressed *ch'i*, and weakness and fever.

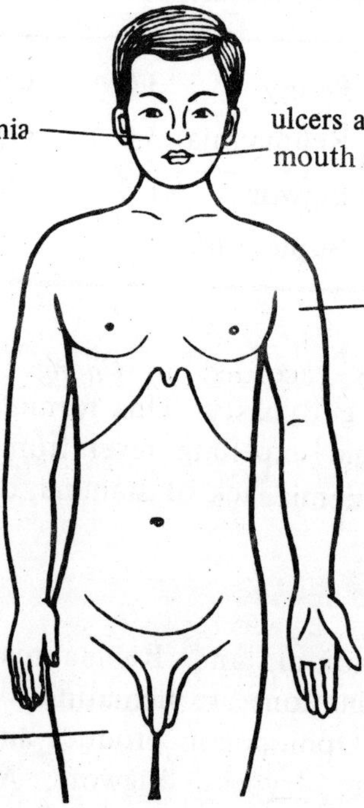

Ching-Tsao-Chiu-Fei-Tang 清燥救肺湯

(Eriobotrya and Ophiopogon Combination)

Ginseng	2.0	Ophiopogon	3.6	Sesame	2.4
Apricot seed	2.0	Eriobotrya	6.0	Gypsum	9.0
Licorice	2.4	Gelatin	2.4		

Ching-tsao-chiu-fei-tang was recorded in the *I men fa lu* (醫門法律) by Yu Chang during the Ching dynasty. This formula is used for treating headache, fever, hacking cough, flushing up, asthma, dry throat, restlessness, thirst, and dryness of the tongue when there is no sputum or tongue fur.

Herbs and Actions
Gypsum and Ophiopogon dispel "internal heat" in the lungs. Apricot seed and Eriobotrya dispel *ch'i* in the lungs. Gelatin and Sesame nourish the lungs. Ginseng and Licorice nourish the *ch'i* and act as sialgogues.

Indications
Acute and chronic infectious diseases, influenza, asthma, hacking cough, and hemoptysis.

Jun-Chang-Tang 潤腸湯

(Linum and Rhubarb Combination)

Rhubarb	2.0	Linum	2.0	*Tang-kuei*	3.0
Persica	2.0	Apricot seed	2.0	*Chih-shih*	2.0
Scute	2.0	Magnolia bark	2.0	Licorice	1.5
Cured rehmannia	3.0		Raw rehmannia		3.0

Jun-chang-tang is recorded in *Wan ping hui chun* (萬病回春) of the Ming dynasty. This formula is used for treating acute and chronic constipation, coarse skin, a sensation of stiffness in the abdomen, flaccidity in the abdominal wall, and dry stools resembling rabbit excrement. It is suitable for the elderly, since even frequent use will not bring about harmful side effects.

Herbs and Actions
Tang-kuei and cured Rehmannia are "warm" in nature, treat "Blood dryness", and help produce new blood. Raw Rehmannia and Scute dispel "blood heat" and nourish "blood dryness". Linum, Apricot seed, and Persica nourish the intestines and remove stagnant *ch'i* and "stagnant blood". *Chih-shih* and Magnolia bark remove gas from the intestine. Rhubarb and Scute dispel intestinal heat and help evacuation.

Indications

Habitual constipation, constipation in the elderly, and constipation due to hypertension, arteriosclerosis, and chronic nephritis.

Discrimination

Ma-tzu-jen-wan (Apricot Seed and Linum Formula): constipation, deficiency of body fluid frequent urination, floating and harsh pulse.

Weak conformation

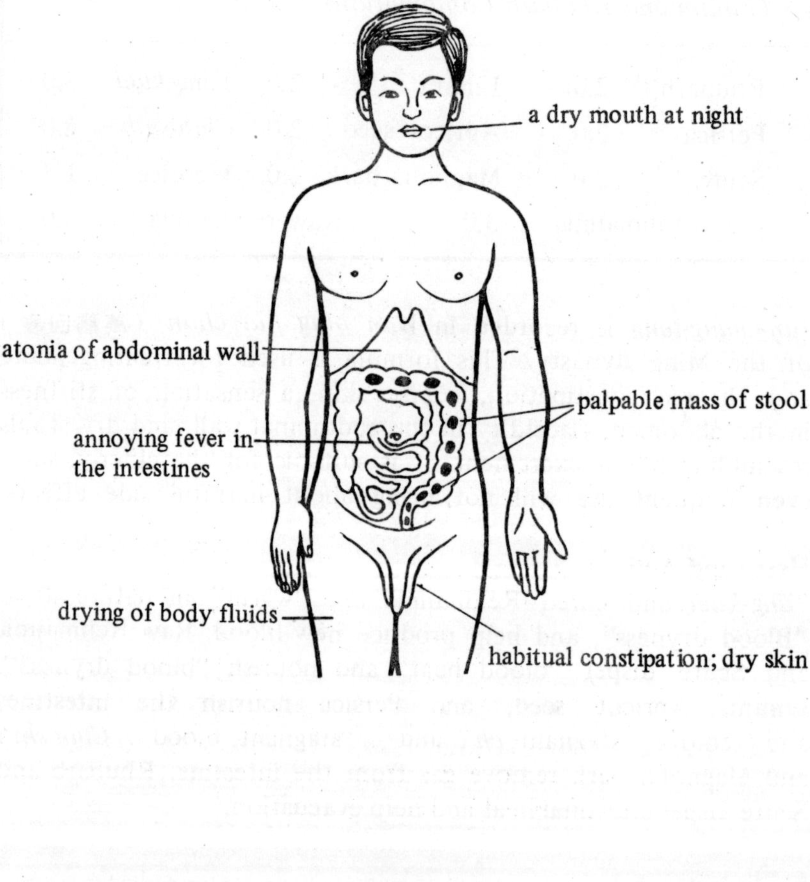

Ma-Tzu-Jen-Wan 麻子仁丸

(Apricot Seed and Linum Formula)

Linum	5.0	Rhubarb	4.0	Peony	2.0
Magnolia bark	2.0	Apricot seed	2.0	*Chih-shih*	2.0

Ma-tzu-jen-wan is recorded in Chinese medical works *Shang han lun* (On General Diseases) and *Chin kuei yao lueh* (Summaries on Household Drugs) by Chang Chung-ching (A.D. 142-220) of the Han dynasty. This formula is suitable for gastrointestinal heat, dry stool, frequent urination, floating pulse, hemorrhoids, and constipation. It is good for the elderly and those with a delicate constitution and dry skin.

Herbs and Actions

Rhubarb, *Chih-shih,* and Magnolia bark of *Hsiao-cheng-chi-tang* (Minor Rhubarb Combination) relieves intense gastrointestinal heat and help smooth evacuation. Linum and Apricot seed are nutritive. Peony relieves constipation.

Indications

Habitual constipation, constipation in the elderly, nocturia, constipation due to atrophic kidney, and hemorrhoids.

Discrimination

Ta-cheng-chi-tang (Major Rhubarb Combination): constipation, firm fever, abdominal hardness and fullness, submerged firm pulse, and black tongue fur.
Ta-huang-kan-tsao-tang (Rhubarb and Licorice Combination): constipation, firm fever, and acute conditions.
Jun-chang-tang (Linum and Rhubarb Combination): habitual and obstinate constipation. This formula is very nourishing.

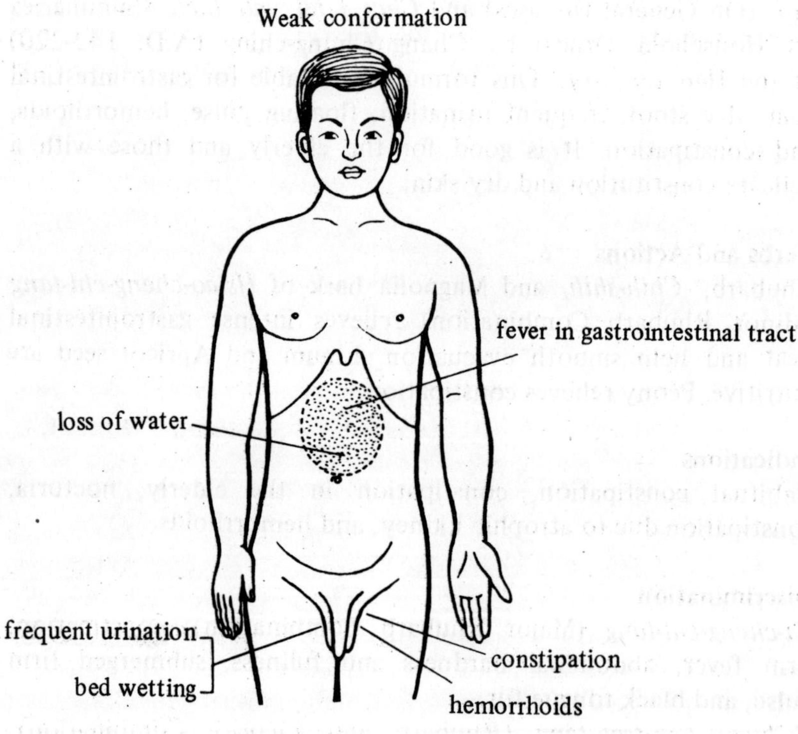
Weak conformation
fever in gastrointestinal tract
loss of water
frequent urination
bed wetting
constipation
hemorrhoids

Mai-Men-Tung-Tang 麥門冬湯

(Ophiopogon Combination)

Ophiopogon	10.0	Pinellia	5.0	Oryza	5.0
Jujube	3.0	Ginseng	2.0	Licorice	2.0

Mai-men-tung-tang was recorded in the Chinese medical work, *Chin kuei yao lueh* (金匱要略) during the Han dynasty. This formula is used for treating flushing up, flushed face, dry and irritated throat, spasmodic coughing, hoarseness, dry mouth, and a floating-sinking pulse.

Herbs and Actions

Ophiopogon removes flushing up. Pinellia dispels stagnant *ch'i* and also removes flushing up. Ginseng is a tonic. Licorice dispels stagnant *ch'i*. Jujube nourishes the chest and relieves flushing up. Oryza is a tonic and stomachic.

Indications

Bronchitis, bronchial, asthma, pneumonia, laryngitis, pertussis, tuberculosis of the pharynx, respiratory tuberculosis, hoarseness, diabetes, hypertension, and arteriosclerosis.

Discrimination

Pan-hsia-hou-pu-tang (Pinellia and Magnolia Combination): sore throat, obstruction of *ch'i*, stagnant water in the stomach.
Chu-yeh-shih-kao-tang (Bamboo Leaf and Gypsum Combination): flushing up of *ch'i*, gasping, severe dryness.
Chih-kan-tsao-tang (Baked Licorice Combination): cough, dryness, gasping, palpitations, stagnancy, weak conformation.
Ling-kan-chiang-wei-hsin-tang (Hoelen and Asarum Combination): cough, wet cough, chills, submerged pulse.
Yueh-pei-chia-pan-hsia-tang (*Ma-huang,* Gypsum, and Pinellia Combination): cough; flushing up of *ch'i*; no dryness or discomfort of the throat; floating, big, and firm pulse.
Ching-fei-tang (Platycodon and Fritillaria Combination): chronic diseases, frequent cough, constant congestion.

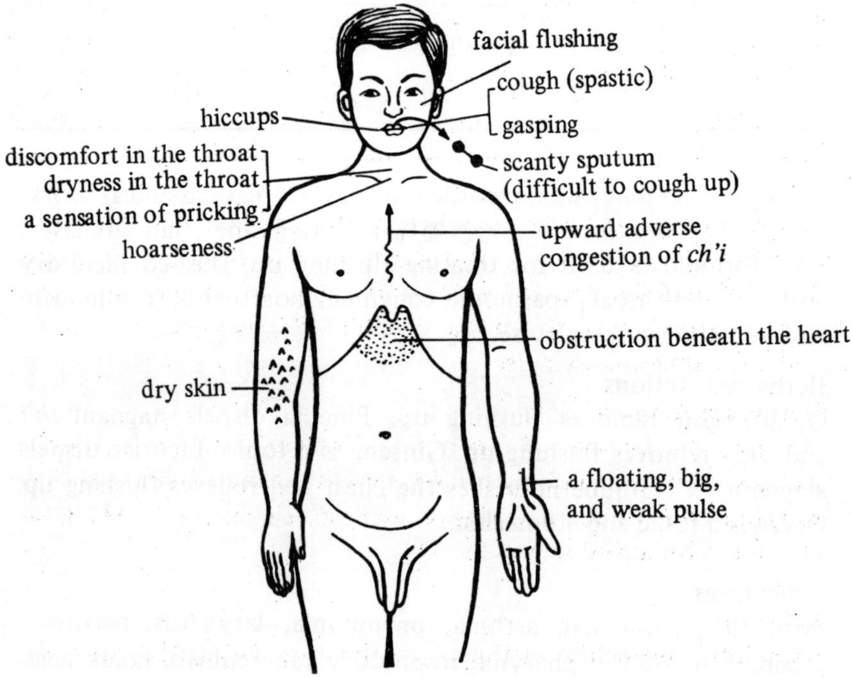

Mai-Men-Tung-Yin-Tzu 麥門冬飲子 *(Ophiopogon and Trichosanthes Combination)*					
Ophiopogon	7.0	Ginseng	2.0	Pueraria	3.0
Rehmannia	4.0	Hoelen	6.0	Schizandra	1.0
Anemarrhena	3.0	Bamboo leaves	1.0	Licorice	1.0
Trichosanthes root	2.0				

Mai-men-tung-yin-tzu is recorded in *Hsuen ming lun* (宣明論). This formula is used for treating thirst due to diabetes, and for polyuria, underweight, coarse skin, lack of vigor, coughing of those with diabetes or tuberculosis, or night cough of the elderly.

Herbs and Actions

Trichosanthes root relieves dryness and acts on sputum and thirst. Anemarrhena and Rehmannia moistens the "blood dryness". Pueraira treats thirst. Schizandra is a salivant and treats coughing. Bamboo leaves is an expectorant which relieves asthma and thirst. Ophiopogon and Licorice relieve cough. Ginseng nourishes the *ch'i* and acts as a salivant. Hoelen is an expectorant.

Indications

Chronic bronchitis, and tuberculosis, coarse skin due to diabetes.

Discrimination

Mai-men-tung-tang (Ophiopogon Combination): cough; thick, sticky sputum; dry skin; dry throat; flushing up of *ch'i*, and obstruction beneath the heart.

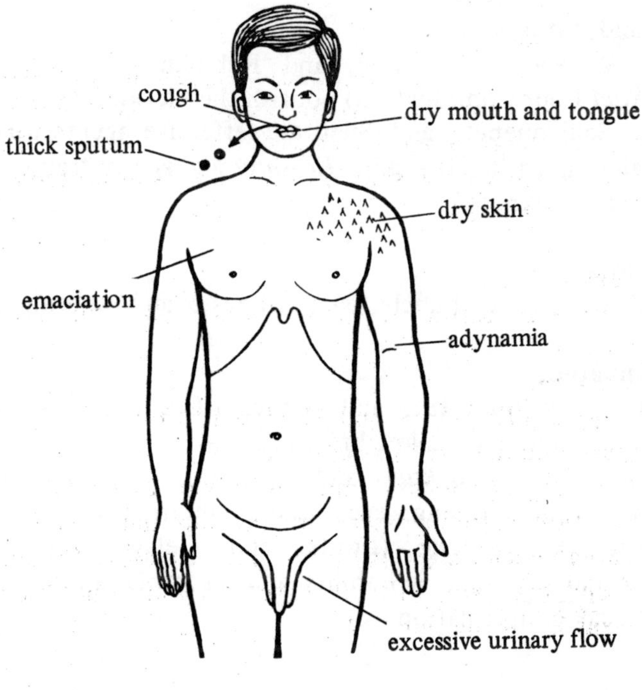

Tang-Kuei-Yin-Tzu 當歸飲子

(Tang-kuei and Tribulus Combination)

Tang-kuei	5.0	Peony	3.0	Cnidium	3.0
Tribulus	3.0	Siler	3.0	Rehmannia	4.0
Ho-shou-wu	2.0	Schizonepeta	1.5	Astragalus	1.5
Licorice	1.0				

Tang-kuei-yin-tzu is recorded in *Chi sheng fang* (濟生方) by Yen Yung-ho of the Sung dynasty. This formula is used for treating dermal itching due to "blood weakness", "blood dryness", and "wind heat". It is also given for anemia, coarse skin, insufficient skin secretions and severe itching. It is suitable for skin diseases in those of delicate constitution and the elderly.

Herbs and Actions

Tang-kuei, Peony, Cnidium, and Rehmannia of *Szu-wu-tang* (*Tang-kuei* Four Combination) nourish the blood. Tribulus relieves itching. Schizonepeta and Siler are effective agents carbuncles. Astragalus nourishes the skin. *Ho-shou-wu* is a nutrient. Licorice helps "*ch'i* weakness"

Indications

Dermal itching, carbuncle, skin disease, and chronic eczema.

Discrimination

Wen-ching-yin (*Tang-kuei* and Gardenia Combination): pruritus; blood fever; and dry, yellow-brown skin.

Hsiao-feng-san (*Tang-kuei* and Arctium Formula): pruritus, much secretion, scabbing, severe itching, internal fever.

Huang-lien-ah-chiao-tang (Coptis and Gelatin Combination): pruritus and dry skin, irritability and insomnia, and blood fever, with a weak conformation.

Weak conformation

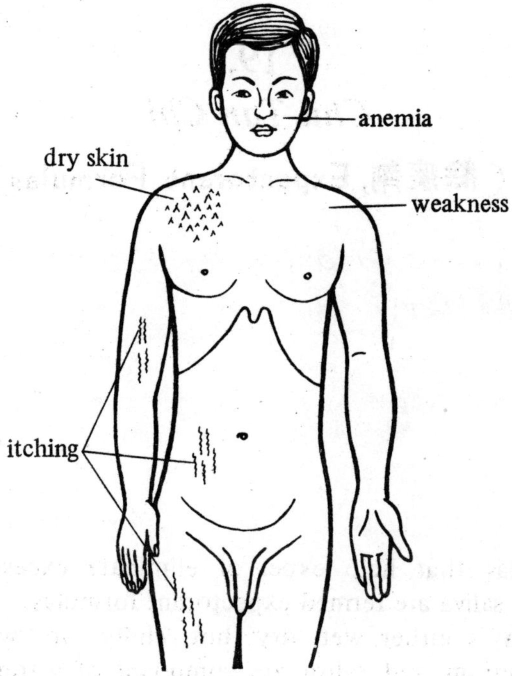

19.

Chu Tan Chi

(除痰劑, Expectorant Formulas)

Formulas that help expel or eliminate excessive sputum (mucus) and saliva are termed expectorant formulas.

Sputum is either wet, dry, hot, chilly, or "windy." Substantially sputum and saliva are composed of water and so are also known as "water toxin." Water toxin results from a functional disturbance in the spleen and kidenys, but most commonly in the spleen. Hence, most expectorants are spleen-healing formulas.

Excessive mucus or saliva either tickles or blocks the trachea, causing a cough and an increase in the generation and secretion of sputum.

Therefore, therapeutically an expectorant is often combined with a cough suppressant in order to bring about a favorable effect.

Chai-Hsien-Tang 柴陷湯

(Bupleurum and Scute Combination)

Bupleurum	5.0	Pinellia	5.0	Scute	3.0
Ginseng	2.0	Jujube	3.0	Ginger	3.0
Trichosanthes seed	3.0	Coptis	1.5	Licorice	1.5

Recorded in *Shen shih tsun sheng shu* (沈氏尊生書) of the Ching dynasty. A combination of *Hsiao-chai-hu-tang* (Minor Bupleurum Combination) and *Hsiao-hsien-hsiung-tnag* (Minor Trichosanthes Combination). Used for treating suppressed distention in the chest, chest pains due to coughing or deep breathing, viscous sputum, rapid respiration, recurrent chills and fever, a bitter taste in the mouth, a yellow coating on the tongue, and loss of appetite.

Herbs and Actions

Pinellia and Ginger are expectorants and increase vitality. Coptis and Scute are anti-inflammatives and antipyretics. Bupleurum removes chest distention. Trichosanthes seed is an antipyretic, expectorant, antitussive (reducing severity of coughing), and analgesic. Ginseng, Licorice, and Jujube increase gastric function.

Indications

Bronchitis, pneumonia, hepatitis, pleurisy, and the common cold.

Discrimination

Hsiao-chai-hu-tang (Minor Bupleurum Combination): obstruction and fullness in the chest, alternating chills and fevers, without chest pain, nor thick sputum, nor difficult expectoration.

Chih-So-Erh-Chen-Tang 枳縮二陳湯

(Chih-shih and Cardamon Combination)

Pinellia	2.0	Hoelen	3.0	*Chih-shih*	1.5
Cardamon	1.5	Citrus	2.0	Cyperus	2.0
Magnolia bark	2.0	Corydalis	2.0	Fennel	1.0
Dried ginger	1.0	Saussurea	1.0	*Tsao-tou-kou*	1.0
Raw ginger	1.5	Licorice	1.0		

Chih-so-erh-chen-tang was recorded in the *Wan ping hui chun* (萬病回春) during the Ming dynasty. This formula is used for treatıng severe vomiting caused by excessive sputum and "water poisoning" in the chest as well as pain in the chest and back.

Herbs and Actions

Erh-chen-tang (Citrus and Pinellia Combination) nourishes the spleen and stomach, and eliminates "moist sputum". Fennel, Corydalis, Cyperus, and Ginger dispel chills and ease pain. *Chih-shih,* Cardamon, Magnolia bark, Saussurea, and *Tsao-tou-kou* increase vitality and dispel excessive sputum.

Indications

Gastritis, stomachache, gastric distention, dyspepsia, gastric ulcer, intercostal neuralgia, cardiac neuralgia, and angina pectoris.

Discrimination

Kua-lu-hsieh-pai-pai-chiu-tang (Trichosanthes, Vinegar, and Bakeri Combination): pain in the chest and back, asthma, and congestion.
Kua-lu-hsieh-pai-pan-hsia-tang (Pinellia and Bakeri Combination): chest pain, vomiting, asthma.
Chih-shih-hsieh-pai-kuei-chih-tang (*Chih-shih,* Bakeri, and Cinnamon Combination): spasmodic pain in the hypochondrium, shoulders and back; flushing up, asthmatic coughing.

Ta-chai-hu-tang (Major Bupleurum Combination): pain beneath the heart, thoraco-costal distress, firm conformation.
Chien-chin-tang-kuei-tang (*Tang-kuei* Combination): cardiac-abdominal colia pain which radiates to the shoulders and back, hernia colic, chill conformation.

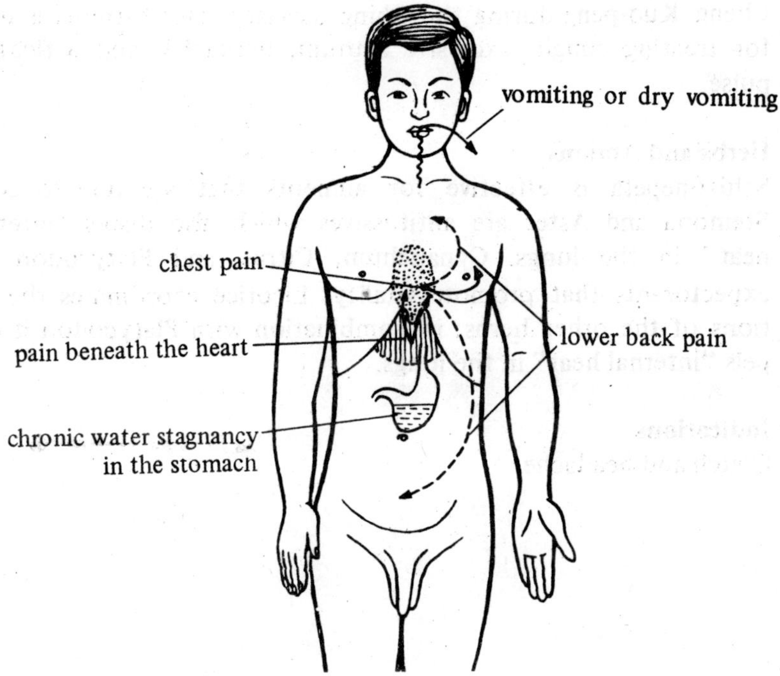

Chih-Sou-San 止嗽散

(Platycodon and Schizonepeta Formula)

Platycodon	9.0	Schizonepeta	4.5	Aster	9.0
Stemona	9.0	Cynanchum	9.0	Licorice	3.0
Citrus	3.0				

Chih-sou-san was recorded in *I hsueh hsin wu* (醫學心悟) by Cheng Kuo-peng during the Ching dynasty. This formula is used for treating cough, excessive sputum, headache, and a floating pulse.

Herbs and Actions

Schizonepeta is effective for ailments that are due to cold. Stemona and Aster are antitussives which also dispel "internal heat" in the lungs. Cynanchum, Citrus, and Platycodon are expectorants that promote vitality. Licorice coordinates the actions of the other herbs; in combination with Platycodon it dispels "internal heat" in the lungs.

Indications

Cough and headache.

Chin-Fei-Tsao-San 金沸草散

(Schizonepeta and Pinellia Formula)

Inula	3.0	Peucedanum	3.5	Asarum	3.0
Hoelen	1.8	Schizonepeta	4.5	Pinellia	1.5
Licorice	1.0	Jujube	1.0	Ginger	1.0

Chin-fei-tsao-san is recorded in *I fang chi chieh* (醫方集解) of the Ching dynasty. This formula is used for treating catarrh, dizziness, productive cough, and rhinitis. It is effective for chest distention, asthma, and headache due to a common cold.

Herbs and Actions
Schizonepeta is a diaphoretic and carminative. Peucedanum and Inula increase expectoration. Pinellia is a dessicant and expectorant. Asarum relieves chills and dispels sputum. Hoelen acts as a diuretic. Licorice, Ginger and Jujube are nutritives which also regulate *ch'i*.

Indications
Common cold, cough, bronchitis, and bronchial asthma.

Ching-Fei-Tang 清肺湯

(Platycodon and Fritillaria Combination)

Scute	2.0	Platycodon	2.0	Morus	2.0
Apricot seed	2.0	Gardenia	2.0	Asparagus	2.0
Fritillaria	2.0	Citrus	2.0	Jujube	3.0
Bamboo	2.0	Hoelen	3.0	*Tang-kuei*	3.0
Ophiopogon	3.0	Schizandra	0.5	Ginger	0.5
Licorice	1.0				

Ching-fei-tang is mentioned in a Chinese medical dictionary *Wan ping hui chun* (A.D. 1587) of the Ming dynasty as a treatment for chronic respiratory diseases. These diseases arise from internal heat in the respiratory organs which causes chronic inflammation, fever, sputum, and severe cough. Other symptoms are abundant viscid sputum, dry mouth, persistant cough, sore and itching throat, and hoarseness.

Herbs and Actions

Scute and Gardenia remove internal heat in the chest. *Tang-kuei* and Licorice nourish the blood and sedate flushing up. Asparagus, Ophiopogon, and Schizandra nourish the lungs, remove internal heat in the lungs, and cure cough with sputum. Fritillaria, Apricot seed, Morus, Platycodon, Citrus, Hoelen, Bamboo, Jujube and Ginger coordinate and improve the effects of other herbs.

Indications

Chronic bronchitis, laryngitis, pneumonia, tuberculosis, bronchodilation, bronchial asthma and cardiac asthma.

Discrimination

Mai-men-tung-tang (Ophiopogon Combination): cough, the yielding of less but sticky sputum, and severe flushing up of *ch'i*.
Hsiao-ching-lung-tang (Minor Blue Dragon Combination): cough with copious, thin sputum.

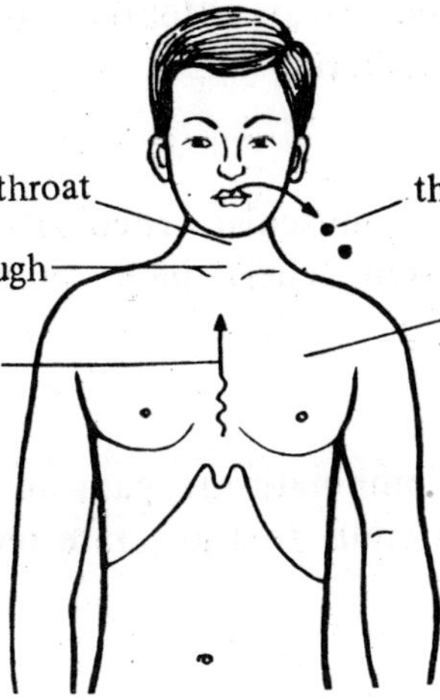

Ching-Shih-hua-Tan-Tang *(Pinellia and Arisaema Combination)*					**清濕化痰湯**
Pinellia	4.0	Hoelen	4.0	Arisaema	3.0
Atractylodes	4.0	Scute	3.0	Citrus	2.5
Chianghuo	1.5	Angelica	1.5	Brassica	1.5
Ginger	3.0	Licorice	1.5	Bamboo sap	1.5

Ching-shih-hua-tan-tang is recorded in *Wan ping hui chun* (萬病回春) of the Ming dynasty. This formula is used for treating generalized pain, paralysis tenacious sputum, chest pain, shoulder stiffness, stridor, cough and arthralgia.

Herbs and Actions

Pinellia, Hoelen, Atractylodes, and Citrus are expectorants *Chianghuo* treats rheumatism and arthralgia. Arisaema is an expectorant and treats rheumatism. Angelica improves blood circulation. Brassica nourishes the *ch'i* and treats pain due to swelling. Ginger treats ailments due to cold. Licorice coordinates the actions of the other herbs and acts as an antitussive and analgesic. Bamboo sap treats "febrile sputum". Scute is an antiphlogistic and antipyretic.

Indications

Intercostal neuralgia, muscular rheumatism, swollen lymph gland, gastric distention, chest pain, chills in the back, and shoulder stiffness.

Discrimination

I-yi-jen-tang (Coix Combination): pain in the arms and legs, numbness, winds and chills that generate fever, and rheumatism.

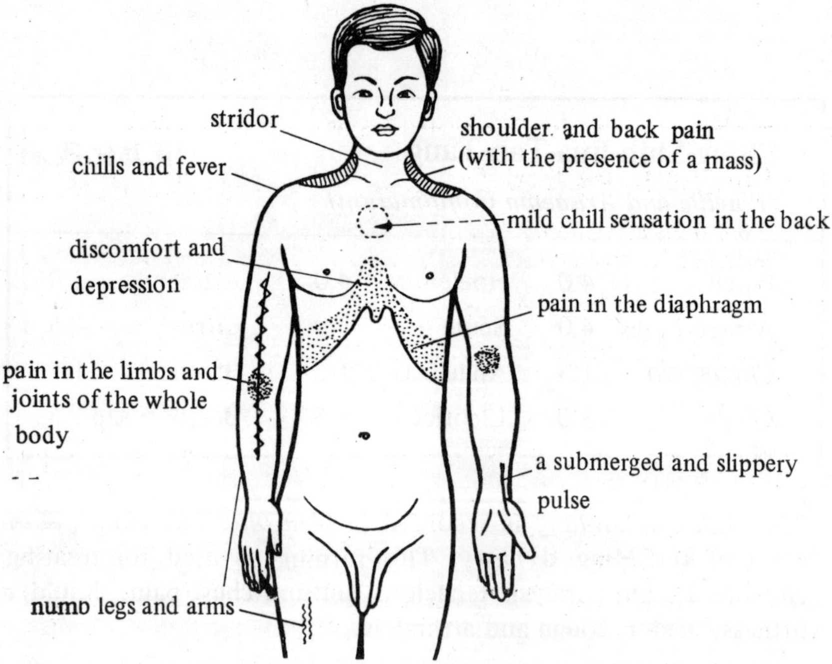

Erh-Chen-Tang 二陳湯

(Citrus and Pinellia Combination)

Citrus	4.0	Pinellia	5.0	Hoelen	5.0
Licorice	1.0	Ginger	3.0		

Erh-chen-tang is recorded in the *Tai ping huei min ho chi chu fang* (太平惠民和劑局方). This formula is used for treating patients with copious watery sputum, vertigo, palpitations, discomfort in the stomach, occasional fever, a sinking-weak pulse, and vomiting and nausea due to stagnant water in the stomach.

Herbs and Actions

This formula nourishes the spleen and stomach and dispels moist sputum. Pinellia dispels moist sputum. Hoelen improves metabolism and eliminates sputum. Citrus is used as an expectorant. Licorice nourishes the spleen and the stomach. Ginger promotes elimination of stagnant food and sputum.

Indications

Vomiting, nausea, vertigo, headache, eclampsia, stagnant *ch'i*, hangover, apoplexy, gastroptosis, and nervous diseases.

Discrimination

Liu-chun-tzu-tang (Six Major Herb Combination): chiefly *ch'i* weakness with congestion as the subordinate symptom.
Erh-chen-tang (Citrus and Pinellia Combination): congestion with *ch'i* weakness as the subordinate symptom.

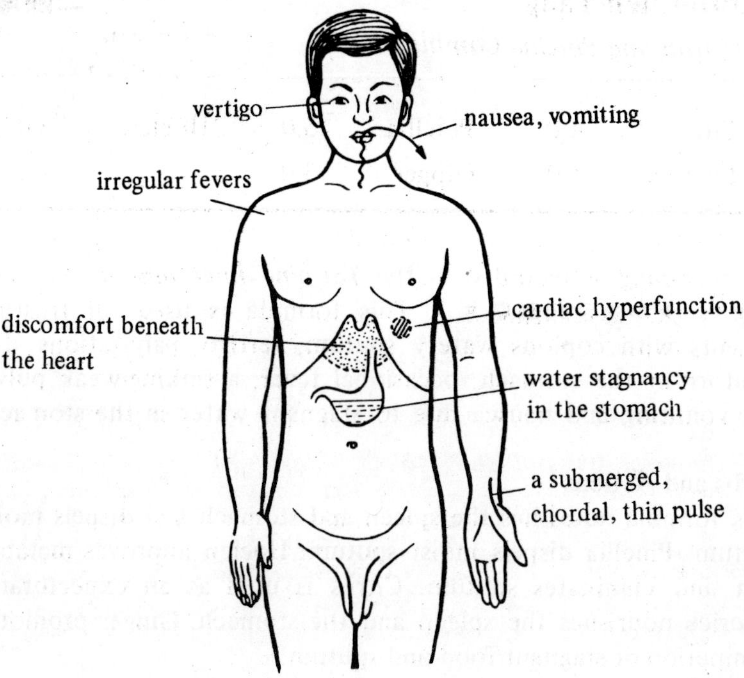

Hsiang-Sheng-Po-Ti-Wan *(Gasping Formula)*				**響聲破笛丸**	
Forsythia	2.5	Platycodon	2.5	Licorice	2.5
Rhubarb	1.0	Cardamon	1.0	Cnidium	1.0
Terminalia	1.0	Catechu	2.0	Mentha	4.0

Hsiang-sheng-po-ti-wan was recorded in the *Wan ping hui chun* (萬病回春) during the Ming dynasty. This formula is used for treating hoarseness due to overexertion of the vocal cords.

Herbs and Actions

Forsythia, Platycodon, and Cnidium are antiphlogistics which cool the blood and reduce swelling and suppuration. Catechu is an antitussive that alleviates hoarseness due to sore throat. Terminalia is an antipyretic and refrigerant. Cardamon is an expectorant and stimulant. Mentha is a refrigerant that soothes the throat. Rhubarb is an antiphlogistic and antipyretic. Licorice coordinates the actions of the other herbs.

Indications
Hoarseness and discomfort in the throat.

Kua-Lou-Chih-Shih-Tang 栝樓枳實湯

(Trichosanthes and Chih-shih Combination)

Tang-kuei	3.0	Hoelen	3.0	Fritillaria	3.0
Platycodon	2.0	Citrus	2.0	Scute	2.0
Cardamon	1.0	Saussurea	1.0	Licorice	1.0
Gardenia	1.0	*Chih-shih*	1.0	Ginger	2.0
Bamboo sap	1.0	Trichosanthes seed	2.0		

Kua-lou-chih-shih-tang was recorded in the *Wan ping hui chun* (萬病回春) during the Ming dynasty. This formula is used for treating viscid sputum, dry mouth, chest pains, chest distention, wheezing, cough, and dark-colored urine. It is especially effective for severe coughing in the morning.

Herbs and Actions
Gardenia and Scute are antiphlogistics and antipyretics that dispel "internal heat" in the liver. *Tang-kuei* and Licorice nourish the blood and dispel "internal heat" in the chest and stomach. Trichosanthes seed and Fritillaria are expectorants; when combined with Bamboo sap and Ginger, they dispel stagnant sputum. *Chih-shih,* Platycodon, Citrus, Cardamon, Saussurea, and Hoelen dispel "internal heat" and remove stagnant *ch'i* and stagnant sputum.

Indications

Acute and chronic bronchitis, pneumonia, pleurisy, intercostal neuralgia, asthma, pulmonary emphysema, tuberculosis, smoker's cough, arteriosclerosis, and dyspepsia.

Discrimination

Hsiao-hsien-hsiung-tang (Minor Trichosanthes Combination): sticky sputum, hardness with pain when palpated beneath the heart, and floating and slippery pulse.

Tzu-yin-chiang-huo-tang (Phellodendron Combination): cough, yin-weakness fever, weak and quick pulse, and no chest pain.

Chuan-szu-chun-tzu-tang (Magnolia and Citrus Combination): asthmatic cough, weak conformation, cold feet, flushing up.

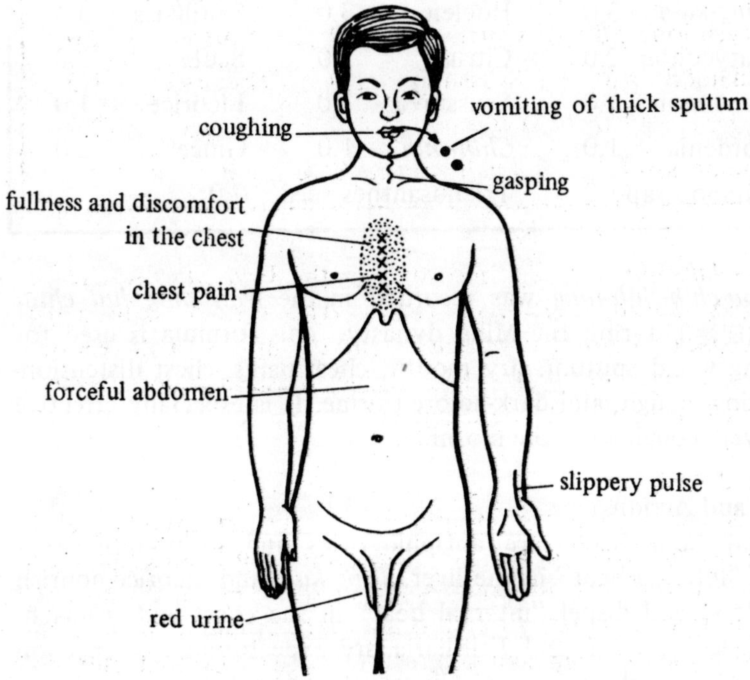

Li-Ke-Tang 利膈湯

(Pinellia and Gardenia Combination)

Pinellia	8.0	Aconite	0.5-1.0	Gardenia	3.0

Invented by Genyi of Nagoya, Japan. Used for treatment of structure at the middle of the esophagus resulting in dysphagia (difficulty in swallowing); vomiting; sticky sputum; and thirst. Suitable for those who have an obstructed and painful feeling in the throat, dysphagia, and trouble swallowing food. After taking this formula most patients will spit out a glue-like sputum, experience immediate relief in the chest, and discover that the difficulty with swallowing has been completely eliminated.

Herbs and Actions

Pinellia treats vomiting caused by sputum stagnancy, relieves water stagnation, calms up-rushing air and gas, and expels moist sputum. Gardenia relieves thoracic suppressed fever, relieves distention, and calms moving gas and air. Aconite restores yang and warms the uterus.

Indications

Esophageal cancer, gastric cancer, esophageal stenosis, esophageal polyps, throat obstructions, and pain.

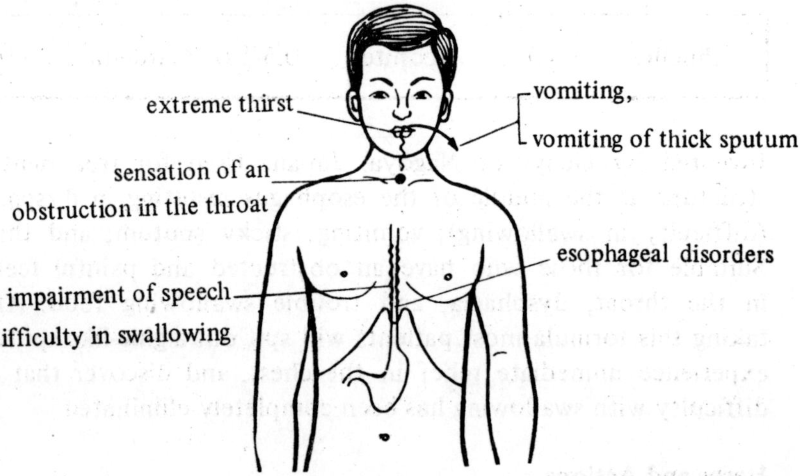

Ling-Kan-Chiang-Wei-Hsin-Hsia-Jen-Tang 苓甘薑味辛夏仁湯

(Hoelen and Schizandra Combination)

Hoelen	4.0	Licorice	2.0	Ginger	2.0
Schizandra	3.0	Pinellia	4.0	Asarum	2.0
Apricot seed	4.0				

Ling-kan-chiang-wei-hsin-hsia-jen-tang is recorded in *Chin kuei yao lueh* (金匱要略) of the Han dynasty. This formula is used for treating stridor, cough, dropsy, tendency towards anemia, sunken and weak pulse, chills in the hands and feet, severe chills, headache, generalized pain, and delicate constitution without fever.

Herbs and Actions

Hoelen dispels "stagnant water" in the stomach and is effective for dysuria and palpitation. Pinellia coordinates the actions of

Hoelen. Apricot seed removes "stagnant water" in the chest and relieves asthma, difficulty in breathing, and edema. Schizandra is an astringent and antitussive. Asarum removes "stagnant water", and relieves coughing due to "water *ch'i*" beneath the heart. Ginger dispels "water poisoning" and removes "stagnant water". Licorice coordinates the actions of the other herbs.

Indications
Acute and chronic bronchitis, bronchial asthma, pulmonary emphysema, edema, ascites, chronic nephritis, atrophic kidney, pleurisy, pulmonary edema, beriberi, and cardiac asthma.

Discrimination
Hsiao-ching-lung-tang (Minor Blue Dragon Combination): asthmatic cough, external fever, edema, slobbering, floating and weak pulse.
Ma-hsing-kan-shih-tang (*Ma-huang* and Apricot Seed Combination): mild asthma with no external fever.

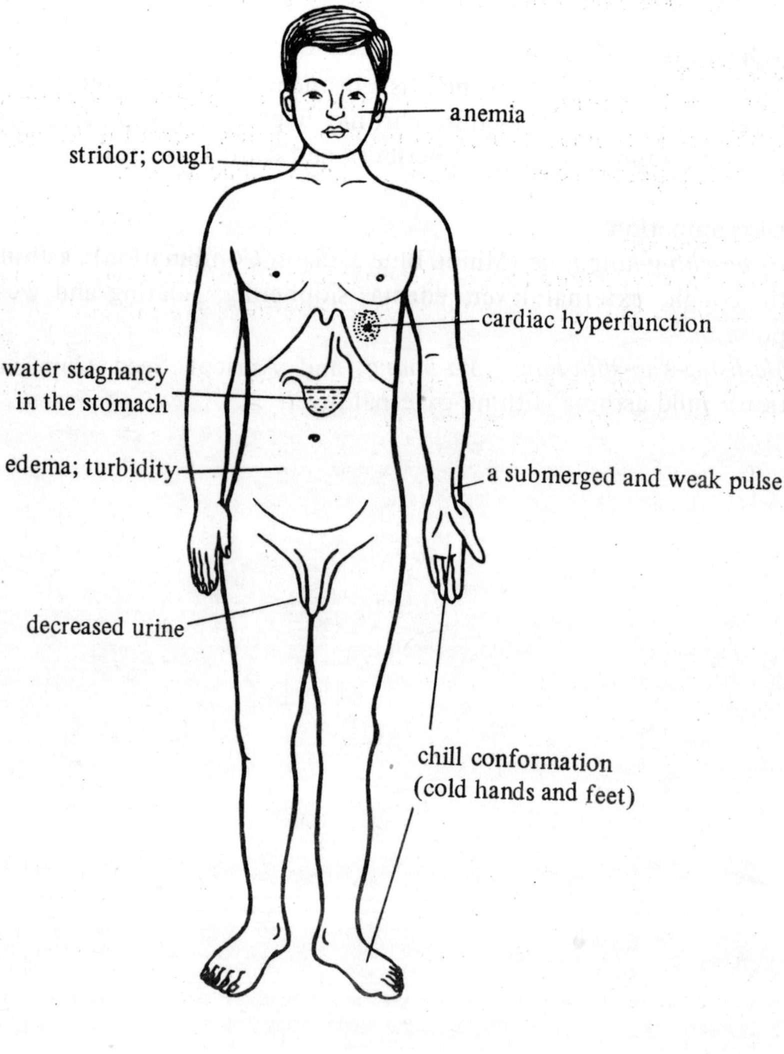
anemia
stridor; cough
cardiac hyperfunction
water stagnancy
in the stomach
edema; turbidity
a submerged and weak pulse
decreased urine
chill conformation
(cold hands and feet)

Meng-Shih-Kuen-Tan-Wan 礞石滾痰丸

(Lapis and Scute Formula)

Lapis	12.0	Aquilaria	4.5	Rhubarb	9.0
Scute	9.0				

Meng-shih-kuen-tan-wan is recorded in *I fang chi chieh* (醫方集解) of the Ching dynasty. This formula is used for treating those in a coma or those with a firm fever and long-standing congestion, epilepsy, mental illness, irrationality, cough with thick sputum, distention in the chest, vertigo, constipation, yellow and thick tongue fur, slippery and quick pulse. It acts as an antiphlogistic and expectorant, causing excretion of the accumulated sputum and expulsion of the impurities and toxins by way of the intestines. Because of the properties of this formula, pregnant women and those of delicate constitution should be careful when using it so that the normal *ch'i* may not be disturbed.

Herbs and Actions

Lapis expels stale sputum. Rhubarb is bitter and cold in nature; it purges the body of deep-seated impurities and toxins via the intestines. Scute relieves the heat of the *shang-chiao* (upper abdomen). Aquilaria coordinates the actions of the other herbs.

Indications

Acute gastritis, trachitis, bronchitis, excessive secretion accompanying pharyngitis, firm fever with long-standing congestion, tenacious sputum, and various symptoms of tuberculosis.

Ning-Sou-Wan 寧嗽丸

(Fritillaria and Platycodon Formula)

Platycodon	2.0	Dendrobium	2.0	Fritillaria	2.0
Perilla fruit	2.0	Pinellia	2.0	Hoelen	2.0
Mentha	1.5	Morus	1.5	Licorice	0.5
Wheat sprouts	1.0	Apricot seed	1.5	Orange peel	1.0

Ning-sou-wan was recorded in the Chinese governmental medical text, *Chung kuo kuo yao ku yeou cheng fang hsuan chi* (中國國藥固有成方選輯). This formula is good for treating both acute and persistent cough, excessive sputum, and fever.

Herbs and Actions

Orange peel, Hoelen, Platycodon, Fritillaria, Morus, and Apricot seed are expectorants, antitussives, and antipyretics that dispel "internal heat" in the lungs. Perilla seed is an antitussive and expectorant, effective for asthma and flushing up. Pinellia is a sedative and expectorant that relieves nausea. Wheat sprouts improve the function of the spleen. Mentha is a refrigerant. Dendrobium dispels "internal heat" from the spleen and stomach and acts as a stomachic. Licorice coordinates the action of the other herbs.

Indications

Cough, common cold with phlegm, tracheitis, and acute and chronic bronchitis with cough.

Pan-Hsia-Pai-Chu-Tien-Ma-Tang 半夏白朮天麻湯

(Pinellia and Gastrodia Combination)

Pinellia	3.0	Atractylodes	3.0	Citrus	3.0
Hoelen	3.0	Malt	2.0	Gastrodia	2.0
Ginger	2.0	Astragalus	1.5	Ginseng	1.5
Alisma	1.5	Phellodendron	1.0	*Shen-chu*	2.0

Pan-hsia-pai-chu-tien-ma-tang was recorded in the *Pi wei lun* (脾胃論) by Li Tung-yuan during the Yuan dynasty. This formula is used for treating recurrent headaches, gastrointestinal weakness, stagnant water, water poisoning, vomiting, vertigo, cold feet, and fatigue.

Herbs and Actions

Ginseng and Astragalus nourish the stomach. Pinellia, Atractylodes, Citrus, and Hoelen dispel ascites. Malt and *Shen-chu* improve the functioning of the spleen and stomach. Ginger nourishes the stomach and stops vomiting. Phellodendron and Alisma dispel "internal heat" from the kidneys and bladder. Gastrodia is a sedative effective for relieving vertigo.

Indications

Recurrent headaches and vertigo, compulsive sleeping after eating, weakness of the hands of feet, hypertension due to gastrointestinal weakness, headache and vertigo due to hypotension, abdominal distention. gastroptosis, and sinusitis.

Discrimination

Wu-chu-yu-tang (Evodia Combination): vomiting, headache, vertigo, anxiety, flushing up, "cold water toxin", slightly forceful abdomen, submerged pulse.

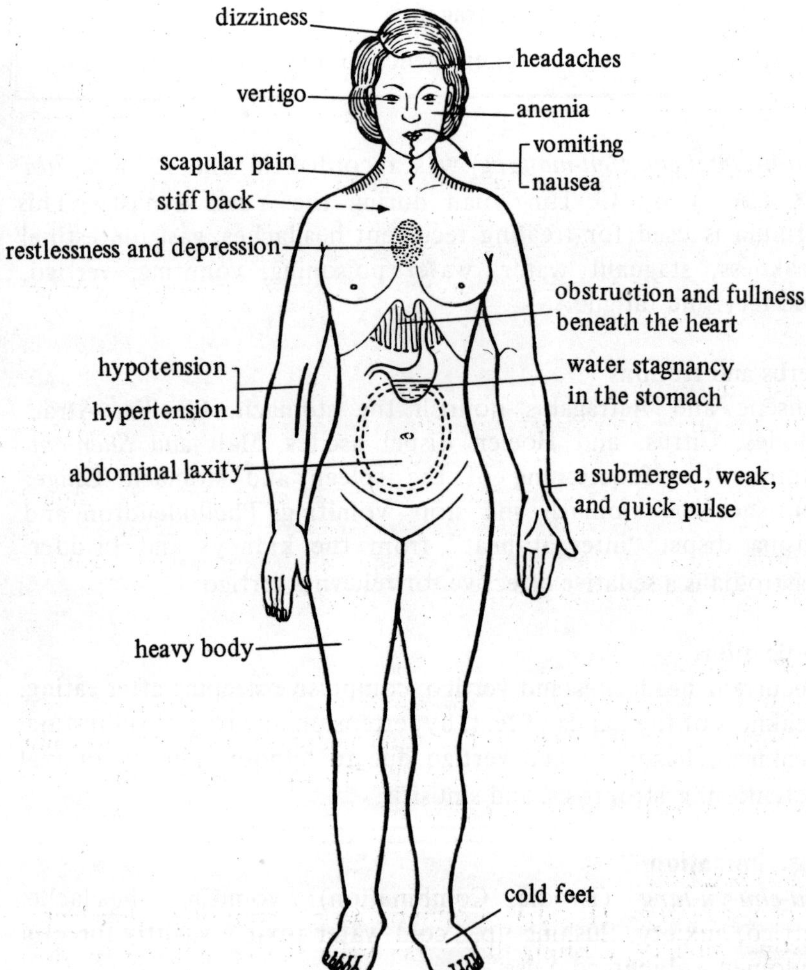
dizziness
headaches
vertigo
anemia
vomiting
nausea
scapular pain
stiff back
restlessness and depression
obstruction and fullness beneath the heart
hypotension
hypertension
water stagnancy in the stomach
abdominal laxity
a submerged, weak, and quick pulse
heavy body
cold feet

Tun-Sou-San 頓嗽散

(Morus and Platycodon Formula)

Bupleurum	5.0	Platycodon	3.0	Scute	3.0
Morus	3.0	Gardenia	2.5	Licorice	1.0
Gypsum	5.0				

Tun-sou-san is an experimental formula from Japan. This formula is mainly used for a hot cough, dry cough due to lack of sputum, severe cough with abundant sputum, and pertussis.

Herbs and Actions

Bupleurum coordinates with Scute to relieve chest distention, acting as an antiphlogistic and detoxifier. Morus and Platycodon remove heat from the lungs. Licorice increases vitality. Gardenia relieves anxiety and pain in the chest. Gypsum dispels external and internal heat and acts as a refrigerant and antipyretic.

Indications

All types of coughs, including that which is due to the common cold, pertussis, and bronchitis.

20.
Chu Chung Chi
(驅蟲劑, Anthelmintic Formulas)

Formulas that dispel parasitic worms are named *chu chung chi*.

An anthelmintic either dispels or kills parasitic worms living in the alimentary tract. People suffering from parasites often have a swollen and aching belly; loss of appetite or a voracious appetite, often favoring peculiar foods; and irregular bowel movements. As the condition continues the patient may become withered and yellow and emaciated. Depending on the type of parasites, anthelmintics are classified as ascaricide, (agent that kills nematodes), taeniacide (agent that kills tapeworms), oxyuricide (agent that kills pinworms), and ankylostomiacide (agent that kills hookworms).

Kan-Tsao-Fen-Mi-Tang 甘草粉蜜湯

(Licorice, Minium, and Honey Combination)

Licorice	2.0	Minium	1.0	Honey	4.0

From in *Chin kuei yao lueh* (金匱要略). Used for ascariasis (infestation of the intestines by roundworms) which recurs at regular intervals and causes the infested individual to slobber and have abdominal pain. If the disease has not been cured by the use of ordinary ascaricides, this formula can then be taken.

Herbs and Actions
Minium, an ascaricide, is a potent poison and should not be taken in large amounts or too frequently. Licorice and Honey lure the worms to ingest the poison. The poison begins to take effect the moment the sweet taste disappears and the ascaris are killed thereby.

Indications
Ascariasis, intense abdominal pain caused by the use of ascaricides.

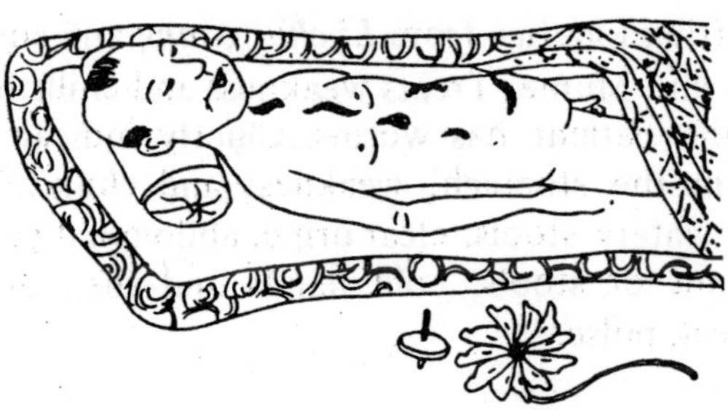

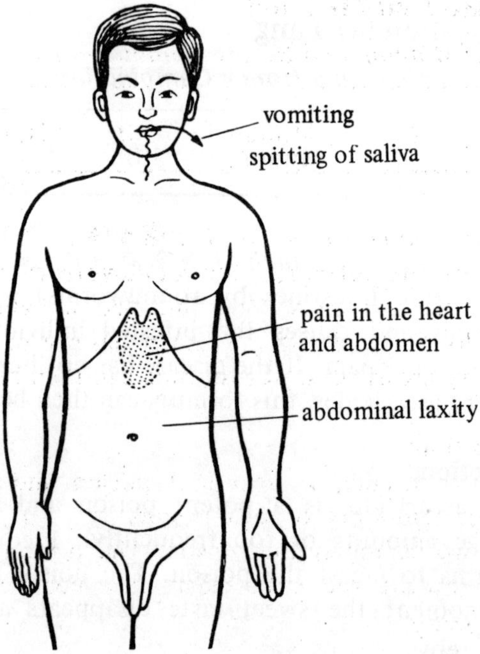

Li-Chung-An-Huei-Tang 理中安蛔湯

(Ginseng and Zanthoxylum Combination)

Ginseng	1.5	Atractylodes	5.0	Hoelen	6.0
Mume	2.0	Zanthoxylum	1.5	Ginger	1.5

Made by omitting Licorice from *Li-chung-tang* and adding Hoelen, Zanthoxylum and Mume. Treats weakness and chills in the middle torso when the patient has worms. Chiefly indicated for insufficient yang in the stomach, weakness and chills of the spleen and stomach, watery stools, clear urine, abdominal pains with gas, worms in vomit or stools, cold hands and feet, and a whitish tongue and weak pulse.

Herbs and Actions

Ginseng, dry Ginger, Atractylodes and Hoelen warm and nourish yang in the middle torso, and in the spleen and stomach. Incorporation of Zanthoxylum and Mume causes the expulsion of worms by means of their acrid and sour nature. As the worms are eliminated and the spleen and stomach regain their yang, the disease heals spontaneously.

Indications

Ascariasis in those having a weak stomach, vomiting, and cold limbs.

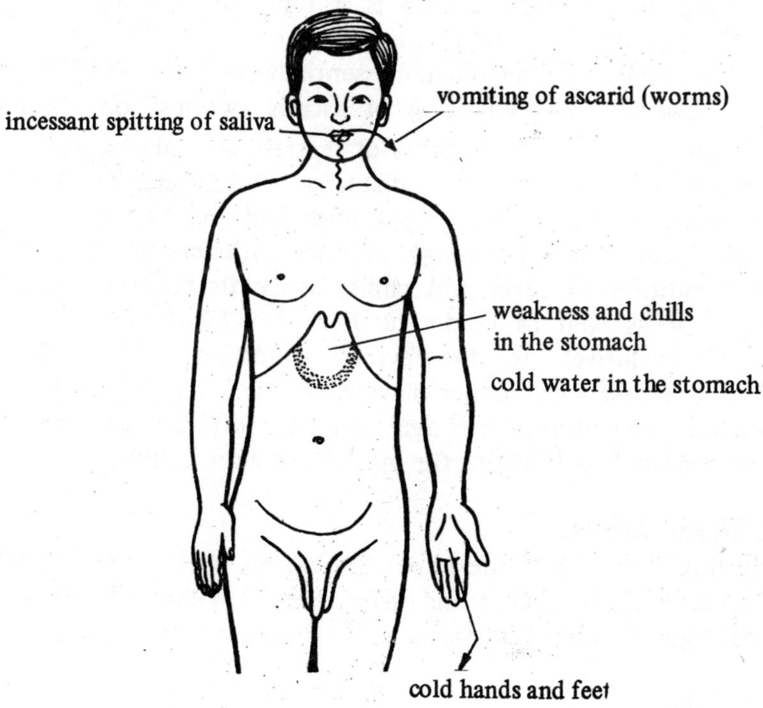

Lien-Mei-An-Huei-Tang 連梅安蛔湯

(Picrorrhiza and Mume Combination)

Picrorrhiza	3.0	Omphalia	9.0
Phellodendron	2.4	Mume	2 seeds
Zanthoxylum	10 pieces	Areca seed	2 seeds

Anthelmintics kill or dispel worms and should be selected to agree with the condition. Some conditions are of the cold type, others of the feverish type, and still others a combination of cold and fever. This formula is a representative anthelmintic for the feverish condition caused by excessive heat in the liver and the stomach. It is indicated essentially for parasitic abdominal pain, anorexia, and vomiting of ascaris (worms) on ingestion of food; or for the symptoms of distress and adverse chills accompanied by a ruddy face, disturbed functioning of the heart, dry mouth, reddish tongue, quick pulse, and somatic fever.

Wu-mei-wan (Mume Formula), another anthelmintic, is used for the condition of fever and chills; hence its constituents comprise hot as well as cold-natured herbs. *Lien-mei-an-huei-tang* is used exclusively for the feverish condition and is composed of heat-cleansing components which purge fever of the liver and stomach. *Li-chung-an-huei-tang* typifies formulas for the cold type condition as it warms the insides and expels chills.

Herbs and Actions

Zanthoxylum and Mume expel the worms. Picrorrhiza and Phellodendron clean hepatic and stomach fever. Omphalia and Areca seed augment the anthelmintic activity.

Indications

Ascariasis, stomatitis, intestinal hernia.

Wu-Mei-Wan 烏梅丸

(Mume Formula)

Mume	3.0	Asarum	3.0	Aconite	3.0
Cinnamon	3.0	Phellodendron	3.0	Ginseng	3.0
Tang-kuei	2.0	Zanthoxylum	5.0	Ginger	5.0
Coptis	7.0				

Wu-mei-wan is recorded in *Shang han lun* (傷寒論) of the Han dynasty. This formula is used for treating recurrent abdominal pain, anxiety due to stress, chills in the hands and feet due to ascariasis, and vomiting, severe diarrhea, and pain beneath the heart.

Herbs and Actions

Mume is an anthelmintic, detoxifier, refrigerant, and astringent. Zanthoxylum treats intestinal spasms and acts to improve the anthelmintic action of Mume. Asarum and Cinnamon coordinate with the action of Aconite to improve metabolism and blood circulation. Ginseng is a tonic which increases appetite and relieves vomiting and diarrhea. *Tang-kuei* is a sedative, blood tonic, and nutritive. Coptis and Phellodendron are stomachics, sedatives, and inflammatives.

Indications

Ascariasis, gastritis, indigestion, gastric ulcer, intestinal colic, chronic diarrhea, neurosis, insomnia, and blood disease.

Discrimination

Lien-mei-an-huei-tang (Picrorrhiza and Mume Combination): chills due to infection with worms, strong fever in the liver and stomach, red facial complexion, and dry mouth.

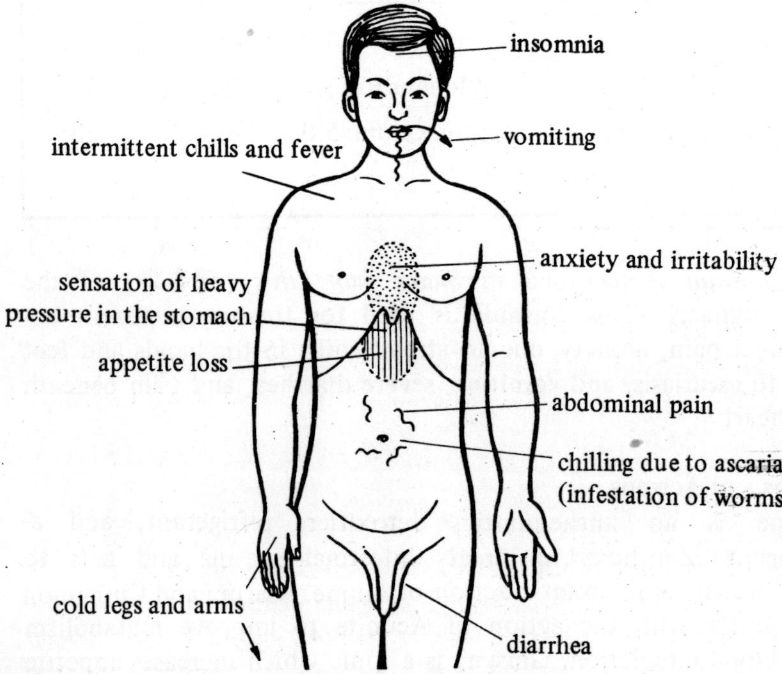
insomnia
vomiting
intermittent chills and fever
anxiety and irritability
sensation of heavy pressure in the stomach
appetite loss
abdominal pain
chilling due to ascariasis (infestation of worms)
cold legs and arms
diarrhea

21.

Ching Chan Chi

(經産劑, Gyneco-obstetric Formulas)

Formulas for women that treat abnormal menstruation and leukorrhea, increase fertility, and ease pregnancy and childbirth problems are collectively termed *ching chan chi.*

Prophylaxis, diagnosis, and treatment of women's diseases are different from men's. Abnormal or irregular menstruation or amenorrhea yellow and red types. Problems associated with pregnancy include vomiting, fetal agitation, eclampsia, and edema. Labor may give rise to many kinds of medical problems, all of which are treated with these types of formulas.

An-Tai-Yin 安胎飲（保產無憂方）

(Tang-kuei and Parsley Combination)

Magnolia bark	2.0	Artemisia	2.0	Cnidium	4.5
Schizonepeta	2.4	*Tang-kuei*	4.5	Fritillary	3.0
Cuscuta	3.0	Astragalus	2.4	*Chianghuo*	1.5
Licorice	1.5	*Chih-ko*	1.8	Peony	6.0
Ginger	1.0				

An-tai-yin is recorded in the *Yen fang hsin pien* (驗方新編) during the Ching dynasty. This formula is used for treating pernicious vomiting, watery sputum, anxiety due to stress, a feeling of heaviness in the head, vertigo, sudden pain in the waist and abdomen, and hemorrhaging. It is also effective in stopping false labor.

Herbs and Actions
Tang-kuei, Cnidium, and Peony nourish the blood and are effective for stopping false labor. Magnolia bark relieves flushing up. Ginger improves gastric function. Magnolia bark and Ginger are antiemetics and appetizers. *Chih-ko* and Fritillary dispel stagnant sputum. Astragalus and Artemisia check pain in the midline and abdomen. Schizonepeta is a hemostatic, and it relieves rheumatism. *Chianghuo* is an analgesic. Cuscuta eases childbirth. Licorice is a detoxifier and tonic.

Indications
False labor, difficult labor, pain in the waist and abdomen during pregnancy, and habitual abortion.

Discrimination
Chiao-ai-szu-wu-tang (Gelatin and Artemisia Four Combination): fetal agitation, bleeding during pregnancy, abdominal pain.

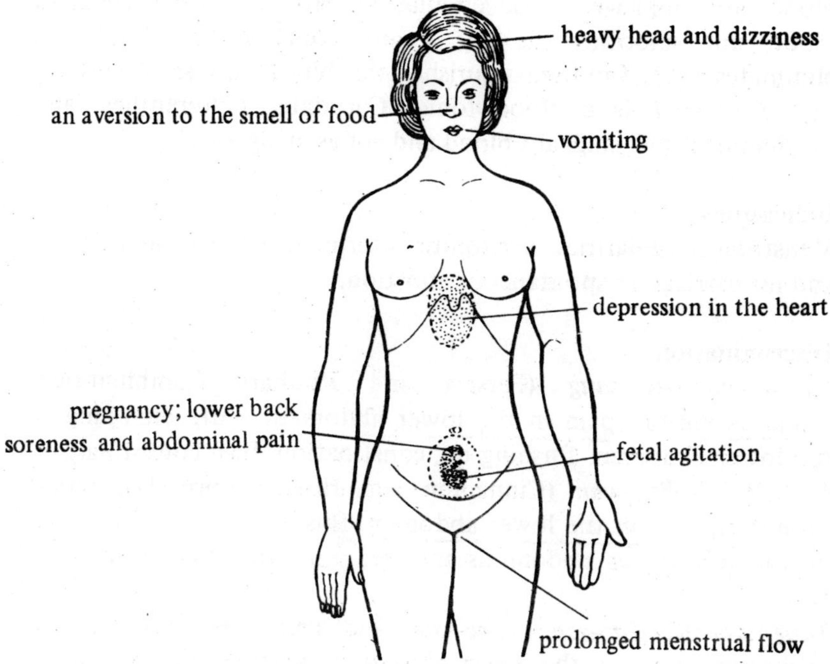

Che-Tsung-Yin 折衝飲

(Cinnamon and Persica Combination)

Moutan	3.0	Cnidium	3.0	Peony	3.0
Persica	5.0	Cinnamon	3.0	*Tang-kuei*	5.0
Carthamus	1.0				

Che-tsung-yin is recorded in *Chan lun* (產論) by Kagawa Genyetsu of Japan. This formula is used for treating lower abdominal pain due to stagnant blood, pain in the pelvis, symptoms caused by stagnant blood during pregnancy, and pain during menstruation.

Herbs and Actions

Cinnamon improves blood circulation. Persica removes stagnant blood, and improves blood circulation. Moutan relieves stagnant blood, and smoothes the *ch'i.* Peony nourishes the blood, and eliminates pain. Cnidium nourishes the blood, and smoothes the *ch'i. Tang-kuei* is a blood tonic. Corydalis, Achyranthes, and Carthamus dispel stagnant blood and act as analgesics.

Indications

Menstrual irregularities, peritonitis, uterine inflammation, ovaritis, and miscarriage or spontaneous abortion.

Discrimination

Tao-ho-cheng-chi-tang (Persica and Rhubarb Combination): blood occlusion, pain in the lower abdomen, acute cramping in the lower abdomen, flushing up, constipation, firm conformation.

Kuei-chih-fu-ling-wan (Cinnamon and Hoelen Formula): blood occlusion, pain in the lower abdomen, flushing up, vertigo, spasm in the left rectus abdominis muscle, somewhat firm conformation.

Tang-kuei-shao-yao-san (*Tang-kuei* and Peony Formula): blood occlusion, pain in the lower abdomen, anemia, chills, a weak conformation.

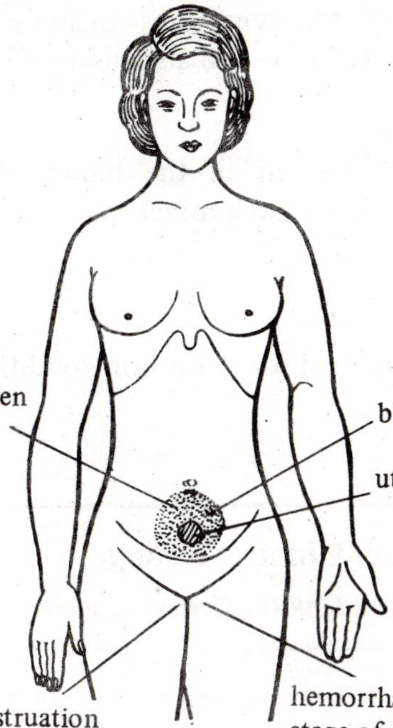

Chih-Shih-Shao-Yao-San *(Chih-shih and Peony Formula)*	**枳實芍藥散**
Chih-shih 3.0 Peony 3.0 (administered with barley congee)	

Recorded in *Chin kuei yao lueh* (金匱要略). Postpartum abdominal pain is differentiated into weak and firm types. If the abdominal pain is not accompanied by distress and distention, internal weakness is indicated and the pain is of the weak type. If distress and distention are present making it impossible for the patient to lie down, the pain is of internal firmness. This firm conformation is the result of postartum hemostasis (stagnation of blood) and pneumastasis (stagnation of air) and must be treated with this formula in order to move the obstructed air and blood. Consequently all the symptoms–including abdominal pain, irritability, and distention–will also disappear.

Herbs and Actions
Chih-shih moves the air in the blood. Peony harmonizes the blood and alleviates abdominal pain. Barley congee soothes gastric air.

Indications
Postpartum abdominal pain of a firm condition.

Chiung-Kuei-Chiao-Ai-Tang 芎歸膠艾湯

(Tang-kuei and Gelatin Combination)

Tang-kuei	4.0	Cnidium	3.0	Peony	4.0
Licorice	3.0	Artemisia	3.0	Rehmannia	5.0
Gelatin	3.0				

Chiung-kuei-chiao-ai-tang was first mentioned in the ancient Chinese medical text, *Chin kuei yao lueh* (金匱要略 A.D. 205, Summaries on Household Drugs) of the Han dynasty. This formula is a tonic and hemostatic and is used to treat bleeding, stagnant blood, anemia, weak arms and legs, pain in the lower limbs, and habitual abortion. It is contraindicated for patients with fever and a flushed face.

Herbs and Actions
Cnidium dispels stagnant blood. Gelatin, Licorice, *Tang-kuei*, Rehmannia, and Peony are blood tonics that nourish the uterus. Artemisia is an astringent and hemostatic which also nourishes the uterus. Gelatin and Artemisia are important components for preventing miscarriage.

Indications
Uterine bleeding, endometritis, uterine cancer, habitual abortion, menorrhagia, rectal bleeding, hemorrhoidal bleeding, intestinal bleeding, hematuria, bleeding due to injuries, hemoptysis, hemopthalmia, purpura, and anemia.

Discrimination
Szu-wu-tang (*Tang-kuei* Four Combination): anemia.
Tang-kuei-shao-yao-san (*Tang-kuei* and Peony Formula): anemia, spasms in left rectus abdominis muscle, water toxin, no hemorrhaging.
Huang-tu-tang (*Fu-lung-kan* Combination): anemia in a person leaning toward a yin conformation.
Kuei-chih-fu-ling-wan (Cinnamon and Hoelen Formula): hemorrhaging, resistance and pain in the abdomen, and a forceful abdomen.
Wen-ching-yin (*Tang-kuei* and Gardenia Combination): anemia, uterine hemorrhaging, and dry skin together with hot flashes.
Huang-lien-chieh-tu-tang (Scute and Coptis Combination): gastrointestinal hemorrhaging when the person has strong vitality.
Jen-sheng-tang (Ginseng and Ginger Combination): stomach hemorrhaging, pain in the upper abdomen, chills, and fatigability.

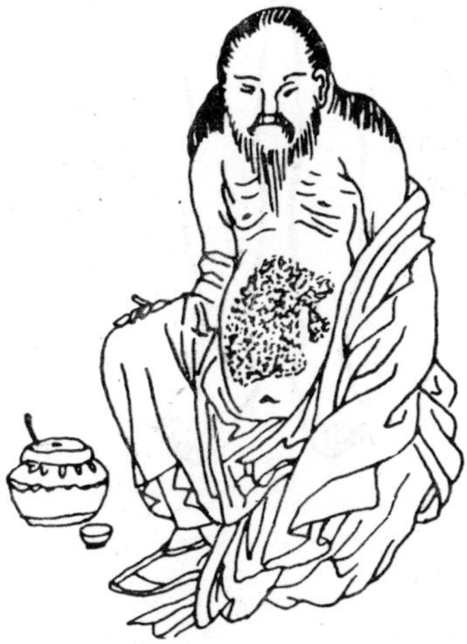

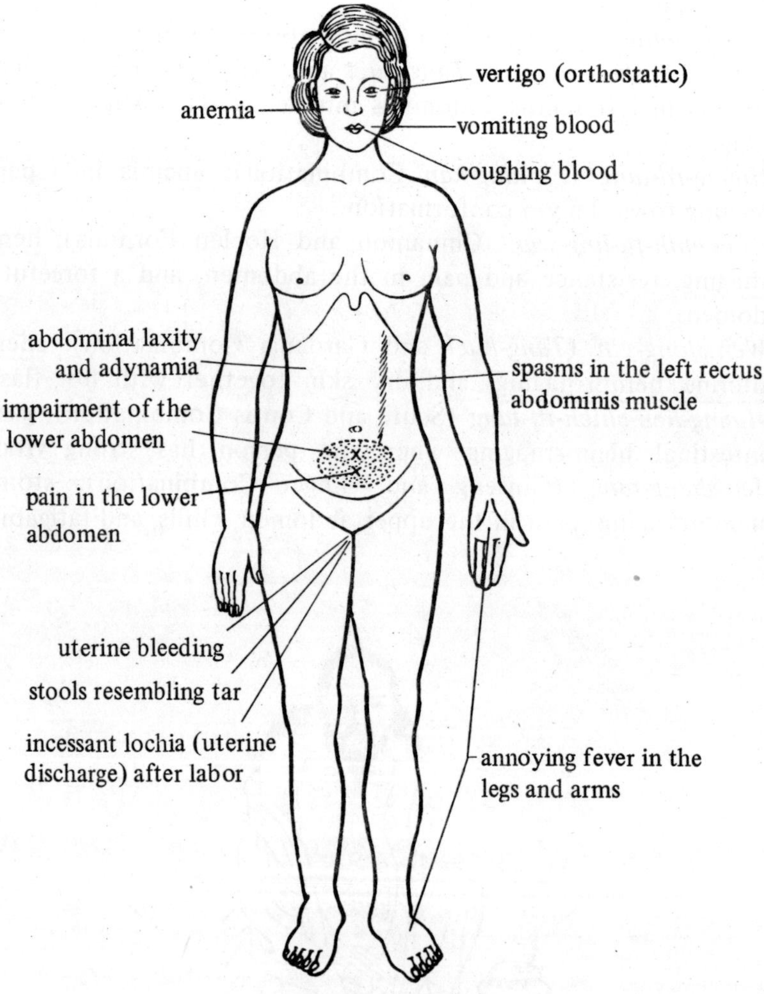
vertigo (orthostatic)
anemia
vomiting blood
coughing blood
abdominal laxity and adynamia
spasms in the left rectus abdominis muscle
impairment of the lower abdomen
pain in the lower abdomen
uterine bleeding
stools resembling tar
incessant lochia (uterine discharge) after labor
annoying fever in the legs and arms

Chiung-Kuei-Tiao-Hsieh-Yin 芎歸調血飲

(Cnidium and Rehmannia Combination)

Tang-kuei	2.0	Cnidium	2.0	Rehmannia	2.0
Atractylodes	2.0	Hoelen	2.0	Citrus	2.0
Lindera	2.0	Cyperus	2.0	Moutan	2.0
Leonurus	1.5	Jujube	1.5	Licorice	1.0
Ginger	1.5				

Chiung-kuei-tiao-hsieh-yin is recorded in *Wan ping hui chun* (萬病回春) of the Ming dynasty. This formula is used for treating all postpartum diseases, weakness of vitality and blood, weakness of the spleen and stomach, loss of appetite, sweating, dry throat, anxiety, asthma, abdominal pain, chest distention, vertigo, and tinnitus. It is suitable for anemia, lochia, and postpartum diseases.

Herbs and Actions

Tang-kuei, Cnidium, and Rehmannia nourish the blood. Hoelen, Atractylodes, Citrus, and Licorice nourish the spleen and stomach. Lindera and Cyperus regulate the *ch'i* and improve the blood circulation. Ginger and Jujube nourish the stomach.

Indications

Postpartum fever, postpartum headache, tinnitus, palpitations, vertigo, flushing up, climacteric disorders, beriberi, and menstrual irregularities.

Discrimination

Pa-chen-tang (*Tang-kuei* and Ginseng Eight Combination): weakness in *ch'i* and blood; relatively hotter-natured herbs are used than those in *Shih-chuan-ta-pu-tang.*

Shih-chuan-ta-pu-tang (Ginseng and *Tang-kuei* Ten Combination): weakness in *ch'i* and blood, anemia, fatigability, dry skin, weak conformation.

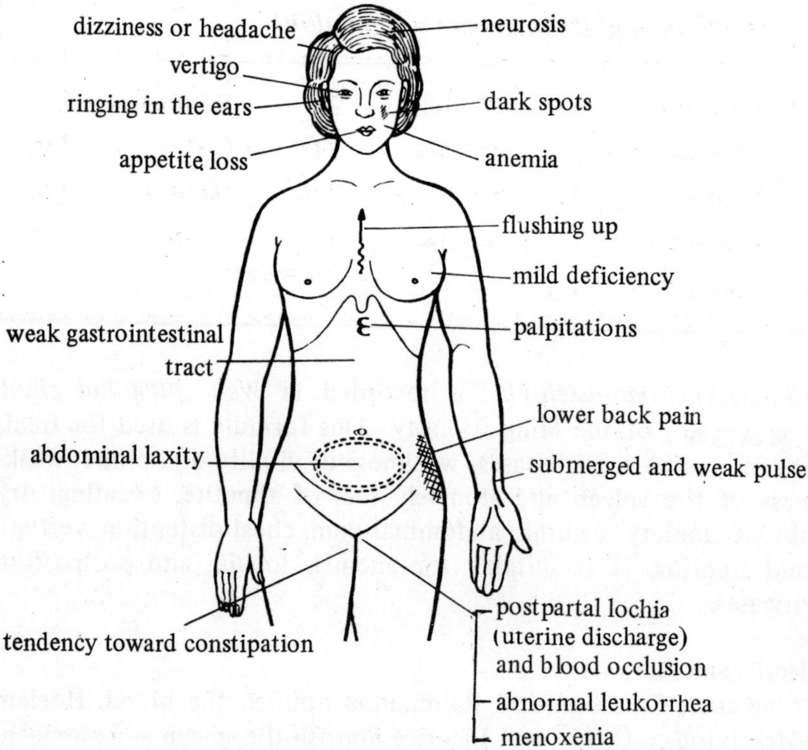

Hsia-Yu-Hsieh-Tang 下瘀血湯

(Persica and Eupolyphaga Combination)

Rhubarb	16.0	Eupolyphaga	21.0	Persica	7.0

Recorded in *Chin kuei yao lueh* (金匱要略). Treats abdominal pain in postpartum women caused by blood occlusion. It is indicated for incessant uterine discharge following childbirth that results in such turgidity and pain in the lower abdomen that the patient can't be touched. The way to treat such a condition is to use a formula such as this one that combats rigidity, breaks up accumulations, and removes palpable, obstructed masses. For the condition of amenorrhea resulting from blood occlusion and obstruction, this formula is also used.

Herbs and Actions
Persica and Eupolyphaga activate occluded blood and remove the occlusion. Rhubarb purges fever and discharges occlusion. In combination these components purge fever and remove occlusion.

Indications
Incessant uterine discharge after labor; abdominal pain that is so severe the patient cannot tolerate pressure on the abdomen; dysmenorrhea or menoxenia; and all the diseases derived therefrom, as well as menopausal abdominal pain and turgidity.

Discrimination
Tang-kuei-sheng-chiang-yang-zou-tang (*Tang-Kuei,* Ginger, and Mutton Combination) treats postpartum abdominal pain, anemia, chills and cramps.
Chih-shih-shao-yao-san (*Chih-shih* and Peony Formula) treats postpartum abdominal pain, respiratory obstruction and stagnation of blood that causes pain, as well as distention in the abdomen that makes it painful or impossible for the patient to lie down.

Po-Tzu-Jen-Wan 柏子仁丸

(Biota and Achyranthes Formula)

Biota	2.0	Achyranthes	2.0	Selaginella	2.0
Lycopus	8.0	Dipsacus	8.0	Rehmannia	4.0

Po-tzu-jen-wan is recorded in *Fu jen ta chuan liang fang* (婦人大全良方) of the Sung dynasty. This formula is used for treating anemia with fever, menstrual irregularity, anxiety, and amenorrhea. It is suitable for irregular menstruation and amenorrhea accompanying tuberculosis.

Herbs and Actions
Biota tranquilizes the nerves and the heart. Selaginella and Lycopus promote good blood circulation and relieve amenorrhea. Rehmannia acts as a tonic. Achyranthes regulates the menses and stimulates the circulation of the blood. Dipsacus is a hemostatic.

Indications
Menstrual irregularity, amenorrhea.

Pu-Kung-Ying-Tang 蒲公英湯

(Dandelion Combination)

Dandelion	8.0	*Tang-kuei*	6.0	Dioscorea	4.0
Cyperus	3.0	Moutan	3.0		

Pu-kung-ying-tang was recorded in the Japanese medical work, *Fang yu ni* (方輿輗) by Arimochi Keiri and Hachiya Bunkyo. It is used for treating agalactia.

Herbs and Actions
Dandelion, the major herb in this formula, is a lactagogue. Moutan nourishes the blood. Dioscorea is a general tonic. Cyperus dispels stagnant blood and acts as an emmenagogue. *Tang-kuei* nourishes the blood and treats blood disorders in women.

Indications
Agalactia.

Sheng-Hua-Tang 生化湯

(Tang-kuei and Ginger Combination)

Tang-kuei	2.4	Cnidium	9.0	Persica	4.0
Ginger	1.5	Licorice	1.5		

Recorded in *Fu ching chu nu ko* (傅青主女科) by Fu Ching-chu of the Ching dynasty. Used for treating postnatal bleeding, stagnant blood, abdominal pain due to uterine constriction, and postnatal infection.

Herbs and Actions
Tang-kuei nourishes the blood, Cnidium increases vitality, Persica dispels stagnant blood, Ginger eases pain, and Licorice coordinates the actions of the other herbs.

Indications
Postnatal bleeding and abdominal pain.

Shih-Hsiao-San 失笑散

(Pteropus and Bulrush Formula)

Pteropus	3.0	Bulrush	3.0

Shih-hsiao-san is recorded in *Tai ping huei min ho chi chu fang* (太平惠民和劑局方) of the Ming dynasty. This formula is used for treating menstrual irregularity and pain during menstruation due to stagnant blood; postpartum bleeding; abdominal pain; and stagnant blood and swelling pain due to external injuries.

Herbs and Actions

Bulrush nourishes the blood and dispels stagnant blood. Pteropus removes stagnant blood and eliminates pain.

Indications
Abdominal pain in women, postpartum bleeding, pain beneath the heart, and pain due to external injuries.

Tang-Kuei-San 當歸散

(Tang-kuei Formula)

Tang-kuei	1.5	Peony	3.0	Cnidium	3.0
Atractylodes	1.5	Scute	3.0		

Recorded in *Chin kuei yao lueh* (金匱要略) of the Han dynasty. Used primarily to cleanse fevers and prevent spontaneous abortions; hence it is given to pregnant women who have deficient blood and a fever and who show signs of aborting. It also eases difficult labor. Regular taking of the formula aids development of the fetus, prevents various gynecological diseases, and alleviates postpartum problems.

Herbs and Actions
Atractylodes nourishes the spleen and strengthens the intestines. Scute cleanses fever in the intestines. *Tang-kuei* and Cnidium remove obstructed blood. Peony also purges a fever of the blood and blood vessels.

Indications
Habitual spontaneous abortion; overactive, unsecured fetus; and postpartum problems.

Tang-Kuei-Shao-Yao-San 當歸芍藥散

(Tang-kuei and Peony Formula)

Tang-kuei	3.0	Peony	4.0	Hoelen	4.0
Atractylodes	4.0	Cnidium	3.0	Alisma	4.0

Tang-kuei-shao-yao-san was first mentioned in an ancient Chinese medical work *Chin kuei yao lueh* (A.D. 205, Summaries on Household Drugs) of the Han dynasty. This formula is used to ease abdominal pain during pregnancy and various other abdominal aches in women. It can cure men as well as women of weak conformation with anemia, pallor, general lassitude, and pain in the lower abdomen, waist, and heart. It is also effective for conditions without abdominal pain but with symptoms of heaviness in the head, vertigo, tinnitus, lumbago, chilled feet, and palpitation. However, the patient suffering from nausea, vomiting, and loss of appetite should not take this formula.

Herbs and Actions

Tang-kuei, a hematinic and nutritive, synthesizes the actions of the herbs and eases pain. Atractylodes is a diuretic. Cnidium increases vitality and nourishes the blood. Hoelen dispels inner fluid accumulation and is compatible with Atractylodes and Alisma.

Indications

1. Pregnancy Disorders: edema, habitual abortion, premature rupture of the membrane, hemorrhoids, abdominal pain, cystitis, and lumbago.
2. Postpartum weakness.
3. Menstrual irregularity, difficult menstruation, and female disorders.
4. Chronic nephritis, menoplegia, vascular disease, and beriberi.

Discrimination

Hsiao-chien-chung-tang (Minor Cinnamon and Peony Combina-

tion): abdominal pain but no chilling and water toxin.
Tang-kuei-chien-chung-tang (*Tang-kuei,* Cinnamon, and Peony Combination): abdominal pain, lower back pain at night, floating pulse, no cold feet or water toxin.
Pan-hsia-hou-pu-tang (Pinellia and Magnolia Combination): mental distress and sore throat.
Kuei-chih-fu-ling-wan (Cinnamon and Hoelen Formula): pain in the lower abdomen, irregular menses, firm conformation, no symptoms of a water conformation.
Chiung-kuei-chiao-ai-tang (Gelatin and *Tang-kuei* Combination): pain in the lower abdomen, anemia; this formula chiefly treats hemorrhages.
Tang-kuei-szu-ni-chia-wu-chu-yu-sheng-chiang-tang (*Tang-kuei,* Evodia, and Ginger Combination): severe and painful chilling in the hands and feet, submerged and minute pulse.
Pa-wei-wan (Rehmannia Eight Formula): anemia, lassitude, numbness in the lower abdomen or cramping.
Wen-ching-tang (*Tang-kuei* and Evodia Combination): pain in the lower abdomen, infertility, annoying fever in the palms, dry mouth.
Chia-wei-hsiao-yao-san (Bupleurum and Peony Formula): mild fever, mental instability, insomnia, mild thoraco-costal distress in the abdomen.
Tao-ho-cheng-chi-tang (Persica and Rhubarb Combination): firm conformation, flushing up, acute cramping in the lower abdomen.

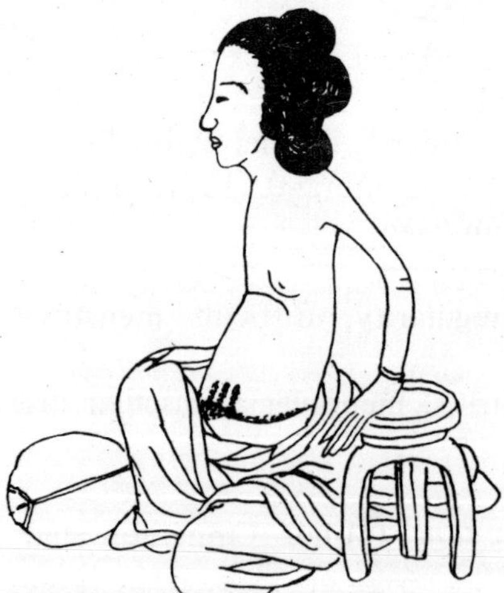

Yin weakness conformation

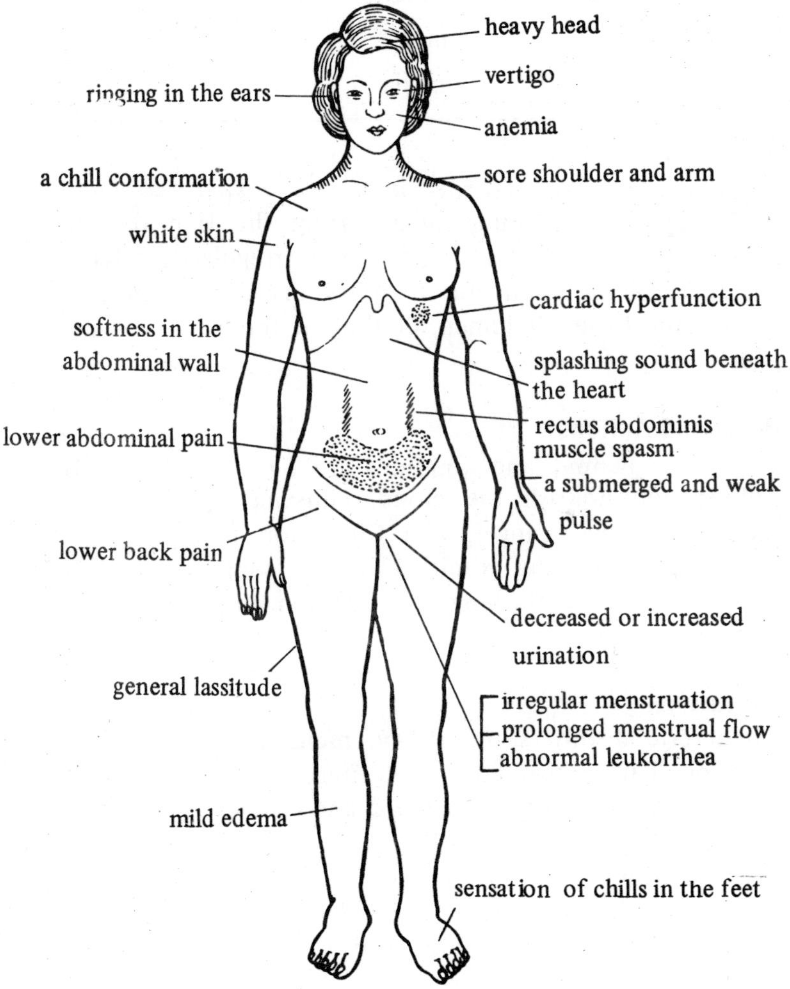

Wen-Ching-Tang 溫經湯

(Tang-Kuei and Evodia Combination)

Evodia	1.0	*Tang-kuei*	3.0	Cnidium	2.0
Ginseng	2.0	Cinnamon	2.0	Gelatin	2.0
Moutan	2.0	Ginger	1.0	Peony	2.0
Licorice	2.0	Pinellia	5.0	Ophiopogon	5.0

Wen-ching-tang was recorded in the *Chin kuei yao lueh* (金匱要略) by Chang Chung-ching during the Han dynasty. This formula is used for treating menstrual irregularity, uterine bleeding, fever in the palms due to stress, dry lips and mouth, distention in the lower abdomen, chilling at the waist, and abdominal pain.

Herbs and Actions

Tang-kuei, Peony, and Cnidium are blood tonics. Gelatin and Ophiopogon nourish the blood. Ginseng and Licorice nourish the *ch'i.* Evodia, Ginger, and Cinnamon relieve chills. Pinellia stops leukorrhea and vomiting and, in conjunction with Ophiopogon, decreases flushing up. Moutan dispels stagnant blood in the lower abdomen.

Indications

Climacteric disorders, infertility, menstrual irregularity, uterine bleeding, leukorrhea, pubescent uterus, habitual abortion, emotional disorders, frostbite, eczema, and calluses and corns.

Discrimination

Tang-kuei-chien-chung-tang (*Tang-kuei,* Cinnamon, and Peony Combination): annoying fever, warm feet, dry mouth and throat, stinging pain in the abdomen.

San-wu-huang-chin-tang (Scute Three Herb Combination): annoying fever in the arms and legs.

Tang-kuei-shao-yao-san (*Tang-kuei* and Peony Formula): infertility, chills, annoying fever in the palms, no dry mouth and lips.

Pa-wei-wan (Rehmannia Eight Formula): annoying fever, annoying fever in the soles of the feet, extreme thirst, numbness beneath the umbilicus.

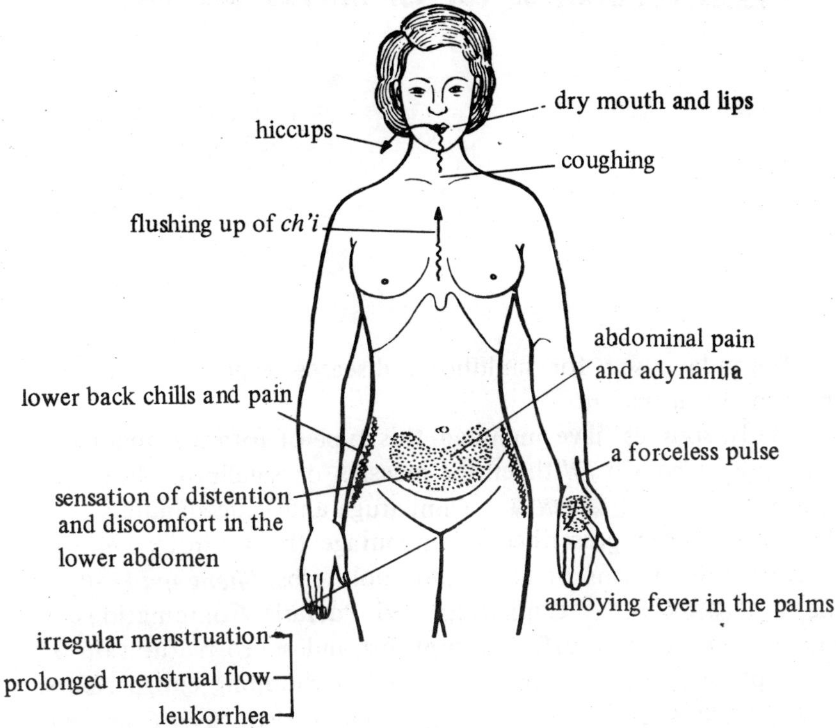

22.

Tou Ma Chi

(痘麻劑, Formulas for Childhood Diseases)

Formulas used for childhood diseases, especially measles, are termed *tou ma chi.*

Many sources have included this type of formula under the term *chieh piao chi.* With either measles or smallpox *Hsuan-tu-fa-piao-tang* (宣毒發表湯 , Cimicifuga and Peucedanum Combination) is often prescribed to encourage the toxin to come to the surface by means of acrid and cool herbs; *Sheng-ma-ko-ken-tang* (升麻葛根湯 , Cimicifuga and Pueraria Combination) is used to disperse the surface symptoms and speed maturation of the eruptions. In the event of pertussis (whooping cough), *San-ao-tang* (三拗湯, *Ma-huang*, Licorice, and Apricot Seed Combination) is used to clear the lungs and to ease muscle aching. *Ma-hsing-kan-shih-tang* (麻杏甘石湯 , Apricot Seed and *Ma-huang* Combination) is used to cleanse the lungs by means of acrid and cool herbs. Some literature also includes acute and chronic infantile tetanus in this chapter.

Smallpox and measles are quarantined contagious diseases which must be reported to the authorities; these formulas must be used with care.

Hsuan-Tu-Fa-Piao-Tang 宣毒發表湯

(Cimicifuga and Peucedanum Combination)

Cimicifuga	1.5	Pueraria	9.0	Peucedanum	6.0
Apricot seed	6.0	Platycodon	4.5	*Chih-ko*	2.4
Schizonepeta	3.0	Siler	6.0	Akebia	6.0
Mentha	1.5	Forsythia	9.0	Arctium	9.0
Lophatherum	6.0	Licorice	3.0		

This formula is most commonly used to speed the ripening of measles. It acts also as a lung-cleanser and an antidote. It was first recorded in *Tou chen jen tuan lu* (痘疹仁端錄 , A Compendium on Pox and Measles) written by Hsu Chien of the Ming dynasty. It is given in the initial stage when the measles have not yet thoroughly and completely erupted.

Actions and Herbs
Cimicifuga and Pueraria relax the muscles and ripen measles; Peucedanum cleans the lungs and dissolves sputum, and when combined with Apricot seed, Platycodon, and *Chih-ko,* it purges the lungs and descends the *ch'i*; Siler and Schizonepeta disperse the "wind and chill evils"; Mentha, acrid and cool, disperses "wind" and cleans fever toxins. Forsythia reduces fever and promotes fluid generation; Arctium, Platycodon, and Licorice act jointly to clean the lungs, loosen congestion, and benefit the throat; Lophatherum eliminates fever and distress: Akebia reduces fever and renders diuresis.

Indications
The initial stage of measles when the eruptions have yet to break out. The patient's conformation exhibits fever. mild chillphobia, stuffy and runny nose, cough, hyperemic eyelids, copious tearing, lassitude, scarce and yellow urine, reddish and raised finger whorls, and diarrhea. The measles-ripening effect of this formula is superior to that of *Sheng-ma-ko-ken-tang.*

San-Ao-Tang 三拗湯

(Ma-huang, Licorice, and Apricot Seed Combination)

Ma-huang	5.0	Apricot seed	5.0	Licorice	5.0

Recorded in *Tai ping huei min ho chi chu fang* (太平惠民和劑局方 *Tai ping huei min* Pharmacopeia). Used to treat common colds, stuffy nose, headaches, hoarseness, vertigo, lassitude, cough with copious sputum, thoracic distention, and gasping.

Herbs and Actions

This formula is made by abstracting Cinnamon from *Ma-huang-tang* (*Ma-Huang* Combination). It works as an acrid, warm, yang-channeling diaphoretic (increases perspiration). Used exclusively for clearing the lungs, arresting coughs, it is named *San-ao-tang. Ma-huang* dispels wind and chill toxins and clears the lungs and calms asthmatics; Apricot seed relieves and calms respiration and helps *Ma-huang* relieve asthma;Licorice harmonizes the various herbs.

Indications

Common cold, chronic bronchitis, bronchial asthma, cough.

Sha-Sheng-Mai-Tung-Tang 沙參麥冬湯

(Adenophora and Ophiopogon Combination)

Adenophora	9.0	Polygonatum	6.0	Licorice	3.0
Morus leaves	4.5	Dolichos (raw)	4.5	Ophiopogon	9.0
Trichosanthes root	4.5				

Taken from *Wen ping tiao pien* (溫病條辨). Cleans and nourishes the lungs and stomach, promotes salivation, and lubricates or moistens aridity. Good for a dry throat and thirst when the fluid secretion of the lungs and stomach has been inhibited. It is also used for a fever and a hacking cough with little production of sputum. Moreover, it is given during the terminal stage of infantile measles when the macules are gradually disappearing and the fever is subsiding. It increases the appetite and recuperates the spirit.

Herbs and Actions

Adenophora and ophiopogon both clean and nourish the lungs and the stomach. Polygonatum and Trichosanthes root promote salivation and relieve thirst. Raw Dolichos and raw Licorice benefit respiration and reinforce the interior; the dulcet flavor of Licorice harmonizes the stomach and, in conjunction with Morus leaves, disperses the arid fever.

Indications

Cough, bronchitis, dry throat, thirst, and the final stage of infantile measles.

Sheng-Ma-Ko-Ken-Tang 升麻葛根湯

(Cimicifuga and Pueraria Combination)

Pueraria	5.0	Peony	3.0	Licorice	1.5
Cimicifuga	2.0	Ginger	2.0		

Sheng-ma-ko-ken-tang is recorded in the Chinese medical text, *Tai ping huei min ho chi chu fang* (太平惠民和劑局方) during the Sung dynasty. This formula is used for treating headache, fever, generalized pain, and measles.

Herbs and Actions

Cimicifuga, Pueraria, and Ginger are detoxifiers that dispel "internal heat". Peony is an astringent, antispasmodic, analgesic, and antipyretic. Licorice coordinates the action of the other herbs.

Indications

Influenza, measles, scarlet fever, chickenpox, epistaxis, hemophthalmia, tonsillitis, and skin diseases.

Discrimination

Ko-ken-tang (Pueraria Combination): chillphobia, fever, headaches, no sweating, severe stiffness in the neck and back.
Ta-ching-lung-tang (Major Blue Dragon Combination): Chillphobia, fever, generalized pain, and vexation and irritativeness.

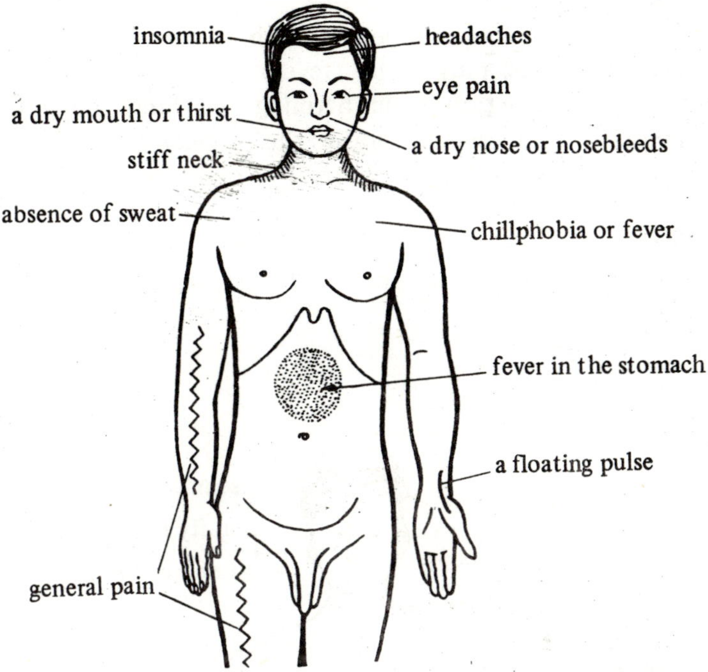

Ting-Li-Ta-Tsao-Hsieh-Fei-Tang *(Lepidium and Jujube Combination)*			葶藶大棗瀉肺湯
Lepidium	1.0	Jujube	6.0

Recorded in *Chin kuei yao lueh* (金匱要略). Treats pulmonary furunculosis at the initial stage when the patient has profuse saliva and sputum clogging the passages, an asthmatic cough that renders lying down impossible, thoracic fullness and distention, tumidity in the face as well as in the whole body, a stuffy and runny nose, and an inability to smell. All these are symptoms of incipient suppurative pulmonary furunculosis indicating a "full-heteropathy" and a very firm conformation.

This formula opens and drains the lungs.

Herbs and Actions

Lepidium is bitter, cold, slippery and sharp in nature. It opens and drains the lungs, purges fire (fever) and expels sputum. To prevent its violent action from harming the lungs, Lepidium is subordinated to Jujube which soothes the stomach and harmonizes the action of Lepidium so that normal respiration is not harmed.

Indications

Pulmonary gangrene, pulmonary abscess, putrid bronchitis, bronchial asthma.

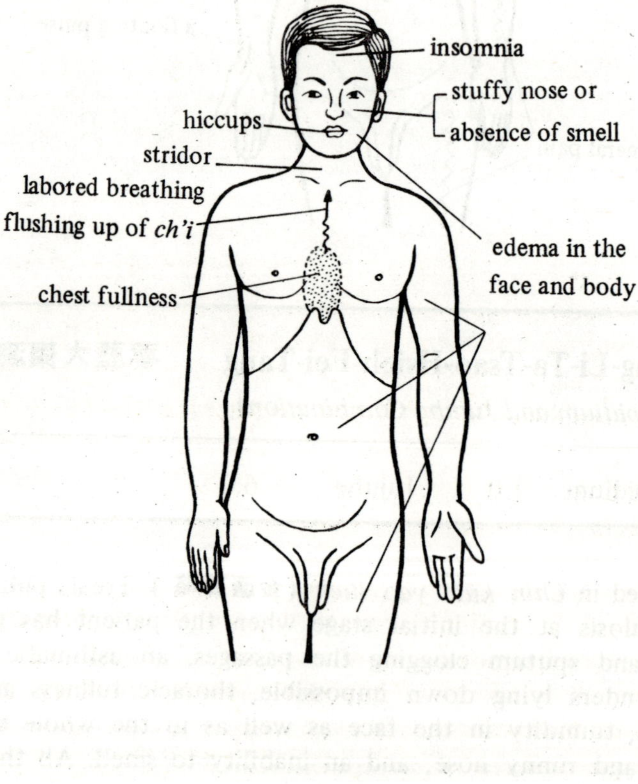

23.
Ming Mu Chi
(明目劑, Eye Formulas)

Formulas that treat ocular diseases are called *ming mu chi.*

The development of ophthalmology as an independent branch of Chinese herbal medicine began during the Sung dynasty. Its therapeutics include internal, external, and surgical treatments. Internal treatment for eye ailments is based on the theoretical concept of there being a relationship between the eyes, the viscera, and the meridians. Localized pathological changes of the eyes are treated by external and surgical methods. The eye is divided into five regions, each called a *lun.* For example, the pupil is the water *lun* and the iris is the wind *lun.* Based on the diagnostic findings, an appropriate internal treatment is selected to adjust the visceral conditions or to attack injurious toxin. Then external treatment is coordinated to the internal treatment. Internal treatment is not only suitable for the eye diseases that arise from visceral or meridian disorders, but also is useful in treating eye diseases caused by epidemic infection or external injuries. Chinese herbal medicine often uses the wind-dispersing, fever-reducing, fire-purging, poison-detoxicating, or liver-supplementing, kidney-benefiting methods to effectively treat eye diseases.

Chi-Chu-Ti-Huang-Wan 杞菊地黃丸

(Lycium, Chrysanthemum, and Rehmannia Formula)

Rehmannia	6.0	Cornus	3.0	Moutan	3.0
Alisma	3.0	Dioscorea	3.0	Hoelen	3.0
Chrysanthemum	1.0	Lycium fruit	1.0		

The origin of this formula is not known although it is recorded in *Tang tou ko chueh* (湯頭歌訣) and *The Grand Lexicon of Chinese Medicine*. It nourishes yin; enriches the blood; benefits the liver; and treats dilation of blood vessels (hyperemia), swelling and pain of the eyes, dizziness and blurring of sight after long use, tearing on contact with wind, photosensitivity (abnormal intolerance to light), vertigo, night sweats, tidal fever, and the loss of muscle power in the feet.

Herbs and Actions

Composed of *Liu-wei-ti-huang-wan* (Rehmannia Six Formula) plus Lycium fruit and Chrysanthemum. *Liu-wei-ti-huang-wan* nourishes yin and supplements the kidneys; Lycium fruit has strengthening and analgesic actions; Chrysanthemum has febrifuge and sedative effects and is effective in treating hyperemia, swelling, and pain in the eyes.

Indications

Hyperemia, swelling and pain in the eyes, dizziness and blurring of vision, tearing, and photosensitivity.

Hsi-Kan-Ming-Mu-Tang 洗肝明目湯

(Gardenia and Vitex Combination)

Tang-kuei	1.5	Peony	1.5	Cnidium	1.5
Rehmannia	1.5	Scute	1.5	Gardenia	1.5
Forsythia	1.5	Siler	1.5	Cassia seed	1.5
Coptis	1.0	Mentha	1.0	*Chianghuo*	1.0
Schizonepeta	1.0	Vitex	1.0	Gypsum	3.0
Chrysanthemum	1.0	Platycodon	1.0	Licorice	1.0
Tribulus	1.0				

Hsi-kan-ming-mu-tang was recorded in the *Wan ping hui chun* (萬病回春) during the Ming dynasty. This formula is used for treating eye ailments in those of strong conformation who have inflammation, congestion, swelling, and pain. It is suitable for keratitis and conjunctivitis.

Herbs and Actions

Tang-kuei, Peony, Cnidium, and Rehmannia of the *Szu-wu-tang* (*Tang-kuei* Four Combination) nourish the blood and eyes. Coptis, Scute, and Gardenia are antipyretics, *Chianghuo,* Siler, Platycodon, Schizonepeta, and Mentha are detoxifiers. Cassia seed dispels "wind heat" and relieves eye ailments. Gypsum is an antipyretic. Vitex cools the blood and is effective for opthalmia. Chrysanthemum dispels "internal heat" in the liver, nourishes the eyes, and clears nebula. Tribulus dispels "wind heat" and nourishes the eyes. Licorice coordinates the actions of the other herbs.

Indications

Sclerosing keratitis, keratitis, scleritis, iritis, and glaucoma.

Discrimination

Pa-wei-ti-huang-wan (Rehmannia Eight Formula): cataracts, weak legs and feet, chills in the lower back.

Tzu-sheng-ming-mu-tang (Scute Combination): weakness from prolonged illness, *ch'i* and blood weakness, tired eyes and astigmatism.

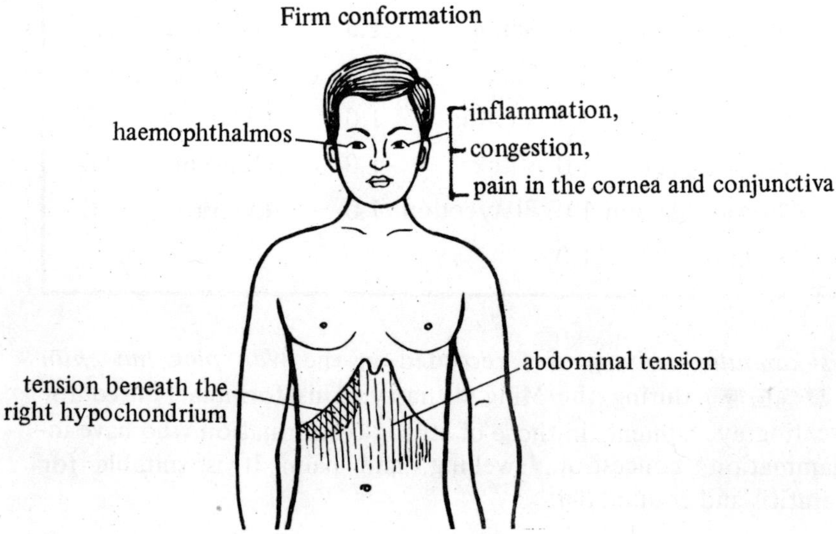

Tzu-Sheng-Ming-Mu-Tang *(Chrysanthemum Combination)*				**滋腎明目湯**	
Tang-kuei	3.0	Peony	3.0	Cnidium	3.0
Platycodon	1.5	Ginseng	1.5	Gardenia	1.5
Coptis	1.5	Angelica	1.5	Vitex	1.5
Licorice	1.5	Chrysanthemum	1.5	Juncus	1.5
Tea	1.5	Raw rehmannia	3.0		
Cured rehmannia		3.0			

Tzu-sheng-ming-mu-tang was recorded in the *Wan ping hui chun* (萬病回春) during the Ming dynasty. This formula is used for treating cataract and also visual defects due to a delicate constitution or lingering disease. It should be taken frequently.

Herbs and Actions

Tang-kuei, Peony, Cnidium, and Rehmannia of *Szu-wu-tang* (*Tang-kuei* Four Combination) nourish the blood and eyes. Chrysanthemum nourishes the eyes, dispels "internal heat" in the liver, and is effective for nebula. Vitex cools the blood and treats ophthalmia. Coptis and Gardenia dispel "internal heat". Ginseng and Licorice nourish the spleen and stomach and increase vitality. Angelica is used to treat headaches and eye ailments. Platycodon reinforces the actions of the other herbs. Juncus nourishes the spleen and acts as an antipyretic and diuretic. Tea is a diuretic and stimulant.

Indications

Visual defects, asthenopia, and cataract.

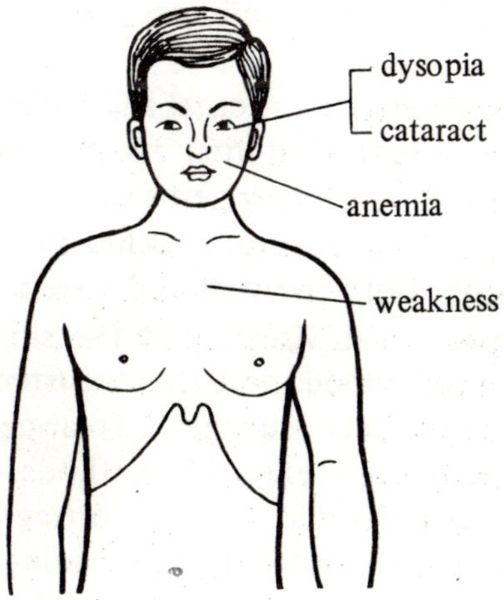

24.
Yung Yang Chi
(癰瘍劑, Carbuncle-dermatosis Formulas)

Formulas that cleanse fever, detoxicate poisons, deflate swelling, soften hardening, and eliminate carbuncles are called *yung yang chi*.

Yung yang chi formulas treat internal and external carbuncles as well as various dermatoses. Internal factors include injuries caused by the seven emotions or by ingestion of acrid, hot, baked, or barbecued foods. External factors include the six excesses and all external wounds. Both internal and external factors can cause disharmony between the viscera and the skin, coagulation and stagnancy of *ch'i* and blood, and the occurrence of various carbuncular or dermatological changes. Treatment for these diseases includes internal and external methods. The internal method of treatment includes *tuo* (托 supporting), *pu* (補 supplementing), and *hsiao* (消 dissolving), depending on the stage of the disease. The external method acts directly on the lesion. Whatever method used, the formulas indicated are essentially antidotal, antiphlogistic, and fever-purging, and chiefly act to circulate and nourish the blood.

Descriptive terms are attached to the illustrative figure accompanying each formula. The terms are arranged clockwise beginning at the top of each figure.

Chieh-Keng-Tang 桔梗湯

(Platycodon Combination)

Platycodon	2.0	Licorice	3.0

Chieh-keng-tang is recorded in the *Shang han lun* (傷寒論) of the Han dynasty. This formula is used for treating suppuration, cough with thick phlegm, pain in the throat due to swelling, pus mixed with blood, severe chills, shivering, chest distention, and dry throat.

Herbs and Actions

Platycodon is a detoxifying agent. Licorice is also a detoxifying agent which nourishes the muscle.

Indications

Gangrene of the lungs, lung abscess, acute bronchitis, and tonsillitis.

Discrimination

Chieh-keng-pai-san (Platycodon and Croton Formula): cough and congested chest, purulent sputum, mild symptoms, strong vitality.
Kan-tsao-tang (Licorice Combination): sore throat but no cough and purulent sputum; aims chiefly at pain.

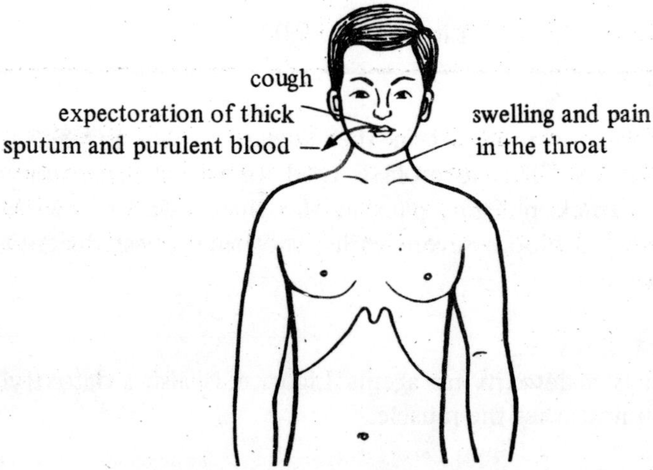

Chien-Chin-Nei-Tuo-San 千金內托散

(Astragalus and Platycodon Formula)

Ginseng	2.5	*Tang-kuei*	3.0	Astragalus	2.0
Cnidium	2.0	Siler	2.0	Platycodon	2.0
Magnolia bark	2.0	Cinnamon	2.0	Angelica	1.0
Licorice	1.0				

Recorded in *Wan ping hui chun* (萬病回春) of the Ming dynasty. Used for treating carbuncles, suppurating skin, delicate constitutions, pain, and polyps.

Herbs and Actions

Ginseng, *Tang-kuei*, Cnidium, and Angelica are tonics. Cinnamon and Astragalus dispel internal poison. Platycodon and Siler are detoxifiers and anti-inflammatives. Magnolia bark is a stomachic. Licorice coordinates the actions of the other herbs.

Indications
Carbuncles, hemorrhoids, periproctitis, suppurative mastitis, lymphadenitis, and suppurative otitis media.

Discrimination
Kuei-chi-chien-chung-tang (*Tang-kuei* and Astragalus Combination): purulence; conformation weaker than *Chien-chin-nei-tuo-san* conformation.
Tuo-li-hsiao-tu-yin (Gleditsia Combination): purulence with mild weak fever condition.

Chih-Tou-Chung-I-Fang 治頭瘡一方

(Forsythia and Lonicera Formula)

Forsythia	3.0	Cnidium	3.0	Siler	2.0
Atractylodes	3.0	Lonicera	2.0	Carthamus	1.0
Schizonepeta	1.0	Licorice	1.0	Rhubarb	0.5

Chih-tou-chung-i-fang, a reliable formula used in Japan, is effective for treating children who have lesions on the head accompanied by itching and desquamation as well as inflammation and suppuration on the face, neck, armpits, and genital areas. This formula should be used frequently.

Herbs and Actions
Forsythia and Lonicera are used to treat severe ulcers. Siler is an antipyretic and smoothes the stagnant *ch'i*. Schizonepeta dispels stagnant blood and treats boils. Carthamus removes stagnant blood. Atractylodes removes moisture. Cnidium improves the actions of the other herbs. Rhubarb treats constipation. Licorice relieves acute symptoms.

Indications
Eczema on the head in children, and inflammatory dermatitis.

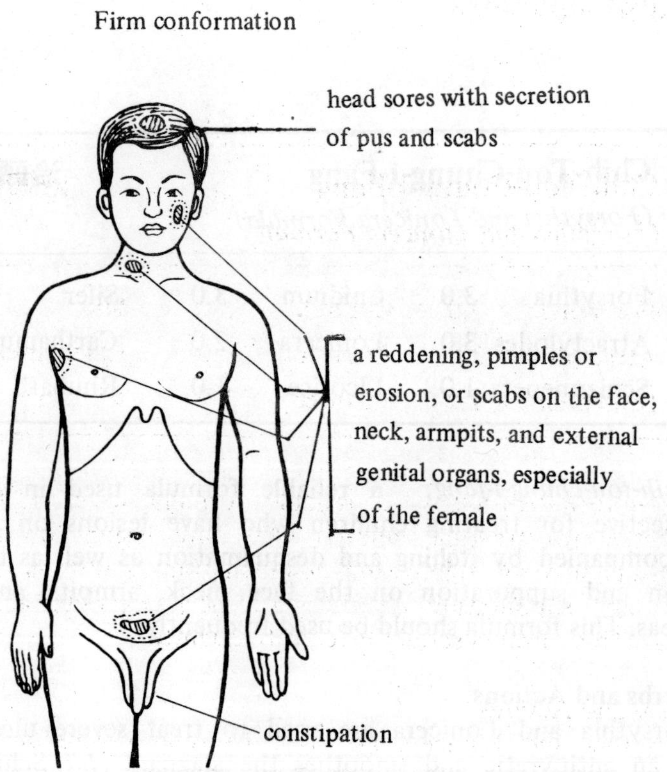
Firm conformation
head sores with secretion of pus and scabs
a reddening, pimples or erosion, or scabs on the face, neck, armpits, and external genital organs, especially of the female
constipation

Ching-Chieh-Lien-Chiao-Tang 荊芥連翹湯

(Schizonepeta and Forsythia Combination)

Tang-kuei	1.5	Peony	1.5	Cnidium	1.5
Scute	1.5	Gardenia	1.5	Forsythia	1.5
Siler	1.5	Schizonepeta	1.5	*Chih-ko*	1.5
Platycodon	2.0	Angelica	2.0	Bupleurum	2.0
Licorice	1.5	Phellodendron	1.5	Licorice	1.5
Coptis	1.5	Mentha	1.5	Rehmannia	1.5

Recorded in *Wan ping hui chun* (萬病回春) of the Ming dynasty. Used for treating otitis, rhinitis, and suppuration. It is effective for people with glandular constitutions who have dark-brown skin, a tight pulse, and abdominal tension.

Herbs and Actions

Tang-Kuei, Cnidium, and Peony nourish the blood. Schizonepeta, Siler, and *Chih-ko* are antipyretic and detoxifying agents. Forsythia and Platycodon suppress suppuration. Scute and Gardenia are anti-inflammatives and antipyretics. Bupleurum removes stagnant heat in the liver. Angelica is a carminative, and licorice coordinates the actions of the other herbs.

Indications

Otitis media, nasal suppuration, rhinitis, tonsillitis, nosebleeds, tuberculosis, acne, and baldness.

Discrimination

Chai-hu-ching-kan-tang (Bupleurum and Rehmannia Combination): for teenagers.

Lung-tan-hsieh-kan-tang (Gentiana Combination): a wet fever in the liver meridian. This formula is usually given to youths.

Hsiao-chai-hu-tang (Minor Bupleurum Combination): thoraco-costal distress.

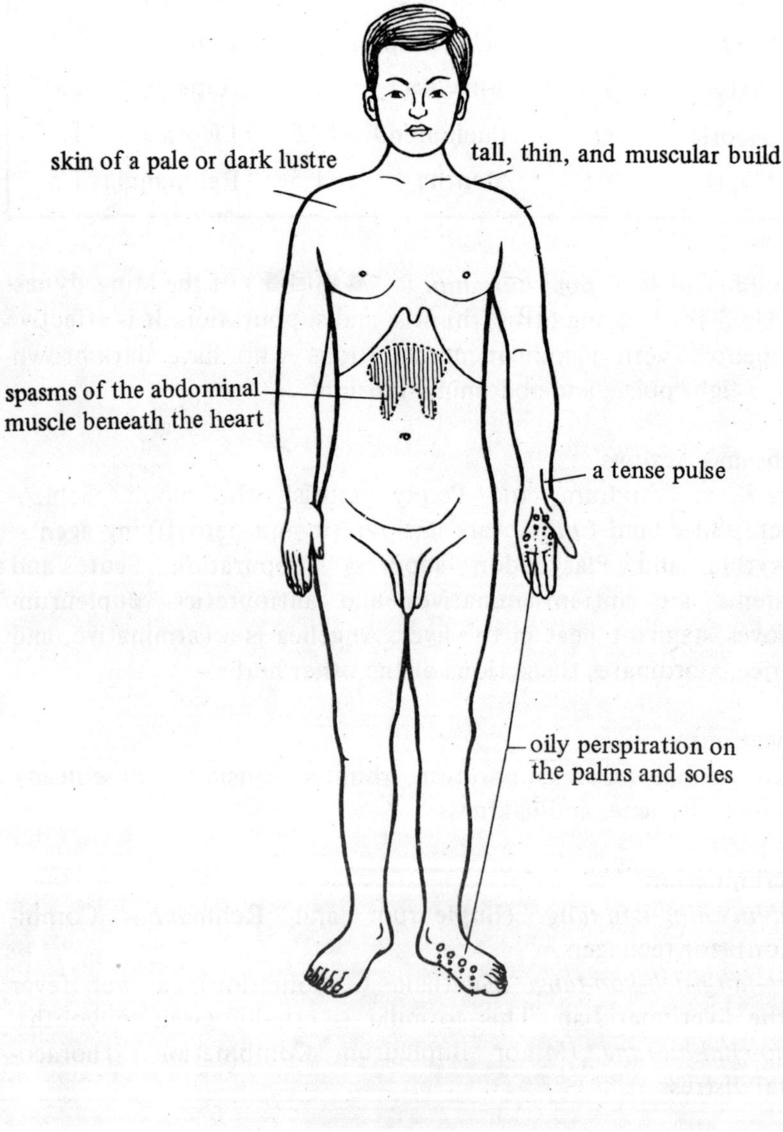
skin of a pale or dark lustre
tall, thin, and muscular build
spasms of the abdominal muscle beneath the heart
a tense pulse
oily perspiration on the palms and soles

Ching-Fang-Pai-Tu-San 荆防敗毒散

(Schizonepeta and Siler Formula)

Schizonepeta	1.5	Siler	1.5	*Chianghuo*	1.5
Tuhuo	1.5	Bupleurum	1.5	Mentha	1.5
Peucedanum	1.5	Platycodon	1.5	Forsythia	1.5
Chih-ko	1.5	Cnidium	1.5	Lonicera	1.5
Licorice	1.0	Ginger	1.0		

Ching-fang-pai-tu-san is recorded in the Chinese medical work of the Ming dynasty *Wan ping hui chun* (萬病回春). This formula is used for treating suppuration accompanied by severe chills, fever, headache, muscle spasms, inflammation, swelling, pain, and congestion.

Herbs and Actions

Bupleurum, Peucedanum, Ginger, and Mentha are carminatives. Schizonepeta, Siler, *Chianghuo,* and *Tuhuo* are detoxifiers and analgesics. Forsythia, Platycodon, Cnidium, and Lonicera are antiphlogistics and depuratives that relieve suppuration and swelling. *Chih-ko* dispels stagnant *ch'i*. Licorice coordinates the actions of the other herbs.

Indications

Carbuncles, pustules, boils, mastitis, urticaria, scabies, eczema, sinusitis, syphilis, dermatitis, and conjunctival disorders.

Discrimination

Tuo-li-hsiao-tu-yin (Gleditsia Combination): suppuration and regressing inflammatory congestion.

Chien-chin-nei-tuo-san (Astragalus and Platycodon Formula) suppuration; a weak conformation after prolonged illness; and deteriorated vitality.

Ching-Shang-Fang-Feng-Tang-Chia-I-Yi-Jen 清上防風湯加薏苡仁

(Siler and Coix Combination)

Schizonepeta	1.5	Coptis	1.5	Mentha	1.5
Chih-shih	1.5	Licorice	1.5	Gardenia	3.0
Cnidium	3.0	Scute	3.0	Forsythia	3.0
Angelica	3.0	Platycodon	3.0	Siler	3.0
Coix	3.0				

This formula is made by adding Coix to the Siler Combination. The purpose of Coix is to increase the therapeutic effect of Siler Combination, especially when treating facial vesicles.
Shen shih tsun sheng shu (1773 A.D.) of the Ching dynasty, records: "*Ching-shang-fang-feng-tang* purges the anxiety and inner heat of the upper body and cures facial boils and heat diseases." Hence, it is used for tense pulse, anhidrosis, oliguria, constipation, flushing of the face, inner heat, and boils on the face and head.

Herbs and Actions

Coix, Scute, and Gardenia purge inner heat. Siler, Platycodon, and Mentha promote diaphoresis and detoxification. Forsythia and *Chih-shih* relieve swelling and eliminate pus. Angelica, Cnidium, and Licorice coordinate and improve the effects of other herbs. And Coix has antiphlogistic, pus-purging, and analgesic effects.

Indications

Head and facial boils, vesicles, eczema, facial flushing, conjunctivitis, red nose, otitis media, gingivitis, and favus.

Discrimination

Ching-fang-pai-tu-san (Schizonepeta and Forsythia Formula): is suitable for a relatively milder condition than a *Ching-shang-fang-feng-tang-chia-i-yi-jen*.

Fang-feng-tung-sheng-san (Siler and Platycodon Formula): firmer conformation than *Ching-shang-fang-feng-tang-chia-i-yi-jen* with severe fever and constipation.

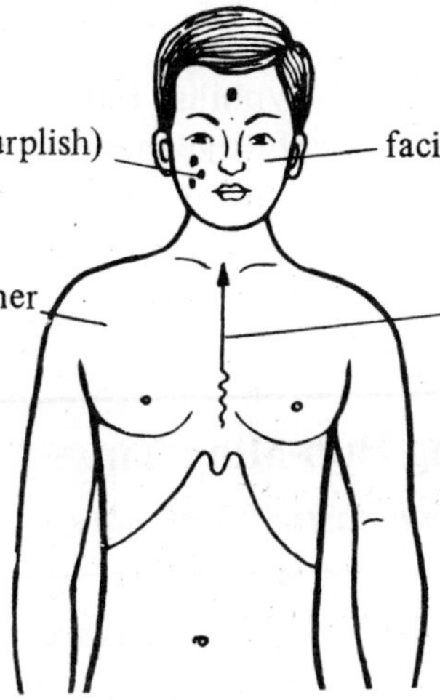

Hsiang-Chun-Chieh-Tu-Chi 香川解毒劑

(Smilax and Akebia Combination)

Smilax	4.0	Akebia	4.0	Cnidium	3.0
Lonicera	3.0	Licorice	1.0	Rhubarb	1.0
Hoelen	5.0				

A family prescription of the Kakawas in Japan. Suitable for common syphilis, dermatoses, and gonorrhea: chiefly indicated for syphilitic sores, inguinal bubo, chancre, second and third stage syphilis, fistula, syphilitic eruption, and various syphilitic symptoms.

Herbs and Actions
Smilax detoxifies and aids the excretion of moisture. Akebia

purges fever and causes urination. Cnidium and Lonicera are antiphlogistic and clean the blood. Rhubarb is an anti-inflammative and purgative. Hoelen aids diuresis and strengthens the spleen. Licorice harmonizes the various components.

Indications

Initial induration of syphilis, bubo, syphilid (any skin eruption due to syphilis), syphilitic neuralgia, syphilitic keratitis, and gonorrhea.

Hsien-Fang-Huo-Ming-Yin 仙方活命飲

(Angelica and Mastic Combination)

Anteater scales	3.0	Licorice	3.0	Mastic	3.0
Angelica	3.0	Peony	3.0	Fritillaria	3.0
Siler	3.0	Myrrh	3.0	*Tang-kuei*	3.0
Gleditsia spine	3.0	Lonicera	9.0	Citrus	9.0
Trichosanthes root	3.0				

Hsien-fang-huo-ming-yin is recorded in *Wai k'o fa hui* (外科發揮). This formula is used for treating carbuncles, swelling, inflammation and pain in an infected area, and suppurative dermatitis.

Herbs and Actions

Lonicera, Licorice, Trichosanthes root, and Fritillaria are antipyretics and detoxifiers. *Tang-kuei* and Peony nourish the blood and remove stagnant blood. Mastic and Myrrh remove stagnant blood and eliminate pain. Siler and Angelica are antiphlogistics. Anteater scales and Gleditsia are antiphlogistics. Citrus removes "stagnant *ch'i*"

Indications

Carbuncles, swelling ulcers, boils and acne.

Firm conformation

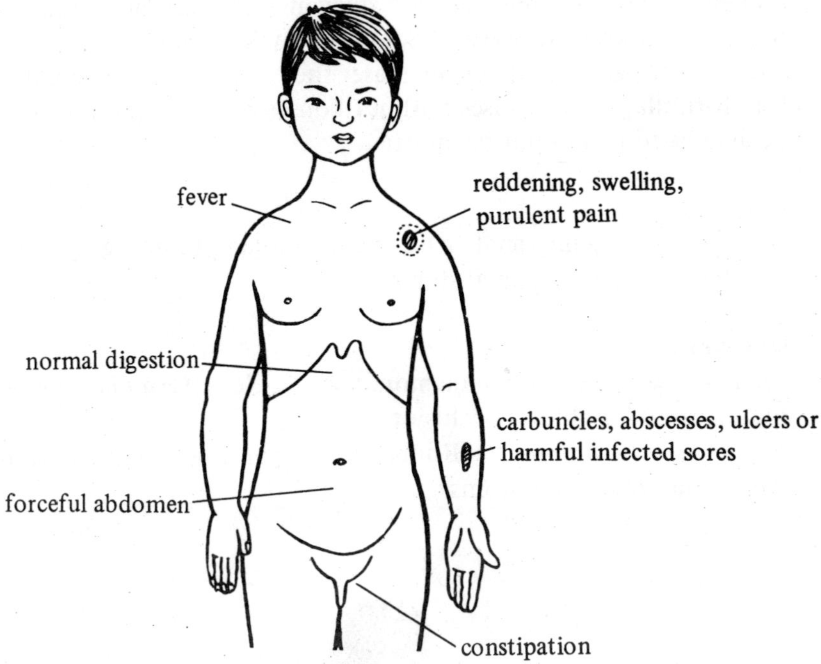

I-Tzu-Tang *(Cimicifuga Combination)*					乙字湯
Cimicifuga	1.5	Bupleurum	5.0	*Tang-kuei*	6.0
Licorice	2.0	Scute	3.0	Rhubarb	1.0

I-tzu-tang is an experimental formula developed by Hara Nan-you, a famous doctor of the Tokugawa era in Japan. Later, Mr. Asata used *Tang-kuei* instead of Jujube in the formula, and it produced better results. This formula is a specific for hemorrhoids. It is effective for those having constipation with bleeding and severe local pain.

Herbs and Actions

Bupleurum and Cimicifuga remove moist heat in the lower abdomen. *Tang-kuei* and Licorice alleviate hemorrhoidal pain and promote smooth evacuation. Scute removes intestinal heat. Those with constipation should increase the amount of Rhubarb in this formula, and in cases without constipation, Rhubarb should be decreased in amount or omitted.

Indications

Hemorrhoidal pain, anal ache, hemorrhoidal bleeding, prolapse of the rectum, and vaginal itching.

Discrimination

Kuei-chih-fu-ling-wan (Cinnamon and Hoelen Formula): hemorrhoids caused by blood occlusion.
Ta-huang-mu-tan-pi-tang (Rhubarb and Moutan Combination): severe and acute symptoms.

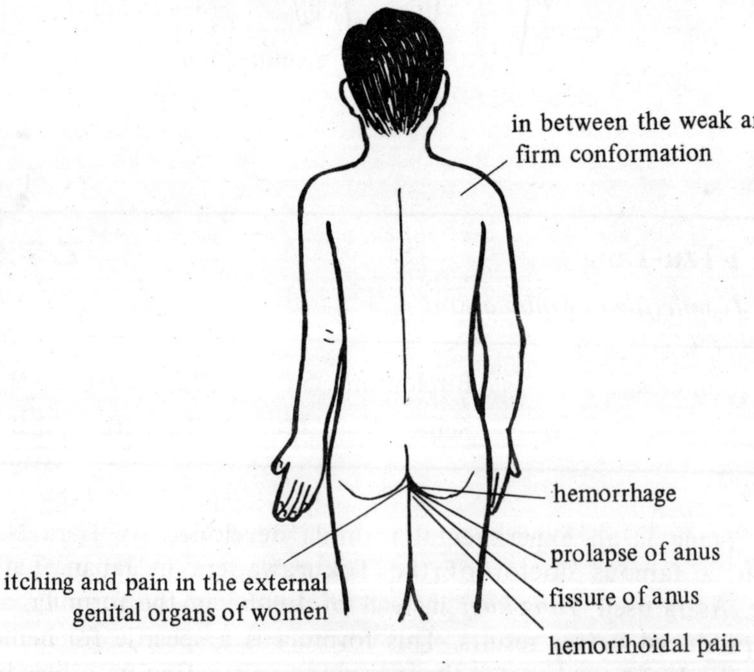

I-Yi-Fu-Tzu-Pai-Chiang-San 薏苡附子敗醬散

(Coix, Aconite, and Thlaspi Formula)

Coix	10.0	Aconite	0.5-1.0	Thlaspi	3.0

Recorded in *Chin kuei yao lueh* (金匱要略). For intestinal furunculosis and a weak-yin conformation. (Intestinal furunculosis is equivalent to appendicitis). The targets of treatment are deteriorated and weakened stamina without fever; skin pallor, especially that of the abdomen, that is as dry as fish scales and exhibits a scleroderma state; cramps in the abdominal muscles; and an abdominal wall that is soft and completely without resistance.

Herbs and Actions
Coix is for all kinds of tumors and ulcerations because it promotes the absorption and excretion of pus. Thlaspi is also effective in dissolving tumors or abscesses. Aconite stimulates metabolic action and accelerates absorption.

Indications
Appendicitis, focal peritonitis, suppurative inflammation in accessory organs, hemorrhoidal fistula, palm keratosis, fungal diseases, verruca, leukorrhea.

Discrimination
Ta-huang-mu-tan-pi-tang (Rhubarb and Moutan Combination) is indicated for intestinal furunculosis, a firm-fever conformation, fever, spontaneous sweating, constipation, and a tense pulse. *Wei-ching-tang* (Phragmites Stem Combination) is indicated for coarse and harsh skin, mild fever, cough, distress, and distention.

Weak yin conformation

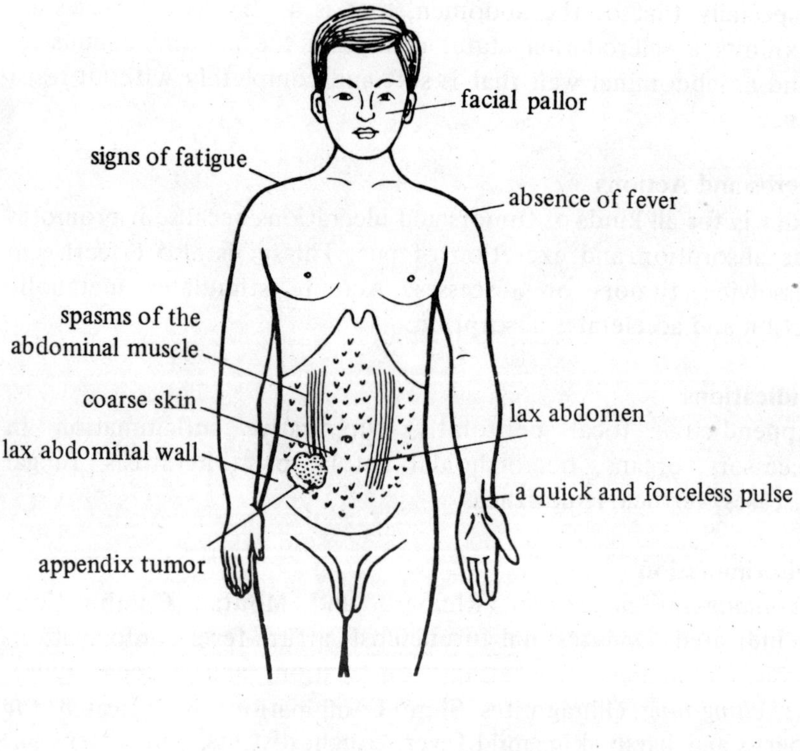

Lo-Shih-Shu 樂適舒

(W. T. T. C.)

Coix	10	Wisteria	10	Trapa	10
Terminalia	10				

Lo-shih-shu is a water soluble ointment manufactured by Sun Ten Pharmaceutical Works Co., Ltd., and Nagakura Pharmaceutical Co. According to a study by Professor Nagayama of Chiba university, W. T. T. C. has a 40% cure rate for gastric cancer and rectal cancer. The pharmacological effects of this formula inhibit the growth of cancer cells and prevent metastasis after cancer surgery.

Herbs and Actions

Coixenolide, an extract of Coix, inhibits the actions of cancer cells, and also acts as an antipyretic, analgesic, and antispasmodic. Trapa is a sedative and astringent. Wisteria is a stomachic and antiphlogistic. Terminalia acts as an antipyretic, detoxifier, and tonic.

Indications

Inflammation, suppuration, dysuria, edema, arthralgia, pain, and muscle spasms.

Pa-Wei-Tai-Hsia-Fang 八味帶下方

(Tang-kuei and Eight Herb Formula)

Tang-kuei	5.0	Cnidium	3.0	Hoelen	3.0
Akebia	3.0	Citrus	2.0	Lonicera	1.0
Rhubarb	1.0	Smilax	4.0		

A commonly used formula recorded in *Ming chia fang hsuan* (名家方選) by Hirai Yoshing of Japan. Used for treating leukorrhea (discharge from the vagina) with "moist heat," mild anemia, subacute inflammation, and congestion.

Herbs and Actions

Smilax and Lonicera detoxify and dispel internal heat. *Tang-kuei and* Cnidium nourish the blood. Hoelen, Akebia, and Citrus dispel moist heat and water poison. In cases without constipation Rhubarb should be omitted.

Indications

If leukorrhea is accompanied by "strong heat," the patient should instead take *Lung-tan-hsieh-kan-tang* (Gentiana Combination).

Discrimination

Lung-tan-hsieh-kan-tang (Gentiana Combination): leukorrhea, yellow leukorrhea, firm conformation, tension in the liver meridian.

Ta-huang-mu-tan-pi-tang (Rehmannia and Moutan Combination): leukorrhea, yellow leukorrhea, firm conformation, inflammation with apparent congestion.

Chia-wei-hsiao-yao-san (Bupleurum and Peony Formula): leukorrhea, white leukorrhea, weak conformation, emotional instability.

Ching-hsin-lien-tzu-yin (Lotus Seed Combination): leukorrhea, watery white leukorrhea, weak conformation, anemia.

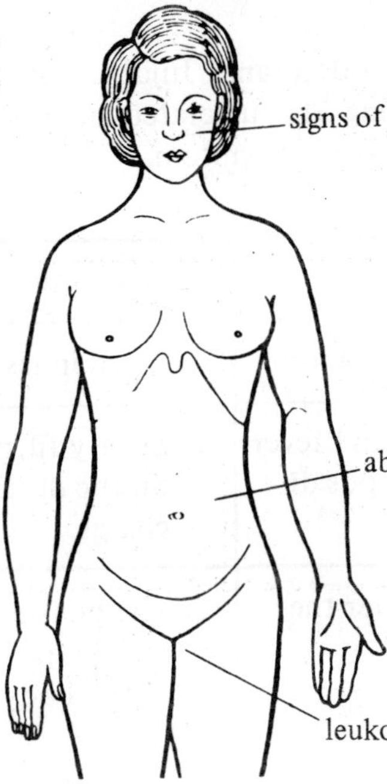

Pai-Nung-San 排膿散

(Platycodon and Chih-shih Formula)

Chih-shih	5.0	Peony	5.0	Platycodon	2.0

Recorded in *Chin kuei yao lueh* (金匱要略) of the Han dynasty. Used for treating suppuration, inflammation, ulceration, harndess in the upper abdomen, and abdominal spasms.

Herbs and Actions

Chih-shih relieves stiffness and tension in the affected area. Peony stimulates blood circulation and removes stagnant blood. Platycodon removes suppuration.

Indications

Carbuncles, boils, lymphadenitis, gangrene, tonsillitis, suppuration, pyorrhoea, otitis externa, hemorrhoids, periproclitis, and mastitis.

Discrimination

Pai-nung-tang (Platycodon and Jujube Combination): Suppuration; it is used during the ulcerated and pus discharge period, scanty infiltration, chronic symptom.

Pai-nung-san	*Pai-nung-tang*
1. Closed in lesion and nature.	1. Open in lesion and nature.
2. Severe infiltration and fever sensation, difficult pus discharge	2. Scanty filtration sensation, on the duration of pus discharge.
3. The pus deeply under the skin.	3. The pus discharge is occurring on the trachea and the surface of the body.

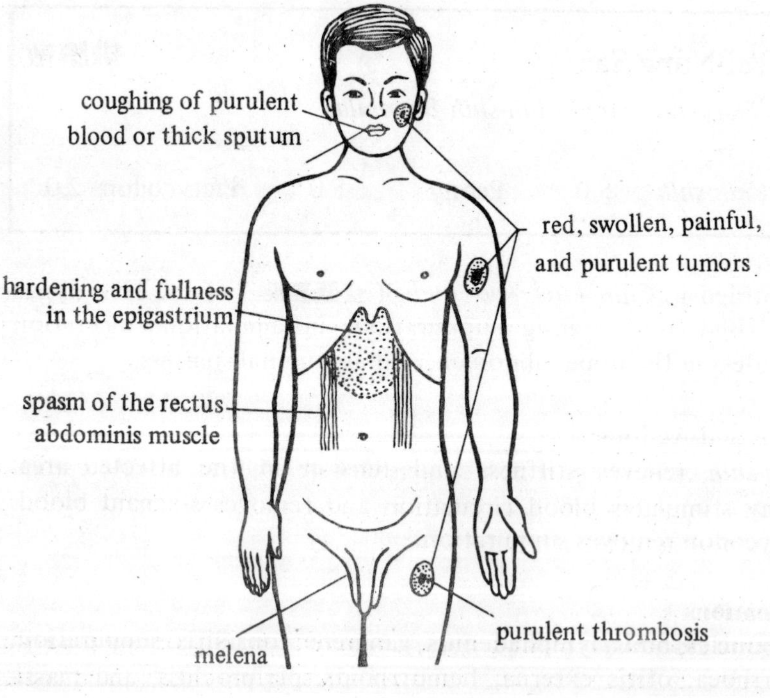

Pai-Nung-Tang *(Platycodon and Jujube Combination)*					**排膿湯**
Licorice	3.0	Platycodon	4.0	Jujube	6.0
Ginger	3.0				

Pai-nung-tang is recorded in *Chin kuei yao lueh* (金匱要略) of the Han dynasty. This formula is used for treatment during the initial stages of infection in which there is swelling, muscular tension in the infected area, and slight suppuration.

Herbs and Actions
Platycodon can prevent suppuration and also dispel pus. Licorice and Jujube relieve acute symptoms and, in combination with Ginger, can improve the actions of the other herbs.

Indications
Carbuncle, suppurative ulcer, otitis media, nasal suppuration, pyorrhea, hemorrhoids, tonsillitis, lung abscess, and lung gangrene.

Discrimination
Pai-nun-san (Platycodon and *Chih-shih* Formula): suppuration, severe edema and coagulation.
Huang-chi-chien-chung-tang (Astragalus and Peony Combination): suppuration with thin pus; severe, weak conformation.

Po-Chou-San 伯州散

(Eriocheir and Viper Formula)

Eriocheir	1.0	Cervus horn	1.0	Viper	1.0

Po-chou-san is an experimental formula in Japan. It has been used for treating subacute or chronic suppurative diseases, pain due to swelling, and purulent discharge. It also acts as a tonic, stimulant, hemostatic, and antiphlogistic. Those having active tuberculosis and malignant tumors should not take this formula.

Herbs and Actions

Viper is a stimulant, tonic, and analgesic, and it increases the elimination of pus. Eriocheir dispels stagnant blood, and nourishes the muscle. Cervus horn is an antipyretic, improves blood circulation, and reduces swelling.

Indications

Carbuncles, mastitis, Lymphadenitis, periproctitis, hemorrhoids, otitis media, gangrene in the bones, ulcers on the legs, and external injuries.

Discrimination

Pai-nung-san (Platycodon and *Chih-shih* Formula): suppuration, initial inflammation, congestion, swelling, and severe pain. This formula cannot be used in conjunction with *Po-chou-san.*

Pai-nung-tang (Platycodon and Jujube Combination): suppuration, chronic symptoms; this formula can be used with *Po-chou-san.*

Chien-chin-nei-tuo-san (Astragalus and Platycodon Formula): suppuration. It is better to give this formula with *Po-chou-san* when pus is discharging.

Tuo-li-hsiao-tu-yin (Gleditsia Combination): suppuration. This formula is to be used with *Po-chou-san*.

San-Tsung-Kuei-Chien-Tang 散腫潰堅湯

(Forsythia and Laminaria Combination)

Tang-kuei	1.5	Peony	1.5	Bupleurum	1.5
Scute	1.5	Coptis	1.5	Forsythia	1.5
Phellodendron	1.5	Platycodon	1.5	Gentiana	1.5
Anemarrhena	1.5	Pueraria	1.5	Scirpus	1.5
Zedoaria	1.5	Laminaria	1.5	Seaweed	1.5
Cimicifuga	1.5	Ginger	1.5	Licorice	1.5
Trichosanthes root	1.5				

San-tsung-kuei-chien-tang is recorded in *Wan ping hui chun* (萬病回春) of the Ming dynasty. This formula is used for treating swollen lymph glands, goiter, carbuncles, acute inflammation, and suppurative ulcers.

Herbs and Actions

Tang-kuei is a nutritive tonic. Peony and Scute dispel "blood heat". Bupleurum and Gentiana dispel "moist heat". Cimicifuga cures severe ulcers. Seaweed treats carbuncles. Laminaria is an expectorant and softens hardened tissues. Forsythia removes stagnant blood. Platycodon is a detoxifier and anti-inflammative. Coptis dispels internal heat. Scirpus and Zedoaria are analgesics which also nourish the *ch'i*. Trichosanthes root is an antipyretic and detoxifier. Pueraria relieves spasms due to stagnant blood. Ginger improves blood circulation. Licorice coordinates the actions of the other herbs.

Indications

Carbuncles and lymphadenitis in the neck.

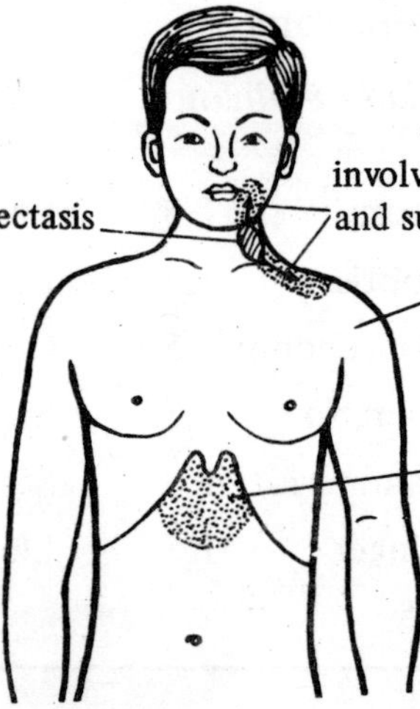

Shih-Wei-Pai-Tu-Tang 十味敗毒湯

(Bupleurum and Schizonepeta Combination)

Bupleurum	3.0	Ginger	1.0	Siler	2.0
Tuhuo	2.0	Hoelen	2.0	Platycodon	3.0
Schizonepeta	1.0	Cnidium	3.0	Licorice	1.0
Cherry bark	3.0				

The original prescription of *Shih-wei-pai-tu-tang* was first modified by Hanaoko Seichiu (a famous Japanese Surgeon) based on his own experience. Asata S. later added Forsythia, after which the formula became a well known remedy for dermatological disorders. Recently, Dr. Yakazu D., an authority on Chinese medicine, stated that this formula is especially effective for eczema, pimples, and urticaria. Better results are obtained in the treatment of suppuration and in nourishing the skin when Coix is added to the basic formula.

Herbs and Actions

This formula is detoxicative and can reinforce liver function.

Bupleurum and Ginger promote diaphoresis. *Tuhuo*, Siler, and Hoelen cure arthritis and rheumatism. Platycodon and Cnidium increase the flow of the urine and stop suppuration. Schizonepeta and Cherry bark are detoxicatives. Licorice synthesizes the actions of other herbs.

Indications

Carbuncles, furuncles, boils, lymphadenitis, mastitis, dermatitis, urticaria, eczema, acne, hordeolum, allergic ophthalmia, nasal suppuration, otitis media, and otitis externa.

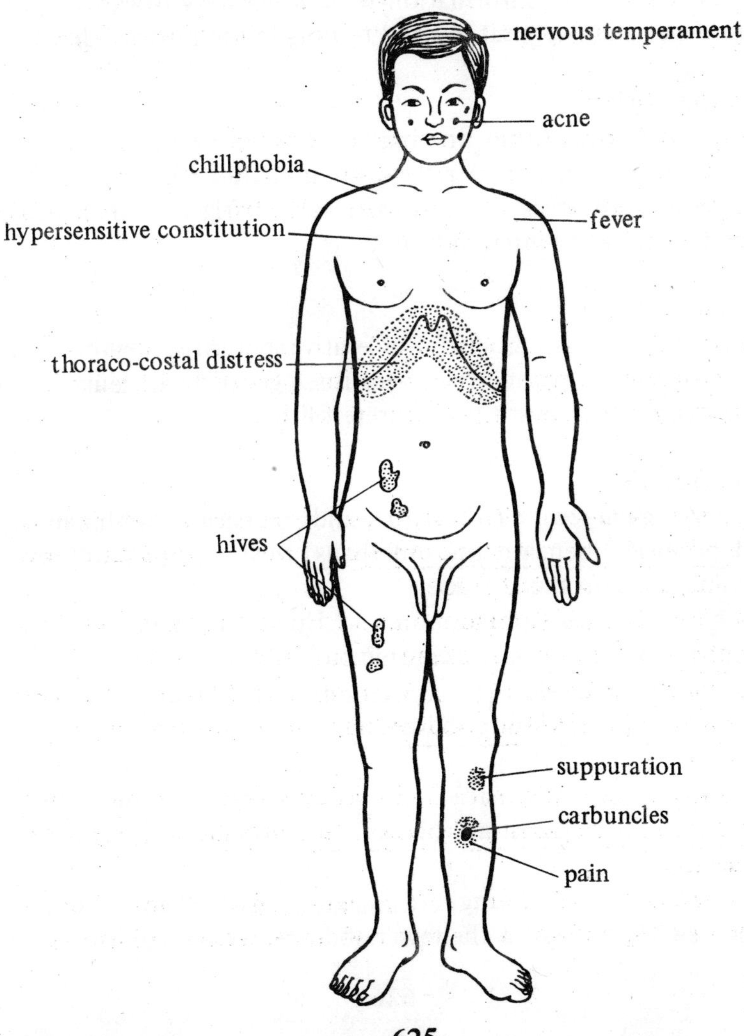

Ta-Huang-Mu-Tan-Pi-Tang 大黃牡丹皮湯

(Rhubarb and Moutan Combination)

Rhubarb	2.0	Moutan	4.0	Benincasa	6.0
Mirabilitum	4.0	Persica	4.0		

Ta-huang-mu-tan-pi-tang is recorded in the *Chin kuei yao lueh* (金匱要略) of the Han dynasty. This formula is used for treating those of strong conformation with a tendency towards constipation, fever and suppuration, and tumors in the lower abdomen.

Herbs and Actions

Rhubarb and Mirabilitum, the major components in this formula, dispel "internal heat" and relieve inflammation. Benincasa is an antipyretic. Moutan is an antipyretic and refrigerant that dispels stagnant blood and "internal heat".

Indications

Periproctitis, colitis, proctitis, ulcerative enteritis, hemorrhoids. rectal prolapse, perimetritis, testitis, gonorrhea, leukorrhea, peritonitis, pyelitis, cystitis, and ureteroliths.

Discrimination

Tao-ho-cheng-chi-tang (Rhubarb and Persica Combination): blood occlusion beneath the umbilicus; flushing up; acute lower abdominal pain on the left side.

Kuei-chih-fu-ling-wan (Cinnamon and Hoelen Formula): swelling mass in the lower abdomen—chronic but mild condition.

I-yi-fu-tzu-pai-chiang-san (Coix, Aconite, and Thlaspi Formula): swelling mass in the lower abdomen, dry skin, pus present, quick pulse.

Hsia-yu-hsieh-tang (Persica and Eupolypaga Combination): occluded blood stagnating beneath the umbilicus, suppressed menstruation.

Kuei-chih-chia-shao-yao-tang (Cinnamon and Peony Combination): swelling mass in the lower abdomen, weak conformation,

weak pulse.
Ta-chien-chung-tang (Major Zanthoxylum Combination): swelling mass in the lower abdomen, abdominal pain, uneasy peristalsis, gas, weak pulse.

Firm conformation

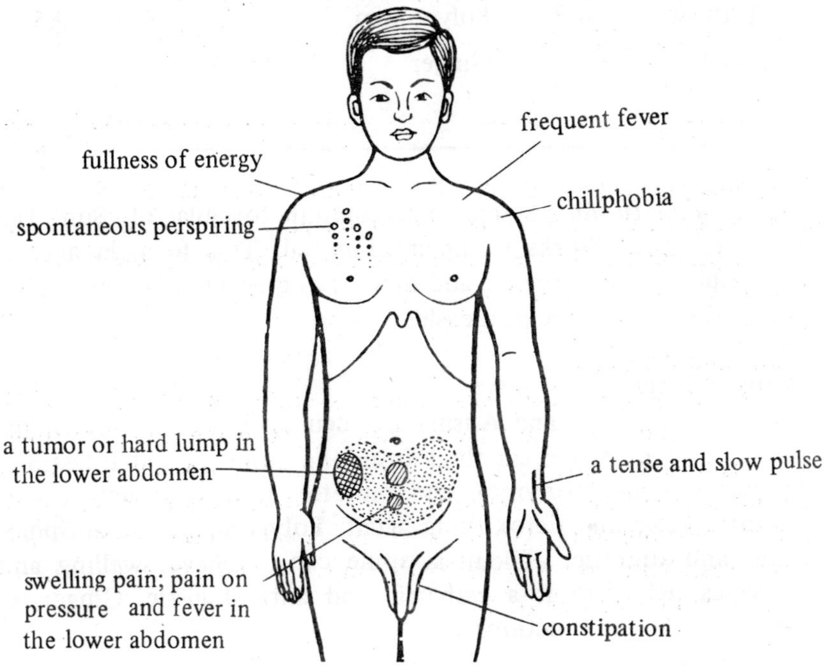

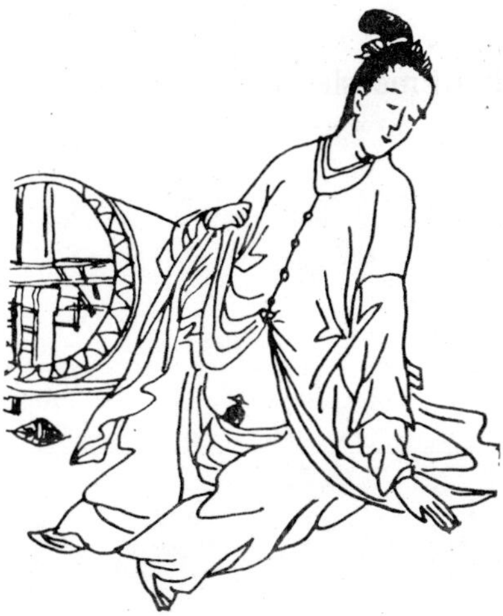

Teng-Hua-Pai-Tu-San 燈花敗毒散

(Ludwigia Formula)

Ludwigia	5.0	Hoelen	2.5	Rhubarb	1.0
Lithospermum	2.5	Polygonum	3.0	Polyporus	2.5
Gleditsia spine	3.0	Ginger	0.5	Alisma	2.5

Teng-hua-pai-tu-san is an experimental formula of Sun Ten Pharmaceutical Works Company Limited. This formula acts as an antiphlogistic, diuretic, and detoxifying agent. It is very effective in the initial stage of measles.

Herbs and Actions

Hoelen, Polyporus, and Alisma are regulators of the body fluids; they also remove excess fluid from the stomach and intestines. Ludwigia is an antipyretic and diuretic. Lithospermum acts as an antipyretic and detoxifying agent. Polygonum is an antiphlogistic and diuretic. Gleditsia spine can relieve swelling and abscesses. Rhubarb is a cathartic and antiphlogistic. Ginger regulates metabolic functions.

Indications

Pruritis, especially of measles.

Teng-Lung-Tang 騰龍湯

(Moutan and Persica Combination)

Moutan	4.0	Persica	4.0	Benincasa	5.0
Atractylodes	4.0	Coix	8.0	Licorice	1.0
Rhubarb	1.5	Mirabilitum	5.0		

A familial formula from the Takenada Fumisuke's of Japan, which was recorded in *Han fang chu fang chieh shuo* (漢方處方解說). Used for treating inflammation and swelling pain in the lower abdomen. In case of severe hemorrhoidal pain, the amounts of Rhubarb and Mirabilitum are increased. If there is no constipation and severe pain, the Rhubarb and Mirabilitum are decreased or omitted.

Herbs and Actions

Persica nourishes the blood and dispels stagnant blood. Moutan removes stagnant blood and stimulates blood circulation. Benincasa also dispels stagnant blood. Coix removes suppuration and stagnant blood. Licorice and Atractylodes help stomach *ch'i*.

Indications

Periproclitis, testitis, prostatitis, peritonitis, endometritis, uterine tumor, and the initial stage of uterine cancer.

Discrimination

Ta-huang-mu-tan-pi-tang (Rhubarb and Moutan Combiantion): inflammation in the lower abdomen; the conformation is generally the same as *Teng-lung-tang*. However, *Teng-lung-tang* is for acute conditions and decreased urine.

Chang-yung-tang (Coix and Persica Combination): chronic inflammation in the lower abdomen.

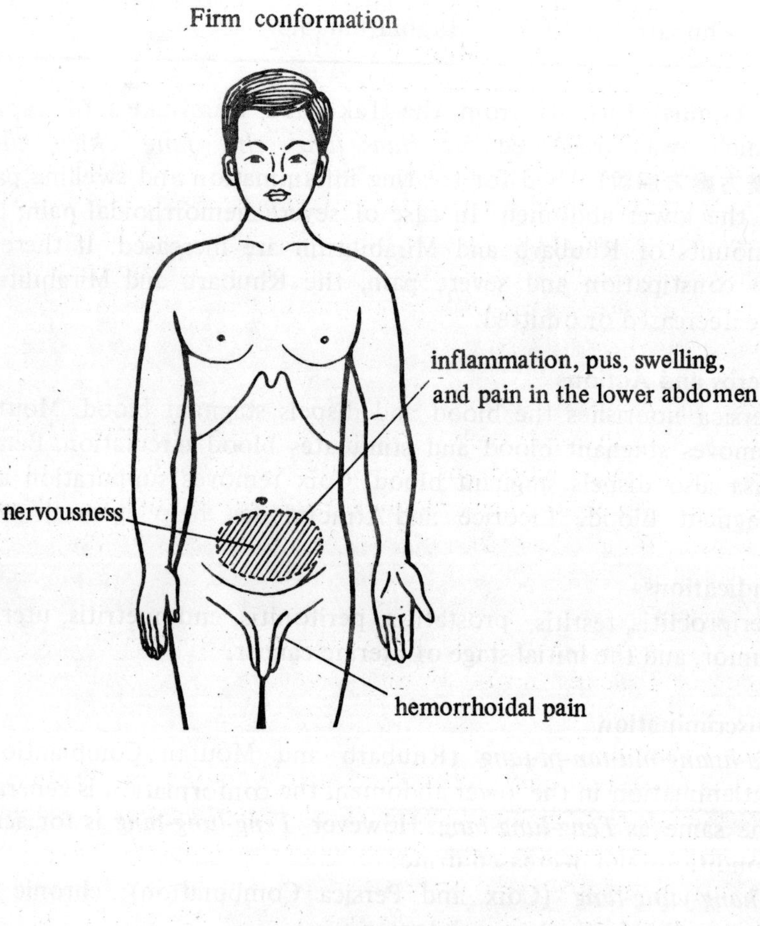
Firm conformation
inflammation, pus, swelling, and pain in the lower abdomen
nervousness
hemorrhoidal pain

Tuo-Li-Hsiao-Tu-Yin 托裏消毒飲

(Gleditsia Combination)

Ginseng	3.0	Cnidium	3.0	Platycodon	3.0
Atractylodes	3.0	Peony	3.0	*Tang-kuei*	5.0
Hoelen	5.0	Licorice	1.0	Gleditsia	2.0
Angelica	1.0	Astragalus	1.5	Lonicera	1.0

Recorded in *Wan ping hui chun* (萬病回春) of the Ming dynasty. Used for patients of a somewhat delicate constitution for treating suppuration with fever. In the initial stage of inflammation and congestion, patients with good vitality should use *Ko-ken-tang* (Pueraria Combination) or *Shih-wei-pai-tu-tang* (Bupleurum and Schizonepeta Combination). In the later stages the patient should use *Tuo-li-hsiao-tu-yin.* Patients with a delicate constitution should use *Chien-chin-nei-tuo-san* (Astragalus and Platycodon Formula).

Herbs and Actions

Tang-kuei, Peony, and Cnidium nourish the blood. Ginseng, Atractylodes, Hoelen, and Licorice nourish the *ch'i.* Lonicera aids suppuration while Platycodon, Angelica, and Gleditsia complete the process. Astragalus nourishes the muscles.

Indications

Carbuncles, suppurative lymphadenitis, gangrene, and otorrhoea (a discharge from the external auditory meatus).

Discrimination

Chien-chin-nei-tuo-san (Astragalus and Platycodon Formula): prolonged suppurative diseases of weak conformation that have depleted the patient's physical strength.

Tzu-Ken-Mu-Li-Tang 紫根牡蠣湯

(Lithospermum and Oyster Shell Combination)

Tang-kuei	5.0	Peony	3.0	Cnidium	3.0
Oyster shell	4.0	Rhubarb	1.5	Cimicifuga	2.0
Astragalus	2.0	Licorice	1.0	Lonicera	1.5
Lithospermum	3.0				

Tzu-ken-mu-li-tang is recorded in *Mei li hsin shu* (黴癘新書) by Katakura Tsurure of Japan. This formula is used for treating recalcitrant swelling ulcer of unknown cause and malignant skin diseases.

Herbs and Actions

Lithospermum can relieve "blood heat" and treat resistent tinea and severe ulcers. Lonicera and Cimicifuga dispel "heat poisoning" and treat ulcers. Astragalus nourishes the blood and muscle, and dispels pus. *Tang-kuei,* Peony, and Cnidium are hemotonics. Rhubarb helps evacuation. Licorice coordinates the actions of the other herbs.

Indications

Breast cancer, mastitis, lymphadenitis in the neck, gangrene in the lungs, syphilitic skin lesions.

Discrimination

Hsiao-chai-hu-tang-chia-chien-fang: enlargement of cervical lymph-node—either acute or tubercular in nature.
Hsiang-chuan-chieh-tu-chi-chia-chien-fang: syphilis and symptoms caused by syphilis.

Weak conformation

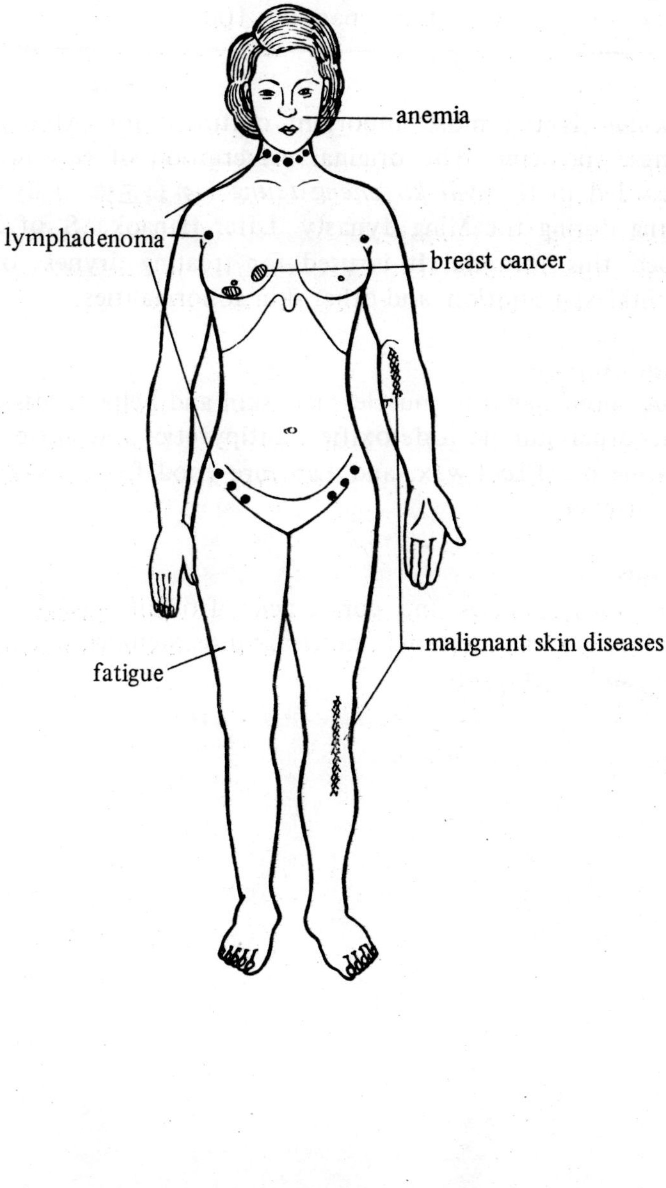

Tzu-Yun-Kao 紫雲膏

(Lithospermum Ointment)

Sesame oil	1000	*Tang-kuei*	100	Lard	25
Flava wax	380	Lithospermum	100		

Tzu-yun-kao is the most important ointment for external use in Chinese medicine. The original prescription of this formula was recorded in the *Wai ko cheng tzung* (外科正宗) by Chen Shih-kung during the Ming dynasty. Later Hanaoka S. of Japan developed this formula. It is used for treating dryness of the skin, wrinkles, ulceration, and other skin abnormalities.

Herbs and Actions

Tang-kuei nourishes the muscles and skin and helps to discharge pus. Lithospermum is a detoxifier, antipyretic, and antiphlogistic. Sesame oil, Flava wax, and Lard are good for external uses as skin softeners.

Indications

Eczema, tinea, calluses and corns, acne, frostbite, prickly heat, body odor, alopecia, external injuries, burns, hemorrhoids, rectal prolapse, and ulcerations.

WHERE YOU CAN BUY CHINESE HERB FORMULAS

In Southeast Asia, approximately one billion people use Chinese herb formulas. In Hong-Kong. Singapore, the Republic of Korea, Japan, and the Republic of China, Chinese herb stores dot the cities and countryside. For instance, although Taiwan is only one sixth the size of California, it supports eight thousand Chinese herb stores.

The ingredients for all the prescriptions mentioned in this book may be obtained in Chinese herb stores, but the herbs must be bought individually and then prepared at home before use. Under the direction of the author, Sun Ten Pharmaceutical Works Co., Ltd. of Taiwan 25 years ago began to scientifically produce concentrated herb granules and powder in accordance with the highest standards. The resultant products are much more convenient and effective than the home decoctions.

Today the Sun Ten Pharmaceutical Works Co., Ltd. of Taiwan is the most important source of scientifically prepared Chinese herbal formulas. Its products can be bought in Chinese herb stores in the Chinese sections of the major cities of the United States. The following organizations will provide information about Chinese medicine.

1) **Brion Corporation**
12020-B Centralia Road, Hawaiian Gardens
California 90716

2) **Sun Ten Pharmaceutical Works Co., Ltd.**
114, Chung-Ching South Road, Section 3
Taipei, Taiwan 107

3) **Junkoh Medicinal Industry Co., Ltd.**
2-4-8 Uehara, Shibuyaku
Tokyo 151, Japan

BIBLIOGRAPHY

Chang shih yi tung (張氏醫通 , Chang's Mastery of Medicine). This book was written by Chang Lu of the Ching dynasty. A sixteen-volume collection, it contains prescriptions and essays of earlier physicians and follows the same order of presentation as the book *Cheng chih chuen sheng* (證治準繩 , Rules of Conformation and Therapy) by Wang Keng-tang. Prescriptions and their indications were taken from Hsueh Chi's *Yi an* (醫案 , Medical Documents) and Chang Chieh-ping's *Ching yueh chuan shu* (景岳全書, Ching Yueh's Book Series). Chang's own notes and commentary add richness and creativity to the collection.

Chan lun (產論 , A Treatise on Parturition). This four-volume book was written by the Japanese physician Kagawa Genyetsu in 1937.

Cheng chih chuen sheng (證治準繩, Rules of Conformation and Therapy). This source was completed by Wang Keng-tang in A.D. 1602 (Ming dynasty). It comprises 120 volumes organized into six categories: miscellaneous diseases; classified formulas; febrile diseases; tumors; pediatrics; and gynecology. The compilation is highly reputed for its excellent summary of all prominent medical writings before the Ming dynasty. It covers diseases, symptoms, therapy, and formulas.

Chiao cheng fang yu ni (校正方輿輗, A Correction of the Cross Bars of a Square Carriage). This book by Arimochi Keiri in 1853 is divided into fifteen volumes. Because of the author's vast clinical experience, moderate approach, and clear descriptions, this book is one of the best references for ancient and modern prescriptions.

Chien chin yao fang (千金要方, Precious Major Formulas). In A.D. 652 Sun Szu-miao of the Tang dynasty wrote these thirty volumes, organized into 31 classes and 223 sub-classes. The contents includes theories relating to various branches of medicine including acupuncture and moxibustion, plus detailed descriptions of the nature, administration, and efficacy of medicinals. *Chien chin yao fang* is regarded as one of the most important sources of Chinese medical history.

Chien tien fang han (淺田方函, Asada's Prescriptions). This book, written by Asada S. in 1878, summarizes ancient Japanese prescriptions, current prescriptions, and imperial prescriptions, in all, 616 formulas. Based on his practical experience, Asada commented on each of the formulas.

Ching yueh chuan shu fa hui (景岳全書發揮, The Development of Ching Yueh's Complete Works). This four-volume work was written by Yao Chiu who later changed his name to Yeh Kuei. Yeh is famous for his clinical experiments and for introducing the diagnostic procedures of examination of the tongue and teeth. Another of his contributions was the discovery of the difference between *tinea versicolor* (chronic superficial infection of the skin) and *pityriasis alba* (eczema of unknown origin). Yeh's popular book is based primarily on the writings of Chang Ching-yueh but criticizes Chang's heavy reliance on supplementation therapy.

Chi sheng fang (濟生方, Life Preserving Prescriptions). These eight volumes were compiled by Yen Yung-ho during the Sung dynasty. Each volume is prefaced with an essay followed by specific prescriptions.

Chou hou pei chi fang (肘後備急方, A Pocket Book of Emergency Prescriptions). This book written by Ko Hung (A.D. 281-341) is divided into fifty-one categories describing recognizable contagious diseases. The prescriptions listed are simple and the herbs easily obtained. Since these formulas have demonstrable therapeutic effects, the book serves as an excellent guide for the layman.

Chung-kuo kuo-yao ku yeou cheng-fen hsuan-chi (中國國藥固有成方選輯, A Selection of the Traditional Prescriptions of Chinese Medicine). Chinese pharmacology has a long history. Hundreds of thousands of prescriptions for pills, powders, ointments, plasters, and pellets are recorded in ancient and modern books. Their contents are so mixed and complex that prescriptions with the same name may have different components and indications. To eliminate this confusion, the Ministry of the Interior convened its Chinese Herb Medicine Committee to integrate the prescriptions contained in *The Encyclopedia of Chinese Medical Science* (中國醫學大辭典) and *A Collection of Pills, Powders, Ointments, and Pellets* (丸散膏丹集成). Hence *A Selection of the Traditional Prescriptions of Chinese Medicine* (中國國藥固有成方選輯) was published in 1967 to serve as the authoritative reference for the manufacture and sale of Chinese medicinals.

Fu Ching-chu nu k'o (傅青主女科, Fu Ching-chu's Gynecology), This book was written by Fu Ching-chu (1607-1684). The prescriptions cited dynamically illustrate the matching of master and servant herbs. Fu's theories are clearly and simply stated; the prescriptions--mostly plant simples--were in contemporary use and based on empirical evidence. Fu--who mastered internal medicine, gynecology, and pediatrics--was a prolific writer.

Fu jen ta chuan liang fang (婦人大全良方, Women's Encyclopedia of Efficacious Prescriptions). This book, written by Chen Tzu-ming of the Sung dynasty and completed in 1237, is composed of twenty-four volumes and divided into nine categories. The first three categories on gynecology cover normal menstrual physiology, various gynecological disorders and diseases, and sterility. The final six categories on obstetrics discuss fetal formation and development, diseases occurring during pregnancy, and conditions pertaining to labor and nursing. In addition, there are detailed descriptions on pre- and postnatal diseases, their diagnosis and treatment, and drugs indicated and contraindicated during pregnancy.

Hsiao erh yao cheng chih chueh (小兒藥證直訣, The Key to Pediatric Prescriptions). Chien I (1035-1117) was the first Chinese pediatrician. His student Yen Hsiao-chung wrote this three-volume study on pediatrics. Volume One contains treatments based on pulse diagnosis. The second volume follows the chronological development of twenty-three children. Volume Three describes relevant formulas and their applications. This work was highly valued formerly and is still used today as a reference.

Hsuan ming lun (宣明論, Interpretation of Prescriptions). Originally named *Yi fang ching yao hsuan ming lun* (醫方精要宣明論, Interpretation of the Essentials of Medical Prescriptions), this book was written by Liu Wan-su (A.D. 1120-1200) in the Chin Yuan period. The special features of this work in fifteen volumes are its assignment of cause on the basis of *Nei ching* (Classic of Internal Medicine) and its classification of disease into seventeen types; for each disease more than ten prescriptions are given. Since the author insisted on the use of cold and cool herbs to diminish fire, most of the treatments are for purging fire. Many people respect his ideas and refer to him as the founder of the *Han Liang Pai* School, literally meaning "The Cold School."

Hsueh shih yi an (薛氏醫案 Hsueh's Medical Cases). This book was completed by Hsueh Chi (A.D. 1522-1566) during Emperor Chia ching's reign in the Ming dynasty. The book is divided into seventy-eight volumes and sixteen categories according to the topics of surgery, internal medicine, and so on. Throughout the work are descriptions of the author's own therapeutic experiences. Although the treatments and prescriptions tend to be rigid and unimaginative, the accuracy of the list of ingredients in compliance with the origin or cause of disease makes this a collection of lasting value.

Jen chai chih chih (仁齋直指, Good Men Give Instruction). This book, written by Yang Shih-ying during the Sung dynasty and completed in A.D. 1264, is divided into twenty-six volumes and seventy-nine articles. An appendix added by Chu Chung-cheng of the Ming dynasty follows each article.

Ju men shih chin (儒門事親, Caring for Parents). The author Chang Tzu-ho, one of the four greatest scholars of the Chin and Yuan dynasties, insisted that "attack" therapy was the only way to treat disease. The inducement of sweating, vomiting, and purging are recognized methods in the world today, but they were greatly disputed and opposed in his day. The book fills fifteen volumes. Although the contents are poorly organized, the subject matter is a major contribution to the study of internal medicine.

Ku chin yi chien (古今醫鑑, A Mirror for Ancient and Modern Medicine). Kung Hsin of the Ming dynasty began this sixteen-volume work and his son, Kung Ting-hsien completed it. Unfortunately, the son duplicated much of the material.

Lan shih mi tsang (蘭室秘藏, Secret Collection of the Orchid House). This book written by Li Tung-yuan (A.D. 1180-1251) is divided into three volumes and covers twenty-one categories. The chief discussions are on drinking, eating, working, and fatigue, plus such things as *hsin fu pi* (cardio-abdominal distention) and *wei kuan tung* (stomach disorders). According to the author, disease stems from disorders of the spleen or stomach since these two organs are the center of nutrition and physiological activities. His concepts laid the foundation for the *pu tu* nutrition theory and have contributed greatly to medical science.

Liang fang chi yeh ho pi (良方集腋合璧, A Collection of the Best Remedies). Dating from the Ching dynasty, this book represents the collaborative efforts of Wu Chung, Hsieh Yuan-ching, and other contemporary physicians who annotated clinically effective prescriptions. At first entitled *Chi yeh* (集腋, collection), it was later enlarged by Wang Ching-hsiao who retitled it *Liang fang chi yeh ho pi*.

Mai yin cheng chih (脈因證治 , Pulses, Causes, Conformations, and Treatments). This book composed of our volumes was written by Chu Chen-hen (1281-1358) of the Yuan dynasty. It opens with a discussion on pathology and follows with prescriptions and treatments. The style is similar to that of *Ho fa chi yao* (活法機要, The Essentials of Lively Methods) but goes into greater detail and is more descriptive.

Mei li hsin shu (黴癘新書 , A New Study of Dermatomycosis and Pellagra). In 1786 Katakura Tsurure wrote two volumes, one on dermatomycosis (fungal infections of the skin) and the other on pellagra (dermatitis). Both volumes contain case histories and detailed descriptions on etiology, symptoms, and therapeutic formulas. This book laid the foundation for the use of dermatological herbs in Japan.

Ming chia fang hsuan (名家方選 , A Selection of Famous Physicians' Prescriptions). This collection of prescriptions was compiled in 1807 by Hirai Yoshing, a Japanese physician.

Ming yi chih chang (明醫指掌 , Physicians' Guide Book). This work was written by Huang Pu-chung and later revised and enlarged to ten volumes by Shao Ta in 1502. The book covers disease etiology and detailed information on individual disease in poetic form, giving explanations and pulses but no prescriptions.

Nei wai shang pien huo lun (內外傷辨惑論, Identification of Internal and External Diseases). This book written by Li Tung-yuan in 1247 is divided into three volumes. It puts forth Li's theory that *nei shang* (internal injury) is caused by an insufficiency or imbalance of *yin, yang, han* (cold), and *je* (heat). Li thought *nei shang* to be the cause of all disease, thus all disease basically comes from a weak spleen and stomach. Therefore, the therapy for all disease is maintenance of a sound spleen and stomach.

Pen shih fang (本事方 , Factual Prescriptions). The complete title of this work is *Lei cheng pu chi pen shih fang*(類證普濟本事方).

The ten volumes written by Hsu Shu-wei during the Sung dynasty are based on the author's own clinical experience. He recorded case histories giving details of his patients' disorders and the prescriptions he gave them.

Pen ts'ao yen yi (本草衍義, An Exposition of the Herbals). In 1119 Kou Tzung-shih completed what is considered the best reference on the medicinal use of herbs. The three-volume herbal was compiled from two earlier sources, *Chia Yu pu tsu pen ts'ao* (嘉祐補注本草 , Chia Yu's Herbal with Notes) and *Ta Kuan Ching shih cheng lei pei chi pen ts'ao* (大觀經史證類備急本草,Ta Kuan's Emergency Herbal of Classical Historical Conformation and Classifications). Kou criticized former writers' theories and opinions when they differed from his own views and experience. He also labeled medicinals as good or inferior.

Pi wei lun (脾胃論 , A Treatise on the Spleen and Stomach). The author, Li Kao, also known as Tung-yuan, was born during the Chin dynasty (1181-1251), and was a student of Chang Chieh-ku. He followed Chang's teachings but preferred prescriptions that ascended yang and supplemented vitality. Kao supported the theory of the five primary elements. He wrote in this three-volume treatise, "The spleen belongs to the earth, and the earth is the origin of all things." Thus, all disease results from damage to the spleen or stomach. The best cure is to restore health to the spleen and stomach through supplementing prescriptions. Historically, Li is regarded as the founder of the *Pu Tu* School (supplementing earth).

San yin chi yi ping cheng fang lun (三因極一病證方論, Triple Treatment–Disease, Conformation, and Prescription). This eighteen-volume work, written by Chen Yen of the Sung dynasty was completed in A.D. 1174. According to his theory, disease is internal, external, or neither internal nor external in origin. Internal cause are linked to the seven emotions which affect the viscera in relation to weakness, firmness, the six fatigues, and the six exhaustions. External causes are associated with the wind, cold, heat, and moisture, in other words environmental factors. Wounds caused by accidents, poisonous insect and animals bites make up the third category.

Shang han liu shu (傷寒六書, Six Essays on Febrile Diseases). This book was written by Tao Hua of the Ming dynasty. It contains six essays on *shang han* (febrile diseases). The listing of prescriptions is poorly ordered and many of them have been discredited by more recent medical practitioners.

Shang han lun (傷寒論); *Chin kuei yao lueh* (金匱要略 , Essay on Febrile Diseases; Outlines of the Golden Shelf). Originally these two books were combined into one called *Shang han tsu ping lun* (傷寒卒病論, A Treatise on the Treatment of Diseases Derived from *Shang Han*). They were written in A.D. 196 by Chang Chung-ching during the Han dynasty. Wang Su-ho later revised the material and divided it into two books: *Shang han lun* (傷寒論) and *Chin kuei yao lueh* (金匱要略). The term *shang han* refers to all kinds of febrile diseases. *Chin kuei yao lueh* deals with the treatment of various diseases and disorders including metabolic, neurological, and gynecological problems. The book presents the pathology, diagnosis, treatment, and administration of herbal formulas in great detail and is regarded as the most definitive work on Chinese medicine.

Shên shih tsun sheng shu (沈氏尊生書, Shen's Way to Ensure a Healthy Life). In 1773 Shen Chien-lu (Ching dynasty) completed this seventy-two volume work. Shen classified diseases into more than 300 categories. Each disease is presented according to cause, development, and diagnostic procedure by pulse. Guide words help the reader determine differences in conformation and the selection of pill or powder form for proper treatment of a given disease. This collection is an important reference for physician and layman alike.

Shih fang ko kua (時方歌括, Current Prescriptions in Lyrical Form). This book was written by Chen Nien-tsu of the Ching dynasty in about 1801. Its 108 formulas compiled from then existing prescriptions are classified into twelve categories according to their actions--expelling, passing, supplementing,and purging; and their characteristics--light, heavy, slippery, harsh, dry, moist, cold, and hot. Each prescription was written in poetic form so that they could be easily memorized. The text is footnoted, thus providing literary sources for the material.

Shih yi te hsiao fang (世醫得效方, Efficacious Prescriptions from Our Forbearers). In nineteen volumes, this book was written by Wei Yi-lin of the Yuan dynasty. Wei compiled traditional formulas from the earliest period of Chinese medicine up to his great-great grandfather's generation. This collection covers every branch of medicine. Perhaps most valuable of all is Volume Eighteen on orthopedics and wounds caused by swords and arrowheads.

Shou shih pao yuan (壽世保元, Prolong Your Life and Protect Your Body). This book was written in 1615 by Kung Ting-hsien during the Ming dynasty. The five volumes of this work are an addendum to Kung's previous writings: *Ku chin yi chien* (古今醫鑑, The Mirror of Ancient and Present Medical Science), *Wan ping hui chun* (萬病回春, Recovery from Myriad Diseases), *Chung hsing hsien fang* (種杏仙方, The Divine Prescriptions from Apricot Plantings), *Yun lin shen kou* (雲林神彀, Divine Rules of the Cloud Forest) and *Lu fu chin fang* (魯府禁方 , Secret Prescriptions of King Lu's Mansion).

Tai ping huei min ho chi chu fang (太平惠民和劑局方, Medical Dictionary of the Sung Dynasty). There were many famous physicians during the Sung dynasty. Consequently, it was a prolific period for medical literature. The government's involvement in editing and publishing books on herbal formulas led to the establishment of an official pharmacopeia. During the Yüan Fang era of Emperor Shen Tzung, all notable and prominent physicians from the nation were asked to submit their empirically effective prescriptions to the Royal Pharmacy to be tested. Then during Emperor Huei Tzung's reign (1107-1110), Chen Shih-wen and Pei Tzung-yuan were ordered to write and edit the pharmacopeia. The result was this medical dictionary of five volumes.

Tan chi hsin fa (丹溪心法, Tan Chi's Logical Diagnoses). Written by Chu Tan-chi of the Yuan dynasty (A.D. 1281-1385), this book is composed of five volumes organized into 100 categories. Externally contracted diseases, internal injuries, gynecology, and pediatrics are some of the subjects covered. The author's biography, written by his students, contains information gathered from his talks about medical theory. This work is the most complete and detailed of Tan's writings.

Tang tou ko chueh (湯頭歌訣, Lyrical Prescriptions). This book was written by Wang Ang during the Ching dynasty (A.D. 1664-1911). Divided into twelve categories, it contains two hundred poems of more than three hundred prescriptions. The poems are simple, easy to understand, and logical. The prescriptions were taken from the works of Chang Chung-ching (A.D. 142-220) and that of physicians of later generations. It was written in lyrical form in order that the prescriptions could be easily learned and memorized by beginning practitioners.

Wai k'o shu yao (外科樞要 , The Essentials of Surgery). Hsueh Chi, who lived during the Ming dynasty, wrote this four-volume treatise on surgical techniques. Volume One covers abscesses and ulcers and various conformations. Volumes Two and Three describe diseases, giving first a theoretical discussion of the pathology, diagnosis and treatment, and then case histories of cured patients. The fourth volume lists prescriptions for abscess and ulcer conformations. It also contains illustrations of *chien chien hsueh* (the shoulder apex, a location of the body where acupuncture and moxibustion are applied) and *chou chien hsueh* (the elbow apex).

Wai k'o cheng tzung (外科正宗 , Orthodox Surgery). Chen Shih-kung of the Ming dynasty wrote these twelve volumes on surgery. Discussed are 160 categories which include every kind of surgical disease, as well as various common diseases, with details regarding their etiology, symptoms, and cures. The more than thirty illustrations pinpoint the location of injury in severe surgical cases. These volumes provide an excellent introduction to the study of surgery.

Wai tai mi yao (外臺秘要, "Secret Measures" as Written Outside the Ministry). This forty-volume collection compiled by Wang Tao in A.D. 752 (Tang dynasty) contains theories of pathology and conformation, and medicinal formulas. These volumes are invaluable as a medical resource because each citation is throughly referenced and many lost books are listed.

Wan ping hui chun (萬病回春, The Recovery from Myriad Diseases). This book was written in 1587 by Kung Ting-hsien during the Ming dynasty. The eight volumes contain discussions on internal organs and the characteristics of various medicinals and causes, treatments, and prescriptions. Kung drew his material from earlier writers and added his own views and opinions to theirs.

Wen je ching wei (溫熱經緯 , The Essentials of Warmth and Heat). This five-volume book was written by Wang Shih-hsiung of the Ching dynasty. The first topic, *nei ching* (internal meridians), is discussed in the chapter "*Fu chi wen je pen*" (Controlling *Ch'i* with Respect to Warmth and Heat). Wang reiterates the theories of Chang Chung-ching, Chen Tsu-kung, and Hsueh Hsueh according to his own interpretation. This compilation that Wang mastered so clearly reflects warm and hot diseases.

Wen ping tiao pien (溫病條辨 , Discrimination of Warm Diseases). This six-volume treatise was written by Wu Tang of the Ching dynasty. The unique feature of this work is the postulation of the theory of the three *chiao's* (zones) which holds that disease starts at the upper *chiao*, the lungs, then migrates to the stomach and intestines, the middle *chiao*, and finally progresses to a more serious stage and injures the yin at the very interior, the lower *chiao*. Quite different from the disease theory of the *Shang han lun* (傷寒論) by Chang Chung-ching, it is none the less important as a creative contribution to clinical and therapeutic practice.

Yang yi ta chuan (瘍醫大全, A Complete Book on Abscesses). This book was written by Ku Shih-ch'eng of the Ching dynasty. It begins with a review of the *Nei ching* (內經 , The Yellow Emperor's Classic of Internal Medicine) followed by detailed description on pulses and related meridians. The book, having adopted the ancestral sages' writings and their precious prescriptions and secret ways, is classified according to subject and provides clear and precise descriptions of carbuncles and abscesses. This collection, in forty volumes, serves as a vital resource for medical students.

Yen fang hsin pien (驗方新編, A New Compilation of Efficacious Prescriptions). This sixteen-volume book is the work of Pao

Hsiang-ao of the Ching dynasty. Like contemporary medical books, this compilation is by far the easiest to use because of its orderly and systematized listing of simple prescriptions. For this reason it is very popular.

Yi chien fang (易簡方, Easy and Simplified Prescriptions). This book was written by Wang Shuo of the Sung dynasty to bring together various Chinese medical theories and prescriptions that evolved over the centuries. Included prescriptions had to have clinical evidence of their therapeutic value. The author carefully described how to use the many common prescriptions thus making them readily accessible for emergency use.

Yi fang chi chieh (醫方集解, A Collection of Interpretations of Medical Prescriptions). This twenty-three volume medical encyclopedia was compiled by Wang Ang (Wang Jen-an) during the Ching dynasty. Divided into twenty-one disease types, it contains information on etiology, pulse conditions, viscera, meridians, diagnostic procedures, conformations, and prescriptions, as well as herbs that are contraindicated.

Yi fang kao (醫方考, A Prescription Reference). This six-volume work was written by Wu Kun of the Ming dynasty. It is arranged by disease in twelve categories and contains 700 prescriptions. This collection has been very popular outside China.

Yi hsueh hsin wu (醫學心悟, Insightful Medicine). Cheng Chung-ling of the Ching dynasty completed this work in 1732. The six volumes serve as a valuable clinical guide. Discussed are the eight ways of treatment--perspiring, vomiting, discharging or purging, harmonizing, clarifying, supplementing, and diminishing--in a concise, clear style. Cheng was very selective and went to great lengths to correct prevailing misconceptions in the areas of gynecology, surgery, and miscellaneous disease.

Yi hsueh ju men (醫學入門, An Introduction to Medicine). This book, comprising seven volumes, was written by Li T'ing of the Ming dynasty. Seeking to systematize Chinese medical literature, Li gathered together the writings of earlier physicians and rewrote them. The order of the material is from the simple to the complex, forming a "ladder book" for beginning medical practitioners.

Yi meng fa lu (醫門法律, Clinical Methods and Rules). This highly regarded twelve-volume book was written by Yu Chang of the Ching dynasty in 1580. Theoretical information prefaces each discussion, followed by clinical rules and methods. This work was primarily intended to instruct physicians of limited experience and training in the proper methods of treating patients.

Yi tzung chin chien (醫宗金鑑, The Golden Mirror of Medical Science). During the reign of Emperor Chien Lung (A.D. 1736-1797) of the Ching dynasty, the author Chien Tou-pao was ordered to compile this book of seventy-four volumes. The first seventeen volumes are a revision of the *Shang han lun tzu* (傷寒論註, Interpretation of the *Shang han lun*), the next eight volumes are a revision of *Chin kuei yao lueh tzu* (金匱要略註 Interpretation of the *Chin kuei yao lueh*). Revisions of other medical writings include *Ming yi fang lun* (名醫方論, Treatise on Famous Prescriptions), *Shih chen yao chueh* (四診要訣, Outlines of the Four Methods of Diagnosis), and *Yuan chi yao chueh* (運氣要訣, Outlines of Phase Energetics). Thirty-five volumes outline various branches of medicine, and the final four volumes are a condensation of *Insightful Orthodox Osteology* (正骨心法要旨). Based on Wu Chien's manuscripts (whose debates and comments were modest and righteous), this work is a valuable medical encyclopedia.

INDEX

A

Achyanthes and Plantago Formula 247
Aconite and G.L. Combination 313
Aconite and Oryza Combination 285
Aconite Combination 288
Aconite, Ginseng, and Ginger Combination 287
Adenophora and Ophiopogon Combination 593
Agastache Formula 100
Alisma and Hoelen Combination 483
Alisma Combination 511
Anemone Combination 187
Anemarrhena, Phellodendron, and Rehmannia Formula 230
Angelica and Mastic Combination 612
Aquilaria and Gastrodia Combination 370
Aquilaria and Perilla Formula 399
Apricot Seed and Linum Formula 535
Apricot Seed and Perilla Formula 46
Arctium Combination 169
Areca and Evodia Combination 397
Areca Seed and Chaenomeles Formula 465
Areca Seed Combination 470
Aster Combination 273
Astragalus and Aconite Formula 453
Astragalus and Atractylodes Combination 218
Astragalus and Cinnamon Five Herb Combination 235
Astragalus and Platycodon Formula 604
Astragalus and Tortoise Shell Formula 236
Astragalus and Zizyphus Combination 275

Astragalus Combination 293
Atractylodes and Aconite Combination 309
Atractylodes and Arisaema Combination 474
Atractylodes and Cardamon Combination 376
Atractylodes and Hoelen Combination 493
Atractylodes and Pueraria Formula 228
Atractylodes and Setaria Combination 461
Atractylodes Combination 523
Aurantium and Bamboo Combination 374

B

Baked Licorice Combination 529
Bamboo and Ginseng Combination 90
Bamboo and Hoelen Combination 114
Bamboo Leaves and Gypsum Combination 220
Biota and Achyranthes Formula 581
Bos and Curcuma Formula 330
Bos and Musk Formula 332
B.P. and Six Major Herb Combination 225
Bupleurum and *Chih-shih* Formula 112
Bupleurum and Cinnamon Combination 117
Bupleurum and Citrus, Pinellia Formula 346
Bupleurum and Dragon Bone Combination 340
Bupleurum and Evodia Combination 432
Bupleurum and Hoelen Combination 464
Bupleurum and Peony Formula 87
Bupleurum and Pinellia Combination 197
Bupleurum and Pueraria Combination 35
Bupleurum and Rehmannia Combination 160
Bupleurum and Schizonepeta Combination 624
Bupleurum and *Tang-kuei* Formula 94
Bupleurum, Cinnamon, and Ginger Combination 85
Bupleurum and Scute Combination 543
Bupleurum Formula 343

C

Capillaris and Hoelen Formula 521
Capillaris Combination 519

Cardamon and Fennel Formula 366
Cardamon Combination 104
Chianghuo and Turmeric Combination 444
Chianghuo Combination 38
Chih-shih and Cardamon Combination 544
Chih-shih and Peony Formula 575
Chih-shih, Bakeri, and Cinnamon Combination 373
Chin-chiu and Bupleurum Combination 231
Chin-chiu and Tortoise Shell Formula 232
Chrysanthemum Combination 600
Cimicifuga and Peucedanum Combination 591
Cimicifuga and Pueraria Combination 594
Cimicifuga Combination 613
Cinnabar Formula 343
Cinnamon, Aconite, and Ginger Combination 305
Cinnamon and Aconite Combination 302
Cinnamon and Anemarrhena Combination 450
Cinnamon and Angelica Formula 452
Cinnamon and Astragalus Combination 55
Cinnamon and Atractylodes Combination 304
Cinnamon and D.D.O. Combination 353
Cinnamon and Dragon Bone Combination 351
Cinnamon and Ginseng Combination 306
Cinnamon and Hoelen Formula 423
Cinnamon and *Ma-huang* Combination 61
Cinnamon and Peony Combination 60
Cinnamon and Persica Combination 573
Cinnamon and Pueraria Combination 58
Cinnamon Combination 63
Cinnamon Five Herb Combination 179
Cinnamon, Magnolia, and Apricot Seed Combination 54
Cinnamon, Peony, and Rhubarb Combination 124
Citrus and Crataegus Formula 212
Citrus and Perilla Combination 377
Citrus and Pinellia Combination 551
Clematis and Carthamus Formula 454
Clematis and Stephania Combination 429
Clove and Hoelen Combination 509
Clove and Kaki Combination 407
Cnidium and Moutan Combination 531

Cnidium and Rehmannia Combination 579
Cnidium and Tea Formula 40
Coix, Aconite, and Thlaspi Formula 615
Coix Combination 489
Coptis and Gelatin Combination 97
Coptis and Rehmannia Formula 168
Coptis and Rhubarb Combination 190
Coptis and Scute Combination 175
Coptis Combination 98
Croton and Apricot Seed Combination 136
Croton and Hematite Formula 156
Cyperus and Cluster Combination 207
Cyperus and Perilla Formula 41
Cyperus, Perilla, and Citrus Formula 382

D

Dandelion Combination 582
Dianthus Formula 502
Dioscorea Combination 266
Dragon Bone and Oyster Shell Combination 355

E

Elsholtzia Combination 221
Elsholtzia Ten Combination 222
Eriobotrya and Ophiopogon Combination 532
Eriocheir and Viper Formula 622
Eucommia and Achyranthes Formula 274
Evodia and Pinellia Combination 411
Evodia Combination 325

F

Forsythia and Laminaria Combination 623
Forsythia and Lonicera Formula 605
Forsythia and Rhubarb Formula 180
Four Major Herb Combination 264
Fritillaria and Platycodon Formula 560
Fu-lung-kan Combination 420

G

Galanga and *Chih-shih* Combination 391
Gambir Formula 386
Gardenia and Hoelen Formula 514
Gardenia and Phellodendron Combination 469
Gardenia and Soja Combination 162
Gardenia and Vitex Combination 599
Gardenia, Ginger, and Soja Combination 162
Gardenia, Licorice, and Soja Combination 161
Gasping Formula 552
Gelatin and Aristolochia Combination 258
Gelatin and Artemisia Four Combination 417
Gentiana Combination 181
Ginger and Hoelen Combination 491
Ginseng and Astragalus Combination 255
Ginseng and Atractylodes Formula 260
Ginseng and Ginger Combination 295
Ginseng and Gypsum Combination 183
Ginseng and Longan Combination 425
Ginseng and Mentha Formula 48
Ginseng and Perilla Combination 126
Ginseng and *Tang-kuei* Formula 241
Ginseng and *Tang-kuei* Ten Combination 262
Ginseng and Zanthoxylum Combination 566
Ginseng and Zizyphus Formula 270
Ginseng, Astragalus, and Pueraria Combination 238
Ginseng, Longan, and Bupleurum Combination 416
Ginseng Nutritive Combination 239
Ginseng Rhizome Combination 135
Ginseng Stomach Combination 209
G.L. and Aconite Combination with Ginseng 311
Gleditsia and Asarum Formula 336
Gleditsia Combination 631
G.P. and Ginseng Formula 385
Gypsum Combination 185
Gypsum, Coptis, and Scute Combination 125

H

H.A. and Licorice Combination 480

Hoelen and Akebia Combination 499
Hoelen and Alisma Combination 205
Hoelen and Areca Combination 519
Hoelen and Cuscuta Formula 360
Hoelen and Jujube Combination 467
Hoelen and Polyporus Formula 358
Hoelen and Schizandra Combination 556
Hoelen, Atractylodes, and Areca Combination 508
Hoelen Combination 486
Hoelen Five Herb Formula 516
Hoelen, G.L. and Aconite Combination 283
Hoelen, Licorice, and Jujube Combination 495
Hoelen, Licorice, and Schizandra Combination 496

I

Inula and Hematite Combination 384

J

Jujube Combination 144

K

Kaki Combination 404
Kaolin and Limonite Combination 358
Kaolin and Oryza Combination 362

L

Lapis and Scute Formula 559
Lepidium and Jujube Combination 595
Licorice, Aconite, and Ginger Pulse Combination 323
Licorice and Aconite Combination 298
Licorice and Ginger Combination 300
Licorice and Hoelen Combination 479
Licorice and Jujube Combination 347
Licorice Combination 349
Licorice, Minium, and Honey Combination 565
Lily Combination 253

Lindera and Cyperus Formula 369
Lindera Formula 409
Linum and Rhubarb Combination 533
Lithospermum and Oyster Shell Combination 632
Lithospermum Ointment 634
Loadstone and Rehmannia Formula 272
Lonicera and Forsythia Formula 83
Lotus and Citrus Combination 204
Lotus Seed Combination 164
Lotus Stamen Formula 359
Ludwigia Formula 628
Lycium, Chrysanthemum, and Rehmannia Formula 598
Lycium Formula 237

M

Ma-huang, Aconite, and Licorice Combination 74
Ma-huang and Apricot Seed Combination 68
Ma-huang and Asarum Combination 72
Ma-huang and Atractylodes Combination 70
Ma-huang and Cimicifuga Combination 79
Ma-huang and Coix Combination 66
Ma-huang and Ginkgo Combination 407
Ma-huang and Ginseng Combination 448
Ma-huang and Gypsum Combination 526
Ma-huang and Magnolia Combination 401
Ma-huang and Morus Formula 47
Ma-huang and Peony Combination 447
Ma-huang Combination 76
Ma-huang, Forsythia, and Phaseolus Combination 497
Ma-huang, Gypsum, and Pinellia Combination 525
Ma-huang, Licorice, and Apricot Seed Combination 592
Magnolia and Alisma Combination 504
Magnolia and Atractylodes Combination 505
Magnolia and Ginger Formula 212
Magnolia and Hoelen Combination 512
Magnolia and Saussurea Combination 290
Magnolia Five Combination 380
Magnolia Flower and Gypsum Combination 174
Magnolia Flower Formula 175
Magnolia Seven Combination 121

Magnolia Three Combination 379
Major Blue Dragon Combination 81
Majon Bupleurum Combination 128
Major Rhubarb Combination 145
Major Siler Combination 457
Major Zanthoxylum Combination 315
Mantis Formula 361
Melon Pedicle Formula 134
Minor Blue Dragon Combination 43
Minor Bupleurum Combination 91
Minor Cinnamon and Peony Combination 291
Minor Pinellia and Hoelen Combination 487
Minor Rhubarb Combination 141
Minor Trichosanthes Combination 142
Morus and Chrysanthemum Combination 78
Morus and Lycium Formula 173
Morus and Platycodon Formula 563
Moutan and Persica Combination 629
Mume Formula 569
Musk and Catechu Formula 415

O

Ophiopogon and Asarum Combination 443
Ophiopogon and Trichosanthes Combination 538
Ophiopogon Combination 537

P

Peony and Licorice Combination 108
Peony Combination 428
Peony, Licorice, and Aconite Combination 310
Perilla Fruit Combination 405
Persica and Eupolyphaga Combination 580
Persica and Rhubarb Combination 435
Phellodendron Combination 199
Picrorrhiza and Mume Combination 568
Pinellia and Arisaema Combination 549
Pinellia and Gardenia Combination 555
Pinellia and Gastrodia Combination 561

Pinellia and Ginger Combination 110
Pinellia and Ginseng Six Combination 254
Pinellia and Licorice Combination 103
Pinellia and Magnolia Combination 395
Pinellia, Atractylodes, and Agastache Formula 214
Pinellia Combination 105
Platycodon and *Chih-shih* Formula 619
Platycodon and Croton Formula 140
Platycodon and Fritillaria Combination 548
Platycodon and Jujube Combination 621
Platycodon and Schizonepeta Formula 546
Platycodon Combination 603
Polyporus Combination 472
Pteropus and Bulrush Formula 582
Pueraria and Carthamus Combination 422
Pueraria and Magnolia Combination 50
Pueraria Combination 51
Pueraria, Coptis, and Scute Combination 122
Pueraria Flower Combination 211
Pueraria Nasal Combination 37

R

Rehmannia and Akebia Formula 196
Rehmannia and Gypsum Combination 201
Rehmannia and Lonicera Formula 188
Rehmannia and Schizandra Formula 226
Rehmannia Eight Formula 250
Rehmannia Six Formula 245
Rhinoceros and Antelope Horn Formula 337
Rhinoceros and Rehmannia Combination 170
Rhinoceros and Succinum Formula 331
Rhubarb and Aconite Combination 150
Rhubarb and *Kan-sui* Combination 148
Rhubarb and Leech Combination 437
Rhubarb and Licorice Combination 152
Rhubarb and Mirabilitum Combination 154
Rhubarb and Moutan Combination 626
Rhubarb Combination 194
Rhubarb, Ginger, and Croton Formula 144

S

Saussurea and Cardamon Combination 234
Saussurea and Coptis Formula 171
Schizonepeta and Forsythia Combination 607
Schizonepeta and Pinellia Formula 547
Schizonepeta and Siler Formula 609
Scute and Cimicifuga Combination 189
Scute and Licorice Combination 95
Scute Combination 271
Scute Three Herb Combination 192
Siler and *Chianghuo* Combination 227
Siler and Coix Combination 610
Siler and Licorice Formula 172
Siler and Platycodon Formula 119
Siler and Veratrum Formula 134
Six Major Herb Combination 242
Smilax and Akebia Combination 611
Stephania and Astragalus Combination 477
Stephania and Carthamus Combination 455
Stephania and Ginseng Combination 500
Stephania and Hoelen Combination 475
Styrax Formula 335
Sweet Combination 177

T

Tang-kuei and Anemarrhena Combination 506
Tang-kuei and Arctium Formula 445
Tang-kuei and Astragalus Combination 267
Tang-kuei and Atractylodes Combination 427
Tang-kuei and Carthamus Combination 438
Tang-kuei and Cimicifuga Combination 167
Tang-kuei and Cyperus Formula 394
Tang-kuei and Eight Herb Formula 618
Tang-kuei and Evodia Combination 588
Tang-kuei and Gambir Combination 415
Tang-kuei and Gardenia Combination 439
Tang-kuei and Gelatin Combination 576
Tang-kuei and Ginger Combination 583

Tang-kuei and Ginseng Eight Combination 248
Tang-kuei and Jujube Combination 321
Tang-kuei and Magnolia Formula 130
Tang-kuei and Parsley Combination 572
Tang-kuei and Peony Formula 585
Tang-kuei and Persica Combination 419
Tang-kuei and Rehmannia Combination 259
Tang-kuei and Tribulus Combination 540
Tang-kuei, Cinnamon, and Peony Combination 317
Tang-kuei Combination 281
Tang-kuei, Evodia, and Ginger Combination 319
Tang-kuei Formula 584
Tang-kuei Four Combination 432
Tang-kuei, Ginger, and Mutton Combination 269
Tang-kuei Sixteen Herb Combination 402
Tokoro Combination 503
Trichosanthes and *Chih-shih* Combination 553
Trichosanthes, Bakeri, and Pinellia Combination 389
Trichosanthes, Bakeri, and Vinegar Combination 388
Tuhuo and Vaeicum Combination 459

V

Vitality Combination 278

W

W.T.T.C. 617
Wu-tou and Cinnamon Combination 327

X

Xanthium Formula 196

Z

Zanthoxylum Combination 280
Zizyphus Combination 355

CHINESE INDEX

A

An-chung-san 366 安中散
An-kung-niu-huang-wan 330 安宮牛黄丸
An-tai-yin 572 安胎飲

C

Chai-hsien-tang 543 柴陷湯
Chai-hu-chia-lung-ku-mu-li-tang 340 柴胡加龍骨牡蠣湯
Chai-hu-ching-kan-tang 160 柴胡清肝湯
Chai-hu-kuei-chih-kan-chiang-tang 85 柴胡桂枝乾薑湯
Chai-hu-kuei-chih-tang 117 柴胡桂枝湯
Chai-ko-chieh-chi-tang 35 柴葛解肌湯
Chai-ling-tang 464 柴苓湯
Chai-shao-liu-chun-tzu-tang 225 柴芍六君子湯
Che-tsung-yin 573 折衝飲
Chen-chi-tien-hsiang-san 369 正氣天香散
Chen-hsiang-tien-ma-tang 370 沈香天麻湯
Chen-wu-tang 278 眞武湯
Chi-chu-ti-huang-wan 598 杞菊地黄丸
Chi-li-san 415 七厘散
Chi-ming-san 465 雞鳴散
Chi-pi-tang 204 启脾湯
Chi-wei-tu-chi-wan 226 七味都氣丸
Chi-wu-chiang-hsia-tang 415 七物降下湯
Chia-wei-hsiao-yao-san 87 加味逍遙散
Chia-wei-kuei-pi-tang 416 加味歸脾湯

Chia-wei-pa-hsien-tang 227 加味八仙湯
Chiao-ai-szu-wu-tang 417 膠艾四物湯
Chieh-chi-shu-chiao-tang 280 解急蜀椒湯
Chieh-keng-pai-san 140 桔梗白散
Chieh-keng-tang 603 桔梗湯
Chien-chin-nei-tuo-san 604 千金內托散
Chien-chin-tang-kuei-tang 281 千金當歸湯
Chien-chung-tang 467 堅中湯
Chien-shih-pai-chu-san 228 錢氏白朮散
Chih-cho-ku-pen-wan 358 治濁固本丸
Chih-kan-tsao-tang 529 炙甘草湯
Chih-pao-tan 331 至寶丹
Chih-po-pa-wei-wan 231 知蘗八味丸
Chih-shih-chih-yu-yu-liang-tang 358 赤石脂禹餘糧湯
Chih-shih-hsieh-pai-kuei-chih-tang 373 枳實薤白桂枝湯
Chih-shih-shao-yao-san 575 枳實芍藥散
Chih-so-erh-chen-tang 544 枳縮二陳湯
Chih-sou-san 546 止嗽散
Chih-tou-chung-i-fang 605 治頭瘡一方
Chih-tzu-kan-tsao-shih-tang 161 梔子甘草豉湯
Chih-tzu-po-pi-tang 469 梔子蘗皮湯
Chih-tzu-sheng-chiang-shih-tang 162 梔子生薑豉湯
Chih-tzu-shih-tang 162 梔子豉湯
Chin-chiu-fu-lei-tang 231 秦艽扶羸湯
Chin-chiu-pieh-chia-san 232 秦艽鼈甲散
Chin-fei-tsao-san 547 金沸草散
Chin-sou-ku-ching-wan 359 金鎖固精丸
Ching-chien-lien-chiao-tang 607 荊芥連翹湯
Ching-fang-pai-tu-san 609 荊防敗毒散
Ching-fei-tang 548 清肺湯
Ching-hsin-lien-tzu-yin 164 清心蓮子飲
Ching-je-pu-chi-tang 167 清熱補氣湯
Ching-je-pu-hsieh-tang 531 清熱補血湯
Ching-pi-tang 37 清鼻湯
Ching-shang-chuan-tung-tang 443 清上蠲痛湯
Ching-shang-fang-feng-tang-chia-i-yi-jen 610 清上防風湯加薏苡仁
Ching-shih-hua-tan-tang 549 清濕化痰湯
Ching-shu-i-chi-tang 218 清暑益氣湯
Ching-tsao-chiu-fei-tang 532 清燥救肺湯

Ching-wei-san 168 清胃散
Ching-yin-li-ke-tang 169 清咽利膈湯
Chiu-ping-wu-fu-tang 470 九檳吳茯湯
Chiu-wei-chiang-huo-tang 38 九味羌活湯
Chiung-kuei-chiao-ai-tang 576 芎歸膠艾湯
Chiung-kuei-tiao-hsieh-yin 579 芎歸調血飲
Chu-ju-wen-tan-tang 90 竹茹溫膽湯
Chu-ling-tang 472 豬苓湯
Chu-pi-chu-ju-tang 374 橘皮竹茹湯
Chu-sha-an-shen-wan 343 朱砂安神丸
Chu-yeh-shih-kao-tang 220 竹葉石膏湯
Chuan-chiung-cha-tiao-san 40 川芎茶調散
Chuan-pi-tang 444 蠲痺湯
Chuan-szu-chun-tzu-tang 376 喘四君子湯

E

Erh-chen-tang 551 二陳湯
Erh-chu-tang 474 二朮湯

F

Fang-chi-fu-ling-tang 475 防己茯苓湯
Fang-chi-huang-chi-tang 477 防己黃耆湯
Fang-feng-tung-sheng-san 119 防風通聖散
Fen-hsiao-tang 205 分消湯
Fen-hsin-chi-yin 377 分心氣飲
Fu-ling-hsing-jen-kan-tsao-tang 480 茯苓杏仁甘草湯
Fu-ling-kan-tsao-tang 479 茯苓甘草湯
Fu-ling-szu-ni-tang 283 茯苓四逆湯
Fu-ling-tse-hsieh-tang 483 茯苓澤瀉湯
Fu-ling-yin 485 茯苓飲
Fu-tu-tan 360 茯菟丹
Fu-tzu-keng-mi-tang 285 附子粳米湯
Fu-tzu-li-chung-tang 287 附子理中湯
Fu-tzu-tang 288 附子湯
Fu-yuan-huo-hsieh-tang 419 復元活血湯

H

Hou-pu-chi-wu-tang 121 厚朴七物湯
Hou-pu-wen-chung-tang 290 厚朴温中湯
Hou-pu-san-wu-tang 379 厚朴三物湯
Hou-pu-sheng-chiang-pan-hsia-kan-tsao-jen-sheng-tang 380 厚朴生薑半夏甘草人參湯
Hsi-chiao-ti-huang-tang 170 犀角地黃湯
Hsi-kan-ming-mu-tang 599 洗肝明目湯
Hsia-yu-hsieh-tang 580 下瘀血湯
Hsiang-chun-chieh-tu-chi 611 香川解毒劑
Hsiang-lien-wan 171 香連丸
Hsiang-ju-yin 221 香薷飲
Hsiang-sha-liu-chun-tzu-tang 234 香砂六君子湯
Hsiang-sha-yang-wei-tang 207 香砂養胃湯
Hsiang-sheng-po-ti-wan 552 響聲破笛丸
Hsiang-su-san 41 香蘇散
Hsiao-chai-hu-tang 91 小柴胡湯
Hsiao-cheng-chi-tang 141 小承氣湯
Hsiao-chien-chung-tang 291 小建中湯
Hsiao-ching-lung-tang 43 小青龍湯
Hsiao-feng-san 445 消風散
Hsiao-hsien-hsiung-tang 142 小陷胸湯
Hsiao-hsu-ming-tang 447 小續命湯
Hsiao-ko-ken-tang 58 小葛根湯
Hsiao-pan-hsia-chia-fu-ling-tang 487 小半夏加茯苓湯
Hsiao-yao-san 94 逍遙散
Hsieh-huang-san 172 瀉黃散
Hsieh-pai-san 173 瀉白散
Hsien-fang-huo-ming-yin 612 仙方活命飲
Hsin-i-ching-fei-tang 174 辛夷清肺湯
Hsin-i-san 175 辛夷散
Hsing-chi-hsiang-su-san 382 行氣香蘇散
Hsing-su-san 46 杏蘇散
Hsu-ming-tang 448 續命湯
Hsuan-fu-hua-tai-che-shih-tang 384 旋覆花代赭石湯
Hsuan-tu-fa-piao-tang 591 宣毒發表湯
Hua-kai-san 47 華蓋散
Huan-shao-tan 237 還少丹
Huang-chi-chien-chung-tang 293 黃耆建中湯
Huang-chi-kuei-chih-wu-wu-tang 235 黃耆桂枝五物湯

Huang-chi-pieh-chia-san 236 黃耆鱉甲散
Huang-chin-tang 95 黃芩湯
Huang-lien-ah-chiao-tang 97 黃連阿膠湯
Huang-lien-chieh-tu-tang 175 黃連解毒湯
Huang-lien-tang 99 黃連湯
Huang-tu-tang 420 黃土湯
Huo-hsiang-cheng-chi-san 100 藿香正氣散

I

I-chi-chung-ming-tang 238 益氣聰明湯
I-kan-san 343 抑肝散
I-kan-san-chia-chen-pi-pan-hsia 346 抑肝散加陳皮半夏
I-tzu-tang 494 乙字湯
I-yi-fu-tzu-pai-chiang-san 615 薏苡附子敗醬散
I-yi-jen-tang 489 薏苡仁湯

J

Jen-sheng-pai-tu-san 48 人參敗毒散
Jen-sheng-tang 295 人參湯
Jen-sheng-tang-shao-san 241 人參當芍散
Jen-sheng-yang-wei-tang 209 人參養胃湯
Jen-sheng-yang-yung-tang 239 人參養榮湯
Jun-chang-tang 533 潤腸湯

K

Kan-chiang-jen-sheng-pan-hsia-wan 385 乾薑人參半夏丸
Kan-lu-yin 177 甘露飲
Kan-mai-ta-tsao-tang 347 甘麥大棗湯
Kan-tsao-fen-mi-tang 565 甘草粉蜜湯
Kan-tsao-fu-tzu-tang 298 甘草附子湯
Kan-tsao-hsieh-hsin-tang 103 甘草瀉心湯
Kan-tsao-kan-chiang-tang 300 甘草乾薑湯
Kan-tsao-tang 349 甘草湯
Ko-hua-chieh-hsing-tang 211 葛花解酲湯
Ko-ken-chia-hsin-i-chuan-chiung 50 葛根加辛夷川芎
Ko-ken-hung-hua-tang 423 葛根紅花湯
Ko-ken-huang-lien-huang-chin-tang 122 葛根黃連黃芩湯

Ko-ken-tang 51 葛根湯
Kou-teng-san 386 鈎藤散
Kua-lou-chih-shih-tang 553 栝樓枳實湯
Kua-lou-hsieh-pai-pai-chiu-tang 388 栝樓薤白白酒湯
Kua-lou-hsieh-pai-pan-hsia-tang 389 栝樓薤白半夏湯
Kua-ti-san 134 瓜蒂散
Kuei-chih-chia-fu-tzu-tang 302 桂枝加附子湯
Kuei-chih-chia-hou-pu-hsing-jen-tang 54 桂枝加厚朴杏仁湯
Kuei-chih-chia-huang-chi-tang 55 桂枝加黃耆湯
Kuei-chih-chia-ko-ken-tang 58 桂枝加葛根湯
Kuei-chih-chia-ling-chu-fu-tang 304 桂枝加苓朮附湯
Kuei-chih-chia-lung-ku-mu-li-tang 351 桂枝加龍骨牡蠣湯
Kuei-chih-chia-shao-yao-tang 60 桂枝加芍藥湯
Kuei-chih-chia-shao-yao-ta-huang-tang 124 桂枝加芍藥大黃湯
Kuei-chih-chu-shao-yao-chia-shu-chi-lung-ku-mu-li-tang 353 桂枝去芍藥加蜀漆龍骨牡蠣湯
Kuei-chih-fu-ling-wan 423 桂枝茯苓丸
Kuei-chih-fu-tzu-tang 305 桂枝附子湯
Kuei-chih-jen-sheng-tang 306 桂枝人參湯
Kuei-chih-ma-huang-ko-pan-tang 62 桂枝麻黃各半湯
Kuei-chih-shao-yao-chih-mu-tang 450 桂枝芍藥知母湯
Kuei-chih-tang 63 桂枝湯
Kuei-chih-wu-wu-tang 179 桂枝五物湯
Kuei-pi-tang 425 歸脾湯

L

Li-chung-an-huei-tang 566 理中安蛔湯
Li-ke-tang 555 利膈湯
Liang-chih-tang 391 良枳湯
Liang-ke-san 180 涼膈散
Lien-chu-yin 427 連珠飲
Lien-mei-an-huei-tang 568 連梅安蛔湯
Ling-chiang-chu-kan-tang 491 苓薑朮甘湯
Ling-kan-chiang-wei-hsin-hsia-jen-tang 556 苓甘薑味辛夏仁湯
Ling-kuei-chu-kan-tang 493 苓桂朮甘湯
Ling-kuei-kan-tsao-tang 495 苓桂甘棗湯
Ling-kuei-wei-kan-tang 496 苓桂味甘湯
Liu-chun-tzu-tang 242 六君子湯
Liu-ho-tang 104 六和湯
Liu-wei-ti-huang-wan 245 六味地黃丸

Lo-shih-shu 617 樂適舒
Lung-ku-mu-li-tang 355 龍骨牡蠣湯
Lung-tan-hsieh-kan-tang 181 龍膽瀉肝湯

M

Ma-hsing-i-kan-tang 66 麻杏薏甘湯
Ma-hsing-kan-shih-tang 68 麻杏甘石湯
Ma-huang-chia-chu-tang 70 麻黃加朮湯
Ma-huang-fu-tzu-hsi-hsin-tang 72 麻黃附子細辛湯
Ma-huang-fu-tzu-kan-tsao-tang 74 麻黃附子甘草湯
Ma-huang-lien-chiao-chih-hsiao-tou-tang 497 麻黃連翹赤小豆湯
Ma-huang-tang 76 麻黃湯
Ma-tzu-jen-wan 535 麻子仁丸
Mai-men-tung-tang 537 麥門冬湯
Mai-men-tung-yin-tzu 538 麥門冬飲子
Meng-shih-kuen-tan-wan 559 礞石滾痰丸
Mi-niao-chien 499 泌尿煎
Mu-fang-chi-tang 499 木防己湯

N

Ning-sou-wan 560 寧嗽丸
Niu-che-shen-chi-wan 247 牛車腎氣丸
Niu-huang-ching-hsin-wan 332 牛黃清心丸
Nu-shen-san 394 女神散

P

Pa-chen-tang 248 八珍湯
Pa-cheng-san 502 八正散
Pa-wei-tai-hsia-fang 618 八味帶下方
Pa-wei-ti-huang-wan 250 八味地黃丸
Pai-chu-fu-tzu-tang 309 白朮附子湯
Pai-ho-ku-chin-tang 253 百合固金湯
Pan-hsia-hou-pu-tang 395 半夏厚朴湯
Pan-hsia-hsieh-hsin-tang 105 半夏瀉心湯
Pai-hu-chia-jen-sheng-tang 183 白虎加人參湯
Pai-hu-tang 185 白虎湯
Pai-nung-san 619 排膿散

Pai-nung-tang 621 排膿湯
Pai-tou-weng-tang 187 白頭翁湯
Pai-tu-san 188 敗毒散
Pan-hsia-hsieh-hsin-tang 105 半夏瀉心湯
Pan-hsia-pai-chu-tien-ma-tang 561 半夏白朮天麻湯
Pan-hsieh-liu-chun-tzu-tang 254 半瀉六君子湯
Pao-ho-wan 212 保和丸
Pi-hsieh-fen-ching-yin 503 萆薢分清飲
Pien-chih-hsin-chi-yin 397 變製心氣飲
Ping-wei-san 212 平胃散
Po-chou-san 622 伯州散
Po-tzu-jen-wan 581 柏子仁丸
Pu-chi-chien-chung-tang 504 補氣健中湯
Pu-chi-hsiao-tu-yin 189 普濟消毒飲
Pu-chung-i-chi-tang 255 補中益氣湯
Pu-fei-ah-chiao-tang 258 補肺阿膠湯
Pu-huan-chin-cheng-chi-san 214 不換金正氣散
Pu-kung-ying-tang 582 蒲公英湯
Pu-yin-tang 259 補陰湯

S

San-ao-tang 592 三拗湯
San-ho-san 399 三和散
San-huang-hsieh-hsin-tang 190 三黃瀉心湯
San-huang-shih-kao-tang 125 三黃石膏湯
San-sheng-san 134 三聖散
San-tsung-kuei-chien-tang 623 散腫潰堅湯
San-wu-huang-chin-tang 192 三物黃芩湯
San-wu-pei-chi-wan 144 三物備急丸
Sang-chu-yin 78 桑菊飲
Sang-piao-hsiao-san 361 桑螵蛸散
Sha-sheng-mai-tung-tang 593 沙參麥冬湯
Shang-chung-hsia-tung-yung-tung-feng-wan 452 上中下通用痛風丸
Shao-yao-kan-tsao-fu-tzu-tang 310 芍藥甘草附子湯
Shao-yao-kan-tsao-tang 108 芍藥甘草湯
Shao-yao-tang 429 芍藥湯
Shen-mi-tang 401 神秘湯
Sheng-chiang-hsieh-hsin-tang 110 生薑瀉心湯
Sheng-hua-tang 583 生化湯

Sheng-ling-pai-chu-san 260 參苓白朮散
Sheng-lu-yin 135 參蘆飲
Sheng-ma-ko-ken-tang 594 升麻葛根湯
Sheng-su-yin 126 參蘇飲
Shih-chuan-ta-pu-tang 262 十全大補湯
Shih-hsiao-san 583 失笑散
Shih-liu-wei-liu-chi-yin 402 十六味流氣飲
Shih-pi-yin 505 實脾飲
Shih-shen-tang 79 十神湯
Shih-ti-tang 404 柿蒂湯
Shih-tsao-tang 144 十棗湯
Shih-wei-hsiang-ju-yin 222 十味香薷飲
Shih-wei-pai-tu-tang 624 十味敗毒湯
Shih-wei-tsuo-san 453 十味挫散
Shu-chin-li-an-san 454 舒筋立安散
Shu-ching-huo-hsieh-tang 429 疏經活血湯
Shu-feng-huo-hsieh-tang 455 疏風活血湯
Shu-kan-tang 432 疏肝湯
Su-ho-hsiang-wan 335 蘇合香丸
Su-tzu-chiang-chi-tang 405 蘇子降氣湯
Suan-tsao-jen-tang 355 酸棗仁湯
Szu-chun-tzu-tang 264 四君子湯
Szu-ni-chia-jen-sheng-tang 311 四逆加人參湯
Szu-ni-san 112 四逆散
Szu-ni-tang 313 四逆湯
Szu-shen-tang 266 四神湯
Szu-wu-tang 433 四物湯

T

Ta-chai-hu-tang 128 大柴胡湯
Ta-cheng-chi-tang 145 大承氣湯
Ta-chien-chung-tang 315 大建中湯
Ta-ching-lung-tang 81 大青龍湯
Ta-fang-feng-tang 457 大防風湯
Ta-hsien-hsiung-tang 148 大陷胸湯
Ta-huang-fu-tzu-tang 150 大黃附子湯
Ta-huang-kan-tsao-tang 152 大黃甘草湯
Ta-huang-huang-lien-hsieh-hsin-tang 194 大黃黃連瀉心湯
Ta-huang-mu-tan-pi-tang 626 大黃牡丹皮湯

Tang-kuei-chien-chung-tang 317 當歸建中湯
Tang-kuei-lien-tung-tang 506 當歸拈痛湯
Tang-kuei-pu-hsieh-tang 267 當歸補血湯
Tang-kuei-san 584 當歸散
Tang-kuei-shao-yao-san 585 當歸芍藥散
Tang-kuei-sheng-chiang-yang-zou-tang 269 當歸生薑羊肉湯
Tang-kuei-szu-ni-chia-wu-chu-yu-sheng-chiang-tang 319 當歸四逆加吳茱萸生薑湯
Tang-kuei-szu-ni-tang 321 當歸四逆湯
Tang-kuei-yin-tzu 540 當歸飲子
Tao-chih-san 196 導赤散
Tao-ho-cheng-chi-tang 435 桃核承氣湯
Tao-hua-tang 362 桃花湯
Tao-shui-fu-ling-tang 508 導水茯苓湯
Teng-hua-pai-tu-san 628 燈花敗毒散
Teng-lung-tang 629 騰龍湯
Ti-tang-tang 437 抵當湯
Tiao-wei-cheng-chi-tang 154 調胃承氣湯
Tien-wang-pu-hsin-tan 270 天王補心丹
Ting-chuan-tang 407 定喘湯
Ting-hsiang-fu-ling-tang 509 丁香茯苓湯
Ting-hsiang-shih-ti-tang 407 丁香柿蒂湯
Ting-li-ta-tsao-hsieh-fei-tang 595 葶藶大棗瀉肺湯
Tsang-erh-san 196 蒼耳散
Tse-hsieh-tang 511 澤瀉湯
Tsing-fu-tang 197 淨腑湯
Tsou-ma-tang 136 走馬湯
Tsu-shih-ti-huang-wan 272 磁石地黃丸
Tu-huo-chi-sheng-tang 459 獨活寄生湯
Tun-sou-san 563 頓嗽散
Tung-kuan-san 336 通關散
Tung-mo-szu-ni-tang 323 通脈四逆湯
Tung-tao-san 438 通導散
Tuo-li-hsiao-tu-yin 631 托裡消毒飲
Tzu-hsueh-tan 337 紫雪丹
Tzu-keng-mu-li-tang 632 紫根牡蠣湯
Tzu-sheng-ming-mu-tang 600 滋腎明目湯
Tzu-sheng-tung-erh-tang 271 滋腎通耳湯
Tzu-wan-tang 273 紫菀湯
Tzu-yin-chiang-huo-tang 199 滋陰降火湯
Tzu-yu-kao 634 紫雲膏

Tzu-yuan 156 紫圓

W

Wei-cheng-fang 274 痿症方
Wei-feng-tang 461 胃風湯
Wei-ling-tang 512 胃苓湯
Wen-ching-tang 588 温經湯
Wen-ching-yin 439 温清飲
Wen-tan-tang 114 温膽湯
Wu-chi-san 130 五積散
Wu-chu-yu-tang 325 吳茱萸湯
Wu-lin-san 514 五淋散
Wu-ling-san 516 五苓散
Wu-mei-wan 569 烏梅丸
Wu-pi-yin 519 五皮飲
Wu-tou-kuei-chih-tang 327 烏頭桂枝湯
Wu-yao-shun-chi-san 409 烏藥順氣散

Y

Yang-hsin-tang 275 養心湯
Yen-nien-pan-hsia-tang 411 延年半夏湯
Yin-chen-hao-tang 519 茵陳蒿湯
Yin-chen-wu-ling-san 521 茵陳五苓散
Yin-chiao-san 83 銀翹散
Yu-nu-chien 201 玉女煎
Yueh-pi-chia-chu-tang 523 越婢加朮湯
Yueh-pi-chia-pan-hsia-tang 525 越婢加半夏湯
Yueh-pi-tang 526 越婢湯